Current Clinical Urology

Eric A. Klein, MD, Series Editor
Professor of Surgery
Cleveland Clinic Lerner College of Medicine Head,
Section of Urologic Oncology
Glickman Urological and Kidney Institute
Cleveland, OH

For further volumes:
http://www.springer.com/series/7635

CURRENT CLINICAL UROLOGY

Manoj Monga
Editor

Ureteroscopy

Indications, Instrumentation & Technique

Humana Press

Editor
Manoj Monga
Department of Urology
Stevan B. Streem Center for Endourology
& Stone Disease
Glickman Urological & Kidney Institute
The Cleveland Clinic
Cleveland, OH, USA

Additional material to this book can be downloaded from http://extras.springer.com

ISBN 978-1-4939-6023-1 ISBN 978-1-62703-206-3 (eBook)
DOI 10.1007/978-1-62703-206-3
Springer New York Heidelberg Dordrecht London

Printed on acid-free paper

Humana Press is a brand of Springer
Springer is part of Springer Science+Business Media (www.springer.com)

To my family: Mary, Nate, Miles, Natalie, and Yogi.

Foreword

Ureteroscopy has become an important, universally accepted part of urologic endoscopy. It has grown from an interesting niche procedure to access the distal ureter into a standard procedure offering access throughout the upper urinary tract for visualization and also active interventional procedures. No longer are distal stones the only application. These have grown to include lateralizing hematuria, neoplasms, and obstructions. Even the application for stones has expanded to include larger calculi including full-branched staghorn stones.

The time has come for a current text on ureteroscopy to summarize the development, the applications, and the present status of the procedure. I am happy to be a part of this effort, which includes authors who are first-, second-, and even fourth-generation endourologists.

Ureteroscopy is impossible without the appropriate instruments. The devices continue to evolve in relation to the need, usually resulting in an improvement in performance. It is in these areas that the laser has found its place in urology. The Holmium laser has become indispensable for many therapeutic interventions.

As indications increase for ureteroscopy in more complex situations, the "tips and tricks" of the procedure become even more important. Although all urologists are now familiar with and, probably, perform ureteroscopy, it is always possible to do it better. The sections on technique and complex cases address these issues.

The need for further development is clear. Unlike the rigid cystoscope, which has had only refinements over decades, the ureteroscopes continue to evolve. Many changes can be anticipated, while others may be surprises. All changes are limited by the anatomy of the upper urinary tract and the diseases to be treated.

This volume attempts to define the history of the procedure, the present status of ureteroscopy, and the potential for future development.

Philadelphia, PA, USA — Demetrius H. Bagley, MD, FACS

Preface

Urologists are progressive surgeons, with innovative and inquisitive minds that drive the development of new approaches to traditional challenges. Ureteroscopy has developed in this nurturing environment, since its early inception in the late 1970s to its current position as a mainstay in the armamentarium of minimally invasive approaches to the upper urinary tract. These advances have lead to improved outcomes and decreased surgical morbidity.

The keys to any successful surgical procedure are selecting the right patient, setting the right expectations by appropriate patient counseling and consent, ensuring the availability of the necessary instrumentation, and using a precise and thoughtful technique. Nowhere are these keys more critical than in the delicate maneuvering of a ureteroscope.

Our goal is to provide all urologists with the evidence base one uses to make decisions regarding patient selection and to counsel patients on the risks and benefits of the procedure. Details on instrumentation and technique will be provided from many authors with varying preferences and techniques, such that the reader will be able to glean those "pearls" that will help them the most in their operating room. Lastly, we glimpse to the future, beyond those great strides that have been accomplished to what lies ahead that will help keep urologists at the forefront of endoscopic innovation.

Cleveland, OH, USA — Manoj Monga, MD

Acknowledgement

Connie Walsh for her outstanding editorial guidance and assistance.

Contents

Part VII The Future

Contributors

Corollos Abdelshehid, MD Department of Urology, University of California, Irvine, Irvine, CA, USA

Samih Al-Hayek, MD, FRCS(Urol) Department of Urology, University of Pittsburgh Medical Center, Pittsburgh, PA, USA

Christopher L. Allam, DO Endourology Division, Urology Department, University of Michigan, Ann Arbor, MI, USA

J. Kyle Anderson, MD Department of Urology, University of Minnesota, Minneapolis, MN, USA

Don C. Arnold II, MD Department of Urology, Loma Linda University School of Medicine, Loma Linda, CA, USA

Timothy D. Averch, MD Department of Urology, University of Pittsburgh Medical Center, Pittsburgh, PA, USA

Demetrius H. Bagley, MD, FACS Department of Urology and Radiology,, Thomas Jefferson University, Philadelphia, PA, USA

D. Duane Baldwin, MD Department of Urology, Loma Linda University Medical Center, Loma Linda University School of Medicine, Loma Linda, CA, USA

Naeem Bhojani, MD Urology, Indiana University Health, Indianapolis, IN, USA

Marluce Bibbo, MD, ScD Cytopathology Division, Pathology Department, Thomas Jefferson University, Philadelphia, PA, USA

Vincent G. Bird, MD Minimally Invasive Surgery Division, Urology Department, University of Florida College of Medicine, Gainesville, FL, USA

Minimally Invasive Surgery Division, Urology Department, Shand's Hospital, University of Florida, Gainesville, FL, USA

Jeffrey A. Cadeddu, MD Department of Urology, University of Texas Southwestern Medical Center at Dallas, Dallas, TX, USA

Benjamin K. Canales, MD, MPH Department of Urology, Center for the Study of Lithiasis and Pathological Calcification, University of Florida, Gainesville, FL, USA

Daniel J. Canter, MD Department of Urology, Emory University, Atlanta, GA, USA

Doh Yoon Cha, MD Urology Department, New York Presbyterian Hospital, Columbia University Medical Center, New York, NY, USA

Ben H. Chew, MD, MSc, FRCSC Department of Urologic Sciences, University of British Columbia, Vancouver, BC, Canada

Jane Cho, MD Department of Urology, University of California, Irvine, Irvine, CA, USA

Jacob H. Cohen, MD, MPH Department of Urology, Lenox Hill Hospital, New York, NY, USA

Seth D. Cohen, MD Department of Urology, Lenox Hill Hospital, New York, NY, USA

Seth A. Cohen, MD Urology Division, Surgery Department, U.C. San Diego Health System, San Diego, CA, USA

Michael J. Conlin, MD Urology Division, Surgery Department, Oregon Health & Sciences University, Portland VA Medical Center, Portland, OR, USA

Mitra R. de Cógain, MD Department of Urology, Mayo Clinic, Rochester, MN, USA

John D. Denstedt, MD, FRCSC, FACS Division of Urology, Department of Surgery, The University of Western Ontario, London, ON, Canada

Mihir M. Desai, MD USC Institute of Urology, University of Southern California, Los Angeles, CA, USA

Branden G. Duffey, DO Urology Division, Surgery Department, San Antonio Military Medical Center, San Antonio, TX, USA

Brian Eisner, MD Department of Urology, Massachusetts General Hospital, Harvard Medical School, Boston, MA, USA

Sean P. Elliott, MD Department of Urology, UT, Minneapolis, MN, USA

Stephen Faddegon, MD Department of Urology, UT Southwestern Medical Center, Dallas, TX, USA

Gary J. Faerber, MD Department of Urology, University of Michigan Hospital and Health Systems, Ann Arbor, MI, USA

Kendall J. Feia, MD Department of Urology, University of Minnesota, Minneapolis, MN, USA

Kirsten Foell, MD, FRCSC Division of Urology, Department of Surgery, St. Michael's Hospital, University of Toronto, Toronto, ON, Canada

Gerhard J. Fuchs, MD, FACS Urology Division, Surgery Department, Cedars-Sinai Medical Center, Los Angeles, CA, USA

Andrew Fuller, MBBS Division of Urology, Department of Surgery, The University of Western Ontario, London, ON, Canada

Matthew T. Gettman, MD Department of Urology, Mayo Clinic, Rochester, MN, USA

Matthew H.C. Goh, MBChB, MRCS(Eng), FRCS(Urol) Bristol Urological Institute, Southmead Hospital, Bristol, UK

Zachariah G. Goldsmith, MD, PhD Division of Urologic Surgery, Surgery Department, Duke University Medical Center, Durham, NC, USA

Ricardo D. Gonzalez, BA Department of Urology, Center for the Study of Lithiasis and Pathological Calcification, University of Florida, Gainesville, FL, USA

Michael Grasso III, MD Department of Urology, Lenox Hill Hospital, New York, NY, USA

Department of Urology, Medical College of New York, Valhalla, NY, USA

Joseph A. Graversen, MD Department of Urology, University of California, Irvine, Irvine, CA, USA

Mantu Gupta, MD Urology Department, New York Presbyterian Hospital, Columbia University Medical Center, New York, NY, USANew York Presbyterian Kidney Stone Center, New York, NY, USA

Kelly A. Healy, MD Department of Urology and Radiology, Thomas Jefferson University, Philadelphia, PA, USA

R. John D'A. Honey, MD, FRCSC Division of Urology, Department of Surgery, St. Michael's Hospital, University of Toronto, Toronto, ON, Canada

Elias S. Hyams, MD Brady Urological Institute, Johns Hopkins Medical Institutions, Baltimore, MD, USA

Wahib E. Isac, MD Urology Department, Minimally Invasive Surgery, Cleveland Clinic Foundation, Cleveland, OH, USA

Adam Kaplan, MD Department of Urology, University of California, Irvine, Irvine, CA, USA

Christopher E. Keel, DO Department of Urology, Tulane University School of Medicine, New Orleans, LA, USA

Francis X. Keeley Jr., MD, FRCS(Ed), FRCS(Urol) Bristol Urological Institute, Southmead Hospital, Bristol, UK

Nir Kleinmann, MD Department of Urology and Radiology, Thomas Jefferson University, Philadelphia, PA, USA

Steven G. Koopman, MD Urology Division, Surgery Department, Cedars-Sinai Medical Center, Los Angeles, CA, USA

Amy E. Krambeck, MD Department of Urology, Mayo Clinic, Rochester, MN, USA

Evgeniy Kreydin, MD Department of Urology, Massachusetts General Hospital, Harvard Medical School, Boston, MA, USA

Bodo E. Knudsen, MD, FRCSC Department of Urology, Wexner Medical Center, The Ohio State University, Columbus, OH, USA

Jaime Landman, MD Department of Urology, University of California, Irvine, Irvine, CA, USA

Dirk Lange, MSc(Hon), PhD Department of Urologic Sciences, University of British Columbia, Vancouver, BC, Canada

David A. Leavitt, MD Department of Urology, University of Minnesota, Minneapolis, MN, USA

Dennis J. Lee, MD USC Institute of Urology, University of Southern California, Los Angeles, CA, USA

James E. Lingeman, MD Urology, Indiana University Health, Indianapolis, IN, USA

Michael E. Lipkin, MD Division of Urologic Surgery, Surgery Department, Duke University Medical Center, Durham, NC, USA

Michael A. Liss, MD Department of Urology, University of California, Irvine, Irvine, CA, USA

Achim Lusch, MD Department of Urology, University of California, Irvine, Irvine, CA, USA

Tracy Marien, MD Department of Urology, New York University School of Medicine, New York, NY, USA

Department of Urology, NYU Langone Medical Center, New York, NY, USA

Brian R. Matlaga, MD, MPH Brady Urological Institute, Johns Hopkins Medical Institutions, Baltimore, MD, USA

Joe Miller, MD Urology Department, University of California San Francisco, San Francisco, CA, USA

Thomas E. Milner, PhD Biomedical Engineering Department, The University of Texas at Austin, Austin, TX, USA

Manoj Monga, MD Department of Urology, Stevan B. Streem Center for Endourology & Stone Disease, Glickman Urological & Kidney Institute, The Cleveland Clinic, Cleveland, OH, USA

Michael E. Moran, MD Urology Department, University of Florida, Gainesville, FL, USA

AUA's William P. Didusch Center for Urologic History, Arizona Institute of Urology, Tucson, AZ, USA

Debra Morrison Department of Anesthesiology, University of California, Irvine, Irvine, CA, USA

Stephen Y. Nakada, MD, FACS Department of Urology, University of Wisconsin, Madison, WI, USA

Mark J. Noble, MD Surgery Division, Urology Department, Glickman Urologic Institute, Cleveland Clinic, Cleveland, OH, USA

Kenneth Ogan, MD Department of Urology, Emory University, Atlanta, GA, USA

Zeph Okeke, MD The Arthur Smith Institute for Urology, Hofstra North Shore-Long Island Jewish Health System, New Hyde Park, NY, USA

Kenneth T. Pace, MD, MSc, FRCSC Division of Urology, Department of Surgery, St. Michael's Hospital, University of Toronto, Toronto, ON, Canada

Vernon M. Pais Jr., MD Section of Urology, Department of Surgery, Geisel School of Medicine at Dartmouth, Lebanon, NH, USA

Ryan F. Paterson, MD, FRCSC Department of Urologic Sciences, University of British Columbia, Vancouver, BC, Canada

Margaret S. Pearle, MD, PhD Department of Urology, UT Southwestern Medical Center, Dallas, TX, USA

Renato Nardi Pedro, MD, PhD Ambulatory Surgical Unit, Litotripsy Center, State University of Campinas, Campinas, Sao Paulo, Brazil

Clinica Padre Almeida, Endourology and Kidney Stones Treatment, Campinas, Sao Paulo, Brazil

Richard A.F. Pellatt, MBChB, BA(Hons) Bristol Urological Institute, Southmead Hospital, Bristol, UK

Glenn M. Preminger, MD Division of Urologic Surgery, Surgery Department, Duke University Medical Center, Durham, NC, USA

Jinze Qiu, PhD Biomedical Engineering Department, The University of Texas at Austin, Austin, TX, USA

Ojas Shah, MD Department of Urology, New York University School of Medicine, New York, NY, USA

Department of Urology, NYU Langone Medical Center, New York, NY, USA

Adam B. Shrewsberry, MD Department of Urology, Emory University, Atlanta, GA, USA

Sri Sivalingam, MD, MSc Department of Urology, University of Wisconsin, Madison, WI, USA

Arthur D. Smith, MD The Arthur Smith Institute for Urology, Hofstra North Shore-Long Island Jewish Health System, New Hyde Park, NY, USA

Marshall L. Stoller, MD Urology Department, University of California San Francisco, San Francisco, CA, USA

Roger L. Sur, MD Urology Division, Surgery Department, U.C. San Diego Health System, San Diego, CA, USA

Surgery Department, Uniform Services University of the Health Sciences, San Diego, CA, USA

Nicholas N. Tadros, MD Urology Division, Surgery Department, Oregon Health and Science University, Portland, OR, USA

Yung Khan Tan, MBBS(Melbourne), MRCS(Edin) Department of Urology, University of Texas Southwestern Medical Centre at Dallas, Dallas, TX, USA

Joel M.H. Teichman, MD, FRCS(C) Department of Urologic Sciences, St. Paul's Hospital, University of British Columbia, Vancouver, BC, Canada

Raju Thomas, MD, FACS, MHA Department of Urology, Tulane University School of Medicine, New Orleans, LA, USA

Nikhil Waingankar, MD The Arthur Smith Institute for Urology, Hofstra North Shore-Long Island Jewish Health System, New Hyde Park, NY, USA

Bingqing Wang, BSc Biomedical Engineering Department, The University of Texas at Austin, Austin, TX, USA

J. Stuart Wolf Jr., MD Division of Endourology and Stone Disease, Department of Urology, University of Michigan Health System, Ann Arbor, MI, USA

Part I

Past and Present

1 History of Ureteroscopy

Michael E. Moran

Introduction

Technology is the application of science, engineering to producing products or devices that improve upon mankind's existence. Ureteroscopy has rapidly evolved to become one of the most common procedures performed by the urologist in his/her everyday work life and represents one of urology's remarkable technologies [1]. To fully comprehend ureteroscopy and the urologic applications that will be presented in this textbook, looking backwards in time is essential. The history of this technology is fascinating in its own right and demonstrates the rapidity of impact that the technology can have upon the profession of urology.

Light allows the physician to peer into the interstices of body cavities, with organs and organ systems [2]. The development of light-guided devices underscores the history and development of the ureteroscope [3]. At the dawn of the twentieth century, one early investigator of urologic applications who is better known as the "father of gynecology," Howard A. Kelly, demonstrated the potential of endoscopic evaluation of the urinary tract. Kelly and Curtis F. Burnam from Johns Hopkins published *Diseases of the Kidneys, Ureters and Bladder* in 1914 (Fig. 1.1) [4]. On page 270 of his classic textbook, Kelly noted that "It is our habit in catheterizing ureters in practically all cases to wax the catheter tip before its introduction." This is the era prior to X-rays; there was no fluoroscopy, and only the hopes for illuminated endoscopes. Yet the need for knowledge about what pathology lies within visceral structures existed and the ability of physicians to anticipate pathology rose as autopsies (the word *autopsy* means personal observation) increased in number and were correlated to clinical symptoms. The scratches on the freshly waxed catheters were critical to identify the presence and location of a potential ureteral calculus before other imaging strategies existed. Take this one step further, Kelly also tried to remove the kidneys, bladder, and ureters transvaginally in his patients *post mortem*, in order to better understand their terminal illnesses [5]. The desire to investigate organs inflicted with pathology precedes the ability to actually do so. Next, a fringe idea is developed to actually inspect the organ or the organ system. Typically, the individuals involved are not treated kindly by their peers. The rogue technique is found faulty, typically called cavalier or dangerous. Finally, gradual improvement of the technical systems wins converts and application becomes the norm. F. Mosteller wrote about the gradual introduction of technology in his classic treatise in 1980. New technology has

M.E. Moran, M.D. (✉)
Urology Department, University of Florida, Gainesville, FL, USA

AUA's William P. Didusch Center for Urologic History, Arizona Institute of Urology, 1100 N. El Dorado Place, Tucson, AZ 85715, USA
e-mail: memoran2@juno.com

M. Monga (ed.), *Ureteroscopy: Indications, Instrumentation & Technique*, Current Clinical Urology,
DOI 10.1007/978-1-62703-206-3_1,

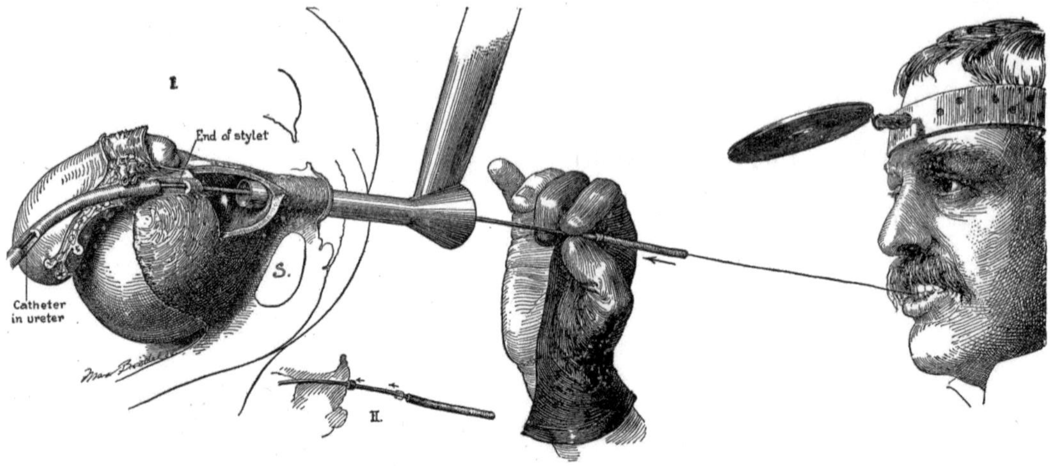

Fig. 1.1 Howard Kelly and his cystoscopic-guided ureteral catheterization using freshly waxed tips. Courtesy of the William P. Didusch Center for Urologic History

an apparent life cycle with five stages: (1) feasibility (technical performance, applicability, safety complications, morbidity, mortality); (2) efficacy (benefit for the patient demonstrated in centers of excellence); (3) effectiveness (benefit for the patient under normal conditions, reproducible with widespread application); (4) costs (benefit in terms of cost-effectiveness); and (5) gold standard [6].

In this historical sojourn, the development of light-guided devices will follow a theme. First, the development of direct and indirect light-guides which forms the basis of all types of endoscopes in medicine, from laparoscopy to colonoscopy and ureteroscopy, will be presented. Second, the methods for delivering better illumination will be pursued. This is closely related to the development of image improvement through rod-lens systems, to the modern utilization of fiber optics. Finally, camera systems allow the urologist to multitask which is so fundamental to modern or historically more accurate, current ureteroscopy [7].

Brief Historical Overview

A quick overview here in the introduction is followed by a more detailed historical development. The word endoscopy is derived from Greek meaning "to examine within." The first lighted examinations were external openings to the gastroenteral tract and the female introitus. Early Roman specula have been unearthed that record the foundations of primitive endoscopy (Fig. 1.2). Early practitioners of medicine realized that viewing a viscus from the inside should provide valuable information in the management of illnesses [8]. Bozzini in 1806 recognized the need to build a direct light to facilitate the examination or the operation of visceral structures [9]. Waxed candles and mirrors provided the illumination for the first endoscope (Fig. 1.3). Daniel Colladon demonstrated light guiding at the University of Geneva in 1841 (Fig. 1.4) [10]. Total internal reflection of light made for a spectacular demonstration and this mechanism was quickly artificially simulated by fellow physicist, Auguste de la Rive, using an electric arc light [3]. Jacques Babinet also took the method to use bent glass rods to examine difficult regions of the oral cavity in 1840 [3]. The Paris Opera began to use the same methods for spectacular stage effects in 1849 "Elias et Mysis" and again in 1853 for Gounod's *Faust* [3].

Desormeaux in 1867 developed "open tube" endoscopy for examination of the genitourinary tract and was the first to identify that lenses serve to condense the light source beam to a narrower brighter region that allows for more intricate

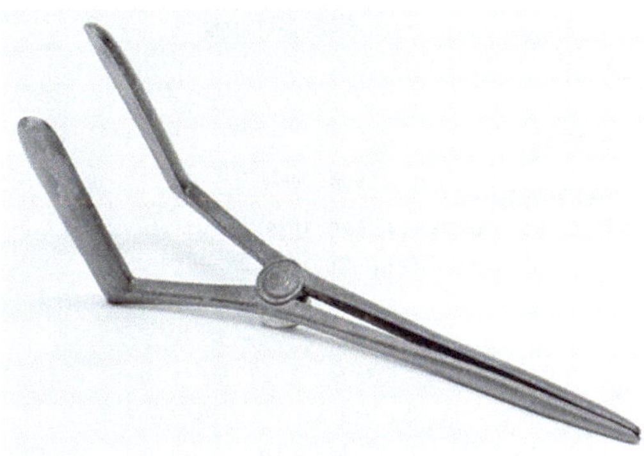

Fig. 1.2 An ancient Roman speculum unearthed at Pompeii. Courtesy of the William P. Didusch Center for Urologic History

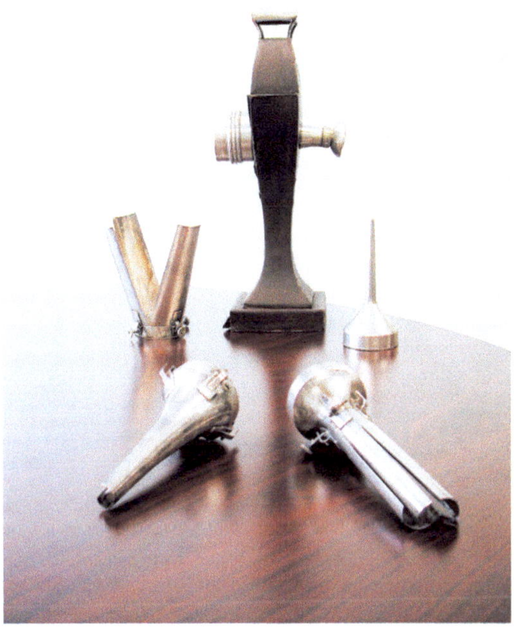

Fig. 1.3 Philip Bozzini's Lichtleiter. Courtesy of the William P. Didusch Center for Urologic History

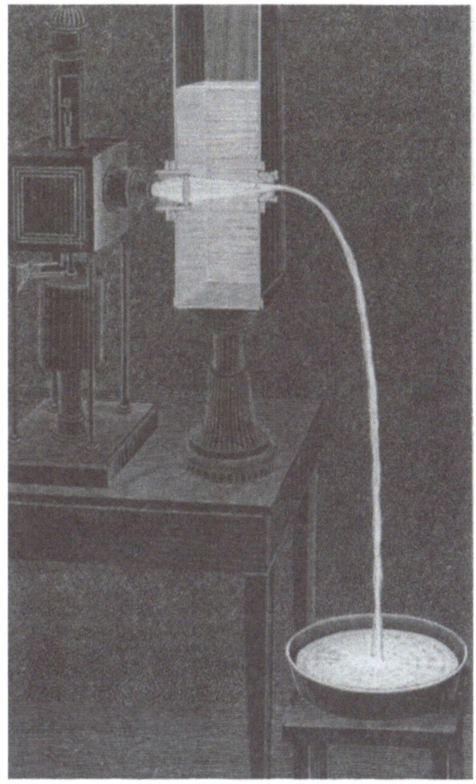

Fig. 1.4 Daniel Colladon's illustration from his "light guide." Courtesy of the William P. Didusch Center for Urologic History

observations [11]. Bevan in 1868 utilized such a device to remove foreign bodies in the esophagus using a ¾ inch diameter, 4 in. length tube with a reflecting mirror [12]. Waldenburg in 1870 lengthened these instruments and referred to them as "telescopes." In 1881, American entrepreneur William Wheeler developed a "light pipe" which he hoped to deliver light to every household, but the incandescent bulb would become his chief rival (Fig. 1.5) [3]. The International Health Exhibition held in South Kensington of 1884 displayed a giant "illuminated fountain" created by Sir Francis Bolton [3]. Stoerk in 1887 designed a right-angled endoscope to allow greater manipulation away from the ocular [12]. In that same year, Charles Vernon Boys developed a method of creating small stretched almost pure silica fibers that could transmit light [13]. Rosenheim in 1895 employed a flexible rubber obturator for safer introduction and easier handling of endoscopes [14]. Kelling in 1897 designed a true flexible scope with small interdigitating metal rings covered by rubber on the outside [15].

Killian in 1898 first used cocaine anesthesia during bronchoscopy [16]. Nitze in 1879 pioneered the first modern endoscope for cystoscopy (Fig. 1.6) [17]. He worked with an optician

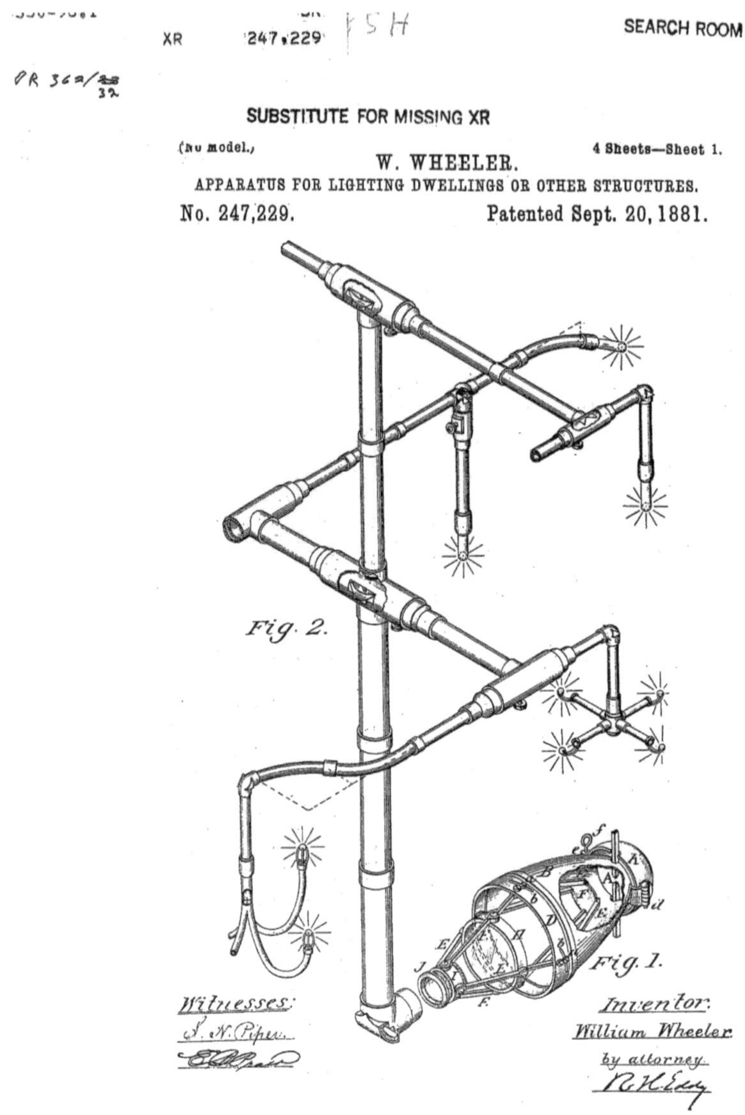

Fig. 1.5 Wheeler's light tubes for bringing lighting into American homes just prior to Edison's incandescent lamp. Courtesy of the William P. Didusch Center for Urologic History

(Beneche), an instrument maker (Leiter), and a dentist (Lesky) to create a 7 mm. deviating prismed endoscope with a liquid cooled glowing wire of platinum [18]. He followed this later with a separate light source, a miniature electric globe (Mignon Lampchen, Fig. 1.7) [19]. In the United States, Otis designed a new cystoscope with telescopic lenses and a distal electric globe. The instrument maker for this scope was Reinhold Wappler (1900) and clearly became the premier optical system of that time. In 1936 Schindler worked with Wolf (an optical physicist) to design the first working flexible endoscope with steel spiral construction and 48 lenses [18]. As early as 1893, Albert Musehold described an apparatus to photograph the endoscopic appearance of the pharynx [20]. Nitze published the first photographic atlas of the pathology of the urinary bladder in 1893 [21]. On December 30, 1926, Clarence Weston Hansell, an RCA engineer, wanted to view

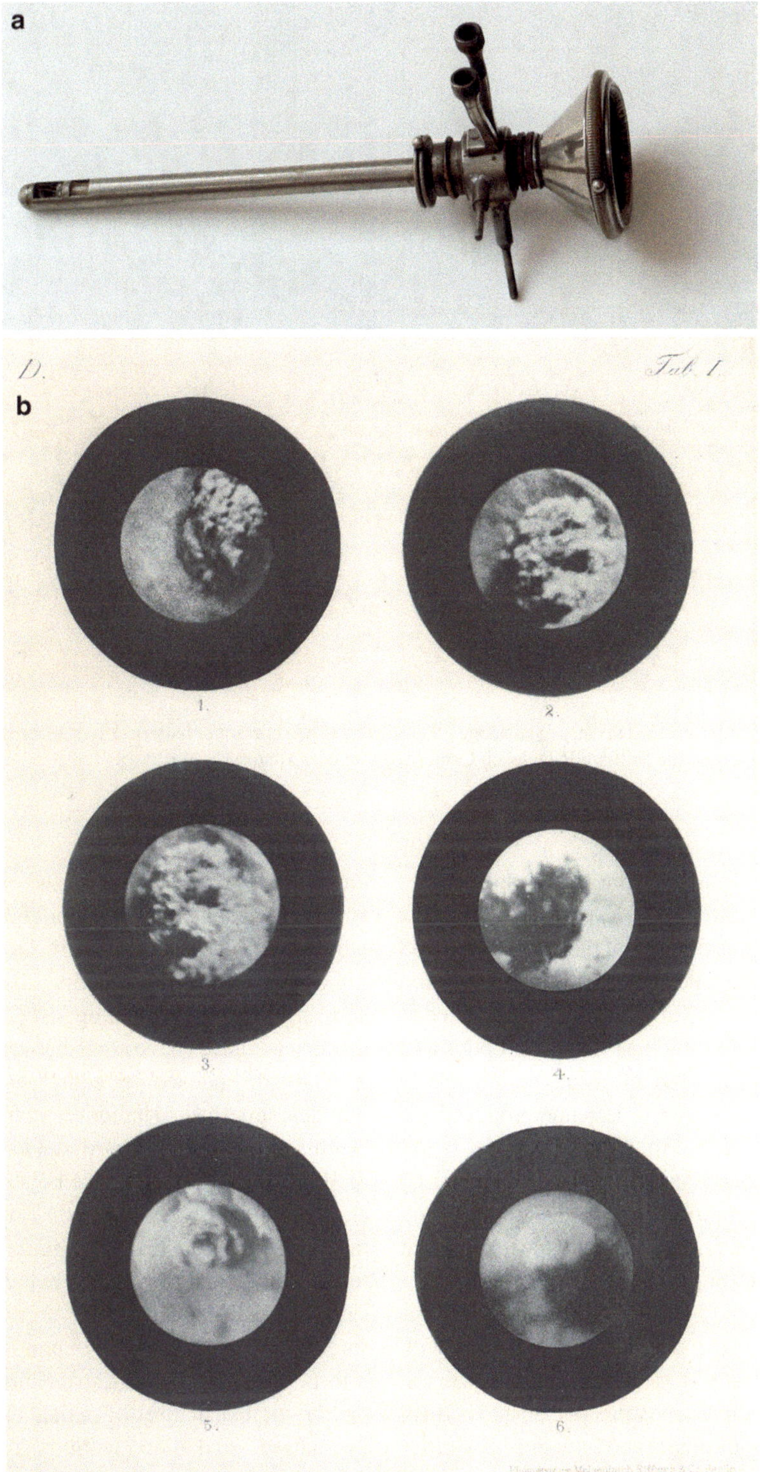

Fig. 1.6 Maximilian Nitze's cystoscope and images from his 1894 book. Courtesy of the William P. Didusch Center for Urologic History

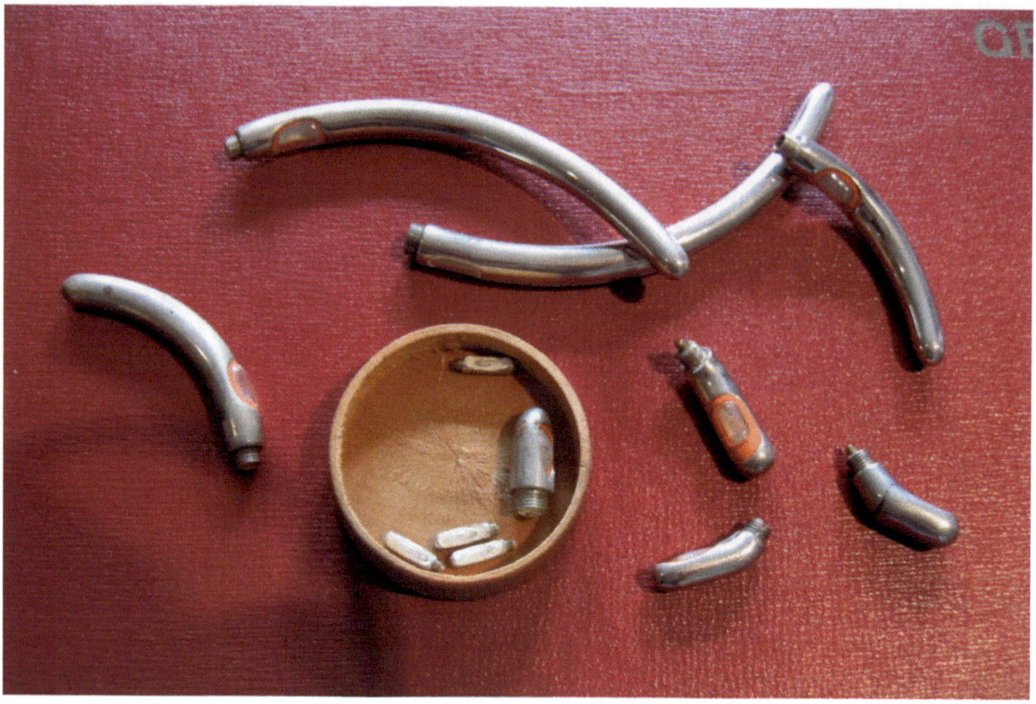

Fig. 1.7 Mignon bulbs utilized in early cystoscopes. These were direct current or battery-driven electrically illuminated endoscopes. Courtesy of the William P. Didusch Center for Urologic History

images from a distance using fiber-optic bundles [22]. Henning and Keihack published the first color photographic pictures of the stomach in 1938 [23] (Rudolf Schindler developed a rigid, then a semirigid gastroscope and Heinrich Lamm tried to reproduce Hansell's findings with fiber optics as a third-year medical student using commercially available optical fiber) [3]. Lejeune produced the first motion pictures of the larynx in 1936.

Abraham Cornelius Sebastian van Heel noted that cladding improved the light transfer and image quality of fiber optics and speculated that it could be used for cystoscopy in a letter he published in *Nature* [24]. Harold Horace Hopkins also published in the same volume of *Nature* with a young graduate student named Narinder S. Kapany, but their fibers were unclad [25]. Basil Hirschowitz (a physician) and Lawrence E. Curtiss (a physics student, later transferred to the American Cystoscope Makers, Inc.) working at the University of Michigan produced a fiber-optic gastroscope which was first tried on Hirschowitz and then presented at the annual meeting of the Optical Society of America in October 1956 in Lake Placid (site of the first digital televised sporting event using fiber optics) [26]. Numerous modern advances have contributed to our modern arsenal of endoscopic equipment (fiber-optic bundles, superheated halide element light sources, electronic charged-coupled devices, CCD, and others) [27, 28]. The need to be able to visualize and eventually operate with tiny endoscopic manipulators is increasingly apparent. This represents the foundations upon which this discussion is based. Advanced ureteropyeloscopic surgery is based entirely upon those pioneer efforts from long ago that strived to better visualize the vital structures of patients suffering with assundried maladies without opening them [29, 30]. The ureters were always present and simply awaited pioneer endoscopists to explore the limits of technology.

Early Endoscopic Development

Most likely, the first instrument described for peering into the recesses of the human body was a rectal speculum. Hippocrates' treatise on fistulas clearly mentions this technique and later, Galen's *Levicom* refers to the catopter which is an anal speculum. Phillip Bozzini (Germany) in 1805 constructed an instrument called "lichtleiter" for the viewing of the openings in the human body [31]. Bozzini's insight into the potential for direct visualization of the body is as amazing as the harsh criticism of his peers regarding his endoscopic adventures utilizing his device. Bozzini's light guide consisted of a housing in which a candle was placed. Open tubes of various sizes and configurations could be placed on one side [9]. He then devised a reflecting mirror between the visual tract and the candle light so that the light would be reflected only toward the targeted organ and not backward into the examiner's eye. The opposite side of the system was the eyepiece. He had published his results in 1806 and began to lecture in 1807 and even tried to have prospective studies of the instrument performed in military hospitals of the time [31]. This development was remarkable in that it was the first use of reflected light as an illumination source. Unfortunately he was censured for his ingenuity since the intended use of the instrument was considered an unnatural act under contemporary mores. Bozzini died at the age of 35 after contracting typhus probably contracted during house calls [9].

Pierre Segalas (France) also reported upon the use of candles and a cone-shaped silver cube to reflect light into the urinary bladder. His refined urethroscope in 1826 was primarily used in female patients which he called "urethro-cystique" [32]. John Fischer from Boston also developed a functional but cumbersome elongated and angled speculum [33]. Anton J. Desormeaux (France) presented the first serviceable endoscope to the Academy of Paris in 1853. The light source for this instrument consisted of a reflected lamp fueled with a mixture of alcohol and turpentine, with which he performed numerous investigations of the urethra and bladder [34].

Other external illumination sources followed; however the next major innovation was to be the development of an independent light source that could be transported into the body cavity being inspected. Julius Bruck (Poland) in 1860 examined the mouth using illumination provided by a platinum wire loop heated by an electric current within a water jacket [35]. This was the first galvanic endoscope and preceded the invention of Edison's filament globe by 20 years. There were numerous other descriptions throughout the remainder of the late nineteenth century on open tube endoscopy procedures including Kussmaul's description of removal of a foreign body from the esophagus using reflected sunlight. Killian in 1898 employed a tube endoscope with illumination via a reflecting head mirror with the assistance of topical cocaine to inspect the bronchus [36].

Maximilian Nitze was a general practitioner who thought that if an instrument could be introduced with ease, minimal pain, and relative safety the endoscopes must be smaller [37]. His idea was to place lenses into the tubes at prescribed distances to focus the image at an ocular. In addition, his early version used a platinum wire in a glass jacket with water cooling methods. He began clinical investigations with this cystoscope in 1877. By 1879, Nitze's design team was aware of Edison's invention of the filament globe and they immediately miniaturized it to fit into the tip of the cystoscopes. The first actual use of the Edison incandescent lamp for cystoscopic application was by Newman (Glasgow, 1883), followed by Nitze (1887), Leiter (1887), and Dittel (1887) [38]. Now the pathway to the ureter and visualization of its pathology became possible.

The Birth of Ureteroscopy

It has now been over a decade since Perez-Castro Ellendt and Martinez-Peneiro first developed a designated rigid ureterorenoscope, almost three decades since Marshall visualized a ureteral calculus with a fiber-optic bundled catheter and almost 6½ decades since H.H. Young and R. McKay (1929) stumbled into the ureter in a child with posterior urethral valves [39]. They reported passing a 9.5 Fr pediatric cystoscope directly up to the renal pelvis of a child. Nearly 50 years later, Tobias Goodman not only passed a 11 Fr. pediatric cystoscope into the ureters, but he also became the first to perform interventional surgery to the upper tracts by fulgurating a low-grade transitional cell carcinoma of the ureter [40]. One year later Lyon dilated the distal ureter to 16 Fr with Jewett sounds to perform ureteroscopy with a 14 Fr resectoscope [41]. This same group first deployed the first purposely built ureteroscopes (13 Fr) for examining the distal ureter [42].

In 1980, Perez-Castro Ellendt and Martinez-Pineiro developed the longer scopes that have allowed visualization of the entire urinary tract, nephroureteroscopy [43]. The first fiber-optic endoscope was developed for the use in gastroenterology by Hirschowitz as previously described in 1957 [26]. Victor Marshall placed a fiberscope antegrade during an open exploration to visualize the pelvis and distal ureter in 1960 [44]. It did not take long for Marshall's colleagues to decrease the size of these fiberscopes and McGovern and Walzak utilized a passive fiber-optic scope transurethrally in the urinary tract in 1962 [44]. Takagi utilized such a scope to visualize the caliceal anatomy in humans in 1968 [45, 46]. Takayasu and colleagues developed and utilized a flexible ureteropyeloscope clinically by 1971 [47].

Throughout this time, urologists have managed to extend the limits of visualized access to the recesses of the urinary tracts. There have been improvements in optical imaging systems, both rod-lens and fiber optic. Illumination systems provide unprecedented color and brightness secondary to halide lamps. Minimization of the trauma of access is the result of smaller and smaller ureterorenoscopes. Finally, by moving the surgeon's eye away from the ocular, video camera systems allow the urologist the freedom to control complex endoscopic interventions. Electronics is now the key to many of these newer innovations. The CCD was invented by George Smith and Willard Boyle at the Bell Laboratory on October 17, 1969, for electronic video recording. This was rapidly applied to fiber-optic technology initially by Welch Allyn in 1983. Japanese makers Olympus, Fuji, and Pentax all introduced video-endoscopy in the early 1980s [48]. Equipment for manipulating ureteral and renal pathology has kept pace with the development of smaller and smaller endoscopes including all of the accoutrements now typically associated with ureteroscopy: guidewires, access sheaths, stents, and baskets [49–59]. The only real question is how small is enough and can high-quality operative instruments allow the endoscopic surgeon to perform necessary interventions in every portion of the urinary tract.

Ureterorenoscopes can be classified by their performance characteristics into rigid, semirigid, and flexible types [60]. Rigid ureteroscopes employ nonflexible optical lens systems. In the past, these have consisted of high-quality glass lenses specially arrayed to magnify the image of an ocular lens. Recent advances in plastic lenses may make these rigid lens systems antiquated before long. Semirigid and flexible ureterorenoscopes utilize fiber-optic bundles to transmit light non-coherently and return the image coherently to an ocular lens. Semirigid scopes are housed usually in a pliable metallic sheath. Since the scope can bend without interference to image transmission it has been referred to as semirigid. Flexible ureterorenoscopes have no rigid outer body. The average size of the adult ureteral orifice without dilatation is roughly 6 FR. Because the tissues are pliable they will usually admit several Fr sizes larger to enter retrograde without dilatation or undue trauma from the endoscope scraping the side walls. Below 9 Fr, it is common industrial practice to refer to a ureterorenoscope as "micro" or "mini."

Finally, the limit of imaging probably depends upon stability of the shaft, the ability of an ocular eye piece to magnify and focus microscopic fiber bundle transmissions, and the ability to simultaneously irrigate and work. Michael Marberger estimates that this limit is approximately 4.8 Fr. This was originally proposed at the World Endourology Congress in Singapore in 1992 [61]. Technology has significantly expanded the potential for miniaturization of flexible ureteroscopes and the continued "downsizing" is perceived by most investigators to be a significant advance to endourology. We have seen that sub-9Fr ureteroscopes have proliferated and that access to the upper tracts via the transurethral route will continue to have an impact upon patients with upper tract pathology. This ability can be seen to be rapidly approaching. There are emerging series of flexible ureteroscopic laser lithotripsy being done under mild sedation in an ambulatory setting without routine placement of stints currently. The scopes themselves are delicate and the "fatigability" of these diminutive instruments drives up the costs of this advancing technology [62]. Regardless of costs, urologists throughout United States and the world are seeking ever-improved methods of dealing with upper tract pathology in a cost-effective, minimally invasive, nonhospital setting [63]. Perhaps robotics and automated microdevices or even autoilluminated human urine can serve as in vivo imaging systems [64]. Alexander Pope once stated, "Be not the first by whom the new are tried, Nor yet the last to lay the old aside."

References

1. Bratslavsky G, Moran ME. Current trends in ureteroscopy. Urol Clin NA. 2004;31(1):181–7.
2. Bragg W. The Universe of Light. New York: Macmillan Co; 1933.
3. Hecht J. In City of Lights: the story of fiber optics. New York: Oxford University Press; 1999.
4. Kelly, Howard A, Curtis F. Burnam. Diseases of the Kidneys. New York: Ureters and Bladder. D Appleton and Co.; (1914)
5. Kelly HA. On a method of post-mortem examination of thoracic and abdominal viscera through vagina, perineum, and rectum, and without incision of the abdominal parietes. The Medical News. 1883;26:733–4.
6. National Institute of Medicine. Assessing medical technologies. Washington, DC: National Academy Press, 1985.
7. Moran ME. Advances in ureteroscopy. Urol Cl NA. 2003;31:xv–xvi.
8. Lang P. Candles to computers: the story of minimally invasive procedures. UWOMJ. 2011;80(1):34–6.
9. Figdor PP. Philip Bozzini: The Beginnings of Modern Endoscopy. Tuttlingen: Verlag Endo-Press; 2002.
10. Colladon D. On the reflections of a ray of light inside a parabolic liquid stream. Comptes Rendus. 1842; 15:800.
11. Desmoreaux AJ. The endoscope and its application to the diagnosis and treatment of affections of the genitourinary passages. Chicago Med J. 1867;24:177–94.
12. Halsted TH. Esophagoscopy, and bronchoscopy, with reports of six cases. NY State J Med. 1908;8(7): 869–74.
13. Stutt RG. Charles Vernon Boys (1855–1944). Obit Notice Fellows Roy Soc. 1944;4(13):771–8.
14. Sircus W, Flisk E, Craigs Z. Milestones in the evolution of endoscopy: a short history. J R Coll Physicians Edinb. 2003;33:124–34.
15. Schollmeyer T, Soyinka AS, Schollmeyer M, Meinhold-Heerlein I. Gerog Kelling (1866–1945): the root of modern day minimal invasive surgery. A forgotten legend? Arch Gynecol Obstet. 2007;276(5):505–9.
16. Zollner F. Gustave Killian, father of bronchoscopy. Arch Otolaryngol. 1965;82(6):656–9.
17. Nitze M. Eine neue Beleuchtungs und Untersuchungs method fur Harnrohre, Harnblase, und Rektum. Wiener Med Wochen. 1879;24:649.
18. Reuter MA, Reuter HJ. The development of the cystoscope. J Urol. 1998;159:638–40.
19. Moran ME. The light bulb, cystoscopy and Thomas Alva Edison. J Endourol. 2010;24(9):1395–7.
20. Musehold A. Stroboskopische und Photographische Studien. Ann des Mal du Larynx Jan. 1893.
21. Nitze MCF. Kystophotograpischer Atlas. Wiesbaden: JF Bergmann; 1894.
22. Brittain JE. Scanning the past. Proc IEEE 1996;84(4).
23. Henning N, Keilhack H. Die gezielte Farben photographie in der Magenhohle. Deutsche Med Wschr. 1938;64:1392–3.
24. vanHeel ACS. A method of transporting optical images without aberrations. Nature. 1954;173:39.
25. Hopkins HH, Kapany NS. A flexible fiberscope, using static scanning. Nature. 1954;173:39–41.
26. Hirschowitz BI. A personal history of the fiberscope. Gastroenterology. 1970;36:864–7.
27. Kieser CW. Introduction of cold light endoscopy. Akt Urol. 2008;39(2):130–4.
28. Epstein M. Endoscopy: developments in optical instrumentation. Science. 1980;210(4467):280–5.
29. Bagley DH. Ureteroscopic surgery: changing times and perspectives. Urol Cl NA. 2004;30(1):1–4.
30. Johnston III WK, Low RK, Das S. The evolution and progress of ureteroscopy. Urol Cl NA. 2004;31(1): 5–13.
31. Bozzini P. Lichtlieter, eine Enfindung zur Auschschauung innere Theiler und Krankheiten. J der Practischen Arzneykunde und Wunderartzney kunst. 1806;24:107–24.
32. Segalas PR. Un moyen d'eclairer 'uretre et la vessie de maniere a voir dans l'interieur de ces organs. Revue Medicale Francaise et de L'etrangere. 1827;1:157–8.
33. Fisher J. Instruments for illuminating dark cavities. Phil J Med. 1827;14:409.
34. Desmormeaux AJ. De l'Endoscopie, instrument proper a' ec lairer certaines cavities interieures de l'economie. Compte rendus de L'Academie des Sciences. 1855;40:692–3.

35. Bruck J. Das Urethroscop und Stomatoscop Durch Galvanisches Gluhlict. Breslau: Marushke and Berendt; 1867.
36. Killian G. Zur Geschicnte der Oesophago und Gastroskopie. Deutsche Zeitschrift fur Chirirgie. 1900;59:499–512.
37. Nitze M. Beitrage zur Endosckopie der mannlichen Hamblase. Arch fur Klinishce Chirurgie. 1881;36: 661–732.
38. Newell OK. The endoscopic instruments of Joseph Leiter of Vienna and the present development of endoscopy. Boston Med. 1887;117:528–30.
39. Young HH, McKay RW. Congenital valvular obstruction of the prostatic urethra. Surg Gynecol Obstet. 1929;48:509.
40. Goodman T. Ureteroscopy with pediatric cystoscope in adults. Urology. 1977;9(4):394.
41. Lyon ES, Kyker JS, Schoenberg HW. Tranurethral ureteroscopy in women: a ready addition to the urological armamentarium. J Urol. 1978;119:35–6.
42. Lyon ES. The birth of modern ureteroscopy: the Albona Jaybis story. J Endourol. 2004;18(6):525–6.
43. Perez-Castro EE, Martinez-Piniero JA. Transurethral ureteroscopy- a current urological procedure. Arch Esp Urol. 1980;33(5):445–60.
44. Marshall VF. Fiber optics in urology. J Urol. 1964;91:110–4.
45. Takagi T, Go T, Takayasu H, Aso Y. A small-caliber fiberscope for visualization of urinary tract, biliary tract, and spinal canal. Surgery. 1968;64:1033.
46. Takagi T, Go T, Takayasu H, Aso Y. Fiberoptic pyeloureteroscopy. Surgery. 1971;70:661.
47. Takayasu H, Aso Y. Recent development for pyeloureteroscopy: guide tube method for tis introduction into the ureter. J Urol. 1974;112:176.
48. Vilardell F. Digestive endoscopy in the second millennium. Thieme, Madrid: From Lichleiter to endoscopy; 2006.
49. Das S. Transureteral ureteroscopy and stone manipulation under direct vision. J Urol. 1981;125:112–3.
50. Huffman JL, Bagley DH, Lyon ES. Treatment of distal ureteral calculi using rigid ureteroscope. Urology. 1982;20(6):574.
51. Huffman JL, Bagley DH, Lyon ES. Extending cystoscopic techniques into the ureter and renal pelvis: experience with ureteroscopy and pyeloscopy. JAMA. 1983;250:2002–5.
52. Goodfiend R. Ultrasonic and electrohydraulic lithotripsy of ureteral calculi. Urology. 1984;23: 5–8.
53. Dretler SP, Watson G, Parrish JA, Murray S. Pulsed dye laser fragmentation of ureteral calculi: initial clinical experience. J Urol. 1987;137:386–9.
54. Webb DR, Kockelburgh R, Johnson WF. The VersaPpulse holmium surgical laser in clinical urology: a pilot study. Minim Invasive Ther. 1993;2: 23–6.
55. Fritzsche P, Moorhead JD, Axford PD, Torrey RR. Urologic applications of andiographic guide wire and catheter techniques. J Urol. 1981;125(6):774–80.
56. Newman RC, Hunter PT, Hawkins IF, Finlayson B. A general ureteral dilator-sheathing system. Urology. 1985;25(3):287–8.
57. Zimskind PD, Fetter TR, Wilkerson JL. Clinical use of long-term indwelling silicone rubber ureteral splints inserted cystoscopically. J Urol. 1967;97(5): 840–4.
58. Gibbons RP, Correa RJJ, Cummings KB, Mason JT. Experience with indwelling ureteral stent catheters. J Urol. 1976;115:22–6.
59. Finney RP. Experience with new double J ureteral catheter stent. J Urol. 2002;167(2 Pt 2):1135–8.
60. Basillote JB, Lee DI, Eichel L, Clayman RV. Ureteroscopes: flexible, rigid, and semirigid. Urol Cl NA. 2004;31(1):21–32.
61. Marberger M. "Needle" ureteroscopes- where are the limits of miniaturization [abstract]. J Endourol. 1992;1–2:46.
62. White MD, Moran ME. Fatigability of the latest generation ureteropyeloscopes [abstract]. J Endourol. 1998;12:S182.
63. Natalin RA, Landman J. Where next for the endoscope? Nat Rev Urol. 2009;6(11):622–8.
64. Moran ME. The history of robotic surgery. In: Hemal AK, Menon M, editors. Robotics in Genitourinary Surgery. London: Springer; 2011. p. 3–24.

Ureteroscopy in 2012: The Scope of the Scope

2

Stephen Faddegon and Margaret S. Pearle

Introduction

Understanding the current and future role of ureteroscopy (URS) in the management of urologic disease requires scrutiny of the current niche that URS fills, examination of utilization trends, and analysis of new and competing technologies. URS has the potential to gain increasing application due to advances in instrumentation, effective dissemination of endourologic techniques, and evidence of more favorable outcomes compared with other treatment modalities. For example, URS is gradually assuming a larger role in the treatment of upper tract urothelial cancer (UTUC) as the importance of renal preservation is further validated and the oncologic results in select patients appear to be comparable to more established treatments [1]. On the other hand, URS appears to be losing ground in the management of primary ureteropelvic junction obstruction (UPJO), increasingly supplanted by laparoscopy, because of the high success rates of the latter. Nevertheless, incisional URS continues to play an important role as salvage therapy for UPJO and as primary therapy for ureteral stricture disease [2].

S. Faddegon, M.D. • M.S. Pearle, M.D., Ph.D. (✉)
Department of Urology, UT Southwestern Medical Center, 5323 Harry Hines Blvd., J8.106, Dallas, TX 75390-9110, USA
e-mail: margaret.pearle@utsouthwestern.edu

Clinical decision-making, however, takes into account not only primary outcomes but also the availability and skill of specialized practitioners, patient and physician preference, and economic considerations. Increasingly, financial concerns must be factored into the therapeutic decision-making equation. From this perspective, URS offers a number of advantages over other minimally invasive treatment modalities, including outpatient treatment, relatively low-cost instrumentation, and a short learning curve.

In this chapter, we aim to identify current utilization patterns for URS and to briefly review treatment outcomes and economic factors that drive treatment decisions. By understanding these driving forces and recognizing emerging technologies both competing and not, we can anticipate the direction of URS in the future.

Utilization Patterns

By far, the most common indication for URS is the management of renal and ureteral calculi. In one institutional series of 1,000 consecutive URS from a tertiary care center, the procedural indication was urolithiasis in 57.9%, diagnostic in 20.6%, urothelial carcinoma in 12.6%, ureteral stricture in 4.4%, and UPJO in 0.8% [3]. As such, URS for urolithiasis is the most well-studied indication from a utilization perspective and thus it will comprise the focus of this section.

Despite significant advances in ureteroscope design and instrumentation during the 1990s, the

M. Monga (ed.), *Ureteroscopy: Indications, Instrumentation & Technique*, Current Clinical Urology,
DOI 10.1007/978-1-62703-206-3_2,

Urologic Diseases in America Project found that the distribution of surgical procedures for stone disease remained relatively stable between 1992 and 2000, with shock wave lithotripsy (SWL) comprising the most commonly performed procedure in all years of study, followed closely by URS. Percutaneous nephrolithotomy (PCNL) and open surgery together comprised less than 5% of procedures. Among Medicare beneficiaries in 1998, SWL, URS, and PCNL comprised 54%, 41%, and 3–4% of procedures, respectively. Commercially insured individuals demonstrated a remarkably similar distribution and trend [4].

On the other hand, Kerble and colleagues reported a 53% increase in URS utilization between 1990 and 1998 at Washington University, St. Louis. Because their institution represents a tertiary care center with a strong Endourology program, however, the generalizability of their institutional findings is limited. However, using data derived from the Health Care Financing Administration (HCFA), a dataset more representative of general practice, they identified an increase in the proportion of surgical stone procedures accounted for by URS, from 14 to 22%, representing a 57% increase between 1992 and 2000 [5]. The discrepancy between the HCFA and UDA datasets in the distribution of surgical stone procedures during this time period is not clear.

Recent analysis of urologist case logs also suggested that URS utilization is increasing at the expense of SWL. Matlaga [6] examined case logs from nearly 3,000 urologists undergoing certification (2004–2008) and recertification (2003–2007) in order to identify trends in the distribution of surgical stone procedures. Since recertification is required every 10 years, these groups of urologists serve as surrogates for temporal trends in the surgical management of stone disease. Matlaga found that recently trained urologists (candidates for initial American Board of Urology certification), arguably the cohort most predictive of future practice patterns, were more likely than successive recertification groups to perform URS than SWL. URS comprised 52% of surgical stone procedures in the certification group compared with 38% and 36.7% in the first and second recertification groups, respectively. Accordingly, SWL use increased from 41 to 57% and 60.5% in the three cohorts, respectively. Moreover, 90% of these newly trained urologists, compared with less than 80% of recertification candidates, reported performing at least one case of URS with lithotripsy [6].

An e-mail survey by Bandi and colleagues [7] supports Matlaga's finding that newly trained urologists are more likely to perform URS than SWL. The authors queried 790 North Central Section AUA members about their practice patterns with regard to surgical stone management. With a response rate of 22% for their survey, they found that SWL was the most commonly performed procedure overall for renal and proximal ureteral calculi, but that URS was more likely to be performed by younger urologists (<5 years in practice) than older urologists (>20 years in practice) [7]. The reasons for this finding are not entirely clear, but likely include increasing exposure to URS during residency, varying referral patterns, and changing treatment paradigms that are disseminated more quickly in academic training centers. Alternatively, Matlaga suggested that perhaps newly trained urologists simply have less busy practices that allow more time to perform URS, a more time-consuming procedure, compared with SWL [6].

Intuitively, the choice to perform URS is also likely to be influenced by the existing practice patterns. Scales and colleagues performed a multivariate analysis to identify factors independently associated with the choice of URS or SWL. Using a Medicare 5% sample, they identified patients with a stone encounter between 1997 and 2007 and found that among 9,358 beneficiaries, URS was performed in 44% and SWL in 56% of cases. Additionally, they determined that the likelihood of a patient undergoing URS rather than SWL was nearly fivefold greater when the provider performed high-volume URS (OR 4.71, 95% CI 4.14–5.36, $p=0.001$). Likewise, when treated at a high-volume URS facility, a patient was 44% more likely to undergo URS than SWL [8].

Although it is apparent that utilization rates differ according to the age of the practitioner, a variety of other nonclinical factors, such as geographic region or patient gender, may also influence practice patterns. Unfortunately, little data is available regarding geographic variation of URS rates. However, Scales and colleagues found that female patients were statistically less likely than males to undergo URS (OR 0.844, $p=0.006$) based on a multivariate analysis of a Medicare 5% sample dataset [8]. The reason for this discrepancy between genders could not be determined from this dataset, and the UDA analysis did not stratify utilization rates of URS by patient gender. Interestingly, theoretical concerns about potential injury to the ovaries in women of child-bearing age undergoing SWL for middle and distal ureteral calculi [9] might be expected to increase URS utilization among female patients. However, Scales and colleagues found the opposite [8].

Utilization rates for URS in the treatment of UTUC have not been systematically analyzed. However, Razdan and colleagues assessed urologist practice patterns regarding the management of UTUC in a 2005 postal survey of 220 urologists. Among the respondents (38% response rate), 80% practiced in an academic medical center, likely reflecting a sampling bias. Among the respondents, 70% indicated that URS was their surveillance tool of choice after endoscopic management of UTUC. For the treatment of low-grade, superficial renal pelvic tumors, 77% responded that laser ablation was their treatment of choice. In contrast, most respondents (73%) preferred to treat large, high-grade tumors with laparoscopic nephroureterectomy. The survey revealed significant variation among respondents in the preference for treatment of high-grade UTUC in a solitary kidney: 34% favored nephroureterectomy, 30% favored URS, and 27% favored percutaneous ablation [10]. Unfortunately, surveys only reveal what a practitioner says he prefers, not what he actually does, and therefore this tool is of limited value in assessing utilization trends.

Utilization patterns in the management of UPJO have evolved significantly over the past 10–15 years. Although laparoscopic pyeloplasty has become more widely utilized [11], it is unclear whether this trend has impacted utilization rates of retrograde endopyelotomy, or whether it simply reflects decreasing rates of open pyeloplasty and Acucise™ ureteral cutting balloon endopyelotomy. Gerber and colleagues surveyed urologists in 2002 and 2007 using mailing lists from the American Urological Association and the Endourological Society. In the 2002 survey, only 8% and 11–21% of respondents selected retrograde endopyelotomy as the treatment of choice for patients with and without a crossing vessel, respectively. The relatively low rate of laparoscopic pyeloplasty (<14% of respondents) and ureteroscopic endopyelotomy was balanced by more frequent preference for Acucise endopyelotomy and open pyeloplasty. In 2007, 68% of respondents reported that endourology comprised ≤25% of their practice. For patients without a crossing vessel, 43–69% of respondents selected laparoscopic pyeloplasty as their treatment of choice, depending on the degree of hydronephrosis. Only 5 and 20% of respondents preferred retrograde endopyelotomy for the treatment of patients with and without a crossing vessel, respectively [12].

Factors Impacting Ureteroscopy Utilization

Clinical and socioeconomic factors influence the decision as to which surgical modality is selected to treat particular upper tract pathology. While stone, tumor, or stricture characteristics may impact the success rate of a given treatment modality, procedural costs are an increasing consideration, particularly in the setting of comparable outcomes. Competing and emerging technologies may change the balance of treatment modalities and threaten to replace or relegate URS to a salvage procedure for some indications, thereby leading to flux in URS utilization. Finally, nonclinical factors, such as patient demographics and provider bias, may not impact outcomes, yet nonetheless constitute important driving forces behind the trends in utilization of URS.

Clinical Determinants

Urolithiasis

In stone disease, URS has traditionally been favored for the treatment of distal ureteral calculi because of the ease with which distal stones can be accessed with a semirigid ureteroscope. While URS remains the first-line option for distal ureteral stones for many practitioners, the indications for URS have expanded over the years to include proximal and mid ureteral calculi and renal stones. Improved optics, flexible ureteroscopes, miniaturization of instrumentation, and digital technology have made access to the upper ureter and collecting system easier and more reliable [3].

The relative efficacy of URS and SWL for the treatment of ureteral stones depends primarily on stone size, stone location, and stone composition. The AUA Ureteral Stones Clinical Guidelines Panel performed a meta-analysis of clinical trials evaluating the efficacy of URS and SWL for stones in the proximal, middle, and distal ureter. They found no statistically significant difference in the overall stone-free rate for proximal stones treated by URS or SWL (81% versus 82%, respectively). However, while SWL stone-free rates were inversely proportional to stone size (90% for stones <10 mm versus 68% for stones ≥10 mm), URS stone-free rates were size independent (80% versus 79%, respectively). In the mid ureter, stone-free rates were superior for URS compared with SWL (86% versus 73%, respectively), but the advantage of URS was limited to smaller stones (stone-free rate of 91% for URS versus 84% for SWL). Distal ureteral stones were consistently more effectively treated by URS than SWL (94% stone free for URS versus 74% for SWL), and that relationship held true for both smaller stones (97% versus 86%, respectively) and larger stones (93% versus 74%, respectively). While the Panel recommended that both URS and SWL are acceptable first-line treatment options for ureteral calculi, the meta-analysis showed that URS is the procedure associated with the highest stone-free rates in a single procedure in most stratifications examined [13]. Consequently, the role of URS in the management of ureteral stones in all locations is secure.

The use of URS for the management of renal calculi is not new, but is expanding. As long ago as 1990, Fuchs and Fuchs reported a series of 208 patients with intrarenal calculi treated ureteroscopically with a stone-free rate of 87% [14]. Fabrizio and colleagues [15] and Grasso [16] subsequently reported a series of 100 and 228 patients, respectively, treated with URS for renal calculi with "success rates" of 77% and 81%, respectively. With improvements in ureteroscope design and instrumentation, the indications for URS treatment of intrarenal calculi have expanded, and treatment of larger, more complex stones has been reported. Breda and colleagues [17] reviewed 15 patients with single ≥2 cm intrarenal stones who underwent URS and reported an overall stone-free rate of 93.3%, although the mean number of procedures required was 2.3. Grasso and colleagues reported a single session success rate (stone free or <2 mm residual fragments) of 76% for URS treatment of >2 cm stones in 51 patients, increasing to 91% after including a repeat session [18]. While URS in patients with large renal calculi is feasible, it is debatable whether this treatment modality offers a significant advantage over PCNL, which is clearly associated with the higher stone-free rate [19].

The biggest controversy surrounding the management of renal calculi involves small- to moderate-sized stones (<1 cm), where both URS and SWL have demonstrated good success and low morbidity. Unfortunately, the only randomized trial (RCT) comparing the two treatment modalities was limited to lower pole renal calculi. Using strict CT criteria to determine stone-free rates, both treatment modalities were associated with disappointingly low stone-free rates (50% versus 35%, respectively) [20]. Further trials are necessary to compare URS and SWL for comparable sized stones in non-lower pole locations.

Strict assessment of stone-free rates using CT has demonstrated reduced stone-free rates compared to historical series using KUB and/or ultrasound imaging. Portis and associates reported a 59% stone-free rate by CT in 48 patients with 5–15 mm renal calculi evaluated prospectively after URS using a ureteral access sheath and manual stone retrieval [21]. Macejko and coworkers also reported a dismal 35% stone-free rate by CT in a group of patients retrospectively reviewed after URS for renal calculi [22]. These disappointing results underscore the importance of accurate and uniform radiographic assessment of outcomes after treatment of stones using any modality in order to facilitate the decision-making process.

Recent adjuncts to URS and SWL have the potential to change the balance of these two treatment modalities as they compete for first-line treatment of renal calculi. Ureteral access sheaths provide the opportunity for improved intraoperative fragment passage or removal, thereby potentially enhancing URS stone-free rates [23]. The use of manual fragment retrieval via a ureteral access sheath in conjunction with URS has shown a trend toward higher stone-free rates, although statistical significance has not been demonstrated in the single reported RCT [24]. On the other hand, the use of adjuvant pharmacotherapy has been shown to enhance stone-free rates after SWL [25, 26] and URS [27], potentially further altering historical outcomes. Finally, optimizing SWL treatment parameters, such as slowing the rate of shock wave delivery, has been shown to improve stone-free rates [28]. Still, URS provides the most flexibility among the minimally invasive treatment options for renal calculi because it is not limited by patient body habitus, weight, or anticoagulant use [29–32].

Refinement in patient selection has further streamlined the choice of URS versus SWL for renal calculi, and enhanced stone-free rates overall. The use of parameters derived from CT images, such as CT Hounsfield units and skin-to-stone distance, has allowed construction of algorithms to guide treatment selection taking into account stone size, CT Hounsfield units, skin-to-stone distance, stone location, and stone composition [33–35]. Further RCTs, incorporating treatment adjuncts and perhaps new treatment algorithms, are necessary to more accurately compare treatment modalities in their current state.

Diagnostic Ureteroscopy

Diagnostic URS is typically undertaken to investigate a finding of abnormal cytology or upper tract filling defect, or as surveillance following conservative treatment for upper tract urothelial cancer (UTUC). CT urography constitutes the gold standard for the radiographic investigation of UTUC and can detect papillary lesions >5 mm with 96% sensitivity and 99% specificity. However, sensitivity drops to 89% for <5 mm polypoid lesions and to 40% for <3 mm lesions [36]. MR urography has not improved diagnostic accuracy and remains investigational at this time [37]. Furthermore, radiographic imaging cannot detect CIS. As such, URS is still useful for the definitive exclusion or diagnosis of UTUC in these scenarios.

But could advances in imaging render diagnostic URS obsolete? The 2011 EAU guidelines do not require URS for the diagnosis of UTUC, instead requiring only urine cytology, CT urography, and cystoscopy [38]. Indeed, many practitioners proceed to radical nephroureterectomy based on positive cytology and upper tract filling defect alone. Nevertheless, URS enables procurement of a biopsy, which is the only definitive diagnostic tool. Furthermore, tumor grade remains the best predictor of the invasiveness of UTUC and the risk of progression. Until future radiographic techniques can accurately predict tumor stage and grade, URS is likely to remain an important diagnostic tool for UTUC.

Several urine tests are currently under investigation for their role in the diagnosis and prognostication of UTUC. Although no contemporary biomarker or panel of biomarkers can substitute for URS and biopsy for the diagnosis of UTUC, it is conceivable that a highly sensitive urine test, in conjunction with radiographic imaging, could render URS and biopsy unnecessary in select cases.

Cytology is the most widely used urine test, but it has limited sensitivity for detecting low-grade tumors which are often found on surveillance URS following conservative management [39, 40]. Although one small study found that fluorescence in situ hybridization (FISH) test reliably diagnosed UTUC with 100% sensitivity and 90% specificity [41], most studies have shown that the sensitivity of FISH, like urine cytology, diminishes significantly with low-grade tumors [39]. Consequently, these urine tests cannot replace the diagnostic accuracy of URS and biopsy.

There are, however, other urine tests on the horizon that deserve further consideration. ImmunoCyt (Diagnocure, Inc.), for example, reportedly has higher sensitivity for detecting low-grade tumors, although it has been studied primarily in bladder tumors [39] and is still far less accurate than imaging or endoscopy.

While URS undoubtedly facilitates the diagnosis of UTUC, there are significant limitations with regard to tumor visualization and biopsy. Visual inspection has been suggested to be less than 70% accurate in predicting tumor grade [42]. In one study examining the accuracy of endoscopic biopsy for UTUC, 43% of patients were reclassified from low-grade, noninvasive disease to high-grade and/or invasive disease on subsequent biopsy or resection performed at a median of 6 weeks post biopsy [43]. The significantly improved optics of current digital ureteroscopes will likely enhance the diagnostic accuracy of URS. In addition, several adjuncts to URS are currently under investigation to enhance diagnostic accuracy, including endoluminal ultrasound for staging assessment [44], narrow band imaging (NBI) [45], PPD fluorescence to aid in the identification of CIS and small tumors [46], and development of multivariate models which predict tumor stage by combining results of URS, biopsy, and imaging [47].

Serial surveillance URS, along with imaging, is recommended for the follow-up of conservatively managed UTUC but it is costly and resource intensive since it involves use of the operating room and anesthesia. A few centers have attempted to avoid the cost and inconvenience of the operating room by performing diagnostic URS in the office setting, some with protocols that span almost 20 years. While some centers are highly selective with regard to patient candidates for office surveillance URS, choosing those with patulous ureters, Boari flaps, or reimplanted ureters [48], others have shown that routine patients can readily undergo ureteroscopic evaluation in the office. Reisiger and colleagues performed 67 URS in 10 patients who had been treated conservatively for UTUC, identifying recurrences in 7 [49]. Only one patient had more extensive disease than initially recognized on surveillance URS, and no patients subsequently developed invasive disease or metastasis because of missed lesions. These authors described unroofing the ureteral orifice at the time of initial 3-month follow-up URS in the operating room to facilitate passage of the flexible ureteroscope in the clinic, thereby obviating the need for analgesia or sedation [49]. More widespread use of office surveillance URS will likely increase URS utilization in the future.

Upper Tract Urothelial Cancer

Reports of acceptable oncologic control after ureteroscopic resection of low-grade UTUC have led to increasing interest in this minimally invasive treatment modality as first-line therapy. Furthermore, growing concern over the deleterious effects of renal insufficiency resulting from renal loss is likely to result in a surge of nephron-sparing treatment modalities, including ureteroscopic resection/ablation.

The 2011 EAU guidelines subdivide the indications for a nephron-sparing approach into imperative cases (patients with renal insufficiency or a solitary functional kidney) and elective cases (patients with low-grade, low-stage, completely resectable tumors). However, not all of these patients are amenable to ureteroscopic resection because of technical constraints, anatomic location of the tumor (i.e., lower pole calyx), or lack of surgeon experience [38].

Reports of disease-specific survival for URS are favorable, ranging from 81 to 100% for carefully selected patients with follow-up between 35 and 72 months [1, 50–52]. Ipsilateral recurrence rates, however, are significant, ranging from 25 to 93% with a follow-up of 31–72 months [1, 50, 53, 54]. In a recent multi-institutional study of 1,268 patients undergoing radical nephroureterectomy, 5-year cancer-specific survival was 77% in patients treated initially with ureteropic laser ablation compared to 73% in patients who underwent immediate nephroureterectomy ($p=0.365$). Furthermore, multivariate analysis determined that a history of endoscopic ablation was not associated with increased disease recurrence or cancer-specific mortality, implying that endoscopic resection does not compromise future oncologic control [55]. Although highly select patients have favorable outcomes, patients requiring endoscopic resection for imperative indications do worse, with a 5-year cancer-specific survival of only 49% in one series [56].

URS has the advantage of being the least invasive of the minimally invasive treatment options for UTUC. Percutaneous resection is a good alternative when tumor location or size precludes successful ureteroscopic access or treatment. Distal ureterectomy is favored for distal ureteral tumors, particularly when high grade, while partial renal resection is rarely used in the current treatment paradigm [38].

The primary impetus that could drive increased utilization of uretersocopic treatment of UTUC is the mounting evidence of a strong advantage of renal functional preservation. Radical nephroureterectomy has been shown to result in a 25% decline in GFR [57, 58] in a patient population already at risk for preexisting renal dysfunction. Lane and colleagues reported a series of 336 patients undergoing radical nephroureterectomy for whom the mean preoperative GFR of 61.7 mL/min/1.73 m^2 decreased to 47.9 mL/min/1.73 m^2 postoperatively, representing a mean GFR loss of 13.9 ml/min/1.73 m^2 (95% CI 12.4–15.4, $p<0.001$) [58].

This data is further corroborated by a wide body of literature evaluating renal functional loss in patients undergoing nephrectomy for renal cell carcinoma (RCC). Huang and colleagues, for example, reported on renal function outcomes in 662 patients undergoing radical nephrectomy for RCC and found that the 3-year probability of freedom from new-onset GFR<60 mL/min/1.73 m^2 was only 35%, compared to 80% in those undergoing a nephron-sparing approach [59]. Furthermore, GFR is known to be inversely proportional to overall mortality and cardiovascular events. The hazard ratio for death from any cause was 5.9 (95% CI 5.4–6.5) in patients with a GFR <15 mL/min/1.73 m^2 compared to those with a GFR >60 mL/min/1.73 m^2 [60]. These concerns may justify increasing usage of ureteroscopic and percutaneous tumor resection for UTUC, particularly in the setting of low-grade, low-stage disease that can potentially be completely resected. Improvements in technique and instrumentation that facilitate tumor base resection and extraction may also allow less experienced endoscopists to safely adopt this treatment approach.

Ureteropelvic Junction Obstruction and Ureteral Strictures

A number of endoscopic cutting techniques, using both a retrograde and antegrade approach, have been reported to treat UPJO. Retrograde use of the Acucise™ ureteral cutting balloon catheter has been largely supplanted by ureteroscopic laser endopyelotomy due to comparable success rates, a greater safety profile, and lower cost [61]. Nevertheless, endoscopic approaches have been shown to yield inferior outcomes compared with reconstructive techniques [62–64], particularly when long-term success rates are considered. DiMarco and colleagues reported 3- and 10-year recurrence-free survival rates of 63% and 41% for endopyelotomy compared with 85 and 75% for open or laparoscopic pyeloplasty [65]. In the pre-robotic era, endoscopic resection allowed a minimally invasive approach while sparing the morbidity of open surgery and permitting treatment by urologists lacking advanced laparoscopic skills. With the widespread dissemination of the robot, however, minimally invasive dismembered pyeloplasty has become accessible to more urologists and is quickly becoming the favored treatment for UPJO [2]. Even in countries where robots are not economically feasible, laparoscopy is widely considered the standard of care despite being more technically difficult than endoscopic incision [66]. Certain clinical factors such as crossing vessels or massive hydronephrosis may strengthen the preference for dismembered pyeloplasty in some practitioners [11]. Overall, the role of endopyelotomy is likely to continue to dwindle over time as the experience with robotic or laparoscopic pyeloplasty grows.

Despite the advantages of dismembered pyeloplasty in treating primary UPJO, including the higher success rate, ability to concomitantly remove stones, and ability to accommodate crossing vessels or anomalous kidneys, ureteroscopic endopyelotomy retains a small niche in treatment of pyeloplasty failures or patients not amenable to laparoscopic surgery [2]. Butani and associates used strict criteria to select patients for endopyelotomy and reported a 95% success rate at 60 months follow-up in patients without severe hydronephrosis, with strictures <2 cm and with >25% ipsilateral differential renal function [67].

Unlike endopyelotomy, however, ureteroscopic endoureterotomy for the treatment of ureteral strictures remains viable first-line therapy in select cases in which the stricture is short and non-ischemic. Reported success rates range from 55 to 85%, depending on the location, length, and etiology of the stricture [10, 68]. Despite some reports of improved success with adjuvant injection therapies [69], success rates do not yet approach reconstructive modalities.

Ureteroenteric anastomotic strictures comprise a special subgroup of ureteral strictures that pose a risk regardless of approach. Open surgery is fraught with difficulty due to proximity of the great vessels and intense adhesions, although success rates are quite high, ranging from 76 to 92% [70]. On the other hand, endoscopic management usually requires an antegrade approach and involves blind incision in proximity to the great vessels and bowel. Success rates from 50 to 90% have been reported, but appear to diminish with time, with reported success rates as low as 32% at 3 years [69–71].

Nonclinical Determinants

Urolithiasis

The choice of surgical modality for stone removal may be influenced by patient preference, which relies on patient perception of the success and morbidity of the procedure. Several studies have suggested that patients perceive URS as a more morbid procedure than SWL [20, 72]. Bensalah and associates administered the SF-36™ quality of life questionnaire to 155 consecutive consenting patients seen in a specialized stone clinic, and then performed multivariate analysis to identify factors predictive of quality of life. They determined that the number of URS procedures and stent placements were independently associated with mental well-being (mental composite summary), negatively impacting the individual domains of general health, emotional well-being (URS only), role limitation caused by emotional problems (stents only), and energy/fatigue. In contrast, SWL had no influence on quality of life or individual domains [72].

Although stent placement and URS were independently associated with quality of life domains, it is not clear how well URS and stent placement can be separated, since the study by Bensalah did not differentiate URS with or without stent placement. Indeed, Pearle and colleagues suggested that perhaps differences in perceived morbidity associated with SWL and URS for the treatment of lower pole stones may be accounted for by the routine use of ureteral stents after URS. In a randomized trial comparing SWL and URS for the treatment of patients with ≤10 mm lower pole renal calculi, patients undergoing URS required more pain pills postoperatively (mean 14.7 versus 5.6, $p=0.015$) and reported longer convalescence time (15.6 versus 8.1 days, $p=0.006$) than SWL. Furthermore, when asked if they would undergo the same procedure again, only 63% of URS patients said "yes," compared to 90% of SWL patients ($p=0.031$) [20]. Whether the difference in perceived morbidity is related to the use of stents with URS is not clear. However, perhaps due to its non-invasiveness, SWL is perceived by patients as less morbid. Whether patient perceptions and preferences have ultimately influenced URS utilization has not been carefully analyzed.

Upper Tract Urothelial Carcinoma

There is limited data examining nonclinical factors predicting utilization patterns of ureteroscopic ablation although at least one study suggests that surgeon training or preference may be important. In a survey of 84 urologists who were members of either the Society of Urologic Oncologists (SUO) or the Endourological Society (ES), 21% of ES members were comfortable with endoscopic management of high-grade, large distal ureteral tumors, while 100% of SUO members performed distal ureterectomies for this pathologic scenario [10].

Ureteropelvic Junction Obstruction

Nonclinical factors also play into the decision-making process for UPJO. In a 2005 survey of 391 urologists selected from the American Urological Association directory, for instance, surgeon training or experience was the most influential factor in deciding between endopyelotomy or pyeloplasty [11], followed by the expected success rate of the procedure, degree of invasiveness, time required to perform the procedure, and finally the cost. Practitioners in an academic setting were also more likely than those in a nonacademic setting to recommend an endoscopic or laparoscopic procedure versus an open procedure (87.4% versus 79.9%, respectively). A survey of 37 academic endourologists found that these same factors affected their choice of treatment modality. An additional 9% of respondents stated that patient preference influenced their decision [73].

Economic Factors

While URS treatment of upper tract pathology may, in some settings, have clinical advantages over other treatment modalities, economic considerations may also play a role in the decision-making process. Initial and salvage procedure costs, provider compensation, and the risk of requiring a secondary procedure clearly play an important role in current and future utilization patterns of URS. Compared with competing technology (SWL, percutaneous procedures, laparoscopy with or without a robot), URS has relatively low capital costs, is nearly exclusively an outpatient procedure, and has low associated morbidity, making it a highly cost-favorable procedure.

However, procedural cost is not equivalent to cost-effectiveness, since the latter takes into account not only the cost of the procedure but also the success rates, morbidity, and cost of salvage treatment in the event of failure. Evaluating the cost-effectiveness of any procedure is complicated by the lack of generalizability across regions, healthcare systems, or time periods. For example, Chandhoke and colleagues surveyed ten countries and found SWL to be more costly than URS in five countries and less costly in two [74]. Furthermore, the cost of the procedure differs according to whose perspective is being considered (patient, healthcare system, insurance provider, society). Even within the same region, different insurance plans are associated with different cost distributions for patient and provider. Finally, it must be recognized that the most cost-effective strategy does not always translate into higher utilization. Although from a societal perspective selection of the most cost-effective strategy is desirable, other considerations may favor a more costly procedure. For example, SWL has one of the highest physician reimbursements per unit time of any urological procedure [75, 76]. Furthermore, SWL is associated with a separate reimbursable "facility fee," which has encouraged urologists to invest in lithotripters and ambulatory surgical centers [77]. Indeed, between 1993 and 2001, urologist investment in lithotripters grew from 36 to 54%, which some have speculated may account for the higher utilization of SWL compared with URS [77].

The extent to which physician compensation affects URS utilization patterns is unclear. One might expect that compensation patterns would favor SWL use over URS. However, a recent study failed to show a correlation between increasing urologist ownership of lithotripters and utilization rates of URS [78]. Review of the State Ambulatory Surgery Database for Michigan revealed that the number of outpatient URS procedures remained unchanged from the years prior to 2004, the date on which physician lithotripter ownership was permitted, to 3 years later when ownership became widespread. The population of patients undergoing URS, however, did change, shifting toward those who were older, non-Caucasian, had more co-morbidities, and were less likely to have private health insurance [78]. Another multivariable analysis examining factors predictive of URS use also found that facility ownership and the number of local ambulatory surgical centers were not associated with preferential use of SWL [8].

Urolithiasis

Total expenditures for stone management rose 50% (from $1.27 billion to $2.07 billion per year) between 1994 and 2000 [4]. Since URS accounts for 40–50% of procedures performed for stones, it is clear that significant economic resources are allocated to this treatment modality annually.

There are few reports comparing the costs of URS and PCNL. One single-center study concluded that URS was more cost-effective than PCNL for renal calculi ($6,675 versus 19,845, $p<0.0001$), even for stones 2–3 cm in size, because URS was performed on an outpatient basis, and fewer second-stage procedures were required for primary URS than PCNL (1.1 procedures versus 1.6 procedures, respectively, $p=0.003$) [79]. However, in this non-randomized trial, residual fragments were much more likely to be treated after PCNL than after URS, thereby limiting the value of this analysis.

Several cost analyses have compared URS and SWL for the management of renal or ureteral calculi. In most of these studies, URS has been shown to be a more cost-effective treatment modality than SWL for the management of ureteral stones, primarily due to higher SWL retreatment rates [80–83]. In a decision tree analysis that takes into account success rates, procedural costs, and the cost of treatment failures, Lotan and associates [76] showed that URS was more cost-effective than SWL regardless of stone location. In their model, the total cost of SWL ranged from $4729 to $4865, while the total cost of URS ranged from $2,785 to $3,344, depending on stone location. URS was more cost-effective by $1440, $1670, and $1750 for stones in proximal, middle, and distal ureter, respectively. In no scenario did SWL become cost-equivalent with URS, largely because of the large capital cost of the lithotripter [76].

Upper Tract Urothelial Carcinoma

Resources allocated to the management of UTUC are insignificant compared with the expenditures for stone disease, with an estimated $64 million spent in the USA in 2000 for UTUC compared with over $2.1 billion for stone disease [84]. Furthermore, the proportion of that figure allocated to ureteroscopic management of UTUC is negligible. Cost comparison between URS and open/laparoscopic management is problematic because of the significant bias associated with patient selection for these different procedures. However, one study reported 2009 perioperative costs of diagnostic URS, URS laser ablation, and laparoscopic radical nephroureterectomy as $2,961, $5,270, and $21,764, respectively. These authors performed a cost comparison assuming a worst-case scenario of a solitary kidney subjected to either definitive radical nephroureterectomy or to URS resection and surveillance every 3 months. They determined that over a 2-year period of time, upper tract preservation with URS treatment would result in savings of $252,272, primarily due to costs attributable to dialysis and the management of ESRD [85]. While this simplified analysis does not apply to the majority of patients, the cost differential in this case is staggering.

Ureteropelvic Junction Obstruction

A number of cost analyses have been reported comparing treatment modalities for UPJO. Using a decision tree model, Gettman and colleagues sought to identify the most cost-effective treatment for UPJO taking into account the cost of the individual procedures, the success rates, and the cost of treating failures [86]. The overall treatment costs were as follows: retrograde ureteroscopic endopyelotomy (RUE) ($3,842), Acucise™ endopyelotomy ($4,427), antegrade endopyelotomy (AE) ($5,297), laparoscopic pyeloplasty ($7,026), and open pyeloplasty ($7,119). Using two-way sensitivity analyses, RUE proved to be the most cost-effective, although not the most successful, procedure. However, the authors assumed an 84% success rate for RUE based on reports from that time period, which likely represent an overestimate based on long-term studies. However, success rates of open and laparoscopic pyeloplasty were also shown in the DiMarco study to diminish over time, and therefore it is not clear if lowering the success rates of all procedures would alter the outcome of the analysis [65].

Another study determined that Acucise™-endopyelotomy was more costly than open or laparoscopic pyeloplasty based on higher retreatment rates in the Acucise™ cohort [87]. In any analysis, the most cost-effective strategy depends on both the success rate of the procedure and the cost of the initial and salvage procedures. Over the long term, laparoscopic or robotic dismembered pyeloplasty, though costly, may prove to be more cost-effective than endopyelotomy, as the cost of laproscopic/robotic instruments decreases. In the meantime, however, while robot-assisted pyeloplasty is highly effective, it is significantly more costly and is unlikely to prove cost-superior at this time [66].

Conclusions

URS is poised to maintain an important role in the management of upper tract disease well into the future. The utilization of URS for renal and ureteral calculi will continue to be influenced by clinical and socioeconomic factors, although the current trend is toward increased utilization. As nephron-sparing approaches for UTUC have garnered interest due to greater recognition of the detrimental effects of renal insufficiency, ureteroscopic management may play an increasing role in management. However, technological advances are required to ensure reliable tumor resection and accurate staging assessment. Finally, while URS will likely play a diminishing role in the future management of UPJO, endopyelotomy will remain an important salvage therapy and endoureterotomy will continue to be utilized for ureteral stricture disease.

References

1. Zigeuner R, Pummer K. Urothelial carcinoma of the upper urinary tract: surgical approach and prognostic factors. Eur Urol. 2008;53:720–31.
2. Yong D, Albala DM. Endopyelotomy in the age of laparoscopic and robotic-assisted pyeloplasty. Curr Urol Rep. 2010;11:74–9.
3. Krambeck AE, Murat FJ, Gettman MT, et al. The evolution of ureteroscopy: a modern single-institution series. Mayo Clin Proc. 2006;81:468–73.
4. Pearle MS, Calhoun EA, Curhan GC. Urologic diseases in America project: urolithiasis. J Urol. 2005; 173:848–57.
5. Kerbl K, Rehman J, Landman J, et al. Current management of urolithiasis: progress or regress? J Endourol. 2002;16:281–8.
6. Matlaga BR. Contemporary surgical management of upper urinary tract calculi. J Urol. 2009;181:2152–6.
7. Bandi G, Best SL, Nakada SY. Current practice patterns in the management of upper urinary tract calculi in the north central United States. J Endourol. 2008;22:631–6.
8. Scales Jr CD, Krupski TL, Curtis LH, et al. Practice variation in the surgical management of urinary lithiasis. J Urol. 2011;186:146–50.
9. Smith FL, Carper SW, Hall JS, et al. Cellular effects of piezoelectric versus electrohydraulic high energy shock waves. J Urol. 1992;147:486–90.
10. Razdan S, Johannes J, Cox M, et al. Current practice patterns in urologic management of upper-tract transitional-cell carcinoma. J Endourol. 2005;19:366–71.
11. Tan BJ, Rastinehad AR, Marcovich R, et al. Trends in ureteropelvic junction obstruction management among urologists in the United States. Urology. 2005; 65:260–4.
12. Gerber GS. Trends in endourologic practice. J Endourol. 2002;16:347–8.
13. Preminger GM, Tiselius HG, Assimos DG, et al. 2007 Guideline for the management of ureteral calculi. Eur Urol. 2007;52:1610–31.
14. Fuchs M, Fuchs GJ. Retrograde intrarenal surgery for calculus disease: new minimally invasive treatment approach. J Endourol. 1990;4:337–41.
15. Fabrizio MD, Behari A, Bagley DH. Ureteroscopic management of intrarenal calculi. J Urol. 1998;159: 1139–43.
16. Grasso M. Ureteropyeloscopic treatment of ureteral and intrarenal calculi. Urol Clin North Am. 2000; 27:623–31.
17. Breda A, Ogunyemi O, Leppert JT, et al. Flexible ureteroscopy and laser lithotripsy for single intrarenal stones 2 cm or greater–is this the new frontier? J Urol. 2008;179:981–4.
18. Grasso M, Conlin M, Bagley D. Retrograde ureteropyeloscopic treatment of 2 cm. or greater upper urinary tract and minor Staghorn calculi. J Urol. 1998;160:346–51.
19. Chung BI, Aron M, Hegarty NJ, et al. Ureteroscopic versus percutaneous treatment for medium-size (1–2-cm) renal calculi. J Endourol. 2008;22:343–6.
20. Pearle MS, Lingeman JE, Leveillee R, et al. Prospective, randomized trial comparing shock wave lithotripsy and ureteroscopy for lower pole caliceal calculi 1 cm or less. J Urol. 2005;173:2005–9.
21. Portis AJ, Rygwall R, Holtz C, et al. Ureteroscopic laser lithotripsy for upper urinary tract calculi with active fragment extraction and computerized tomography followup. J Urol. 2006;2006(175):2129–33. discussion 33–4.
22. Macejko A, Okotie OT, Zhao LC, et al. Computed tomography-determined stone-free rates for ureteroscopy of upper-tract stones. J Endourol. 2009;23: 379–82.
23. L'Esperance JO, Ekeruo WO, Scales Jr CD, et al. Effect of ureteral access sheath on stone-free rates in

patients undergoing ureteroscopic management of renal calculi. Urology. 2005;66:252–5.
24. Schatloff O, Lindner U, Ramon J, et al. Randomized trial of stone fragment active retrieval versus spontaneous passage during holmium laser lithotripsy for ureteral stones. J Urol. 2010;183:1031–5.
25. Gravina GL, Costa AM, Ronchi P, et al. Tamsulosin treatment increases clinical success rate of single extracorporeal shock wave lithotripsy of renal stones. Urology. 2005;66:24–8.
26. Zhu Y, Duijvesz D, Rovers MM, et al. Alpha-blockers to assist stone clearance after extracorporeal shock wave lithotripsy: a meta-analysis. BJU Int. 2010;106:256–61.
27. John TT, Razdan S. Adjunctive tamsulosin improves stone free rate after ureteroscopic lithotripsy of large renal and ureteric calculi: a prospective randomized study. Urology. 2010;75:1040–2.
28. Semins MJ, Trock BJ, Matlaga BR. The effect of shock wave rate on the outcome of shock wave lithotripsy: a meta-analysis. J Urol. 2008;179:194–7. discussion 97.
29. Dash A, Schuster TG, Hollenbeck BK, et al. Ureteroscopic treatment of renal calculi in morbidly obese patients: a stone-matched comparison. Urology. 2002;60:393–7. discussion 97.
30. Deem S, Defade B, Modak A, et al. Percutaneous nephrolithotomy versus extracorporeal shock wave lithotripsy for moderate sized kidney stones. Urology. 2011;78:739–43.
31. Turna B, Stein RJ, Smaldone MC, et al. Safety and efficacy of flexible ureterorenoscopy and holmium:YAG lithotripsy for intrarenal stones in anticoagulated cases. J Urol. 2008;179:1415–9.
32. Wignall GR, Canales BK, Denstedt JD, et al. Minimally invasive approaches to upper urinary tract urolithiasis. Urol Clin North Am. 2008;35:441–54. viii.
33. Ng CF. The effect of age on outcomes in patients undergoing treatment for renal stones. Curr Opin Urol. 2009;19:211–4.
34. Ng CF, Siu DY, Wong A, et al. Development of a scoring system from noncontrast computerized tomography measurements to improve the selection of upper ureteral stone for extracorporeal shock wave lithotripsy. J Urol. 2009;181:1151–7.
35. Perks AE, Schuler TD, Lee J, et al. Stone attenuation and skin-to-stone distance on computed tomography predicts for stone fragmentation by shock wave lithotripsy. Urology. 2008;72:765–9.
36. Wang LJ, Wong YC, Huang CC, et al. Multidetector computerized tomography urography is more accurate than excretory urography for diagnosing transitional cell carcinoma of the upper urinary tract in adults with hematuria. J Urol. 2010;183:48–55.
37. Takahashi N, Kawashima A, Glockner JF, et al. MR urography for suspected upper tract urothelial carcinoma. Eur Radiol. 2009;19:912–23.
38. Roupret M, Zigeuner R, Palou J, et al. European guidelines for the diagnosis and management of upper urinary tract urothelial cell carcinomas: 2011 update. Eur Urol. 2011;59:584–94.
39. Caraway NP, Katz RL. A review on the current state of urine cytology emphasizing the role of fluorescence in situ hybridization as an adjunct to diagnosis. Cancer Cytopathol. 2010;118:175–83.
40. Messer J, Shariat SF, Brien JC, et al. Urinary cytology has a poor performance for predicting invasive or high-grade upper-tract urothelial carcinoma. BJU Int. 2011;108:701–5.
41. Mian C, Mazzoleni G, Vikoler S, et al. Fluorescence in situ hybridisation in the diagnosis of upper urinary tract tumours. Eur Urol. 2010;58:288–92.
42. El-Hakim A, Weiss GH, Lee BR, et al. Correlation of ureteroscopic appearance with histologic grade of upper tract transitional cell carcinoma. Urology. 2004;63:647–50. discussion 50.
43. Smith AK, Stephenson AJ, Lane BR, et al. Inadequacy of biopsy for diagnosis of upper tract urothelial carcinoma: implications for conservative management. Urology. 2011;78:82–6.
44. Matin SF, Kamat AM, Grossman HB. High-frequency endoluminal ultrasonography as an aid to the staging of upper tract urothelial carcinoma: imaging findings and pathologic correlation. J Ultrasound Med. 2010; 29:1277–84.
45. Traxer O, Geavlete B, de Medina SG, et al. Narrow-band imaging digital flexible ureteroscopy in detection of upper urinary tract transitional-cell carcinoma: initial experience. J Endourol. 2011;25:19–23.
46. Audenet F, Traxer O, Yates DR, et al. Potential role of photodynamic techniques combined with new generation flexible ureterorenoscopes and molecular markers for the management of urothelial carcinoma of the upper urinary tract. BJU Int. 2012;109(4):608–13.
47. Favaretto RL, Shariat SF, Savage C, et al. Combining imaging and ureteroscopy variables in a preoperative multivariable model for prediction of muscle-invasive and non-organ confined disease in patients with upper tract urothelial carcinoma. BJU Int. 2012;109:77–82.
48. Jones JS, Streem SB. Office-based cystoureteroscopy for assessment of the upper urinary tract. J Endourol. 2002;16:307–9.
49. Reisiger K, Hruby G, Clayman RV, et al. Office-based surveillance ureteroscopy after endoscopic treatment of transitional cell carcinoma: technique and clinical outcome. Urology. 2007;70:263–6.
50. Elliott DS, Segura JW, Lightner D, et al. Is nephroureterectomy necessary in all cases of upper tract transitional cell carcinoma? Long-term results of conservative endourologic management of upper tract transitional cell carcinoma in individuals with a normal contralateral kidney. Urology. 2001;58:174–8.
51. Keeley Jr FX, Bibbo M, Bagley DH. Ureteroscopic treatment and surveillance of upper urinary tract transitional cell carcinoma. J Urol. 1997;157:1560–5.
52. Roupret M, Hupertan V, Traxer O, et al. Comparison of open nephroureterectomy and ureteroscopic and percutaneous management of upper urinary tract transitional cell carcinoma. Urology. 2006;67:1181–7.
53. Daneshmand S, Quek ML, Huffman JL. Endoscopic management of upper urinary tract transitional cell carcinoma: long-term experience. Cancer. 2003;98:55–60.
54. Martinez-Pineiro JA, Garcia Matres MJ, Martinez-Pineiro L. Endourological treatment of upper tract

urothelial carcinomas: analysis of a series of 59 tumors. J Urol. 1996;156:377–85.
55. Gurbuz C, Youssef RF, Shariat SF, et al. The impact of previous ureteroscopic tumor ablation on oncologic outcomes after radical nephrouretectomy for upper urinary tract urothelial carcinoma. J Endourol. 2011; 25:775–9.
56. Krambeck AE, Thompson RH, Lohse CM, et al. Imperative indications for conservative management of upper tract transitional cell carcinoma. J Urol. 2007;178:792–6. discussion 96–7.
57. Kaag MG, O'Malley RL, O'Malley P, et al. Changes in renal function following nephroureterectomy may affect the use of perioperative chemotherapy. Eur Urol. 2010;58:581–7.
58. Lane BR, Smith AK, Larson BT, et al. Chronic kidney disease after nephroureterectomy for upper tract urothelial carcinoma and implications for the administration of perioperative chemotherapy. Cancer. 2010;116:2967–73.
59. Huang WC, Levey AS, Serio AM, et al. Chronic kidney disease after nephrectomy in patients with renal cortical tumours: a retrospective cohort study. Lancet Oncol. 2006;7:735–40.
60. Go AS, Chertow GM, Fan D, et al. Chronic kidney disease and the risks of death, cardiovascular events, and hospitalization. N Engl J Med. 2004;351:1296–305.
61. Nahas AR, Shoma AM, Eraky I, et al. Prospective, randomized comparison of ureteroscopic endopyelotomy using holmium:YAG laser and balloon catheter. J Urol. 2006;175:614–8. discussion 18.
62. Ost MC, Kaye JD, Guttman MJ, et al. Laparoscopic pyeloplasty versus antegrade endopyelotomy: comparison in 100 patients and a new algorithm for the minimally invasive treatment of ureteropelvic junction obstruction. Urology. 2005;66:47–51.
63. Rassweiler JJ, Subotic S, Feist-Schwenk M, et al. Minimally invasive treatment of ureteropelvic junction obstruction: long-term experience with an algorithm for laser endopyelotomy and laparoscopic retroperitoneal pyeloplasty. J Urol. 2007;177: 1000–5.
64. Szydelko T, Kopec R, Kasprzak J, et al. Antegrade endopyelotomy versus laparoscopic pyeloplasty for primary ureteropelvic junction obstruction. J Laparoendosc Adv Surg Tech A. 2009;19:45–51.
65. Dimarco DS, Gettman MT, McGee SM, et al. Long-term success of antegrade endopyelotomy compared with pyeloplasty at a single institution. J Endourol. 2006;20:707–12.
66. Eden CG. Minimally invasive treatment of ureteropelvic junction obstruction: a critical analysis of results. Eur Urol. 2007;52:983–9.
67. Butani RP, Eshghi M. Cold-knife retrograde endopyelotomy: a long-term follow-up. J Endourol. 2008;22:657–60.
68. Hafez KS, Wolf Jr JS. Update on minimally invasive management of ureteral strictures. J Endourol. 2003; 17:453–64.
69. Wolf Jr JS, Elashry OM, Clayman RV. Long-term results of endoureterotomy for benign ureteral and ureteroenteric strictures. J Urol. 1997;158:759–64.
70. El-Nahas AR, Shokeir AA. Endourological treatment of nonmalignant upper urinary tract complications after urinary diversion. Urology. 2010;76:1302–8.
71. Watterson JD, Sofer M, Wollin TA, et al. Holmium: YAG laser endoureterotomy for ureterointestinal strictures. J Urol. 2002;167:1692–5.
72. Bensalah K, Tuncel A, Gupta A, et al. Determinants of quality of life for patients with kidney stones. J Urol. 2008;179:2238–43. discussion 43.
73. Marcovich R, Jacobson AI, Aldana JP, et al. Practice trends in contemporary management of adult ureteropelvic junction obstruction. Urology. 2003;62:22–5. discussion 25–6.
74. Chandhoke PS. When is medical prophylaxis cost-effective for recurrent calcium stones? J Urol. 2002;168:937–40.
75. Lotan Y, Cadeddu JA, Roehrborn CG, et al. The value of your time: evaluation of effects of changes in medicare reimbursement rates on the practice of urology. J Urol. 2004;172:1958–62.
76. Lotan Y, Gettman MT, Roehrborn CG, et al. Management of ureteral calculi: a cost comparison and decision making analysis. J Urol. 2002;167:1621–9.
77. Lotan Y, Pearle MS. Economics of stone management. Urol Clin North Am. 2007;34:443–53.
78. Tan HJ, Wolf Jr JS, Hollenbeck BK, et al. Use of ureteroscopy before and after expansion of lithotripter ownership in Michigan. Urology. 2011;78:1287–91.
79. Hyams ES, Shah O. Percutaneous nephrostolithotomy versus flexible ureteroscopy/holmium laser lithotripsy: cost and outcome analysis. J Urol. 2009;182:1012–7.
80. Grasso M, Beaghler M, Loisides P. The case for primary endoscopic management of upper urinary tract calculi: II. Cost and outcome assessment of 112 primary ureteral calculi. Urology. 1995;45:372–6.
81. Kapoor DA, Leech JE, Yap WT, et al. Cost and efficacy of extracorporeal shock wave lithotripsy versus ureteroscopy in the treatment of lower ureteral calculi. J Urol. 1992;148:1095–6.
82. Parker BD, Frederick RW, Reilly TP, et al. Efficiency and cost of treating proximal ureteral stones: shock wave lithotripsy versus ureteroscopy plus holmium:yttrium-aluminum-garnet laser. Urology. 2004;64:1102–6. discussion 06.
83. Wolf Jr JS, Carroll PR, Stoller ML. Cost-effectiveness v patient preference in the choice of treatment for distal ureteral calculi: a literature-based decision analysis. J Endourol. 1995;9:243–8.
84. Litwin MS, Saigal CS (editors). Upper tract urothelial carcinoma. In: Urologic disease in America. Washington, DC: US Government Printing Office; 2007.
85. Pak RW, Moskowitz EJ, Bagley DH. What is the cost of maintaining a kidney in upper-tract transitional-cell carcinoma? An objective analysis of cost and survival. J Endourol. 2009;23:341–6.
86. Gettman MT, Lotan Y, Roerhborn CG, et al. Cost-effective treatment for ureteropelvic junction obstruction: a decision tree analysis. J Urol. 2003;169:228–32.
87. Baldwin DD, Dunbar JA, Wells N, et al. Single-center comparison of laparoscopic pyeloplasty, Acucise endopyelotomy, and open pyeloplasty. J Endourol. 2003;17:155–60.

Part II

Evidence-Based Outcomes for Ureteroscopy and Implications for Patient Selection

Ureteroscopy for Lateralizing Hematuria

3

Nicholas N. Tadros and Michael J. Conlin

Introduction

Improvements in ureteroscopic instrumentation have had a significant effect on our ability to evaluate patients with lateralizing hematuria. In the past, computed tomography (CT), angiography, and various retrograde studies were the only tools available for evaluating patients with possible upper urinary tract abnormalities. With the development of safe and effective ureteroscopy, we can directly inspect the urothelium and no longer need to rely on radiologic imaging studies alone. Ureteroscopy not only allows us to better determine the underlying cause of bleeding in patients with hematuria, but also it has greatly improved our ability to treat these patients.

The first flexible ureteroscopes developed were of limited use because they lacked a working channel, having only visual and illuminating capabilities [1, 2]. As ureteroscopes evolved with the development of working channels and deflection capabilities, their therapeutic role in treating upper urinary tract abnormalities dramatically expanded. Although these therapeutic indications (especially urolithiasis) dominated the early use of ureteroscopes, the addition of working channels and deflection also improved the diagnostic capabilities of ureteroscopes. It is now possible to inspect the entire intrarenal collecting system, and through the working channel we can obtain the fluid for cytology and perform biopsy for any abnormal tissue. The use of ureteroscopy as a diagnostic tool will expand as the imaging capabilities, maneuverability, and durability of ureteroscopes continue to improve. Another significant improvement in ureteroscopes has been the decrease in their diameter over the years. This has increased our ability to perform ureteroscopy without prior ureteral dilation, allowing clearer inspection of the untouched ureteral urothelium [3]. As the invasiveness of ureteroscopy decreases, there will be little reason to rely on radiologic studies alone when one can so safely inspect and sample the urothelium of the upper urinary tract with minimal damage to the surrounding tissues.

This chapter will focus on the diagnostic uses of ureteroscopy, the specific technical nuances of diagnostic ureteroscopy, and current results of ureteroscopy for evaluating lateralizing hematuria.

Indications for Diagnostic Ureteroscopy

Ureteroscopy can be used to diagnostically investigate any condition that may involve the upper urinary tract. Ureteroscopy allows urologists direct urothelial visualization, and fluid and tissue sampling of the upper urinary tract. Any upper

N.N. Tadros • M.J. Conlin (✉)
Division of Urology, Surgery Department, Portland VA Medical Center, OHSU Center for Health & Healing, 3303 SW Bond Avenue, 10th Floor CH10U, Portland, OR 97239, USA
e-mail: conlinm@ohsu.edu

M. Monga (ed.), *Ureteroscopy: Indications, Instrumentation & Technique*, Current Clinical Urology,
DOI 10.1007/978-1-62703-206-3_3, © Springer Science+Business Media New York 2013

urinary tract abnormality that might benefit from these diagnostic interventions should be considered for diagnostic ureteroscopy. Common indications for diagnostic ureteroscopy include evaluating patients with unexplained recurrent or persistent urinary tract infections, persistent positive cytologies, upper urinary tract filling defects, and hematuria [4, 5]. We will discuss these indications, and focus our attention on the ureteroscopic evaluation of lateralizing hematuria.

Upper Urinary Tract Filling Defects

CT urography has largely replaced excretory urography as the most common imaging modality for evaluating patients with hematuria. CT urography can better differentiate radiolucent stones and soft-tissue defects. This has decreased, but not eliminated, the need for diagnostic ureteroscopic evaluation of filling defects. Despite these improvements in upper urinary tract imaging for patients with hematuria, the evaluation of the upper urinary tract filling defects identified on imaging studies remains one of the most common indications for diagnostic ureteroscopy.

Filling defects may include calculi, transitional cell carcinoma, blood clots, benign tumor (e.g., fibroepithelial polyps), extrinsic compression (e.g., crossing vessels), and intrinsic ureteral strictures or ureteropelvic junction (UPJ) obstructions [4].

Direct ureteroscopic inspection alone often provides the diagnosis when evaluating upper urinary tract filling defects [4]. Upper urinary tract calculi are easily distinguishable from soft-tissue lesions, and treatment can be rendered using various stone removal techniques in the same setting. Extrinsic filling defects can often be determined visually with the appearance of compression of the ureter in the absence of any intrinsic mass in the ureteral lumen. When the ureter is extrinsically compressed by a venous structure, the ureteral lumen is distensible during ureteroscopic inspection, whereas extrinsic compression from an artery often results in visible pulsations. Endoluminal ultrasound can also be used in conjunction with ureteroscopic inspection to visualize structures beyond the walls of the ureter to better evaluate causes of extrinsic compression. The presence of ureteral strictures and UPJ obstructions can also be confirmed visually.

With the expanded use of CT urography, most upper urinary tract calculi will be identified prior to ureteroscopy. In this setting, most filling defects will be soft tissue (non-calculus) and should be considered as cancer until proven otherwise. The ureteroscopic appearance of upper tract transitional cell carcinoma is similar to the familiar cystoscopic appearance of bladder-based transitional cell carcinoma. Low-grade urothelial tumors typically have a papillary, fondler appearance. Higher grade tumors can be more sessile and at times may contain calcifications or have a necrotic appearance. Fibroepithelial polyps are typically papillary and may be similar in appearance to transitional cell tumors. However, they can be distinguished from upper urinary tract transitional cell carcinoma as they frequently have a smooth, normal-appearing urothelial surface.

Although upper urinary tract transitional cell carcinoma can often be determined by direct ureteroscopic inspection alone, this should not be the sole basis of its diagnosis. When evaluating any soft-tissue lesion with concern for possible urothelial cancer, the diagnosis should be based not only on visual appearance but also on cytologic evaluation and biopsy [6].

The choice of treatment for upper urinary tract transitional cell carcinoma depends on the location, size, and number of lesions. The most critical factors in deciding the course of treatment are the stage and grade of the tumor. Accurate staging of upper urinary tract transitional cell carcinoma can be difficult. CT scanning alone has been shown inadequate for accurate staging, and the underlying ureteral musculature can seldom be safely sampled ureteroscopically. Fortunately, stage is closely related to tumor grade, and so we are able to rely on accurate grading of the tumor to guide our choice of treatment options [7]. Cytology and biopsy are complementary tools in diagnosing and grading these tumors. Cytologic sampling is specific, but it is less sensitive because most low-grade lesions will be missed. Higher grade transitional cell carcinoma lesions will more likely produce positive cytology results as the tumor cells have lost their cell–cell adhesion capabilities and demonstrate more easily identifiable morphologic changes. Direct ureteroscopic biopsy is generally specific and highly sensitive. Thus, fluid aspirations for cytology and biopsies should be obtained from any suspicious lesion during ureteroscopy.

Hematuria

Evaluating patients with hematuria is one of the most common urologic consultations. Hematuria initially can be divided into glomerular or nonglomerular causes, on the basis of urinalysis alone. Dysmorphic red blood cells, proteinuria, and red blood cell casts would indicate a probable glomerular (medical) cause of the hematuria and the patient should be referred to a nephrologist for evaluation and treatment. Nonglomerular hematuria can be caused by many urologic problems including tumors, stones, and urinary tract infections. Most causes of nonglomerular hematuria are determined with a standard hematuria evaluation, which includes upper urinary tract imaging and cystoscopy. If the hematuria evaluation is negative, additional studies might include complete blood count (CBC), coagulation studies, and platelet function studies to rule out bleeding diathesis. Referral to hematology for definitive evaluation can be done if bleeding diathesis is strongly suspected. A urine sample also should be sent for cytology and culture. If an obvious source of the hematuria cannot be determined through conventional radiologic and hematologic studies, the condition is referred to as *benign essential hematuria*, and if cystoscopically found to originate from only one upper urinary tract, has been called *lateralizing hematuria* [5, 8]. These terms are frequently interchangeable.

Patients with benign essential hematuria can have frequent bouts of gross hematuria with clots and renal colic; otherwise, their long-term course is generally benign. Some will require repeated transfusions. Benign essential hematuria is found equally in men and women. Additional radiologic studies are frequently performed to evaluate patients with benign essential hematuria. Renal arteriography and venography, and magnetic resonance arteriography (MRA) may reveal larger vascular lesions. However, if the patient has already had a quality CT urogram, it is unlikely a significant vascular lesion would be missed. These additional imaging studies are usually of low yield because the most common vascular lesions causing benign essential hematuria are small venous abnormalities and hemangiomas on the urothelial surface [9]. These are seen better on endoscopic inspection of the upper urinary tract and will usually be missed on vascular imaging studies.

Benign Essential Hematuria Etiology and Pathogenesis

Hemangiomas

The most common ureteroscopic findings during an evaluation of benign essential hematuria are renal hemangiomas. Virchow was the first to describe renal hemangiomas during autopsy studies in 1867, suggesting they may be a cause of chronic hematuria [8]. Rare reports of renal hemangiomas causing unexplained hematuria were published over the next century, but it was not until 1941 when Webb-Johnson and Turner-Warwick described two cases of essential hematuria cured by nephrectomy that hemangiomas re-entered the clinical consciousness of the practicing urologist [10]. Renal hemangioma can be large but are typically quite small (<1 cm in diameter), and most commonly occur on the tips of the renal papilla. Some may be microscopic [9]. They may be seen as small red or blue spots, or larger mulberry-like lesions typically found on the papillae. They are equally distributed between men and women, the right and left kidneys, and the upper and lower poles of the kidney. The associated hematuria tends to be spontaneous in onset and intermittent in nature, though massive hemorrhage is possible. Occasionally, clots may be seen as filling defects but most preoperative imaging studies will be negative. Ureteroscopic evaluation and treatment are more successful when the patient is actively bleeding, and when the lesions are discrete rather than diffuse.

Venous Abnormalities

Another common finding during ureteroscopy for benign essential hematuria is venous abnormalities of the calyces. These abnormalities have been described in the literature as renal forniceal hemorrhages, minute venous ruptures, varices, pyelovenous fistula, and hemorrhagic papillitis. Though they may differ slightly, they likely all share a common pathological basis. Anatomic studies in the past have demonstrated a close relationship between the tributaries of the renal vein and the calyceal fornix [11]. These venous sinuses are close to the surface at the calyceal fornix and may erode or rupture through the urothelium [12]. It has been postulated that these venous calyceal fistulas develop following periods of elevated pressure within the intrarenal collecting system [8]. These lesions may be localized or diffuse and are among the more common causes of bleeding in patients with benign essential hematuria.

Nutcracker Syndrome

Lateralizing hematuria can also be caused by venous vascular abnormalities that result in renal venous hypertension (RVH). The "nutcracker" phenomenon is the most commonly reported abnormality. It is caused by venous hypertension of the left kidney due to compression of the left renal vein, usually between the aorta and the superior mesenteric artery [13]. Other variants have been described as well, such as in patients with retroaortic left renal veins [14]. Regardless of the cause of RVH, the pathogenesis of resulting hematuria appears to be the same: formation of venous-calyceal fistulae secondary to disturbances in renal blood flow in the fornices. Diagnosis is generally made by demonstrating venous hypertension during venography studies with a pressure drop beyond the point of compression of the left renal vein. The nutcracker syndrome (NCS) refers to the complex of symptoms that are commonly caused by this phenomenon. Although it may be associated with substantial morbidity, the diagnosis of NCS is often difficult and is commonly delayed because of the substantial variation in presentation [15]. Symptoms can include hematuria, left flank pain, and occasionally left testicular pain due to renal drainage of the left gonadal vein. Rare findings are sometimes present, such as in a small Australian case series where compression of the left renal vein caused prominent left-gonadal-vein reflux, which in turn resulted in lower-limb varicose veins and varicocele formation [16]. Treatment depends on severity and is usually surgical. Occasionally endovascular stenting can ameliorate symptoms, but reimplantation of the left renal vein is often necessary [17]. Renal autotransplantation has also been used successfully to treat patients with NCS.

Loin Pain Hematuria Syndrome

Loin pain hematuria syndrome is another cause of chronic, though usually bilateral, hematuria. Patients with this condition have intermittent pain and microscopic and or gross hematuria as well as occasional low-grade fevers. Although this diagnostic entity somewhat overlaps benign essential hematuria, loin pain hematuria syndrome has no specific anatomic findings and can have a significant psychiatric component, often associated with somatoform disorder. Though the etiology is unknown, it is postulated that it may be associated with thin glomerular basement membrane disease, which causes hemorrhage into the renal tubules resulting in the characteristic flank pain and hematuria [18]. Treatment is mostly supportive and includes pain management and angiotensin converting enzyme inhibitors that are thought to reduce intraglomerular pressure and therefore reduce renal tubular congestion with red blood cells. Renal autotransplantation is advocated by some centers as an effective treatment, but only as a last resort for well screened individuals, symptoms may often recur after transplant [19].

Other Causes

There are other rare causes of essential hematuria that the practicing urologist should be aware of.

Table 3.1 Causes of benign essential hematuria

Vascular causes
Arteriovenous malformations
Renal hemangioma
Renal vein hypertension
Nutcracker syndrome
Renal arteriovenous fistula
Renal arteriopelvic fistula
Nonvascular causes
Bleeding diathesis
Exercise-induced ("march") hematuria
Renal papillary necrosis
Endometriosis
Renal ptosis
Renal tuberculosis
Previous retroperitoneal surgery
Unilateral idiopathic retroperitoneal fibrosis
Loin pain hematuria syndrome

For example, renal tuberculosis can occasionally present as macroscopic hematuria and should be included in the differential diagnosis of lateralizing hematuria, especially in the absence of an obvious cause of the bleeding [20]. Other rare causes include arteriovenous malformations and endometriosis (Table 3.1). Of note, some findings during ureteroscopy such as submucosal erythema and abnormal papillary tips may or may not have specific diagnoses associated with them.

A small number of patients who are evaluated ureteroscopically for hematuria will be found to have transitional cell carcinoma tumor or urolithiasis. In other patients, nothing will be found. Despite no bleeding lesion being found, many studies report successful resolution of the hematuria after ureteroscopy. It has been suggested that this could be due to resolution of unseen venous-caliceal communication because of increased intraluminal pressure during the ureteroscopy or post-procedure inflammation [21, 22]. Results of ureteroscopy for the evaluation and treatment of benign essential hematuria are presented in Table 3.2. Our systematic review of the literature reveals an overall success rate of 90% for the ureteroscopic treatment of patients with benign essential (lateralizing) hematuria [4, 21–33].

Other causes of *bilateral* benign essential hematuria can be confused with lateralizing hematuria. These include march hematuria or exercise-induced hematuria, a rare condition where repeated impacts to the body (particularly the feet, like when a soldier is marching) can cause hemolysis and subsequent hematuria. Severe march hematuria can lead to athlete nephritis, which is likely caused by the hemoglobin load on the kidney. In children, allergy symptoms can rarely present as unexplained hematuria during allergic flares [34]. Diagnostic ureteroscopy can often be avoided if cystoscopic examination reveals bleeding from both ureteral orifices. These conditions often resolve spontaneously.

Diagnostic and Therapeutic Ureteroscopy Technique

Before performing ureteroscopy, a urinalysis with or without culture should be done to ensure that the urine is free from infection. Prophylactic antibiotics should be given prior to instrumentation of the urinary tract. The primary goal of diagnostic ureteroscopy is clear visual inspection of the entire upper urinary tract. Here we present some techniques that will help achieve this goal.

Bleeding from the urinary tract can occur anywhere from the upper pole of the kidney to the urethral meatus. Endoscopic evaluation of these patients begins with careful cystourethroscopy. Special attention is paid to the prostatic urethra in men, which can be a frequent site of benign gross hematuria. The bladder urothelium is carefully and completely inspected and a bladder lavage for cytology is performed. The next cystoscopic step is careful patient inspection for bloody efflux from the ureteral orifices. When gross hematuria is present, this critical step will allow differentiation of unilateral and bilateral hematuria. Bilateral gross hematuria is likely "nonurologic" and a ureteroscopic evaluation may not be helpful.

Ureteroscopy should be performed in a method that minimizes urothelial trauma prior to visualization, as any trauma could be misinterpreted as a potential cause of hematuria (Fig. 3.1). This includes minimizing guidewire trauma. Some authors have reported performing flexible ureteroscopy without a working or a safety guidewire. Some newer flexible ureteroscopes can be introduced into the ureteral orifice under direct

Table 3.2 Results with ureteroscopy for lateralizing hematuria (benign essential hematuria)

Study				Findings					Success (%)			
				Discrete								
Author (first)	Year	*N*	Mean followup (months)	Hemangioma	Minute venous rupture	Other	Diffuse	Nothing seen	Discrete	Diffuse	Nothing seen	Total
Gittes	1981	13		5	0	0	8	0				
Patterson	1984	4	5.5	0	2	0	2	0	2/2	2/2		4/4
McMurtry	1987	8	11	0	4	1	3	0	5/5	1/3		6/8
Kavoussi	1989	8	11	0	0	6	0	2	5/6			5/6
Bagley	1990	32		11	2	3	9	5	12/13	0/4	5/5	17/22
Kumon	1990	12	10.3	4	4	1	1	2	9/9			9/9
Desgrandchamps	1994	8	16	0	0	3	4	1		4/4	0/1	4/5
Nakada	1997	17	60	5	0	6	3	3	9/11		1/3	10/14
Tawfiek	1998	23	8	7	3	5	3	5	14/14	3/3	4/5	21/22
Yazaki	1999	15		1	2	2	1	4				
Mugiya	1999	4		1	0	3	0	0	4/4			4/4
Daneshmand	2002	15	20.2	15	0	0	0	0	11/12			11/12
Mugiya	2007	23	73	2	14	2	0	5	9/9			9/9
Brito	2009	13	26	9	4	0	0	0	13/13			13/13
Mugiya	2010	20	16	4	15	0	0	1	19/19			19/19
Total		215		64	50	32	34	28	112/117 (96%)	10/16 (63%)	10/14 (71%)	132/147 (90%)

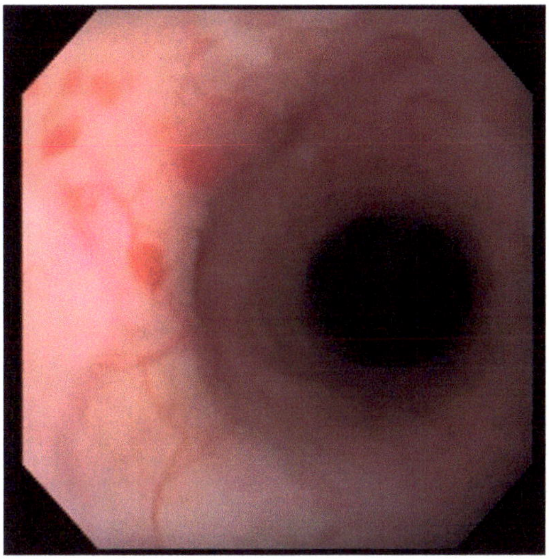

Fig. 3.1 Small area of urothelial abrasion from passage of the ureteroscope. Techniques to minimize this problem will help prevent confusion with potential pathologic lesions

vision without the use of a working guidewire [35]. This technique requires significant expertise and is not possible with all flexible ureteroscopes, in all patients. This technique will likely become less challenging with future generations of ureteroscopes and may soon become the ideal "no touch" method for diagnostic ureteroscopy. However, at this time, it is limited to certain ureteroscopes in the hands of experienced endourologists. For these reasons, we recommend and will review the standard technique of diagnostic ureteroscopy using rigid ureteroscopy and flexible ureteroscopy to inspect the entire upper urinary tract.

Rigid and flexible ureteroscopy provide complimentary access to the entire upper urinary tract [2]. While rigid ureteroscopy allows direct insertion and easy control of the ureteroscope, it does not allow easy access to the ureter superior to the iliac vessels. Without the ability to deflect the tip of a rigid ureteroscope, inspection of the intrarenal collecting system is impossible. Flexible ureteroscopy provides complete access of the entire intrarenal collecting system and upper ureter. However, inspection of the distal ureter is difficult because of buckling of the ureteroscope into the bladder. For this reason, rigid ureteroscopy is performed below the iliac vessels, and flexible ureteroscopy above. This combination of rigid and flexible ureteroscopy provides complete visual inspection of the entire upper urinary tract. When performing ureteroscopy for the evaluation of hematuria, tumor surveillance, or other diagnostic purposes, it is important to recognize that our standard ureteroscopy technique can produce traumatic lesions that may be mistaken for pathology. Care should be taken to minimize this trauma to the ureter during ureteroscopy, as it will interfere with our diagnostic visual inspection. The effort to minimize trauma begins with using the smallest ureteroscope practical to avoid the need for dilation. Direct insertion of a rigid ureteroscope without prior dilation of the intramural ureter allows clean inspection of the distal ureteral mucosa. Avoiding the use of a guidewire during insertion of the rigid ureteroscope will further minimize trauma to the ureter. If a guidewire is needed to obtain access to the ureter, it should be passed no more than 2–3 cm into the ureter, just enough to obtain adequate access for the ureteroscope. This should be done under direct vision to minimize injury to the orifice. Once access is obtained, the ureter is inspected with the rigid ureteroscope from the ureteral orifice to the level of the iliac vessels, taking care to visualize the full circumference of the ureter. Only the least amount of irrigation that will provide adequate distention of the ureter for visualization should be used. This will prevent over-distention of the ureter and intrarenal collecting system. Even minimal over-distention of the collecting system can lead to small areas of urothelial hemorrhage and render the remaining inspection of the ureter for true sources of bleeding pointless. Once the distal ureter is completely inspected to the level of the iliac vessels, further inspection of the proximal ureter requires flexible ureteroscopy. A guidewire is passed through the rigid ureteroscope, only as high as necessary into the ureter to allow placement of the flexible ureteroscope. Preferably, the guidewire is passed only to the level of the ureter that has been inspected with the rigid ureteroscope. The rigid ureteroscope is removed, leaving the guidewire in place, and the flexible ureteroscope is passed over this guidewire to the proximal extent of rigid ureteroscopic inspection. Flexible ureteroscopic inspection is then performed from this point and proceeds proximally, in a retrograde fashion and is generally done without a safety guidewire. Again, this is to avoid trauma to the ureteral urothelium that might interfere with the diagnostic inspection. When using this technique of diagnostic ureteroscopy, we are inspecting a urothelium that is "untouched" either by guidewires or ureteroscopes.

When inspecting the intrarenal collecting system, completeness is ensured through a systematic approach using combined endoscopic and fluoroscopic imaging. Irrigation with dilute contrast allows precise documentation and navigation throughout the intrarenal collecting system. The intrarenal collecting system is inspected from the upper pole moving systematically through the calyces, to the lower pole, and each calyceal inspection is documented fluoroscopically. Care should be taken to avoid over-distention of the intrarenal collecting system to minimize urothelial trauma. Small, subtle urothelial lesions can cause benign essential hematuria. Any trauma, from the guidewire, over-distention, or from the ureteroscope, can prevent accurate visualization of these lesions. Likewise, pre-stenting should be avoided to prevent stent-related inflammation of the urothelium, which will also prevent accurate inspection of the upper urinary tract. As mentioned earlier, a nontraumatic approach to diagnostic ureteroscopy is essential.

There are two goals when performing ureteroscopy for lateralizing hematuria: to determine the cause and to treat any lesion that is present. Ureteroscopy is an endoscopic extension of cystoscopic principles to the upper urinary tract. It allows direct visualization and recognition of pathologic lesions, just as cystoscopy allows visual recognition of calculi, neoplasms, and other bladder lesions. Lesions causing lateralizing hematuria are often easily recognized, but any findings suspicious for malignancy should be sampled appropriately. Transitional cell carcinoma generally has an easily distinguishable appearance. Ureteroscopic sampling for cytologic and pathologic analysis greatly improves our ability to distinguish malignant from benign soft-tissue lesions. Direct irrigation through the ureteroscope with normal saline and aspiration for cytology is done whenever there is the possibility of a malignant lesion. Direct, precise biopsy, guided by ureteroscopic visualization of the lesion, permits a more accurate diagnosis than a brush biopsy guided by fluoroscopy alone (Fig. 3.2). Biopsy of any suspicious lesions can be performed with three French biopsy forceps for sessile lesions, or flat wire baskets for papillary lesions [6].

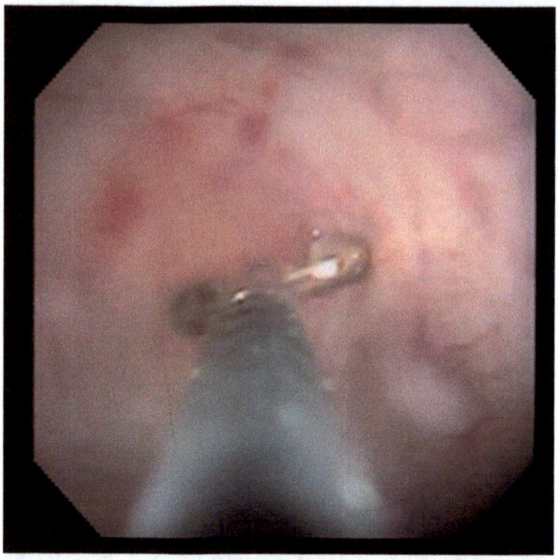

Fig. 3.2 Ureteroscopic biopsy of small renal pelvic papillary tumor

When a source of bleeding is found, it should be fulgurated. This can be performed with either electrocautery delivered with a 2 F blunt tip electrode (30–40 W coagulating current), or the Neodymium/YAG laser. Small tumors can be also biopsied and fulgurated. The holmium/YAG laser can be used, but at a wavelength of 2,100 nm, the laser energy is highly absorbed in water, which results in relatively shallow tissue penetration of 0.4 mm. The holmium laser is primarily ablative, whereas the Neodymium/YAG laser is more coagulative with a tissue penetration of 4–6 mm and is an effective method of management for renal hemangiomas and other vascular lesions (Fig. 3.3). In our review of the literature, discrete lesions are more successfully ureteroscopically treated (96%) than diffuse lesions (63%), which can be more difficult to fully treat.

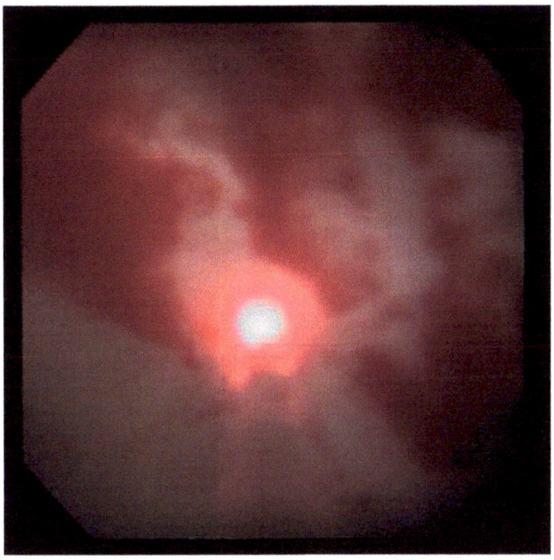

Fig. 3.3 Laser ablation of an area of diffuse pyelitis causing hematuria

Although ureteral stenting after ureteroscopy in general has become less frequent, it is usually required in patients treated for lateralizing hematuria because of their hematuria. Even with identification of a bleeding lesion and successful fulguration, often the hematuria will not resolve for several days after ureteral stent removal. Final determination of success or failure with ureteroscopy for lateralizing hematuria should not be determined until several weeks after ureteral stent removal. Technical considerations during ureteroscopy for lateralizing hematuria are presented in Table 3.3, and Fig. 3.4 presents our approach to the evaluation of patients with benign essential hematuria.

Other Treatments

The mainstay of treatment for essential hematuria is ureteroscopy with or without fulguration of any lesions as described earlier. This is successful in the majority of cases. Before the advent of modern flexible ureteroscopy, installation of 1% silver nitrate solution into the renal pelvis was used with some success to treat hematuria. There has been at least one case report of ureteral stenosis following treatment with silver nitrate, and this treatment should not be considered an option for management of these patients [36]. Oral administration of epsilon aminocaproic acid is a potent antifibrinolytic agent that is used to treat bleeding resulting from a systemic fibrinolytic state, but can also be used to treat hematuria through its action on decreasing urinary fibrinolysis. It has proven relatively safe and effective for the treatment of hematuria in small case series [37, 38]. For prolonged or life threatening bleeding unresponsive to ureteroscopic interventions, total or partial nephrectomy may still be necessary. Fortunately, with the advent of current flexible ureteroscopic instruments and techniques, most of these patients lateralizing hematuria can be evaluated and successfully treated ureteroscopically.

Table 3.3 Technical considerations during ureteroscopy for lateralizing hematuria

1. Evaluate patient when gross hematuria is present
2. Perform complete cystourethroscopy (visualize entire bladder urothelium)
   (a) 30 and 70° lenses
   (b) Flexible cystoscope if needed
3. Bladder lavage for cytology
4. Visualize ureteral efflux
   (a) Localize gross hematuria when present
   (b) If Unilateral, proceed with ureteroscopy
5. Minimize ureteral urothelial trauma
   (a) Direct insertion of rigid ureteroscope without guidewire
   (b) Leave wire through the rigid ureteroscope to the level inspected
   (c) Pass flexible ureteroscope over wire
   (d) Inspect proximally from the level reached with rigid ureteroscope
   (e) Minimize irrigation
6. Systematic inspection of intrarenal collecting system
   (a) Using dilute contrast irrigation and fluoroscopic mapping
7. Aspirate intrarenal urine for cytology
8. Biopsy suspicious lesions
9. Fulgurate bleeding lesions

Conclusion

Lateralizing hematuria is an uncommon clinical problem with poorly understood pathogenesis. It is usually diagnosed after multiple negative

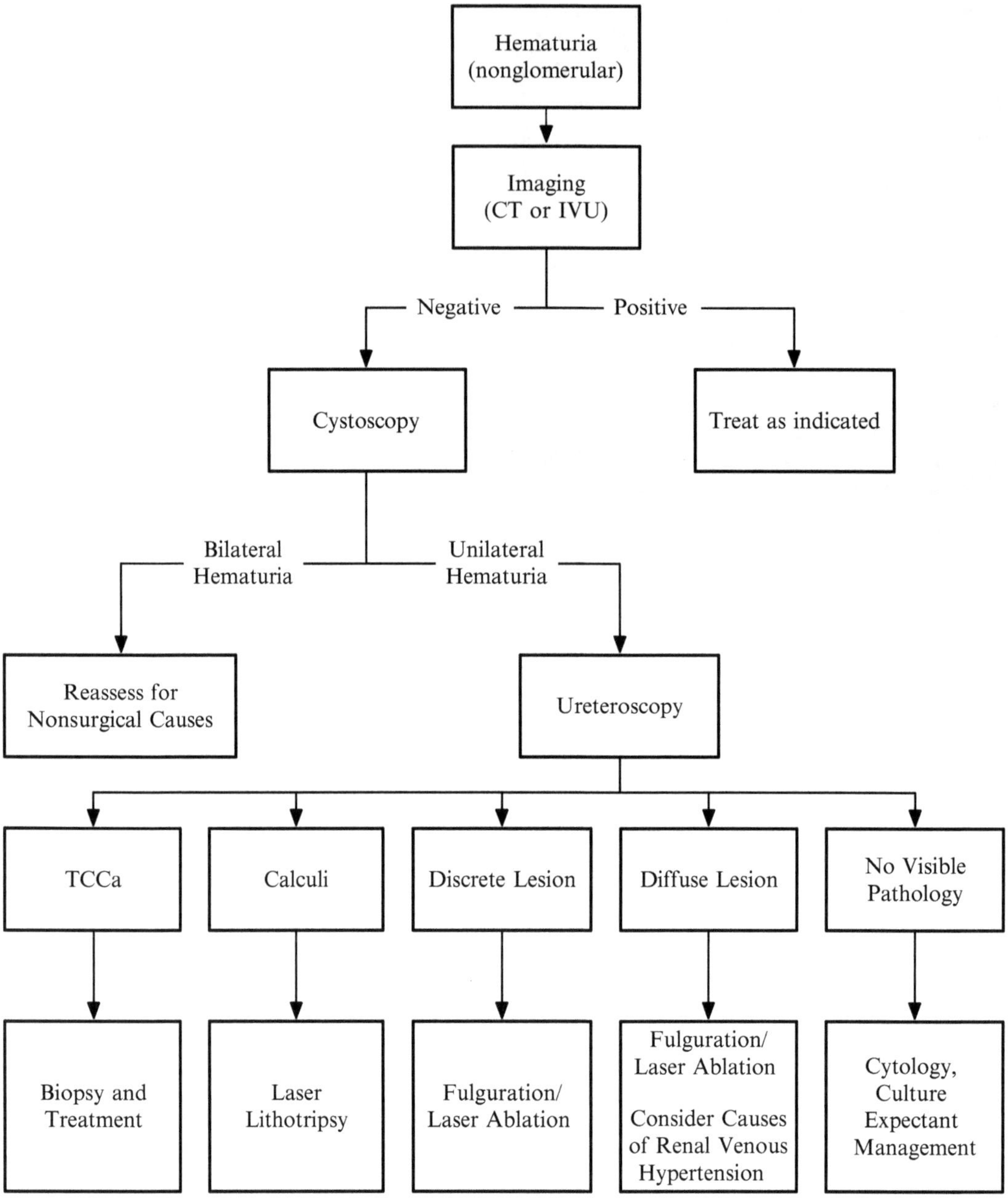

Fig. 3.4 Evaluation of benign essential hematuria

tests and is considered a diagnosis of exclusion. Negative urine culture and cytology, unremarkable imaging studies, and unilateral bleeding seen from a single ureter on cystoscopy are considered the hallmarks of lateralizing hematuria. While it can rarely cause life-threatening hemorrhage, it can often cause significant pain and morbidity. It frequently results in anxiety amongst patients and urologists due to its diagnostic difficulty and repeated investigations. Historically, it was treated with nephrectomy. But improvements in the techniques and instrumentation of ureteroscopy have dramatically improved our ability to evaluate and treat patients with lateralizing hematuria, and ureteroscopy should now be considered the treatment of choice.

References

1. Aso Y, Ohtawara Y, Suzuki K, Tajima A, Fujita K. Usefulness of fiberoptic pyeloureteroscope in the diagnosis of the upper urinary tract lesions. Urol Int. 1984;39(6):355–7.
2. Bagley DH, Huffman JL, Lyon ES. Combined rigid and flexible ureteropyeloscopy. J Urol. 1983;130(2):243–4.
3. Hudson RG, Conlin MJ, Bagley DH. Ureteric access with flexible ureteroscopes: effect of the size of the ureteroscope. BJU Int. 2005;95(7):1043–4.
4. Bagley DH, Allen J. Flexible ureteropyeloscopy in the diagnosis of benign essential hematuria. J Urol. 1990;143(3):549–53.
5. Dooley RE, Pietrow PK. Ureteroscopy for benign hematuria. Urol Clin North Am. 2004;31(1):137–43.
6. Keeley FX, Kulp DA, Bibbo M, McCue PA, Bagley DH. Diagnostic accuracy of ureteroscopic biopsy in upper tract transitional cell carcinoma. J Urol. 1997; 157(1):33–7.
7. Keeley FX, Bibbo M, Bagley DH. Ureteroscopic treatment and surveillance of upper urinary tract transitional cell carcinoma. J Urol. 1997;157(5):1560–5.
8. Rowbotham C, Anson KM. Benign lateralizing haematuria: the impact of upper tract endoscopy. BJU Int. 2001;88(9):841–9.
9. Jahn H, Nissen HM. Haemangioma of the urinary tract: review of the literature. Br J Urol. 1991; 68(2):113–7.
10. Sira W-J, Wt W. "Essential Hæmaturia": are lesions of a renal papilla a frequent cause? Br J Urol. 1941; 13(3):127–34.
11. Fuchs F. Untersuchungen über die innere topographie der niere. Ztschr F Urol Chir. 1925;18:164–80.
12. Low AI, Matz LR. Haematuria and renal fornical lesions. Br J Urol. 1972;44(6):681–91.
13. Beinart C, Sniderman KW, Saddekni S, Weiner M, Vaughan ED, Sos TA. Left renal vein hypertension: a cause of occult hematuria. Radiology. 1982;145(3): 647–50.
14. Lau JL, Lo R, Chan FL, Wong KK. The posterior "nutcracker": hematuria secondary to retroaortic left renal vein. Urology. 1986;28(5):437–9.
15. Kurklinsky AK, Rooke TW. Nutcracker phenomenon and nutcracker syndrome. Mayo Clin Proc. 2010;85(6):552–9.
16. Little AF, Lavoipierre AM. Unusual clinical manifestations of the nutcracker syndrome. Australas Radiol. 2002;46(2):197–200.
17. Rudloff U, Holmes RJ, Prem JT, Faust GR, Moldwin R, Siegel D. Mesoaortic compression of the left renal vein (nutcracker syndrome): case reports and review of the literature. Ann Vasc Surg. 2006;20(1):120–9.
18. Hebert LA, Betts JA, Sedmak DD, Cosio FG, Bay WH, Carlton S. Loin pain-hematuria syndrome associated with thin glomerular basement membrane disease and hemorrhage into renal tubules. Kidney Int. 1996;49(1):168–73.
19. Chin JL, Kloth D, Pautler SE, Mulligan M. Renal autotransplantation for the loin pain-hematuria syndrome: long-term followup of 26 cases. J Urol. 1998;160(4):1232–5. discussion 1235–6.
20. Chan SW, Shalhav AL, Clayman RV. Renal tuberculosis presenting as lateralizing hematuria diagnosis by ureteronephroscopy and selective upper tract urine culture. J Endourol. 1998;12(4):363–4.
21. Tawfiek ER, Bagley DH. Ureteroscopic evaluation and treatment of chronic unilateral hematuria. J Urol. 1998;160(3 Pt 1):700–2.
22. Daneshmand S, Huffman JL. Endoscopic management of renal hemangioma. J Urol. 2002;167 (2 Pt 1):488–9.
23. Brito AH, Mazzucchi E, Vicentini FC, Danilovic A, Chedid Neto EA, Srougi M. Management of chronic unilateral hematuria by ureterorenoscopy. J Endourol. 2009;23(8):1273–6.
24. Desgrandchamps F, Piergiovanni M, Cussenot O, Cortesse A, Benali A, Lesourd A, et al. Exploration and endoscopic treatment of unilateral primary haematuria: is non-specific diffuse pyelitis a real entity? Eur Urol. 1994;26(2):109–14.
25. Gittes RF, Varady S. Nephroscopy in chronic unilateral hematuria. J Urol. 1981;126(3):297–300.
26. Kavoussi L, Clayman RV, Basler J. Flexible, actively deflectable fiberoptic ureteronephroscopy. J Urol. 1989;142(4):949–54.
27. Kumon H, Tsugawa M, Matsumura Y, Ohmori H. Endoscopic diagnosis and treatment of chronic unilateral hematuria of uncertain etiology. J Urol. 1990;143(3):554–8.
28. McMurtry JM, Clayman RV, Preminger GM. Endourologic diagnosis and treatment of essential hematuria. J Endourol. 1987;1(3):145–51.
29. Mugiya S, Ohhira T, Un-No T, Takayama T, Suzuki K, Fujita K. Endoscopic management of upper urinary tract disease using a 200-micron holmium laser fiber: initial experience in Japan. Urology. 1999;53(1): 60–4.
30. Mugiya S, Ozono S, Nagata M, Takayama T, Furuse H, Ushiyama T. Ureteroscopic evaluation and laser treatment of chronic unilateral hematuria. J Urol. 2007;178(2):517–20.
31. Nakada SY, Elashry OM, Picus D, Clayman RV. Long-term outcome of flexible ureterorenoscopy in the diagnosis and treatment of lateralizing essential hematuria. J Urol. 1997;157(3):776–9.
32. Patterson DE, Segura JW, Benson RC, Leroy AJ, Wagoner R. Endoscopic evaluation and treatment of patients with idiopathic gross hematuria. J Urol. 1984;132(6):1199–200.

33. Yazaki T, Kamiyama Y, Tomomasa H, Shimizu H, Okano Y, Iiyama T, et al. Ureteropyeloscopy in the diagnosis of patients with upper tract hematuria: an initial clinical study. Int J Urol. 1999;6(5):219–25.
34. Graham DM, McMorris MS, Flynn JT. Episodic gross hematuria in association with allergy symptoms in a child. Clin Nephrol. 2002;58(5):389–92.
35. Johnson GB, Portela D, Grasso M. Advanced ureteroscopy: wireless and sheathless. J Endourol. 2006;20(8):552–5.
36. Diamond DA, Jeffs RD, Marshall FF. Control of prolonged, benign, renal hematuria by silver nitrate instillation. Urology. 1981;18(4):337–41.
37. Stefanini M, English HA, Taylor AE. Safe and effective, prolonged administration of epsilon aminocaproic acid in bleeding from the urinary tract. J Urol. 1990;143(3):559–61.
38. Nash DA, Henry AR. Unilateral essential hematuria. Therapy with epsilon aminocaproic acid. Urology. 1984;23(3):297–8.

Ureteropelvic Junction Obstruction

4

Mantu Gupta and Doh Yoon Cha

Introduction

Ureteropelvic junction obstruction (UPJO) is defined as a functional impairment of urine flow from the renal pelvis to the ureter. This disease process can be broadly divided into intrinsic or extrinsic causes [1], with most intrinsic causes being congenital. Congenital obstructions can result from an aperistaltic segment of the ureter [1], kinks or valves produced by infoldings of the ureteral mucosa and musculature [2], or true ureteral stricture. However, acquired conditions such as stones, postoperative or inflammatory strictures, or upper tract tumors may also contribute to intrinsic UPJO. In some cases, high insertion of the ureter (Fig. 4.1) can also lead to inadequate drainage of the renal pelvis. Among extrinsic causes of UPJO, "aberrant" or "crossing" vessels have been proposed to be a common etiology. The importance of crossing vessels is controversial. Although crossing vessels are found in the vicinity of the UPJ in 33–79% of patients with UPJO [3], 71% of patients without UPJO also have a vessel within 1.5 cm of the UPJ [4]. Whatever the cause, UPJO warrants prompt attention. The primary aim should be to alleviate symptoms and prevent deterioration of renal function, development of stones or infection, or, rarely, hypertension.

When intervention is indicated, the reference standard has historically been open dismembered pyeloplasty [5]. However, with the advancements in endourological instrumentation, the direction has shifted toward minimally invasive procedures such as endopyelotomy (antegrade and retrograde), laparoscopic pyeloplasty, and robotic pyeloplasty [6]. All minimally invasive procedures share the advantage of short operative time, minimal morbidity, decreased postoperative analgesia, shorter hospital stay, and early recovery [7]. Still, a few questions remain. Which patients should undergo ureteroscopy as the first-line treatment? Are antegrade and retrograde approaches comparable in treatment success? What is the role of endopyelotomy among other minimally invasive procedures? What are the exclusion criteria for endopyelotomy? This chapter focuses on the techniques and clinical results for ureteroscopic endopyelotomy for the management of UPJO.

M. Gupta (✉) • D.Y. Cha
Department of Urology, New York Presbyterian Hospital, New York Presbyterian Kidney Stone Center, Columbia University Medical Center, 161 Fort Washington Avenue 11th floor, New York, NY 10036, USA
e-mail: mg392@columbia.edu

History of Retrograde Approach

The initial concept behind the endourological approach to UPJO can be traced back to Davis and colleagues in 1943 [8]. After a full-thickness incision of the narrow ureteral segment, a stent is placed to allow regeneration of an adequate

M. Monga (ed.), *Ureteroscopy: Indications, Instrumentation & Technique*, Current Clinical Urology,
DOI 10.1007/978-1-62703-206-3_4, © Springer Science+Business Media New York 2013

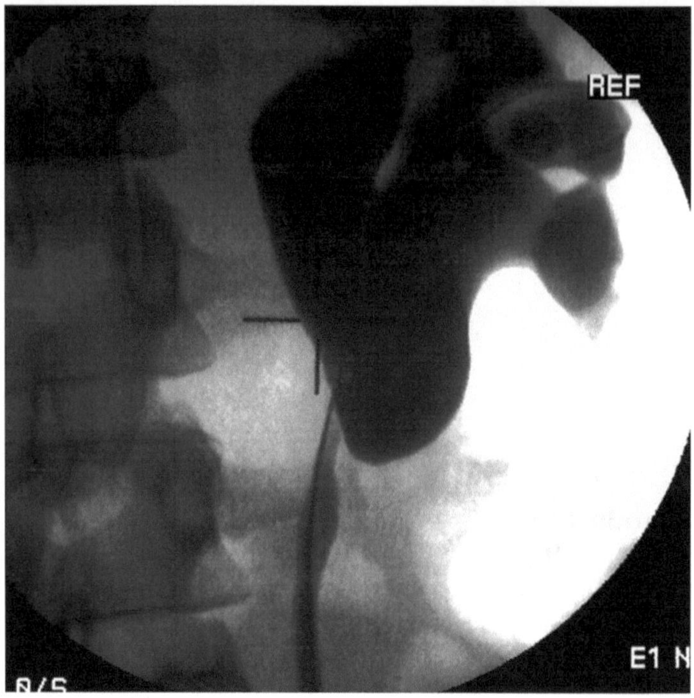

Fig. 4.1 Retrograde pyelogram showing a left ureteropelvic junction (UPJ) obstruction from a high insertion of the left ureter

caliber ureter around the stent. In 1983, Wickham and Kellet described the first ureteroscopic pyelolysis of the UPJ [9]. Bagley et al. reported their combined percutaneous and flexible ureteroscopic procedure approach for the management of an obliterated UPJ in 1985 [10]. As percutaneous renal surgery became more commonplace in the 1980s, antegrade endopyelotomy was introduced by Badlani et al. in 1986 [11] with good success. The retrograde approach became the next logical evolution of the minimally invasive approach in the treatment of UPJO.

The rationale for the introduction of a retrograde approach for endopyelotomy was to make the procedure less invasive by avoiding the potential complications associated with percutaneous renal access. Retrograde endopyelotomy performed with a rigid ureteroscope and electrocautery hook was first reported by Inglis and Tolley in 1986 [12]. The Acucise cutting balloon catheter was then approved by the FDA in 1993 in an effort to simplify retrograde endopyelotomy. This device made it possible for all urologists to perform retrograde endopyelotomy under fluoroscopic control. Thomas et al. [13] reported their experience with pre-stenting to facilitate ureteroscopic endopyelotomy in 1996. Subsequently, a one-stage procedure was described by Soroush and Bagley in 1998 [14]. Failed endopyelotomy did not jeopardize the success of subsequently performed open pyeloplasty [15]. Therefore, endopyelotomy was considered the first-line treatment of UPJO in appropriate clinical situations [6]. Further experience revealed that primary cases of UPJO could be successfully treated [16].

Diagnosis and Preoperative Evaluation

When there is clinical suspicion of UPJO, subsequent radiographic studies should always be performed to confirm the diagnosis. Proper imaging can determine both the anatomic site and the functional significance of obstruction. Renal ultrasound, retrograde pyelography, IVP, diuretic renal scan, Whitaker test, or a combination of them can be used. The diuretic renal scan not only verifies the presence of an obstruction, but also provides quantitative differential renal

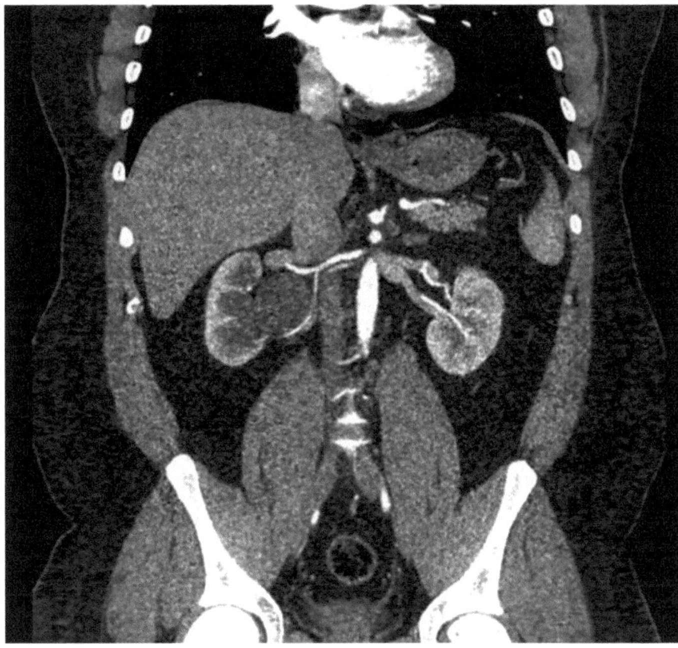

Fig. 4.2 CT angiography demonstrating a right ureteropelvic junction (UPJ) obstruction with a crossing vessel

function, which can direct the selection of the best treatment option. Furthermore, the renal scan facilitates follow-up evaluation of the renal function after treatment. CT angiography (Fig. 4.2) is a common imaging modality, since it provides spatial anatomical information, specifically that of aberrant crossing vessels. A combination of anatomic and functional studies, such as retrograde pyelography and diuretic renal scan, can sometimes be utilized to best plan treatment. For example, retrograde pyelography can both confirm and demonstrate the exact site and nature of obstruction before repair. In most instances, this test is performed at the time of the planned intervention in order to avoid the risk of introducing infection in the setting of obstruction. In the setting of infection or compromised renal function, however, retrograde pyelography and stent placement are indicated emergently for decompression of UPJO. The UPJ can even be evaluated ureteroscopically for pulsations at the time of endopyelotomy. This evaluation can be aided by the use of endoluminal ultrasound [17]. When scheduling operative intervention, risks and benefits of all treatment techniques should be discussed with the patient, since the indications for intervention for UPJO are similar regardless of technique. All the anatomic and functional information should be thoroughly reviewed preoperatively, and all treatments should be individualized. Patients should also be informed that sometimes a secondary intervention may be necessary.

Patient Selection

Although historical success rates with retrograde endopyelotomy have been 10–15% lower than those of open, laparoscopic, or robotic pyeloplasty, it has been noted that success rates can be greatly improved with careful patient selection [16]. Van Cangh et al. reported an overall success rate for endopyelotomy of 73%. However, when patients with both a crossing vessel and a high degree of obstruction were excluded from analysis, the success rate improved to 95%, which is comparable with that of open pyeloplasty [18]. Thus, in an appropriately chosen patient cohort, endopyelotomy still can be a significant and successful minimally invasive option in the treatment of UPJO.

Absolute contraindications include active urinary tract infection, sepsis, and uncontrolled coagulopathy. Relative exclusion criteria are based on a definitive set of clinical parameters that strongly correlate with success rate. Massive hydronephrosis (grade 4), stenosis greater than 2 cm and preoperative ipsilateral renal function <20% have been associated with poor endopyelotomy outcomes [15]. Tan and Smith also noted that total obliteration of the UPJ was also linked with unsatisfactory results [16]. Finally, patients with concurrent renal stones and UPJO and patients with a nephrostomy tube in place should be excluded from the retrograde approach. In these instances, antegrade endopyelotomy should be performed to address both the renal stones and the UPJO in one-stage procedure [16]. Berkman et al. showed that stone removed at the time of antegrade endopyelotomy did not offset success. Overall success rate was reported in 71% of patients undergoing endopyelotomy only and 90% of 41 patients who had simultaneous nephrolithotomy. Also, when adjusting for the severity of preoperative hydronephrosis and/or renal function, simultaneous nephrolithotomy did not decrease the success rate [19]. Patients with poor intrinsic renal function and severely decreased parenchyma should be initially drained by a stent and reevaluated or should be offered a laparoscopic simple nephrectomy for a poorly functioning or nonfunctioning kidney. Patients with massive hydronephrosis, but adequate function (>10–20%), should be treated with dismembered pyeloplasty, either open, laparoscopically, or robot assisted, because of the need for trimming and reduction of the redundant renal pelvis. The presence of massive hydronephrosis can also influence which approach, antegrade or retrograde, should be employed for endopyelotomy. Lam et al. reported that antegrade endopyelotomy was more successful than retrograde endopyelotomy in patients with massive hydronephrosis (66.7 vs. 20.0%) with equal minimal morbidity [20].

Controversy still exists with patients with high insertion of the UPJ in proceeding with retrograde endopyelotomy. Although once considered a contraindication due to initial poor results, there are subsequent published series that documented that high ureteral insertion had no significant impact on the outcome of endopyelotomy [15]. Alternatively, open, laparoscopic, or robotic-assisted pyeloplasty in the case of a known crossing vessel can be offered as a primary treatment modality.

In the past, when the decision was made to proceed with ureteroscopic management of UPJO, a preoperative ureteral stent was placed to drain the obstruction for 1–2 weeks. This maneuver accomplished several important goals. First, it delineated improvement of renal function after drainage and assessed the patient's ability to tolerate an indwelling stent. The latter is an important distinction, given that after retrograde endopyelotomy a stent is typically left indwelling for 6 weeks. Moreover, the stent dilated and straightened the UPJ, stabilized renal function, and facilitated the passage of an ureteroscope at the time of endopyelotomy. Now with smaller, flexible ureteroscopes and laser fibers, this extra step is not necessary and a one-stage procedure can be performed safely and effectively with less morbidity.

Technique

Currently, retrograde ureteroscopic endopyelotomy can be performed in three ways: (1) using a rigid ureteroscope and a cold-knife, electrocautery, or holmium laser incision; (2) using a flexible ureteroscope and electrocautery or laser incision; and (3) using a cutting balloon catheter (Acucise, Applied Medical Resources Corporation, CA). After either general or a spinal anesthesia, the patient is placed in the lithotomy position. Caution is taken so that all pressure points are well padded, and preoperative antibiotics are given.

As ureteroscopic technique has evolved over time, laser energy has largely replaced electrocautery to incise the UPJ. High energy produced by laser provides instant vaporization of tissue for more precise incision, in contrast to low energy produced by electrocautery leading to tissue coagulation and damage to peripheral blood supply. Moreover, the small diameter and flexibility of laser fibers enable their passage through small-diameter semirigid and flexible ureteroscopes, providing more degrees of freedom [6, 21].

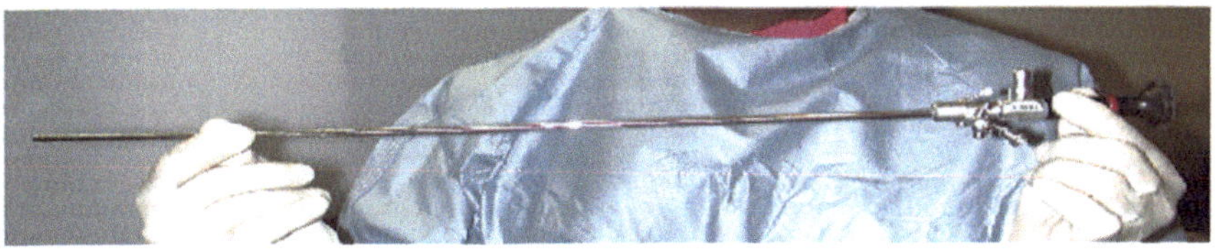

Fig. 4.3 Rigid ureteroscope

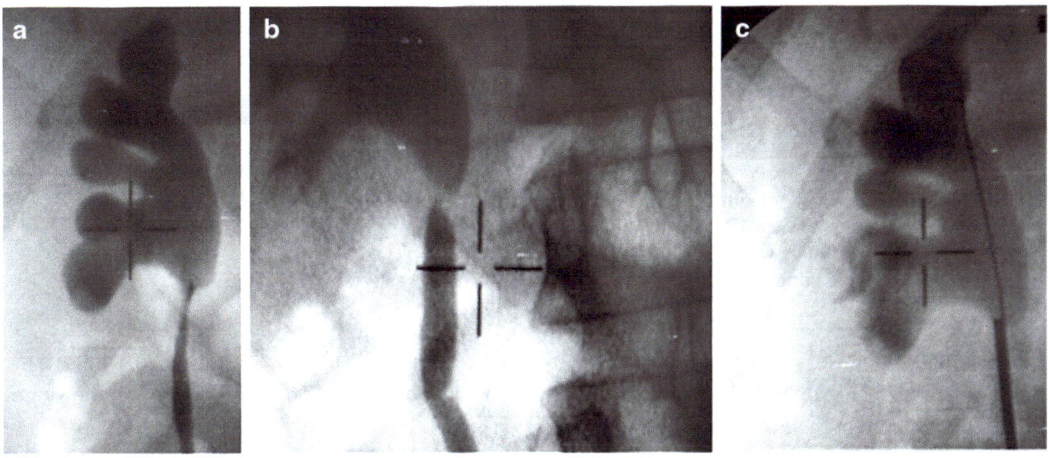

Fig. 4.4 (**a**) Intraoperative fluoroscopy (**a**) showing ureteropelvic obstruction, (**b**) with safety wire placement, and (**c**) confirming position of rigid ureteroscope at the ureteropelvic stenosis

Ureteroscopic Endopyelotomy with Electrocautery

Due to recent advancements in laser technology, the electrocautery technique is not utilized as frequently and will be discussed briefly. In one technique, a 5 F open-ended catheter is placed over a superstiff wire to maintain renal access while preventing conduction of electrical current as with a standard guidewire (Figs. 4.3 and 4.4). The catheter can also serve to continuously drain the renal pelvis of irrigation fluid during the procedure. The ureteroresectoscope is then passed directly alongside the catheter [1]. If there is difficulty accessing the ureteral orifice or ureteral narrowing, these portions can be balloon dilated. Either water or 1.5% glycine solution should be used for irrigation. The UPJ is first inspected for transmitted pulsations and then incised laterally, between 8 and 9 o'clock on the right and between 3 and 4 o'clock on the left [1]. Short, superficial strokes should be performed to avoid bleeding. Any bleeding should be controlled with spot electrocoagulation. A full-thickness incision is carried down to periureteral fat, and performed widely enough so that the scope can easily enter into renal pelvis.

Ureteroscopic Laser Endopyelotomy

Two types of lasers have been described in literature when performing ureteroscopic laser endopyelotomy: neodymium:yttrium aluminum garnet (Nd:YAG) and holmium:YAG (Ho:YAG). The Nd:YAG, with a wavelength of 1,060 μ(mu)m, produces a wider scatter and deeper penetration into tissue than the holmium:YAG. Initial success rate of 85% using the Nd:YAG laser was reported by Renner et al. [22], but a recurrence

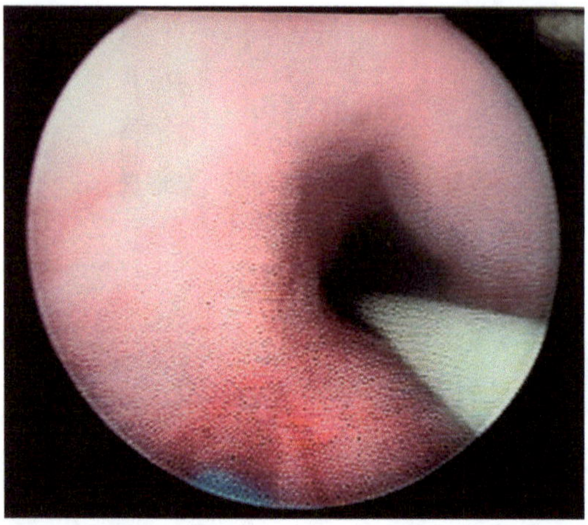

Fig. 4.5 Endoscopic view of ureteropelvic junction (UPJ) obstruction during retrograde laser endopyelotomy. Note the placement of a safety wire and the posterolateral location of the laser fiber during incision

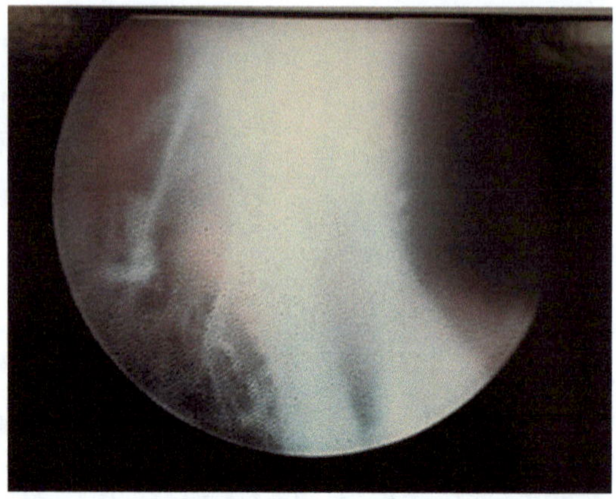

Fig. 4.6 Adventitial fibers noted during laser endopyelotomy. These fibers must be completely taken down to ensure a full-thickness incision

UPJ stenosis rate of 45% was observed by Gallucci et al. [23]. Potential reasons for high recurrence rate lie in the nature of Nd:YAG laser, which relies primarily on thermal coagulation, necrosis, and delayed tissue sloughing. Thus, Biyani et al. concluded that the Nd:YAG was not ideal for laser endopyelotomy [24]. On the contrary, the depth of penetration of the Ho:YAG laser is less than 0.5 mm because of its longer wavelength of 2,100 μ(mu)m. Additionally, tissue absorption of the Ho:YAG laser is more than that of Nd:YAG laser because the Ho:YAG is absorbed by water. These characteristics lead to a rapid rise in tissue temperature which results in prompt vaporization upon tissue contact and coagulation upon near-contact. With the Ho:YAG laser endopyelotomy, a precise incision can be performed with minimal bleeding, because it possesses both ablative and hemostatic properties. Controlled endoscopic incision can be performed because the depth and direction of the incision can be better controlled without scattering tissue [24].

Typically, a 200–300 μm fiber is used with the flexible ureteroscope, while a bigger 365 μm fiber can be used through the semirigid scope. Power setting is set from 0.5 to 1.5 J at the rate of 5–10 Hz when making a full-thickness, lateral, or posterolateral incision (Figs. 4.5 and 4.6). The laser vaporization is started just below the UPJ and advanced proximally through the stenosis until the renal pelvis is reached. All layers are incised until encountering periureteral and peripelvic fat (Fig. 4.7). For hemostasis, the laser beam can be defocused (firing near but without contacting the tissue) to control minor bleeding from the renal pelvis. After the full-thickness incision, subsequent balloon dilation can further ensure complete incision of UPJO, but is not necessary. A double-J ureteral stent is always left in place for 4–6 weeks (Figs. 4.8 and 4.9) [24].

Cutting Balloon Catheter Endopyelotomy

The cutting balloon catheter (Acucise, Applied Medical Resources Corp., CA) features a monopolar electrocautery wire joined with a low-pressure balloon (Fig. 4.10). The balloon is used to define the area of stenosis; radio-opaque markers located on the proximal and distal end of the balloon assist in positioning the cutting wire during the incision. This device was initially developed as a 7 F catheter, but 5 F model was later developed which made preoperative stenting optional. Of note, high-quality fluoroscopic imaging is critical for optimal position of the

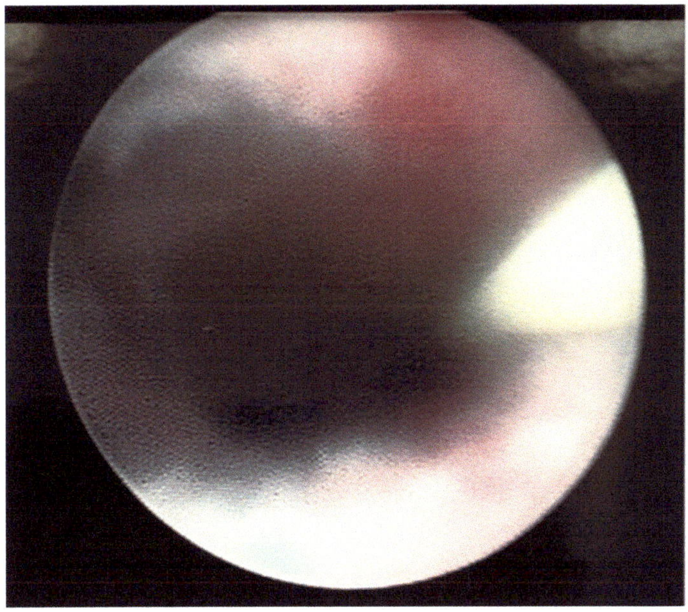

Fig. 4.7 Full-thickness incision shown during laser endopyelotomy

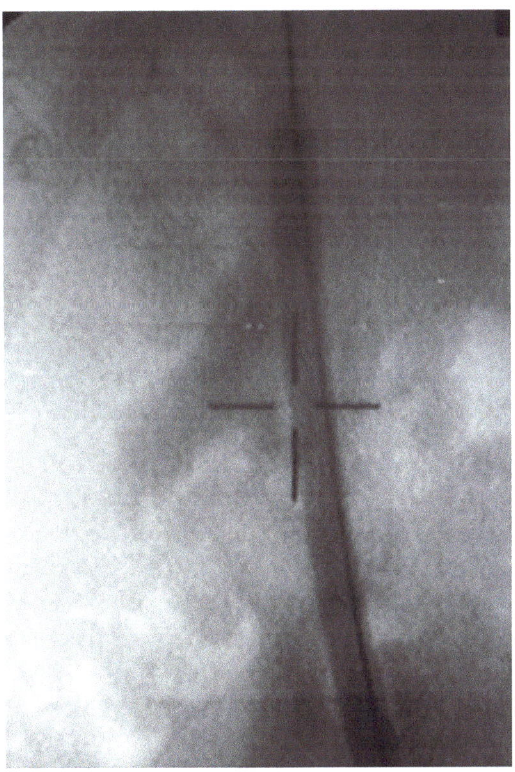

Fig. 4.8 Intraoperative fluoroscopy confirming extravasation after laser endopyelotomy

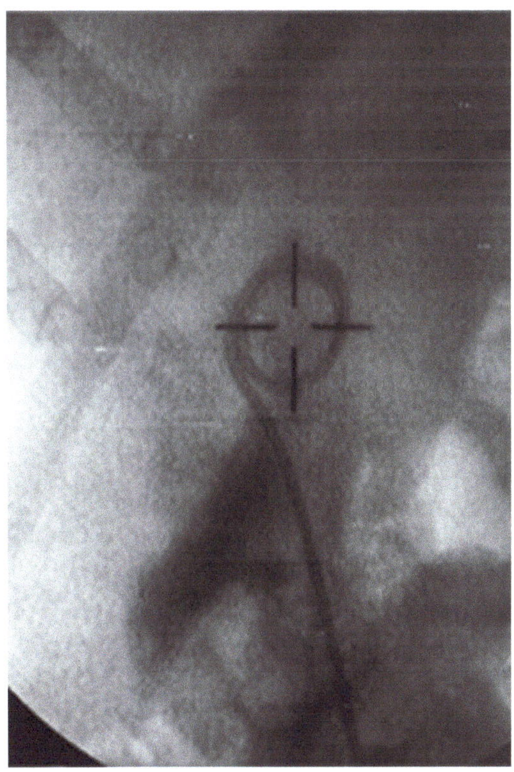

Fig. 4.9 An indwelling double-J stent placement after laser incision of ureteropelvic junction obstruction

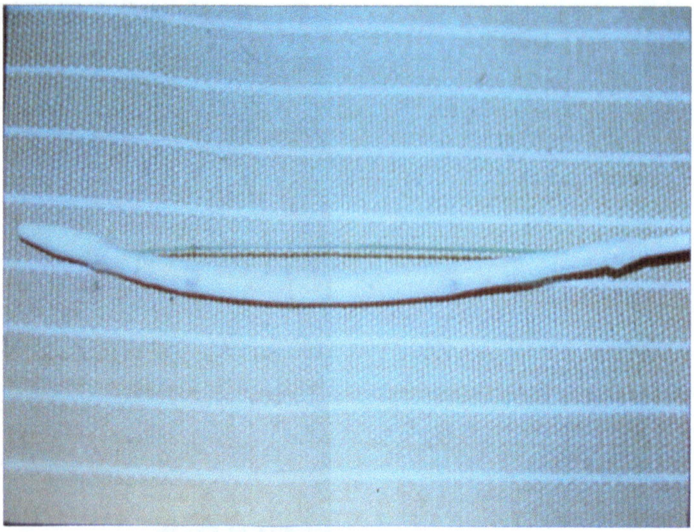

Fig. 4.10 Cutting balloon catheter (Acucise, Applied Medical Resources Corporation, CA)

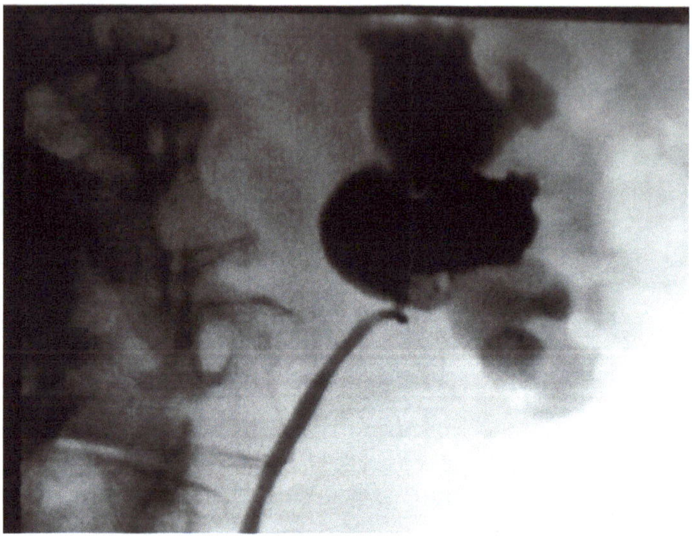

Fig. 4.11 Intraoperative retrograde pyelography showing ureteropelvic obstruction during Acucise endopyelotomy

cutting wire. Before the insertion through the ureteric orifice, the catheter is rotated so that the cutting wire is positioned laterally. Although not an absolute contraindication, the presence of crossing vessels warrants extreme caution with this technique. Evaluation with preoperative CT with angiographic phase is critical in minimizing bleeding complications. Under fluoroscopic guidance, the Acucise catheter is advanced over a guidewire toward the UPJ (Fig. 4.11). The ***balloon is initially inflated with 0.5–1 ml of diluted contrast to ensure correct position demonstrated by characteristic "waist." The monopolar wire is then activated at 75–100 W of pure cut for about 5 s, while additional 2–3 ml of diluted contrast is simultaneously instilled into the balloon. As the balloon inflates, the stricture is incised, noted by the disappearance of the waist of the stricture (Fig. 4.12). If the waist persists, the cutting wire can be reactivated for additional 5 s. After a presumed incision, the inflation of balloon is maintained for about 5–10 min to

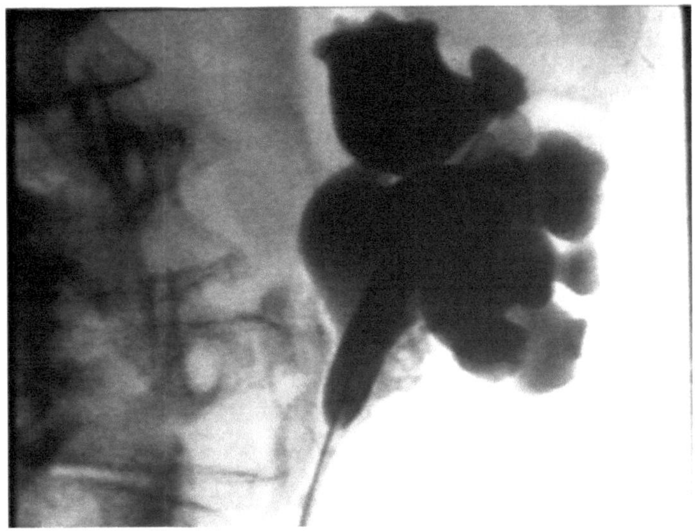

Fig. 4.12 Intraoperative fluoroscopy demonstrating the disappearance of the waist of the stricture during balloon inflation

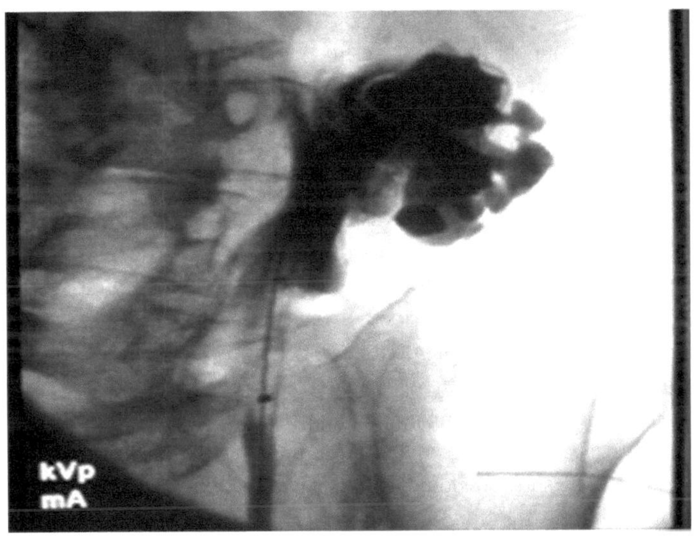

Fig. 4.13 Intraoperative fluoroscopy confirming extravasation after balloon deflation

tamponade any bleeding. The balloon is deflated, and retrograde pyelography is performed through the catheter to confirm extravasation at the incision site (Fig. 4.13). If extravasation is not seen, the UPJ can be directly inspected by a subsequent ureteroscopy. Periureteral fat should be visualized to ensure full-thickness incision (Fig. 4.14). Once this is confirmed, a ureteral stent is placed over the guidewire, transversing the site of UPJ incision. A Foley catheter is then placed for 24–48 h to decompress the bladder. The stent is left in place for 4–8 weeks [25].

Postoperative Management

Most patients undergoing retrograde ureteroscopic endopyelotomy are usually discharged the same day. Oral antibiotics are given at the discretion of the surgeon, while oral antispasmodics

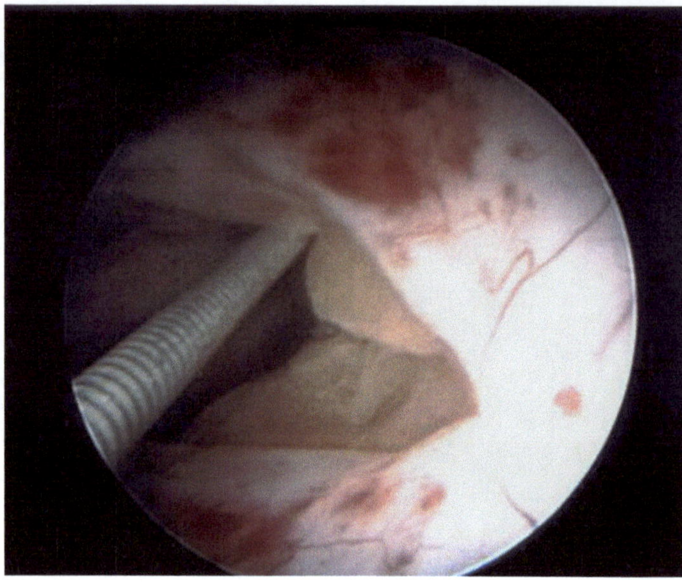

Fig. 4.14 Direct ureteroscopic inspection of the ureteropelvic junction (UPJ) following Acucise endopyelotomy. Periureteric fat is seen clearly after a successful incision

and/or oral anticholinergics are given as needed in the setting of irritative bladder symptoms. The Foley catheter is removed, in office or by the patient, after 24–48 h. The ureteral stent is removed cystoscopically in 4–6 weeks [26]. Endopyelotomy success is measured by improvement in pain symptoms, and in both function and drainage of the involved kidney. Thus, diuretic renal scan should be performed 4 weeks after the ureteral stent removal. Patients can be followed with renal ultrasound or renal scan every 4–6 months during the first year and yearly thereafter or as needed. Of note, follow-up imaging studies may show residual caliectasis and dilation from long-standing obstruction despite functional and symptomatic improvement.

Clinical Results and Complications

Laser Endopyelotomy

The success rates of reported series of retrograde laser endopyelotomy range from 73 to 85% [26, 27]. Longer operative times were reported in early experiences, as well as instances where endoluminal ultrasound was required to perform endopyelotomy. Most patients were discharged on the same day in recently reported series. Early endopyelotomy failures were usually detected within 1 year, and a second minimally invasive procedure was usually successful in relieving obstruction in these cases [28]. Biyani et al. [24] demonstrated that an early success rate of 87.5% decreased to 75% with longer follow-up. Similarly, in the study by Albani et al., 24 of 33 failures after endopyelotomy were diagnosed after 1 year of follow-up [29]. This warrants a long-term follow-up of more than a year, which is recommended to ensure longevity of treatment.

Initially, endopyelotomy was specially indicated for patients who had failed open repair. Geavlete et al. [30] evaluated use of laser retrograde endopyelotomy in cases with recurrent UPJO. Thirty laser procedures were performed, with grade 3 and 4 hydronephrosis (failed pyeloplasty, 17 cases; failed endopyelotomy, 13 cases). Inclusion criteria were absence of renal calculi, stenosis length <2 cm, and absence of massive hydronephrosis (grade 5). Semirigid and flexible endoscopes (Wolf and Storz) and holmium:YAG laser were used. In 11 cases, an indwelling double-J was placed for 2 weeks. An indwelling stent 8/12 F was postoperatively placed for 8 weeks. All cases were evaluated at 6, 12, and 18 months. Ultrasound and retrograde pyelogram were the main follow-up investigations. Follow-up studies revealed a normal UPJ in 9 cases (30%), a reduction of hydronephrosis in 4 cases (13.3%), and no changes of the hydronephrosis in 17 cases (56.6%). Ureteroscopic follow-up evaluation revealed a widely patent UPJ in 13 of 17 cases (76.5%). Success rate at 18 months was 83.3%, with minor complications. Mean follow-up period was 31 months (18–52 months). Thus, laser endopyelotomy may represent an efficient minimally invasive technique in recurrent UPJ stenosis, with a reduced rate of complications, short period of hospitalization, and good anatomical and functional results. In a more recent study evaluating antegrade and retrograde endopyelotomy, Patel et al. reported their experience in 41 patients with secondary UPJO [31]. Of these patients, 14 had failed previous primary open or laparoscopic pyeloplasties, and 20 had iatrogenic etiology from previous renal surgeries. Patients were evaluated by CT, IVP, or diuretic renal scan at 1, 6 months, and 1 year following the procedure. Surgical success was defined as decreased hydronephrosis, improved flow on renal scan, or symptomatic improvement. Success rate was 83.5% (35/41) for endopyelotomy in these cases.

Most complications of laser ureteroscopic endopyelotomy are minor in comparison, and this has further decreased in more recent series [21]. The reported complications of laser endopyelotomy ranged between 8.5 and 12.5% [28]. Bleeding requiring blood transfusion was reported in up to 2% only, and the need for embolization to control severe bleeding was not reported. The reasons include the improvement of ureteroscopic instruments, such as development of smaller semirigid and flexible ureteroscopes with improved visibility, the utilization of laser energy, increasing experience with the procedure, and prior knowledge of crossing vessels via preoperative imaging [27]. Potential complications include bleeding from adjacent aberrant vessels, stent migration through the UPJ incision, and UPJO recurrence. Significant bleeding requiring emergent nephrectomy is another potential complication. A precise and completely lateral incision at the UPJ helps to prevent vascular injury. Minor complications from recent series include stent intolerance, proximal stent migration, minor bleeding, and urinary tract infection [21]. The routine use of antispasmodic and anesthetic drugs after surgery improves symptoms of stent colic in the postoperative period. Most of these complications are alleviated after removal of indwelling ureteral stents. Other postoperative complications included pyelonephritis, perirenal urinoma, or perirenal hematoma, all of which can be managed conservatively [26, 27].

Cutting Balloon Catheter Endopyelotomy

Success rates of cutting balloon catheter endopyelotomy have ranged from 32 to 84% [26]. This discrepancy can be attributed to the different definition of success, and usually, objective evaluation of success was lower than subjective evaluation at the time of follow-up. For example, Sofras et al. [32] reported very low success rates (32%) when they applied strict criteria of objective postoperative evaluation via diuretic renography curve. Improvement of the curve based on the scan was 54%, but when subjective improvement was calculated, the success rate increased to 70%. It was also observed that lower success rates were reported in few series from outside of the US.

Regarding the durability of success, Lechevallier et al. reported that most failures were diagnosed within the first 6 months postoperatively, and repeated Acucise endopyelotomy was performed and successful in 75% of patients who did not have crossing vessels [33]. Nadler et al. noticed that 13% of failures occurred in the second year of follow-up, and open pyeloplasty was not compromised in those patients with previously failed Acucise technique [34].

The overall complications associated with Acucise endopyelotomy ranges from 0 to 34% [35]. Approximately 85% of these complications were minor [36]. Vascular injury requiring blood transfusion ranged from 3 to 6% and most often involved a lower pole accessory renal artery [37]. Bleeding may occur immediately after the incision, or it may be delayed for several days [38].

The necessity for selective renal angiography and embolization of the injured vessel was reported in 3–5.8% of patients. Avulsion of the ureter at the UPJ was reported in one of 45 patients (2.2%) and was successfully managed with open pyeloplasty. Retroperitoneal hematoma was detected in 5.5% of cases [33]. Development of perirenal urinoma was reported in 1–4.5% of cases and was mainly due to transient obstruction of the stent [35, 36]. Percutaneous drainage of urinoma and of the collecting system in association with antibiotics was the suggested management [25]. Acute stent-related problems (obstruction or distal migration) were reported in 3–13% of patients [35]. Postoperative fever and sepsis were reported in 2–22% of cases that were treated with appropriate antibiotics and drainage of any collections [33]. Rupture of the catheter balloon after inflation or breakage of the cutting wire was a rare complication [26].

Based on these reports, it can be concluded that the results of laser endopyelotomy are more reproducible with a narrow range of complications, whereas in the Acucise series, there is a marked discrepancy in success rates and a wide range of complications. The chief advantage of the Acucise procedure is its simplicity. The reason for the inferior results of the Acucise endopyelotomy may be attributed to its blind nature in contrast to the laser technique in which the surgeon can directly visualize the stenosis and depth of the incision. Therefore, extravasation after Acucise endopyelotomy is an important sign of adequate incision [39]. El-Nahas et al. [26] conducted a prospective randomized comparison of retrograde laser and Acucise endopyelotomy. All patients had the same inclusion criteria and the same subjective and objective measurements of success. The incidence of complications was higher with Acucise technique (25% for Acucise vs. 10% for laser). Significant postoperative hematuria developed in the Acucise group that resulted in increased hospital stay and blood loss. Although the Acucise device was developed to allow the general urologist (who did not have advanced endourological skills) to perform endopyelotomy, ureteroscopy was required in 3 of 20 procedures (15%) among the Acucise group. Regarding the outcome, all subjective and objective outcomes of laser endopyelotomy were better than those of the Acucise (85% success for laser vs. 65% for Acucise). However, the difference was not statistically significant. Perhaps, a study containing larger number of patients is needed to confirm these findings.

Conclusions

Adherence to strict endourological principles and direct visualization make retrograde ureteroscopic endopyelotomy a safe and effective treatment modality for UPJO. The ureteroscopic approach has a short learning curve, and can be performed in almost all general hospitals where ureteroscopy is performed. As compared to other treatment options for UPJO, ureteroscopic retrograde endopyelotomy is less invasive, requires less OR time, can be done on an outpatient basis, or with a very short hospital stay. Since ureteroscopic instruments are evolving, the trend continues to favor minimally invasive techniques, and retrograde endopyelotomy will continue to play a significant role in the management of well-selected patient population with UPJO.

References

1. Thomas R, Monga M. Endopyelotomy. Retrograde ureteroscopic approach. Urol Clin North Am. 1998;25:305–10.
2. Maizels M, Stephens FD. Valves of the ureter as a cause of primary obstruction of the ureter: anatomic, embryologic and clinical aspects. J Urol. 1980;123:742.
3. Gupta M, Smith AD. Crossing vessels at the ureteropelvic junction: do they influence endopyelotomy outcome? J Endourol. 1996;10(2):183–7.
4. Sampaio FJB, Favorito LA. Ureteropelvic junction stenosis: vascular anatomical background for endopyelotomy. J Urol. 1993;150:1787–91.
5. Streem SB. Ureteropelvic junction obstruction. Open operative intervention. Urol Clin North Am. 1998;25:331–41.
6. Nakada SY, Johnson M. Ureteropelvic junction obstruction: retrograde endopyelotomy. Urol Clin North Am. 2000;27:677–84.

7. Karlin GS, Badlani GH, Smith AD. Endopyelotomy versus open pyeloplasty: comparison in 88 patients. J Urol. 1988;140:476–8.
8. Davis DM, Stong GH, Drake WM. Intubated ureterotomy: a new operation for ureteral and ureteral pelvic strictures. Surg Gynecol Obstet. 1943;76:513–23.
9. Wickham JEA, Kellet MJ. Percutaneous pyelolysis. Eur Urol. 1983;9:122–4.
10. Bagley DH, Huffman J, Lyon E, McNamara T. Endoscopic ureteropyelostomy: opening the obliterated ureteropelvic junction with nephroscopy and flexible ureteropyeloscopy. J Urol. 1985;133:462–4.
11. Badlani GH, Eshghi M, Smith AD. Percutaneous surgery for ureteropelvic junction obstruction endopyelotomy: techniques and early results. J Urol. 1986;135:26–8.
12. Inglis JA, Tolley DA. Ureteroscopic pyelolysis for pelviureteric junction obstruction. Br J Urol. 1986;58:250–3.
13. Thomas R, Monga M, Klein EW. Ureteroscopic retrograde endopyelotomy for management of ureteropelvic junction obstruction. J Endourol. 1996;10:141–5.
14. Soroush M, Bagley DH. Ureteroscopic retrograde endopyelotomy. Tech Urol. 1998;4:77–82.
15. Gupta M, Tuncay OL, Smith AD. Open surgical exploration after failed endopyelotomy: a 12-year experience. J Urol. 1997;157:1613–9.
16. Tan BJ, Smith AD. Ureteropelvic junction obstruction repair: when, how, what? Curr Opin Urol. 2004;14:55–9.
17. Grasso M, Bagley D. Small diameter, actively deflectable, flexible ureteroscopy. J Urol. 1998; 160:1648–53.
18. Van Cangh PJ, Wilmart JF, Opsomer RJ, et al. Long-term results and late recurrence after endoureteropyelotomy: a critical analysis of prognostic factors. J Urol. 1994;151:934.
19. Berkman DS, Landman J, Gupta M. Treatment outcomes after endopyelotomy performed with or without simultaneous nephrolithotomy: 10-year experience. J Endourol. 2009;23(9):1409–13.
20. Lam JS, Cooper KL, Greene TD, Gupta M. Impact of hydronephrosis and renal function on treatment outcome: antegrade versus retrograde endopyelotomy. Urology. 2003;61(6):1107–11.
21. Conlin MJ, Bagley DH. Ureteroscopic endopyelotomy at a single setting. J Urol. 1998;159:727–31.
22. Renner C, Frede T, Seemann O, Rassweiler J. Retrograde laser endopyelotomy: minimally invasive therapy of ureteropelvic junction obstruction. J Endourol. 1998;12:537–44.
23. Gallucci M, Vincenzoni A, Fortunato P, et al. Retrograde laser endopyelotomy in ureteral pelvic junction (UPJ) stenosis: our experience. Eur Urol. 1999;35:642a.
24. Biyani CS, Cornford PA, Powell CS. Ureteroscopic endopyelotomy with the holmium: YAG laser: mid-term Results. Eur Urol. 2000;38:139–43.
25. Nakada SY. Acucise endopyelotomy. Urology. 2000;55:277–82.
26. El-Nahas AR, Shoma AM, Eraky I, et al. Prospective, randomized comparison of ureteroscopic endopyelotomy using holmium:YAG laser and balloon catheter. J Urol. 2006;175:614–8.
27. Mendez-Torres FR, Urena R, Thomas R. Retrograde ureteroscopic endopyelotomy. Urol Clin North Am. 2004;31:99–106.
28. Giddens JL, Grasso M. Retrograde ureteroscopic endopyelotomy with the holmium: YAG laser. J Urol. 2000;194:1509–12.
29. Albani MJ, Yost AJ, Streem SB. Ureteropelvic unction obstruction: determining durability of endourologic intervention. J Urol. 2004;171:579–82.
30. Geavlete P, Georgescu D, Mirciulescu V, Nita G. Ureteroscopic laser approach in recurrent ureteropelvic junction stenosis. Eur Urol. 2006;51:1542–8.
31. Patel T, Kellner CP, Katsumi H, Gupta M. Efficacy of endopyelotomy in patients with secondary ureteropelvic junction obstruction. J Endourol. 2011;25(4): 587–91.
32. Sofras F, Livadas K, Alivizatos G, et al. Retrograde Acucise endopyelotomy: is it worth its cost? J Endourol. 2004;18:466–8.
33. Lechevallier E, Echazarian C, Ortega JC, et al. Retrograde Acucise endopyelotomy: long term results. J Endourol. 1999;13:575–80.
34. Nadler RB, Rao GS, Pearle MS, et al. Acucise endopyelotomy: assessment of long-term durability. J Urol. 1996;156:1044–98.
35. Gelet A, Combe M, Ramachers JM. Endopyelotomy with the Acucise cutting balloon device. Eur Urol. 1997;31:389–93.
36. Kim FJ, Herrell SD, Jahoda AE, Albala DM. Complications of Acucise endopyelotomy. J Endourol. 1998;12:433–6.
37. Cohen TD, Gross MB, Preminger GM. Long-term follow-up of balloon cautery incision of ureteropelvic junction obstruction. Urology. 1996;47:317–20.
38. Schwartz BF, Stoller ML. Complication of retrograde balloon cautery endopyelotomy. J Urol. 1999;162: 1594–8.
39. Weikert S, Christoph F, Mutller M, et al. Acucise endopyelotomy: a technique with limited efficacy for primary ureteropelvic junction obstruction in adults. Int J Urol. 2005;12:864–8.

Ureteral and Ureteroenteric Strictures

5

Ojas Shah and Tracy Marien

Introduction

The first endoscopic treatment of ureteral stricture disease was described in 1891 when bougies were used to dilate strictures secondary to tuberculosis. Prior to the advent of ureteroscopy in the 1970s the mainstay for treatment for ureteral strictures was open reconstructive surgery and/or nephrectomy [1–4]. The advancement of urologic endoscopic technology and imaging techniques has facilitated minimally invasive options for the management of ureteral and ureteroenteric strictures leading to shorter hospital stays, less morbidity, less blood loss, decreased operative time, and shorter convalescence time. In patients with multiple medical co-morbidities who may not tolerate reconstructive surgery, this may be their only treatment option.

Some reports indicate a lower success rate of open/laparoscopic reconstruction following a failed attempt at endoscopic treatment, therefore decision to proceed with an endoscopic option should be based on the appropriate clinical scenario [5, 6]. Given that endoscopic treatment failure of ureteral and ureteroenteric stricture disease does not preclude open or laparoscopic/robotic reconstruction, the lower rate of morbidity associated with, and the ability to achieve excellent success rates in the setting of suitable patient selection, it is logical to attempt endoscopic management first for the majority of patients before reconstruction.

The aim of this discussion is to present evidence regarding endoscopy, with a focus on ureteroscopy, for the management of ureteral and ureteroenteric strictures. Given the low rate of ureteral stricture diseases and ureteroenteric strictures (with an incidence of 1.9–13% in cases of urinary diversion) most evidence is derived from small retrospective series that lack long-term follow-up [7–22]. We will attempt to present the data in a comprehensive manner and assess the implications of the data for patient selection for endoscopic management of ureteral stricture disease.

Ureteral Strictures

Etiology

A ureteral stricture is a narrowing of the ureteral lumen causing functional obstruction.

Ureteral strictures may be classified as extrinsic or intrinsic, benign or malignant, and iatrogenic or non-iatrogenic. Non-iatrogenic strictures are typically congenital, secondary to infection or stone trauma. Iatrogenic ureteral strictures may result from ureteroscopy, open or laparoscopic

O. Shah, M.D. (✉) • T. Marien
Department of Urology, New York University School of Medicine, 150 E. 32nd Street, 2nd Floor, New York, NY 10016, USA

Department of Urology, NYU Langone Medical Center, New York, NY, USA
e-mail: ojas.shah@nyumc.org

M. Monga (ed.), *Ureteroscopy: Indications, Instrumentation & Technique*, Current Clinical Urology,
DOI 10.1007/978-1-62703-206-3_5,

injury, radiation therapy, urinary diversions, and renal transplantation.

Gynecologic surgery has up to a 4.5% risk of urologic injuries and is responsible for up to 64% of iatrogenic ureteral injuries [23–27]. Ureteral strictures secondary to ureteroscopy occur in up to 19% of cases in early reports of ureteroscopy, with an increased risk when ureteral perforation occurs [28–32]. With the use of smaller instruments, however, several studies have reported a decrease in the rate of post-ureteroscopy stricture to less than 1% [29, 30]. Risk factors for ureteral stricture development following ureteroscopy include stone impaction, large scope size, prolonged case duration, proximal location, perforation, and use of intracorporeal lithotripsy [29–31, 33].

Malignant Ureteral Obstruction

Malignant ureteral strictures are from primary urothelial carcinoma or from extrinsic sources, most commonly ovarian cancer, lymphoma, prostate cancer, testicular cancer, colorectal cancer, and breast cancer. These ureteral obstructions are generally not amenable to ureteroscopic treatment.

When the stricture is from a primary urothelial malignancy, it should be treated with endoscopic resection/ablation, segmental ureterectomy, or nephroureterectomy depending on the extent and grade/stage of the disease to both relieve the obstruction and treat the malignancy. If the primary ureteral tumor cannot be treated curatively secondary to patient and tumor factors, then the patient would likely fail endoscopic treatment of the malignant obstruction [34–36]. Rather, these patients are best managed with ureteral stenting or nephrostomy tube if the patient is symptomatic or in need of improved renal function.

Malignant extrinsic ureteral obstruction (MEUO) secondary to compression from metastatic or locally invasive disease is generally associated with a poor prognosis [37]. In these cases, therapeutic options include ureteral stenting with different techniques and stent sizes versus percutaneous renal drainage. Applied Silhouhette™ stents (Applied Medical, Laguna Hills, CA, USA) and Cook Resonance™ metallic stents (Cook Medical, Bloomington, IN, USA) are stiffer stents commonly used in the management of MEUO, and now several newer stents by ProSurg Inc. (ProSurg, San Jose, CA, USA) (Passage 7.0-Fr and Snake 6.0 to 7.0-Fr) have shown superior resistance to external compression in an ex vivo study [38]. Some studies have found improved patency and improved resistance to external compression with dual ureteral stent placement with stent sizes ranging from 4 to 8 Fr [34–36]. Ultimately (or initially) percutaneous drainage may be required, as ureteral stents tend to fail with disease progression [39, 40].

Techniques for Endoscopic Management of Ureteral Strictures

Prior to undergoing endoscopic treatment for ureteral stricture disease, voided urine culture specimen (and urine culture from nephrostomy tube if present) should be sent. Positive urine cultures should be treated with culture-specific antibiotics prior to intervention and perioperatively to try and sterilize urine as best as possible to minimize risk of infectious complications. Negative urine cultures preoperatively are ideal, but not always achievable, in the setting of indwelling tubes and urinary diversions. Refer to Table 5.1 for a list of equipment that will be helpful to have available before attempting ureteroscopic treatment of ureteral strictures.

Methods to Access the Stricture

Retrograde Technique

Once the patient is anesthetized and placed in the dorsal lithotomy position, a cystoscope is placed in the bladder and the ureteral orifice is cannulated with a 5 Fr open-ended catheter for retrograde pyelography. The retrograde pyelogram will allow further definition of the ureteral

Table 5.1 Instrument and disposables list for ureteroscopic management of ureteral strictures

Equipment list
Cystoscope (rigid and flexible)
Semirigid ureteroscope
Flexible ureteroscope
Nitinol guidewires (0.038″, 0.035″, Amplatz superstiff)
Hydrophilic guidewires—straight and angle-tipped (0.038″, 0.035″, 0.025″)
5 Fr open-ended ureteral catheter
5 Fr angiographic catheter (Berenstein)
Dual-lumen catheter or 8/10 Fr coaxial catheter
Ureteral balloon dilators—multiple sizes and lengths (4–10 cm, 12–18 Fr)
Biopsy devices (cup biopsy, brush biopsy)
Instruments for endoureterotomy (cold-knife, Holmium laser, electrocautery)
Ureteral stents (various sizes and lengths)
Endopyelotomy ureteral stent (various lengths)
Nephrostomy tubes (various sizes)

stricture location, length, and nature (complete versus incomplete obstruction). A Nitinol guidewire is then passed up into the kidney under fluoroscopic guidance with the assistance of the open-ended catheter if needed. If the wire cannot be passed beyond the region of the stricture, a hydrophilic guidewire (angle-tip) can be attempted with the assistance of a 5-Fr open-ended ureteral catheter or angiographic catheter to pass beyond the stricture and up into the kidney. If a wire cannot be passed beyond the strictured area, an option is to complete the case and have a nephrostomy tube placed to relieve the obstructed moiety and plan a possible antegrade approach.

Urologists with more advanced ureteroscopic skills may proceed further in a retrograde manner if feasible and safe. The rigid or flexible ureteroscope can be passed over or adjacent to the working guidewire (or under direct vision) up to the level of the stricture and direct visual inspection of the strictured area can be performed (scope choice based on the stricture location). Via the ureteroscope, a guidewire may be able to be passed through a pinpoint stricture up to the kidney.

Antegrade Technique

An antegrade approach may be preferred with more proximally located strictures, cases in which a retrograde approach was unsuccessful and in cases of concurrent upper tract pathology such as intrarenal calculi. Upper or mid pole calyces are generally preferred to gain straight access to the ureter. Once the patient is anesthetized and placed in the prone position (or supine based on surgeon preference), percutaneous access is achieved if the patient does not already have a nephrostomy tube in place. Antegrade pyelography and fluoroscopy are used throughout the procedure to define anatomy and assist with accessing the region of the ureteral stricture. A guidewire is passed into the kidney under fluoroscopic guidance and if present the nephrostomy tube is removed. A 5-Fr angiographic catheter is passed over the wire and the guidewire is manipulated down the ureter. With the assistance of the angiographic catheter, the wire should able to be passed into the bladder. Similar techniques to the retrograde approach (as noted above) can be used to manipulate the guidewire to obtain access through the level of the stricture and down into the bladder. The wire can then be exchanged for an Amplatz superstiff wire. An 8/10 Fr coaxial catheter is then passed over the superstiff guidewire in order to place two wires down to the bladder (working and safety wires).

If a wire cannot be passed beyond the level of the stricture, a flexible ureteroscope can be passed antegrade over a working guidewire down to the level of the stricture and direct visual inspection of the strictured area can be performed similar to the retrograde approach. Through the ureteroscope, a guidewire may be able to be passed through a pinpoint stricture down to the bladder.

Combined Retrograde/Antegrade Approach

A combined approach can be used for complex ureteral strictures, particularly cases with complete obstruction, when simultaneous antegrade and retrograde access is necessary [41–46]. Several techniques have been described to treat these strictures. In one technique, the patient is placed in the supine position and contrast (with or without indigo carmine) is injected into the percutaneous nephrostomy tube. An ureteroscope is passed retrograde up to the level of the stricture, allowing identification of each end of the stricture under fluoroscopy and direct vision. While studying the stricture under fluoroscopy at various angles, an incision using Holmium laser towards the proximal segment is made and recanalization is verified when indigo carmine/contrast is noted. The incision is carried through to periureteral fat [43]. Hong and associates reported a 75% success rate with 23–67-month follow-up with this technique [43].

Another approach to complete ureteral strictures is the "cut to the light" technique [44]. After percutaneous access is achieved (as described above) the patient is placed in the dorsal lithotomy position and a flexible ureteroscope is passed antegrade to the proximal end of the stricture. Another ureteroscope is passed retrograde to the distal end of the stricture. The light of the scope on the side of intended endoureterotomy is turned off, the instruments are aligned, and the incision is made towards the other illuminated scope taking great care to not laser beyond the level of the stricture to prevent damage to the other ureteroscope. This technique can be helpful in short strictures with complete occlusion of the lumen.

Some authors have described similar techniques but instead of performing endoureterotomy the stiff end of a guidewire is pushed towards the light and the wire will then allow through-and-through access to allow different incision/dilation techniques to be employed [45–47]. Similar results have been reported in small series of complete ureteral obstruction [45–47].

Balloon Dilation and/or Endoureterotomy Technique for Ureteral Strictures

When performing balloon dilation without incision, the balloon is placed in the strictured segment and inflated under fluoroscopic guidance. Successful dilation is achieved once no "waist" is noted on fluoroscopy in the strictured segment. No uniform recommendations exist regarding balloon inflation duration or optimal number of inflations. Our technique typically determines the length of the balloon by the length of the stricture (most commonly using 4 cm dilators). We typically dilate to 15 Fr if the "waist" is effectively dilated with this size and leave the balloon inflated for approximately 1 min.

Several case reports and/or small series also report the use of balloon dilation with cryoplasty; a technique initially developed to treat peripheral vascular stenosis [48, 49]. This system employs a balloon catheter which is expanded and cooled to −10°C using nitrous oxide. The advantage of this technology is that it induces apoptosis in smooth muscle cells and fibroblasts that are generally involved in the scar response/restenosis. Additionally, theoretically by inducing apoptosis instead of necrosis there is a decrease in the amount of cytokines released and thus the inflammatory response, possibly limiting fibrosis/restenosis further [48–50]. Additional studies are needed to assess the safety and efficacy of this technology.

If an endoureterotomy incision is to be performed, it should be made away from periureteral vasculature (Fig. 5.1). Endoluminal ultrasound guidance has also been described to aid in identifying periureteral structures and directing the incision away from the vasculature [51]. The incision can be made using Holmium laser technology, cold-knife, or electrocautery. Our preferred technique uses Holmium laser at settings of 1 J at a rate of 10 Hz. We typically use 365-μm laser fibers when performing semirigid ureteroscopy and 200-μm fibers for flexible ureteroscopy. The advantages of Holmium laser technology for endoureterotomy include the small caliber of the laser, ability to achieve hemostasis with incision, and the depth of penetration is <0.5 mm limiting damage to neighboring blood vessels [52].

Traditionally, endoureterotomy with cold-knife incision uses a flexible, wire-mounted cold-knife that is inserted past the stricture segment under direct visualization or under fluoroscopy

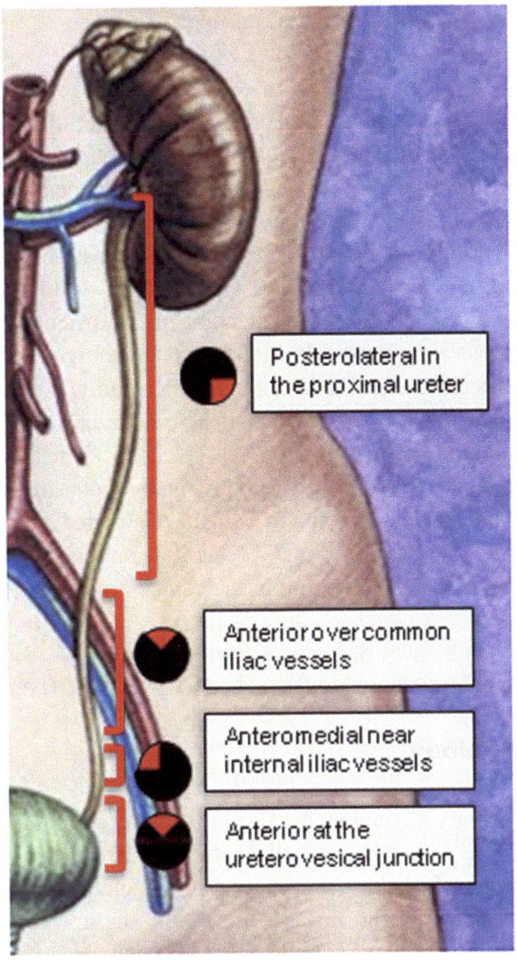

Fig. 5.1 The endoureterotomy incision should be made in the posterolateral portion of the proximal ureter, anteriorly over the iliac vessels, anteromedially over the internal iliac vessels, and then anteriorly over the ureterovesical junction

and pulled through the strictured segment with the use of a rigid ureteroscope (therefore used mostly for distal ureteral strictures) [53]. The lack of hemostatic capability with this technique can be a disadvantage since bleeding can easily obscure visualization. The invention of a blade-mounted guidewire has allowed the procedure to be performed antegrade, retrograde, and under direct vision [52].

Electrocautery incision can be performed with Greenwald Electrodes (2, 3, or 5 Fr) and endoscopic straight or right angle papillotomes (2–3 Fr) [52, 54–56]. These cutting instruments have the advantage of small size and ability to treat more strictures than the cold-knife as well as being able to provide hemostasis in addition to cutting through tissue. However, use of cautery can also lead to risk of scar tissue formation itself [52].

A hot-wire balloon cutting device (Acucise™ – Applied Medical, Laguna Hills, CA) is another option for treatment of ureteral strictures performed endoscopically under fluoroscopic guidance. This device is a combination of monopolar electrocautery and balloon dilation placed cystoscopically under fluoroscopic guidance [57]. The system is inserted into the urinary system over a guide wire either retrograde or antegrade, the balloon is inflated with contrast, the stricture is assessed and incised using electrocautery until the waist of the narrowed segment is gone. The main disadvantage of this method is lack of direct visualization and potential for injury to adjacent structures, especially vasculature resulting in bleeding and possible need for further invasive procedure; therefore we do not recommend this technique based on its risks and potential for complications [58, 59].

Appropriate incision depth is achieved when periureteral adipose tissue is visualized; contrast extravasation can be used to confirm desired incision depth on fluoroscopy. The incision is extended into normal ureteral tissue generally 5 mm proximal and distal to the stricture and in cases of very proximal or very distal strictures, the incision extends into the renal pelvis or into the bladder or urinary diversion, respectively. Balloon dilation can be used prior to the incision to access the strictured area when too tight to pass a ureteroscope through and may allow further characterization of the narrowed segment. Balloon dilation following endoureterotomy can be both therapeutic and diagnostic allowing the surgeon to assess for obliteration of the strictured segment's waist on fluoroscopy [55].

Ureteral Stent Selection

Indwelling ureteral stents placed following dilation and or endoureterotomy have several theoretical functions including scaffolding for healing, maintaining patency, and diversion of urine during the healing process. It is unclear whether larger stents are more effective in maintaining ureteral patency or more likely to cause fibrosis and recurrent strictures [60, 61]. Several prospective porcine models have found no difference in stent size (7 Fr versus 14 Fr) and recurrent stricture rates [62, 63]. One of these series did find a higher infection rate with larger stent size, and given that infection was associated with higher stricture rates, recommended using a smaller stent size [63].

Yu and colleagues found inserting two double J stents more effective than inserting one stent following balloon dilation of ureteral stricture, reporting success rates of 87.8% versus 62.7%, respectively [64]. Razdan and associates reported 80% patency rates on long-term follow-up in patients they considered high risk for failure (i.e., patients with longer strictures and history of radiation therapy) by placing two 6 or 6/8-Fr stents following endoscopic procedure for ureteral stricture [36].

The ideal ureteral stent dwelling duration is also unclear. Many leave indwelling stents for a 6-week period based on animal studies from the 1940s showing 90% muscular regeneration in a ureterotomy defect after 6 weeks [65]. Some porcine series reported increased infection rates with longer dwelling periods [63]. Another porcine model evaluating ideal duration of ureteral stenting found no difference on pathologic healing scores between ureteral stents left in for 1, 3, or 6 weeks and concluded that adequate duration of ureteral stenting following endoureterotomy may be as short as 1 week [66].

We place a double J ureteral stent (our preference is 8-Fr) or endopyelotomy stent (which can be inverted for distal ureteral strictures) for 4–6 weeks (which can be shortened or lengthened based on severity of stricture and operative course). If present, nephrostomy tubes should ideally be left open to drainage for 1–2 days following surgery to maximize drainage, then capped and/or removed after nephrostogram confirms patency. Fluoroscopic guidance should be used when removing a Cope-loop nephrostomy tube to ensure that the indwelling double J ureteral stent position is not affected.

When Endoscopic Treatment of Ureteral Strictures Fail

When balloon dilation and endoureterotomy fail, more invasive techniques may be required to achieve patency or placement of permanent or temporary ureteral stents/nephrostomy tubes with routine changes or nephrectomy. Reconstructive techniques include open, laparoscopic, or robot-assisted laparoscopic resection of the strictured ureteral segment with ureteroureterostomy, transureteroureterostomy, ureterocalicostomy, psoas hitch and/or Boari Flap, ileal transposition, or autotransplantation [67–71]. In cases where the patient's condition precludes major reconstruction, but is symptomatic from the obstructed renal unit, nephrectomy may be the best option if the contralateral renal unit has adequate function.

Ureteroenteric Anastomotic Strictures

Etiology

Urinary diversion has become more commonplace over the last half century in the management of bladder cancer as well as some benign diseases of the urinary tract. One of the most common complications of this procedure is the development of anastomotic strictures. The workup of ureteroenteric strictures includes first ruling out new primary or recurrent malignancy with imaging, cytology, and/or biopsy. The most common benign causes of ureteroenteric strictures are ischemia, ureteral kinking, and inflammation following radiation therapy. The formation of anastomotic strictures may also be related to surgical technique, obesity (theoretically due to shorter ureters to mobilize, higher intraabdominal pressures leading to compromise of the anastomosis, and increased local secretion of cytokines from encroachment of adipose tissue resulting in impaired healing) [14, 19, 21]. The left ureter is at higher risk for ischemia and stricture secondary to more extensive dissection required for mobilization [19]. Non-refluxing ureteral anastomoses are also at higher risk of postoperative stricture [12, 72].

Technique for Endoscopic Management of Ureteroenteric Strictures

Similar preoperative preparation applies to the treatment of ureteroenteric strictures as ureteral strictures as previously described including treatment with culture-specific antibiotics prior to any intervention.

Retrograde Technique

Many urologists are discouraged to attempt retrograde access following urinary diversion given the additional challenge secondary to anatomic distortion even though an antegrade approach may have higher risk of bleeding, infection, and injury to adjacent organs such as the bowel and lungs and is often staged [73, 74]. Finding a ureteral orifice (UO), particularly in the setting of obstruction/stricture at the anastomosis, can be quite challenging in urinary diversions since normal tools to help identify the ureter (intravenous contrast or indigo carmine) will likely not work if the obstruction is high grade. Additionally, the UO can easily be obscured or difficult to locate within a diversion. In our experience, the level of challenge increases from ileal conduits to orthotopic neobladders to continent cutaneous urinary diversions.

Few studies describe the use of retrograde access alone when treating ureteroenteric strictures [6, 55, 75, 76]. Hyams and colleagues describe their experience with retrograde access in patients with urinary diversion in 21 renal units which included 9 cases for ureteroenteric strictures. This technique implements flexible cystoscopy for continent pouches and conduits or a rigid cystoscope for neobladders [76]. The urinary diversion is carefully inspected to identify the UOs based on the operative report's description of the ureteral anastomotic location and what is typically expected with each type of urinary diversion. If the UOs are not readily identifiable, then a loopogram or cystography may be done to help delineate these structures in a patient with refluxing ureteroenteric anastomoses. If the patient has a neobladder with a Studer limb, indigo carmine may be given intravenously while the afferent limb is examined with flexible ureteroscopy [76]. Once the UO(s) of interest is identified, a guidewire is passed up into the kidney as previously described. If this approach fails, a 5-Fr open-ended angiographic catheter with a straight or angle-tip hydrophilic guidewire may be used. A working wire and safety wire should be placed using a dual-lumen catheter, given the challenge of achieving access in these patients. Generally flexible ureteroscopy is used, but rigid ureteroscopy is described for patients with a neobladder and direct access to the UO [76]. This series reported an overall 75% success rate for achieving retrograde access, with orthotopic neobladders having the highest success rate at 90%, followed by ileal conduits (73%) and Indiana pouches being the most difficult (33%) [76].

Antegrade Technique

The antegrade approach is similar to ureteral stricture disease described previously. In rare cases of ureterosigmoidostomy, there has been reports of successful antegrade balloon cautery endoureterotomy and balloon dilation alone for these ureteroenteric anastomotic strictures [77]. This series noted reflux of stool into the collecting system but had no cases of postoperative infections. They did not advocate preoperative bowel preparation, but did recommend a low residue diet while the stent was in place. In our limited experience with ureterosigmoidostomy anastomotic strictures we have had similar results, though employing a bowel preparation in cases where retrograde manipulation will also be performed.

Combined Retrograde/Antegrade Approach

In the case of combined approaches, positioning depends on type of urinary diversion. Patients with ileal conduits and cutaneous continent diversions should be placed in the supine position with access available to the flank region if a nephrostomy tube has been pre-placed. Patients with orthotopic neobladders may be placed in the modified lithotomy position with access to the flank region if a nephrostomy tube has already been placed [78].

One combined technique by Lovaco and colleagues describes intraluminal invagination to better visualize the stricture at the time of endoureterotomy [78]. This method uses an inflated balloon placed percutaneously and dilated in the ureteroenteric stricture while advancing into the urinary diversion to achieve intraluminal invagination. The most distal portion of the stricture is pushed into the urinary reservoir allowing for the stricture to be directly visualized within the intestinal segment and treated with a laser or electrocautery (such as a bugbee or Collin's knife). This approach allows precise control of the incision under direct visualization and away from blood vessels and bowel [78]. This technique can also be extrapolated to be used in a retrograde manner if the ureteral orifice can be identified since this technique allows for a full thickness, full-length incision of the ureteroenteric stricture. At a median follow-up of 51 months (range 2–145) the success rate for endoureterotomy by intraluminal invagination was 80% (20 of 25 ureterointestinal anastomotic strictures) without complications.

Balloon Dilation and/or Endoureterotomy Technique for Ureteroenteric Strictures

Preoperative imaging should be carefully reviewed for nearby vasculature prior to endoureterotomy. Balloon dilation can be used alone or with concurrent endoureterotomy as previously described in ureteral stricture cases with endoureterotomy having higher success for longer strictures. When performing the endoureterotomy, the incision should extend 5 mm to 1 cm proximal to the stricture and extend into the reservoir or urinary conduit. When making the incision, some advocate incising circularly up to three to six times [53]. Some report making the incision posteriorly or laterally [5, 79, 80]. Selection and duration of ureteral stents is similar to ureteral strictures.

Kidney Transplant Ureteral Strictures

Kidneys are the most commonly transplanted organs with over 10,000 transplanted renal units per year in the USA. The most common urological complication following kidney transplantation is ureteral stricture occurring in 3–10% of cases with 80% of the strictures occurring at the ureterovesical junction (UVJ) [29, 81–83]. It is essential to relieve and correct these obstructions promptly in order to preserve graft function.

Endoscopic Techniques for Ureteral Strictures in Transplanted Kidneys

Following immediate decompression with percutaneous nephrostomy drainage and return of baseline renal function, a nephrostogram is performed for treatment planning of transplanted renal units with ureteral stenosis. Prognostic indicators for successful endourological management of these ureteral strictures include diagnosis of stricture a short time after transplantation and previous acute rejection [84]. An antegrade approach is frequently taken secondary to preoperative placement of nephrostomy and challenge of retrograde access, similar to antegrade technique previously described for ureteral strictures.

When taking a retrograde approach, as with ureteroenteric strictures, review of previous surgical reports can help identify the UO, which appears as an irregular region with stippled urothelium [85]. The transplantation technique also impacts the ease with which retrograde access is obtained, some reporting only 59% success when attempting access in patients who underwent the Lich-Gregoir technique versus 100% in those patients who underwent the Leadbetter-Politano method [86]. The rest of the procedure is similar to that previously described.

A combined antegrade/retrograde technique with endoscopic retrograde resection of a bladder window has also been described. This technique allows for direct retroperitoneal visualization and longitudinal incision of the distal ureter when the UO cannot be located on direct vision with or without the use of methylene blue [87]. This approach uses an angiographic catheter to create bladder wall motion to guide resection through the bladder wall with a resectoscope. Full thickness resection of the bladder wall allows entry into the retroperitoneal space and incision into the distal ureter longitudinally with the same resectoscope [87].

In cases where retrograde methods fail and there is a desire to pursue a minimally invasive approach without percutaneous puncture of the transplanted unit, laparoscopic pneumovesicular ureterotomy has also been described [88]. This technique implements laparoscopic surgery in the bladder cavity with pneumovesicum and incision into the stenosed ureter with placement of stent and an indwelling foley catheter for 3 days.

Once access is achieved, balloon dilation can be performed as previously described. When performing endoureterotomy, most describe making the incision anteriorly given that most strictures are located at the UVJ, or further assessment of the vasculature anatomy can be made with imaging and review of the prior operative report before performing endoureterotomy for more proximal strictures [89–91].

If endoscopic management fails other options include open, laparoscopic, or robotic-assisted procedures including ureteral reimplantation, segmental ureterectomy and psoas hitch and/or Boari flap, pyelovesicostomy, vesicocalicostomy, reimplantation with ileal ureter, or implantation of an artificial ureter [92–94]. Long-term ureteral stenting and nephrostomy tubes are also options but should only be considered in exceptional cases as the final solution in these immunosuppressed patients who are at even higher risk for infection [95]. For recurrent and recalcitrant ureteral strictures after kidney transplantation, placement of two double J stents has been shown to be successful [96].

Complications of Treating Ureteral Strictures

Complications from balloon dilation of strictures described in the literature include perirenal hemorrhage, urinary extravasation, hematuria, ureteroenteric fistula (successfully managed with ureteral stent only), fevers, UTIs/sepsis, balloon rupture, ureteral rupture, stent migration, and arteriovenous fistula (that necessitated transplant nephrectomy) [46, 97–102].

Complications from incision, especially when heat is involved, can be a little more complex. Complications with endoureterotomy include perforation, infection/sepsis, large volume intraperitoneal fluid extravasation, bleeding, injury to iliac vessels, urinoma, hyponatremia, ureteroenteric fistula, and stent migration [43, 44, 46, 55–57, 92, 103–109]. The most dangerous complication reported is large vessel injury that has been reported in cases of cold-knife incision and with a hot cutting balloon device [48, 54, 107].

Follow-Up after Ureteroscopic Treatment

When it is time for the stent to be removed, antibiotic prophylaxis should be started the day before stent removal and continue through the day after [110, 111]. There is no standard for postoperative monitoring for recurrence of stricture disease, but several series recommend an aggressive approach with renal scans, intravenous urograms, ultrasound, or CT imaging every 3 months for 2 years with decreasing frequency based on success of the procedure [53, 112]. Most failures occur within the first year; therefore close surveillance initially will prevent renal moiety obstruction and deterioration in renal function [41, 103, 105, 113, 114]. If failure occurs, depending on the condition of the patient and the stricture characteristics, decision will need to be made whether to continue with observation versus chronic stent or nephrostomy tube versus repeat endourologic approach versus ureteral reconstruction procedure or nephrectomy.

Factors Impacting Success Rates of Ureteroscopic Treatment

Renal Function

Decreased ipsilateral renal function is a known risk factor for failure of both endoscopic and open treatments of ureteral stricture disease secondary to low urine flow and decreased patency of stricture [103, 105, 113]. If ipsilateral split function is less than 15% on nuclear renography, strong consideration should be given to nephrectomy versus observation. Wolf and colleagues found that no patient with ipsilateral renal function less than 25% had successful endoureterotomy versus 80% success rate in strictures with ipsilateral function greater than 25% in a series of 47 ureteral strictures [41].

Stricture Length

Shorter ureteral stricture length strongly correlates with higher success rates in most series. Stricture length can usually be broken down into three categories: <1, 1–2, and >2 cm with decreasing ureteroscopic success as stricture length increases. Several series found ureteral stricture length to have statistically significant impact on the success or failure of endourological intervention [6, 41, 53, 98, 105, 113, 115]. One series of 50 patients mostly with benign ureteral stricture (two had ureteroenteric and five had malignant strictures) who underwent various endoscopic treatments found that all patients with strictures >2 cm failed endoscopic management while patients with stricture lengths ≤2 cm experienced 89% success rates [36].

Stricture Location

Multiple studies have reported higher failure rates for strictures located in the mid-ureter [56, 116]. The higher success rates in the proximal and distal ureters may be secondary to the ability to incise into a large cavity such as the renal pelvis or bladder and/or because of the better vascular supply in these segments of the ureter.

Stricture Etiology

Ureteral strictures due to ischemia (such as post-surgical, radiation related, cautery injury) develop significant fibrosis and can lead to lower success rates with endoscopic treatment. One series found that ischemic strictures undergoing laser endoureterotomy had statistically significant lower success rates of 64.7% versus 100% for ischemic versus non-ischemic, respectively [103]. Other series have corroborated these finding of higher failure rates in ischemic stricture disease undergoing ureteroscopic endoureterotomy [56, 105, 106].

Laterality

Unlike ureteral strictures, endoscopic interventions for left-sided ureteroenteric strictures have shown statistically significant lower success rates and trends toward higher failure rates compared to the right side [5, 41, 112, 117–119]. Most theorize that mobilization of the left ureter towards the right side compromises blood supply and results in an ischemic stricture [5].

Stricture Duration

Time from ureteral trauma to stricture formation also correlates with success of endoscopic treatment of ureteral stricture disease in some series [100, 105, 114, 120]. Theoretically, as strictures progress they tend to become more hypovascular and form denser scars with endoscopic treatments. Therefore, earlier intervention in more vascularized tissues should result in higher success rates. One large series reported no significant difference in success rates and stricture duration—however, this series' definition of 24 months as early postoperative period for stricture formation was likely too long of a duration to show a difference as other series reporting more success with earlier identified strictures defined short duration as at least less than 1 year if not even shorter [41].

Stricture Steroid Injection

Reports of increased success rates in the treatment of other stricture diseases such as urethral and gastrointestinal by using concurrent steroids injections at the time of definitive management spurred some to try this method in ureteral stricture disease [121, 122]. Wolf and associates injected triamcinolone into the bed of 22 ureteral and ureteroenteric strictures and compared those to 46 strictures that did not undergo triamcinolone injection; they found statistically significant improved outcomes in those cases that received the steroids [41]. Meretyk and colleagues injected triamcinolone into the bed of a six ureteral strictures following endoureterotomy and had an 80% success rate in this cohort versus 50% in those not treated with steroid injection [56].

Evidence-Based Outcomes

Ureteral Stricture

The largest series evaluating the outcomes of endoureterotomy in patients with benign ureteral stricture disease reports 74–85% success rates with over 2-year follow-up (see Table 5.2) [36, 41, 123]. When looking at studies broken down by treatment type, there is some variation in success rates.

Balloon dilation of benign ureteral strictures has success rates ranging from 0 to 87.8%

Table 5.2 Endoscopic management of benign ureteral strictures

Approach	Study	Number	Stricture length[a] (cm)	Mean follow-up (months)	Success rate (%)
Balloon dilation	Yu[b] [64]	48/57	1.05/0.99	3–15	87.8/62.7[c]
	Anastasescu [97]	12	–	87	75
	Lojanapiwat [106]	18	–	9.7	60
	Myren[d] [125]	40	–	7	85
	Hoe [100]	22	–	12	73
	Beckman [120]	28	–	1–40	79
	Johnson (1987) [114]	24	–	6	62.5
Laser incision	Lin [115]	19	0.85	40.2	52.6
	Gnessin [103]	35	–	27	78.7
	Bach [126]	18	–	12	61.2
	Hibi [127]	17	2.07	60.5	76
	Lane [113]	19	0.9	36	68.4
	Singal [128]	18	–	10.8	76
Cold-knife incision	Erdogru [105]	13	1.3	9	54
	Lojanapiwat [106]	12	–	15.3	75
	Yamada [107]	20	1.9	18	85
Electrocautery incision	Conlin [46]	2	3.75	46	50
	Meretyk [56]	13	3.0	20.4	62
Balloon dilation cautery device	Seseke [57]	15	1.3	15	53
	Knowles [47]	9	–	36	89
Mixed studies	Corcoran[e] [123]	34	1.6	25.2	85
	Razdan[f] [36]	43	–	40.8	74
	Wolf[g] [41]	38	–	28	81.6

[a]Mean or median if given or calculable via provided data
[b]Results given for high pressure/conventional pressure
[c]Success rate represents "overall effectiveness rate," "complete recovery" was 56.1/35.3%
[d]Six patients were dilated more than once
[e]Holmium laser incision in 41% and Balloon dilation in 91%. Some patients underwent repeat procedures
[f]CKI in 4 cases, holmium laser in 17 cases, electrocautery in 21 cases, and dilation in 8 cases
[g]Acucise in 21 cases, electrocautery in 13 cases, non-electrocautery cut in 3 cases, dilation in 1 case

[42, 46, 64, 97, 100, 101, 106, 114, 119, 120, 124, 125]. Series with 20 or more cases report success rates ranging from 54 to 87.8% [64, 100, 101, 114, 120, 125]. The most successful series reports dilation at higher pressures (15 atm), leaving the balloon inflated for 5 min and leaving the stent indwelling for 4 months [64].

Laser endoureterotomy of benign ureteral strictures also achieves high success rates ranging from 52.6 to 78.7% (Table 5.2) [103, 113, 115, 126–128]. A 75% success rate was even reported in one series with an average stricture length of 2.07 cm [127].

Cold-knife incision success rates have declined over time with older series reporting higher success rates than more recent series even in the setting of longer stricture lengths [105, 129]. This may reflect decreasing comfort and familiarity of urologists with this technique versus small study size artifact, which is possible given that other very small series performed in the 1990s report 81–100% success rates with short-term follow-up [42, 44, 46].

Use of electrocautery for ureteral strictures is only reported in a few small retrospective studies performed on relatively long strictures (average lengths of 3.0–3.75 cm) and still demonstrated relatively good success rates of up to 62% [46, 56].

The use of cutting balloons for benign ureteral stricture disease has been sparsely reported in the literature, with only one study having over ten subjects. Success rates are recorded between 40 and 89% [47, 57, 105, 108, 109]. Knowles and associates reported an 89% success rate evaluating nine distal ureteral strictures who required a staged procedure [47].

Incision and balloon dilation alone seem to have comparable success rates for shorter ureteral strictures (<1 cm). The decision to pursue dilation and/or endoureterotomy should be based on surgeon experience, preference, comfort level, and history of patient. However, in our opinion, the length of the stricture in addition to the etiology and location is critical in determining which patient will have success long-term and will be discussed below.

Ureteroenteric Strictures

The success rate for balloon dilation of ureteroenteric strictures in a series of ten or more patients ranges from 5 to 77% with most series reporting a 60% or lower success rates [6, 101, 119, 124, 130–132]. Success rates for laser endoureterotomy of ureteroenteric strictures range from 33 to 87.5% (Table 5.3) [5, 112, 117, 128]. Cold-knife and electrocautery report similar success rates ranging from 52.3 to 80% [53, 55, 78, 130, 133, 134]. Cutting balloon devices have overall success rates of 30–100%, with most series having greater than 50% success rates in this population [57, 92, 108, 109, 112, 135–137]. Unlike ureteral strictures where dilation alone is comparable to endoureterotomy for shorter strictures, in cases of ureteroenteric strictures, incision of the stricture results in higher success rates.

Post-renal Transplant Ureteral Stricture

The success of balloon dilation alone for transplant kidneys with ureteral stricture disease ranges from 0 to 100% [96, 102, 134, 138, 139]. Though only reported in a small number of transplanted renal units with ureteral stricture, laser endoureterotomy offers a promising treatment option with success rates of 67–100% (Table 5.4) [138, 140]. Success rates have been extremely high for electroincision, ranging from 93 to 100% in two small series [134, 135]. Cutting balloon also has very favorable outcomes in these cases with success rates of 83–85% [90, 91]. Endoureterotomy appears to be a very effective treatment for transplant-related ureteral strictures.

Patient Selection Recommendations

There are no absolute factors prohibiting any patient with benign ureteral, ureteroenteric, and kidney transplant-related ureteral strictures to at least undergoing an attempted endoscopic/ureteroscopic procedure before more radical reconstruction or

Table 5.3 Endoscopic management of benign ureteroenteric strictures

Approach	Study	Number	Stricture length[a] (cm)	Mean follow-up (months)	Success rate (%)
Balloon dilation	Nassar [130]	16	–	43	50
	Yagi [131]	13	–	47.1	77
	Ravery [119]	14	1.14	16	61
	Kwak[b] [124]	18	–	6	28
	Shapiro[b] [132]	37	–	–	16
Laser incision	Milhoua [112]	15	1.5	11.5	33
	Laven [5]	16	1–1.5	35	50
	Watterson [117]	24	1.7	22.5	70.8
	Singal [128]	8	–	10.8	87.5
Cold-knife incision	Nassar [130]	21	–	43	52.3
	Poulakis [53]	43	–	38.8	60.5
	Poulakis [133]	22	1.7–2	23.5	74
Electrocautery incision	Lovaco [78]	25	–	51	80
	Meretyk [55]	14	2	28.6	57
	Kramolowsky [134]	7	–	33[c]	71
Balloon dilation cautery device	Boylu [141]	3	~1	12	100
	Seseke [57]	3	3.3	12	100
	Touiti [109]	6	1.42	9.5	50
	Cornud [142]	37	–	25	67.5
	Lin [137]	10	≤2	18–30	30
Mixed	Wolf [41]	30	–	13	32

[a]Mean or median if given or calculable via provided data
[b]Some if not all patients had multiple dilations
[c]For patients with a successful outcome only

Table 5.4 Endoscopic management of kidney transplant-related ureteral strictures

Approach	Study	Number	Mean follow-up (months)	Success rate (%)
Balloon dilation	Kristo [138]	6	24	100
	Benoits [96]	17	–	70
	Kim [139]	10	29	40
	Farah [102]	17	17.8	53
	Voegeli [143]	14	–	79
Laser incision	Gdor [140]	6	58	67
	Kristo [138]	3	24	100
Electrocautery incision	Katz [135]	14	8	93
	Bosma [134]	9	58	100
Balloon dilation cautery device	Schwartz [91]	8	27	83
	Erturk [90]	7	13	85

nephrectomy is performed. Patients most likely to have a successful endoscopic intervention for benign ureteral stricture disease are those with partial, non-ischemic, shorter strictures (<1 cm), without a history of radiation, short interval since onset of stricture, and good ipsilateral renal function >25%. Lack of favorable stricture characteristics does not preclude patients from undergoing minimally invasive intervention, but these patients should be counseled appropriately regarding their higher risk for failure and recurrent stricture and need for a second, possibly more invasive treatment. Patients with minimal ipsilateral renal function should strongly consider observation if they are asymptomatic or nephrectomy if symptoms or recurrent infections occur.

Conclusions

Ureteroscopic endoureterotomy with or without balloon dilation is an effective and low risk therapeutic option that should be the first line of treatment in the majority of patients with ureteral stricture disease. Appropriate patient selection and proper counseling for patients with more complex strictures will result in higher success rates and patient satisfaction.

References

1. Bush IM, Goldberg E, Javadpour N, Chakrobortty H, Morelli F. Ureteroscopy and renoscopy: a preliminary report. Chic Med Sch Q. 1970;30(1):46–9.
2. Goodman TM. Ureteroscopy with pediatric cystoscope in adults. Urology. 1977;9(4):394.
3. Lyon ES, Kyker JS, Schoenberg HW. Transurethral ureteroscopy in women: a ready addition to the urological armamentarium. J Urol. 1978;119(1):35–6.
4. Lyon ES, Banno JJ, Schoenberg HW. Transurethral ureteroscopy in men using juvenile cystoscopy equipment. J Urol. 1979;122(2):152–3.
5. Laven BA, O'Connor RC, Gerber GS, Steinberg GD. Long-term results of endoureterotomy and open surgical revision for the management of ureteroenteric strictures after urinary diversion. J Urol. 2003;170(4 Pt 1):1226–30.
6. DiMarco DS, LeRoy AJ, Thieling S, Bergstralh EJ, Segura JW. Long-term results of treatment for ureteroenteric strictures. Urology. 2001;58(6):909–13.
7. Studer UE, Burkhard FC, Schumacher M, et al. Twenty years experience with an ileal orthotopic low pressure bladder substitute—lessons to be learned. J Urol. 2006;176(1):161–6.
8. Schmidt JD, Hawtrey CE, Flocks RH, Culp DA. Complications, results and problems of ileal conduit diversions. J Urol. 1973;109(2):210–6.
9. Cheng M, Looney SW, Brown JA. Ureteroileal anastomotic strictures after a Bricker ileal conduit: 50 case assessment of the impact of conversion from a slit incision to a "shield shaped" ileotomy. Can J Urol. 2011;18(2):5644–9.
10. Yang WJ, Cho KS, Rha KH, et al. Long-term effects of ileal conduit urinary diversion on upper urinary tract in bladder cancer. Urology. 2006;68(2):324–7.
11. Hetet JF, Rigaud J, Karam G, et al. Complications of Bricker ileal conduit urinary diversion: analysis of a series of 246 patients. Prog Urol. 2005;15(1):23–9. discussion 29.
12. Pantuck AJ, Han KR, Perrotti M, Weiss RE, Cummings KB. Ureteroenteric anastomosis in continent urinary diversion: long-term results and complications of direct versus nonrefluxing techniques. J Urol. 2000;163(2):450–5.
13. Ali-El-Dein B, Shaaban AA, Abu-Eideh RH, El-Azab M, Ashamallah A, Ghoneim MA. Surgical complications following radical cystectomy and orthotopic neobladders in women. J Urol. 2008;180(1):206–10.
14. Muraishi O, Yamashita T, Ishikawa S, Hara Y, Tokue A. Improvement of ureteroileal anastomosis in orthotopic ileal neobladder with modified le duc procedure: short submucosal tunnel technique. J Urol. 2001;165(3):798–801.
15. Arai Y, Taki Y, Kawase N, et al. Orthotopic ileal neobladder in male patients: functional outcomes of 66 cases. Int J Urol. 1999;6(8):388–92.
16. Lugagne PM, Herve JM, Lebret T, Barre P, Mollier S, Botto H. Ureteroileal implantation in orthotopic neobladder with the Le Duc-Camey mucosal-through technique: risk of stenosis and long-term follow-up. J Urol. 1997;158(3 Pt 1):765–7.
17. De Carli P, Micali S, O'Sullivan D, et al. Ureteral anastomosis in the orthotopic ileal neobladder: comparison of 2 techniques. J Urol. 1997;157(2):469–71.
18. Knap MM, Lundbeck F, Overgaard J. Early and late treatment-related morbidity following radical cystectomy. Scand J Urol Nephrol. 2004;38(2):153–60.
19. Kouba E, Sands M, Lentz A, Wallen E, Pruthi RS. A comparison of the bricker versus wallace ureteroileal anastomosis in patients undergoing urinary diversion for bladder cancer. J Urol. 2007;178(3):945–8.
20. Barbieri CE, Schwartz MJ, Boorjian SA, Lee MM, Scherr DS. Ureteroileal anastomosis with intraluminal visualization: technique and outcomes. Urology. 2010;76(6):1496–500.
21. Hautmann RE, de Petriconi RC, Volkmer BG. 25 years of experience with 1,000 neobladders: long-term complications. J Urol. 2011;185(6):2207–12.
22. Evangelidis A, Lee EK, Karellas ME, Thrashert JB, Holzbeierlein JRM. Evaluation of ureterointestinal anastomosis: Wallace vs Bricker. J Urol. 2006; 175(5):1755–8.
23. Ozdemir E, Ozturk U, Celen S, et al. Urinary complications of gynecologic surgery: iatrogenic urinary tract system injuries in obstetrics and gynecology operations. Clin Exp Obstet Gynecol. 2011;38(3): 217–20.
24. Goodno Jr JA, Powers TW, Harris VD. Ureteral injury in gynecologic surgery: a ten-year review in a community hospital. Am J Obstet Gynecol. 1995;172(6):1817–20. discussion 1820–1812.

25. Vakili B, Chesson RR, Kyle BL, et al. The incidence of urinary tract injury during hysterectomy: a prospective analysis based on universal cystoscopy. Am J Obstet Gynecol. 2005;192(5):1599–604.
26. St Lezin MA, Stoller ML. Surgical ureteral injuries. Urology. 1991;38(6):497–506.
27. Selzman AA, Spirnak JP. Iatrogenic ureteral injuries: a 20-year experience in treating 165 injuries. J Urol. 1996;155(3):878–81.
28. Johnson DB, Pearle MS. Complications of ureteroscopy. Urol Clin North Am. 2004;31(1):157–71.
29. Harmon WJ, Sershon PD, Blute ML, Patterson DE, Segura JW. Ureteroscopy: current practice and long-term complications. J Urol. 1997;157(1):28–32.
30. Jeromin L, Sosnowski M. Ureteroscopy in the treatment of ureteral stones: over 10 years' experience. Eur Urol. 1998;34(4):344–9.
31. Carter SS, Cox R, Wickham JE. Complications associated with ureteroscopy. Br J Urol. 1986;58(6):625–8.
32. O'Brien WM, Maxted WC, Pahira JJ. Ureteral stricture: experience with 31 cases. J Urol. 1988;140(4):737–40.
33. Roberts WW, Cadeddu JA, Micali S, Kavoussi LR, Moore RG. Ureteral stricture formation after removal of impacted calculi. J Urol. 1998;159(3):723–6.
34. Liu JS, Hrebinko RL. The use of 2 ipsilateral ureteral stents for relief of ureteral obstruction from extrinsic compression. J Urol. 1998;159(1):179–81.
35. Hamm M, Rathert P. Therapy of extrinsic ureteral obstruction by 2 parallel double-J ureteral stents. Urologe A. 1999;38(2):150–5.
36. Razdan S, Silberstein IK, Bagley DH. Ureteroscopic endoureterotomy. BJU Int. 2005;95 Suppl 2:94–101.
37. Wong LM, Cleeve LK, Milner AD, Pitman AG. Malignant ureteral obstruction: outcomes after intervention. Have things changed? J Urol. 2007;178(1):178–83. discussion 183.
38. Hendlin K, Korman E, Monga M. New metallic ureteral stents: improved tensile strength and resistance to extrinsic compression. J Endourol. 2011;26(3):271–4.
39. Docimo SG, Dewolf WC. High failure rate of indwelling ureteral stents in patients with extrinsic obstruction: experience at 2 institutions. J Urol. 1989;142(2 Pt 1):277–9.
40. Chung SY, Stein RJ, Landsittel D, et al. 15-year experience with the management of extrinsic ureteral obstruction with indwelling ureteral stents. J Urol. 2004;172(2):592–5.
41. Wolf Jr JS, Elashry OM, Clayman RV. Long-term results of endoureterotomy for benign ureteral and ureteroenteric strictures. J Urol. 1997;158(3 Pt 1):759–64.
42. Netto Junior NR, Ferreira U, Lemos GC, Claro JF. Endourological management of ureteral strictures. J Urol. 1990;144(3):631–4.
43. Hong JH, Jeon SS, Lee KS. Result of endoscopic ureteroureterostomy with holmium:YAG laser for complete ureteral obstruction. J Endourol. 2005;19(8):979–83.
44. Lopatkin NA, Martov AG, Gushchin BL. An endourologic approach to complete ureteropelvic junction and ureteral strictures. J Endourol. 2000;14(9):721–6.
45. Egilmez T, Guvel S, Kilinc F, Yaycioglu O, Ozkardes H. Management of complete ureteral obstructions with a transluminal puncture technique. Int Braz J Urol. 2005;31(3):264–8.
46. Conlin MJ, Gomella LG, Bagley DH. Endoscopic ureteroureterostomy for obliterated ureteral segments. J Urol. 1996;156(4):1394–9.
47. Knowles DR, Staiman VR, Gupta M. Long-term results of the treatment of complete distal ureteral stenosis using a cutting balloon catheter device. J Urol. 2001;166(6):2087–90.
48. Orsi F, Penco S, Matei V, et al. Treatment of ureterointestinal anastomotic strictures by diathermal or cryoplastic dilatation. Cardiovasc Intervent Radiol. 2007;30(5):943–9.
49. Heran MKS, Bergen DC, MacNeily AE. The use of cryoplasty in a benign ureteric stricture. Pediatr Radiol. 2010;40(11):1806–9.
50. Yiu WK, Cheng SWK, Sumpio BE. Vascular smooth muscle cell apoptosis induced by "supercooling" and rewarming. J Vasc Interv Radiol. 2006;17(12):1971–7.
51. Bagley DH, Conlin MJ, Liu JB. Device for intraluminal incision guided by endoluminal ultrasonography. J Endourol. 1996;10(5):421–3.
52. El-Nahas AR, Shokeir AA. Endourological treatment of nonmalignant upper urinary tract complications after urinary diversion. Urology. 2010;76(6):1302–8.
53. Poulakis V, Witzsch U, De Vries R, Becht E. Cold-knife endoureterotomy for nonmalignant ureterointestinal anastomotic strictures. Urology. 2003;61(3):512–7. discussion 517.
54. Cornud F, Lefebvre JF, Chretien Y, Helenon O, Casanova JM, Moreau JF. Percutaneous transrenal electro-incision of ureterointestinal anastomotic strictures: long-term results and comparison of fluoroscopic and endoscopic guidance. J Urol. 1996;155(5):1575–8.
55. Meretyk S, Clayman RV, Kavoussi LR, Kramolowsky EV, Picus DD. Endourological treatment of ureteroenteric anastomotic strictures: long-term followup. J Urol. 1991;145(4):723–7.
56. Meretyk S, Albala DM, Clayman RV, Denstedt JD, Kavoussi LR. Endoureterotomy for treatment of ureteral strictures. J Urol. 1992;147(6):1502–6.
57. Seseke F, Heuser M, Zoller G, Plothe KD, Ringert RH. Treatment of iatrogenic postoperative ureteral strictures with acucise endoureterotomy. Eur Urol. 2002;42(4):370–5.
58. Kim FJ, Herrell SD, Jahoda AE, Albala DM. Complications of acucise endopyelotomy. J Endourol. 1998;12(5):433–6.
59. Wagner JR, D'Agostino R, Babayan RK. Renal arterioureteral hemorrhage: a complication of acucise endopyelotomy. Urology. 1996;48(1):139–41.

60. Ramsay JW, Payne SR, Gosling PT, Whitfield HN, Wickham JE, Levison DA. The effects of double J stenting on unobstructed ureters. An experimental and clinical study. Br J Urol. 1985;57(6):630–4.
61. Levine RS, Pollack HM, Banner MP. Transient ureteral obstruction after ureteral stenting. AJR Am J Roentgenol. 1982;138(2):323–7.
62. Moon YT, Kerbl K, Pearle MS, et al. Evaluation of optimal stent size after endourologic incision of ureteral strictures. J Endourol. 1995;9(1):15–22.
63. Soria F, Sanchez FM, Sun F, Ezquerra J, Duran E, Uson J. Comparative study of ureteral stents following endoureterotomy in the porcine model: 3 vs 6 weeks and 7F vs 14F. Cardiovasc Intervent Radiol. 2005;28(6):773–8.
64. Yu HL, Ye LY, Lin MH, Yang Y, Miao R, Hu XJ. Treatment of benign ureteral stricture by double J stents using high-pressure balloon angioplasty. Chin Med J. 2011;124(6):943–6.
65. Davis DM, Strong GH, Drake WM. Intubated ureterotomy; experimental work and clinical results. J Urol. 1948;59(5):851–62.
66. Kerbl K, Chandhoke PS, Figenshau RS, Stone AM, Clayman RV. Effect of stent duration on ureteral healing following endoureterotomy in an animal-model. J Urol. 1993;150(4):1302–5.
67. Matlaga BR, Shah OD, Singh D, Streem SB, Assimos DG. Ureterocalicostomy: a contemporary experience. Urology. 2005;65(1):42–4.
68. Matlaga BR, Shah OD, Hart LJ, Assimos DG. Ileal ureter substitution: a contemporary series. Urology. 2003;62(6):998–1001.
69. Simmons MN, Gill IS, Fergany AF, Kaouk JH, Desai MM. Laparoscopic ureteral reconstruction for benign stricture disease. Urology. 2007;69(2):280–4.
70. Boxer RJ, Fritzsche P, Skinner DG, et al. Replacement of the ureter by small intestine: clinical application and results of the ileal ureter in 89 patients. J Urol. 1979;121(6):728–31.
71. Eisenberg ML, Lee KL, Zumrutbas AE, Meng MV, Freise CE, Stoller ML. Long-term outcomes and late complications of laparoscopic nephrectomy with renal autotransplantation. J Urol. 2008;179(1): 240–3.
72. Shaaban AA, Abdel-Latif M, Mosbah A, et al. A randomized study comparing an antireflux system with a direct ureteric anastomosis in patients with orthotopic deal neobladders. BJU Int. 2006;97(5):1057–62.
73. Michel MS, Trojan L, Rassweiler JJ. Complications in percutaneous nephrolithotomy. Eur Urol. 2007;51(4):899–906. discussion 906.
74. Mousavi-Bahar SH, Mehrabi S, Moslemi MK. Percutaneous nephrolithotomy complications in 671 consecutive patients: a single-center experience. Urol J. 2011;8(4):271–6.
75. Gerber GS, Kuznetzov D, Leef JA, Rosenblum J, Steinberg GD. Holmium: YAG laser endoureterotomy in the treatment of ureteroenteric strictures following orthotopic urinary diversion. Tech Urol. 1999;5(1):45–8.
76. Hyams ES, Winer AG, Shah O. Retrograde ureteral and renal access in patients with urinary diversion. Urology. 2009;74(1):47–50.
77. Eisenberg ML, Lee KL, Stoller ML. Endoscopic management of obstructive complications in ureterosigmoidostomy. Urology. 2007;70(6):1048–52.
78. Lovaco F, Serrano A, Fernandez I, Perez P, Gonzalez-Peramato P. Endoureterotomy by intraluminal invagination for nonmalignant ureterointestinal anastomotic strictures: description of a new surgical technique and long-term followup. J Urol. 2005;174(5):1851–6.
79. Kramolowsky EV, Clayman RV, Weyman PJ. Management of ureterointestinal anastomotic strictures—comparison of open surgical and endourological repair. J Urol. 1988;139(6):1195–8.
80. Cornud F, Mendelsberg M, Chretien Y, et al. Fluoroscopically guided percutaneous transrenal electroincision of ureterointestinal anastomotic strictures. J Urol. 1992;147(3):578–81.
81. Liatsikos EN, Karnabatidis D, Katsanos K, et al. Metal stents for the management of malignant ureteral obstruction. J Endourol. 2008;22(9):2099–100. discussion 2107.
82. Liatsikos EN, Kagadis GC, Karnabatidis D, et al. Application of self-expandable metal stents for ureteroileal anastomotic strictures: long-term results. J Urol. 2007;178(1):169–73.
83. Antimisiaris SG, Siablis D, Liatsikos E, et al. Liposome-coated metal stents: an in vitro evaluation of controlled-release modality in the ureter. J Endourol. 2000;14(9):743–7.
84. Benson AD, Taylor ER, Schwartz BF. Metal ureteral stent for benign and malignant ureteral obstruction. J Urol. 2011;185(6):2217–22.
85. Basiri A, Nikoobakht MR, Simforoosh N, Hosseini Moghaddam SM. Ureteroscopic management of urological complications after renal transplantation. Scand J Urol Nephrol. 2006;40(1):53–6.
86. Basiri A, Simforoosh N, Nikoobakht M, Hosseini Moghaddam MM. The role of ureteroscopy in the treatment of renal transplantation complications. Urol J. 2004;1(1):27–31.
87. Best CD, Bolton DM, Bretan P, Stoller ML. Endoscopic ureteroneocystostomy for post-transplantation ureterovesical junction stenosis. J Endourol. 1994;8(3):213–5.
88. Mongha R, Gupta A, Bansal P, Narayan S, Bera MK. Vesicoscopic ureterotomy: novel technique for management of posttransplant ureteric stricture. Transplant Proc. 2009;41(1):173–6.
89. Bhayani SB, Landman J, Slotoroff C, Figenshau RS. Transplant ureter stricture: acucise endoureterotomy and balloon dilation are effective. J Endourol. 2003;17(1):19–22.
90. Erturk E, Burzon DT, Waldman D. Treatment of transplant ureteral stenosis with endoureterotomy. J Urol. 1999;161(2):412–4.
91. Schwartz BF, Chatham JR, Bretan P, Goharderakhshan R, Stoller ML. Treatment of refractory

kidney transplant ureteral strictures using balloon cautery endoureterotomy. Urology. 2001;58(4): 536–9.
92. Giessing M. Transplant ureter stricture following renal transplantation: surgical options. Transplant Proc. 2011;43(1):383–6.
93. Del Pizzo JJ, Jacobs SC, Bartlett ST, Sklar GN. The use of bladder for total transplant ureteral reconstruction. J Urol. 1998;159(3):750–2.
94. Gowda BDR, Goldsmith P, Ahmad N. Boari flap vesicocalycostomy: a salvage drainage procedure for complete ureteric stricture and pyelocalyceal fistula. Clin Transplant. 2009;23(1):129–31.
95. Borden Jr LS, Pais Jr VM, Assimos DG. Repetitive ureteral stenting for management of transplant graft ureteral obstruction. Int Braz J Urol. 2006;32(2):142–5. discussion 145–146.
96. Benoit G, Alexandre L, Moukarzel M, Yataghene Y, Charpentier B, Jardin A. Percutaneous antegrade dilation of ureteral strictures in kidney transplants. J Urol. 1993;150(1):37–9.
97. Anastasescu R, Merrot T, Chaumoitre K, Panuel M, Alessandrini P. Antegrade percutaneous balloon dilation of ureteral strictures after failed pelviureteric or ureterovesical reimplantation in children. Urology. 2011;77(6):1444–9.
98. Byun SS, Kim JH, Oh SJ, Kim HH. Simple retrograde balloon dilation for treatment of ureteral strictures: etiology-based analysis. Yonsei Med J. 2003;44(2):273–8.
99. ElAbd SA, ElShaer AF, ElMahrouky AS, ElAshry OM, Emran MA. Long-term results of endourologic and percutaneous management of ureteral strictures in bilharzial patients. J Endourol. 1996;10(1): 35–43.
100. Hoe JW. Benign ureteric strictures–management by percutaneous interventional uro-radiological techniques. Ann Acad Med Singapore. 1993;22(5): 670–4.
101. Banner MP, Pollack HM. Dilatation of ureteral stenoses: techniques and experience in 44 patients. AJR Am J Roentgenol. 1984;143(4):789–93.
102. Farah NB, Roddie M, Lord RH, Williams G. Ureteric obstruction in renal transplants: the role of percutaneous balloon dilatation. Nephrol Dial Transplant. 1991;6(12):977–81.
103. Gnessin E, Yossepowitch O, Holland R, Livne PM, Lifshitz DA. Holmium laser endoureterotomy for benign ureteral stricture: a single center experience. J Urol. 2009;182(6):2775–9.
104. Hibi H, Kato K, Mitsui K, et al. Endoscopic ureteral incision using the holmium:YAG laser. Int J Urol. 2001;8(12):657–61.
105. Erdogru T, Kutlu O, Koksal T, et al. Endoscopic treatment of ureteric strictures: acucise, cold-knife endoureterotomy and wall stents as a salvage approach. Urol Int. 2005;74(2):140–6.
106. Lojanapiwat B, Soonthonpun S, Wudhikarn S. Endoscopic treatment of benign ureteral strictures. Asian J Surg. 2002;25(2):130–3.
107. Yamada S, Ono Y, Ohshima S, Miyake K. Transurethral ureteroscopic ureterotomy assisted by a prior balloon dilation for relieving ureteral strictures. J Urol. 1995;153(5):1418–21.
108. Steiner DL, Johns-Putra L, Lyon S. Ureteroplasty with a cutting balloon: a novel approach to ureteric anastomotic strictures. Australas Radiol. 2007; 51(2):143–6.
109. Touiti D, Gelet A, Deligne E, et al. Treatment of uretero-intestinal and ureterovesical strictures by acucise balloon catheter. Eur Urol. 2002;42(1):49–54. discussion 55.
110. Ramaswamy K, Shah O. Antibiotic prophylaxis after uncomplicated ureteroscopic stone treatment: is there a difference? J Endourol. 2011;26(2):122–5.
111. Wolf Jr JS, Bennett CJ, Dmochowski RR, Hollenbeck BK, Pearle MS, Schaeffer AJ. Best practice policy statement on urologic surgery antimicrobial prophylaxis. J Urol. 2008;179(4):1379–90.
112. Milhoua PM, Miller NL, Cookson MS, Chang SS, Smith JA, Herrell SD. Primary endoscopic management versus open revision of ureteroenteric anastomotic strictures after urinary diversion—single institution contemporary series. J Endourol. 2009; 23(3):551–5.
113. Lane BR, Desai MM, Hegarty NJ, Streem SB. Long-term efficacy of holmium laser endoureterotomy for benign ureteral strictures. Urology. 2006;67(5): 894–7.
114. Johnson CD, Oke EJ, Dunnick NR, et al. Percutaneous balloon dilatation of ureteral strictures. AJR Am J Roentgenol. 1987;148(1):181–4.
115. Lin CM, Tsai TH, Lin TC, et al. Holmium: yttrium-aluminum-garnet laser endoureterotomy for benign ureteral strictures: a single-centre experience. Acta Chir Belg. 2009;109(6):746–50.
116. Smith AD. Management of iatrogenic ureteral strictures after urological procedures. J Urol. 1988; 140(6):1372–4.
117. Watterson JD, Sofer M, Wollin TA, Nott L, Denstedt JD. Holmium: YAG laser endoureterotomy for ureterointestinal strictures. J Urol. 2002;167(4): 1692–5.
118. Laven BA, O'Connor RC, Steinberg GD, Gerber GS. Long-term results of antegrade endoureterotomy using the holmium laser in patients with ureterointestinal strictures. Urology. 2001;58(6):924–9.
119. Ravery V, de la Taille A, Hoffmann P, et al. Balloon catheter dilatation in the treatment of ureteral and ureteroenteric stricture. J Endourol. 1998;12(4): 335–40.
120. Beckmann CF, Roth RA, Bihrle 3rd W. Dilation of benign ureteral strictures. Radiology. 1989;172(2): 437–41.
121. Tavakkoli Tabassi K, Yarmohamadi A, Mohammadi S. Triamcinolone injection following internal urethrotomy for treatment of urethral stricture. Urol J. 2011;8(2):132–6.
122. Mazdak H, Izdapanahi MH, Ghalamkari A, et al. Internal urethrotomy and intraurethral submucosal

injection of triamcinolone in short bulbar urethral strictures. Int Urol Nephrol. 2010;42(3):565–8.
123. Corcoran AT, Smaldone MC, Ricchiuti DD, Averch TD. Management of benign ureteral strictures in the endoscopic era. J Endourol. 2009;23(11):1909–12.
124. Kwak S, Leef JA, Rosenblum JD. Percutaneous balloon catheter dilatation of benign ureteral strictures: effect of multiple dilatation procedures on long-term patency. AJR Am J Roentgenol. 1995;165(1):97–100.
125. Myren CJ, Nielsen KD, Madsen M, Nielsen HV. Balloon dilatation of ureteral strictures. Scand J Urol Nephrol. 1993;27(2):251–3.
126. Bach T, Geavlete B, Herrmann TW, Gross AJ. Retrograde blind endoureterotomy for subtotal ureteral strictures: a new technique. J Endourol. 2008;22(11):2565–70.
127. Hibi H, Ohori T, Taki T, Yamada Y, Honda N. Long-term results of endoureterotomy using a holmium laser. Int J Urol. 2007;14(9):872–4.
128. Singal RK, Denstedt JD, Razvi HA, Chun SS. Holmium:YAG laser endoureterotomy for treatment of ureteral stricture. Urology. 1997;50(6):875–80.
129. Schneider AW, Conrad S, Busch R, Otto U. The cold-knife technique for endourological management of stenoses in the upper urinary tract. J Urol. 1991;146(4):961–5.
130. Nassar OA, Alsafa ME. Experience with ureteroenteric strictures after radical cystectomy and diversion: open surgical revision. Urology. 2011;78(2):459–65.
131. Yagi S, Goto T, Kawamoto K, Hayami H, Matsushita S, Nakagawa M. Long-term results of percutaneous balloon dilation for ureterointestinal anastomotic strictures. Int J Urol. 2002;9(5):241–6.
132. Shapiro MJ, Banner MP, Amendola MA, Gordon RL, Pollack HM, Wein AJ. Balloon catheter dilation of ureteroenteric strictures: long-term results. Radiology. 1988;168(2):385–7.
133. Poulakis V, Witzsch U, de Vries R, Becht E. Antegrade percutaneous endoluminal treatment of non-malignant ureterointestinal anastomotic strictures following urinary diversion. Eur Urol. 2001;39(3):308–15.
134. Bosma RJ, van Driel MF, van Son WJ, de Ruiter AJ, Mensink HJ. Endourological management of ureteral obstruction after renal transplantation. J Urol. 1996;156(3):1099–100.
135. Katz R, Pode D, Gofrit ON, et al. Transurethral incision of ureteroneocystostomy strictures in kidney transplant recipients. BJU Int. 2003;92(7):769–71.
136. Boyvat F, Aytekin C, Colak T, Firat A, Karakayali H, Haberal M. Memokath metallic stent in the treatment of transplant kidney ureter stenosis or occlusion. Cardiovasc Intervent Radiol. 2005;28(3):326–30.
137. Lin DW, Bush WH, Mayo ME. Endourological treatment of ureteroenteric strictures: efficacy of acucise endoureterotomy. J Urol. 1999;162(3):696–8.
138. Kristo B, Phelan MW, Gritsch HA, Schulam PG. Treatment of renal transplant ureterovesical anastomotic strictures using antegrade balloon dilation with or without holmium:YAG laser endoureterotomy. Urology. 2003;62(5):831–4.
139. Kim JC, Banner MP, Ramchandani P, Grossman RA, Pollack HM. Balloon dilation of ureteral strictures after renal transplantation. Radiology. 1993;186(3):717–22.
140. Gdor Y, Gabr AH, Faerber GJ, Wolf Jr JS. Holmium:yttrium-aluminum-garnet laser endoureterotomy for the treatment of transplant kidney ureteral strictures. Transplantation. 2008;85(9):1318–21.
141. Boylu U, Oommen M, Raynor M, Lee BR, Blank B, Thomas R. Ureteroenteric anastomotic stricture: novel use of a cutting balloon dilator. J Endourol. 2010;24(7):1175–8.
142. Cornud F, Chretien Y, Helenon O, et al. Percutaneous incision of stenotic uroenteric anastomaoses with a cutting balloon catheter: long-term results. Radiology. 2000;214(2):358–62.
143. Voegeli DR, Crummy AB, McDermott JC, Jensen SR. Percutaneous dilation of ureteral strictures in renal transplant patients. Radiology. 1988;169(1):185–8.

Transitional Cell Cancer

6

Matthew H.C. Goh, Richard A.F. Pellatt, and Francis X. Keeley Jr.

Epidemiology

Transitional cell carcinoma of the upper urinary tract (UUT-TCC) is relatively uncommon and accounts for 5–10% of urothelial tumors [1–4]. The annual incidence is 1–2 cases per 100,000 people in the Western population. The peak incidence occurs in patients of 70–80 years and is three times more prevalent in men. Tumors of the renal pelvis and calyces are twice as common as ureteral tumors with concurrent bladder cancer occurring in 8–13% of cases [5, 6].

Risk Factors and Genetics

The most important risk factor is smoking which increases the relative risk from 2.5 to 7 [7, 8]. Occupational exposure to aromatic amines in the dye, textiles, rubber, petrochemicals, and coal industries confers an estimated risk of 8.3 with a latency period of 20 years. The average duration of aromatic amine exposure required for development of UUT-TCC is 7 years [7, 9]. Prolonged use of the analgesic phenacetin, radiation exposure, and cyclophosphamide chemotherapy are other risk factors, not to mention a history of lower tract TCC.

Patients with hereditary nonpolyposis colorectal carcinoma (HNPCC) syndrome have an increased prevalence of UUT-TCC [10]. UUT-TCC is likely to be hereditary if the patient is below 60 years of age and/or has a history or family history of HNPCC [11, 12]. The tumor suppressor gene p53 is over-expressed in UUT-TCC, and staining for p53 may be a useful aid in initial diagnosis combined with ureteroscopy and cytology [13].

Presentation

The most common presenting symptom is hematuria, either non-visible or visible. This is followed by flank pain due to tumor obstruction or clot colic. Flank pain does not correlate with locally advanced disease or worse prognosis as is the case with bladder cancer. A lumbar mass is present in 10–20% of patients [2, 14]. Approximately 15% of patients are asymptomatic and are diagnosed incidentally following radiological imaging for other reasons. Patients may present with symptoms and signs of locally advanced or metastatic disease, such as a flank mass, anorexia, weight loss, malaise, fatigue, fever, and bone pain.

M.H.C. Goh, M.B.Ch.B., M.R.C.S. (Eng.), F.R.C.S. (Urol) (✉) • R.A.F. Pellatt, M.B.Ch.B, B.A. (Hons)
F.X. Keeley Jr., M.D., F.R.C.S. (Ed.), F.R.C.S. (Urol)
Bristol Urological Institute, Southmead Hospital, Bristol, UK
e-mail: matthew.goh@nhs.net

M. Monga (ed.), *Ureteroscopy: Indications, Instrumentation & Technique*, Current Clinical Urology,
DOI 10.1007/978-1-62703-206-3_6,

Diagnosis

The diagnosis of UUT-TCC is based on urinary cytology, cystoscopic evaluation of the bladder mucosa, and imaging of the upper tracts whereby a firm diagnosis will only be achieved in a minority of patients. Thus, the majority of patients require further investigations such as retrograde studies, selective ureteral cytology, as well as the reference standard of upper tract endoscopy and biopsy [10].

Urinary Cytology and Cystoscopy

In the absence of bladder pathology, a positive urine cytology is highly suggestive of UUT-TCC [5]. Urinary cytology alone has poor sensitivity for low-grade disease, but detection rates approach 100% for advanced disease (G3 tumors and carcinoma in situ) [10]. Given its low sensitivity of UUT-TCC, urine for cytological analysis should be taken directly from the upper tract rather then from a voided specimen [5].

Radiological Imaging

Computed tomography urography (CTU) is the current gold standard radiological investigation of the upper urinary tract and has superseded intravenous urography (IVU) [15–18]. One study demonstrated that in 86 patients with a negative IVU, 8 small renal neoplasms were detected on CT [19]. CTU has a sensitivity of 96% and specificity of 99% for polypoid lesion of 5–10 mm. The sensitivity decreases to 89% and 40% for polypoid lesions <5 and <3 mm, respectively [7, 12]. CTU can detect thickening of the wall of the renal pelvis or ureter but there is difficulty identifying flat lesions [5]. CT is the standard for assessing disease stage, with extensive local invasion on CT corresponding to histological findings, but with relative insensitivity for lower stage lesions [20].

For patients who cannot undergo a CTU, magnetic resonance urography (MRU) can be performed [21]. The use of gadolinium contrast, however, is contraindicated in patients with severe renal impairment (creatinine clearance <30 ml/min) because of the risk on nephrogenic systemic fibrosis which can be fatal. For tumors <2 cm, the detection rate with contrast is 75% [22].

Retrograde Ureteropyelography

Diagnostic accuracy increases from 75% with retrograde ureteropyelography to 90% when combined with ureteroscopy. In the series of 92 patients with UUT-TCC, only 25% of recurrences were detected on retrograde ureteropyelography with the remaining 75% detected endoscopically [23].

Diagnostic Ureteroscopy and Biopsies

The gold standard for diagnosis of UUT-TCC is upper tract endoscopy and biopsy. A flexible ureteroscope can reach the renal cavities in 95% of cases, thus allowing visual inspection and obtaining biopsies and selective cytology [24]. Inspection alone accurately predicts low- and high-grade lesions in roughly 75% of all UUT-TCC cases. Biopsy of the lesion allows for a formal diagnosis and prognostic information. Improved biopsy techniques and better specimen handling techniques have significantly improved diagnostic accuracy [23]. Tumor biopsies are taken with a flat wire stone basket or cold cup biopsy forceps. Multiple biopsies are recommended, particularly if small biopsy forceps are used. Specimens are usually minute and special care should be taken when placed in fixative [25]. Pathological techniques include Cytospin cytocentrifugation and cell blocks to maintain architecture [23].

In a study by Keeley et al., the use of ureteroscopic biopsy as a diagnostic tool for staging and grading tumors improved diagnostic accuracy from 60% (using cytology, IVU/CT, and retrograde pyelography) to 69% using ureteroscopic biopsy in conjunction with traditional methods [26]. The accurate staging and grading of tumors is essential in determining patient prognosis.

The current best practice is to use the triad of ureteral urine sampling, direct ureteroscopic inspection, and ureteroscopic biopsies in grading UUT-TCC and determining disease severity. Suspicion of high-grade, high-stage disease should be aroused by grade 2/3 TCC on biopsy combined with malignant cell cytology.

Staging and Grading

The Union Internationale Contre le Cancer (UICC) TNM and American Joint Committee on Cancer (AJCC) staging systems are available with the TNM system most commonly used (Table 6.1). The World Health Organization (WHO) grading classification is shown in Table 6.2. The newer classification of 2004 stratifies tumors according to risk potential and has taken into account evidence in molecular biology and histological data in distinguishing potential tumor growth and also between noninvasive tumors. In the upper urinary tract, there are almost no tumors of low malignant potential [4, 27, 28].

In contrast to the lower urinary tract, accurate staging of tumors of the upper tract is limited to tumor grade as depth cannot be assessed as biopsies do not usually provide deep or full-thickness specimens. Tumor grade, however, correlates well with the pathological grading and staging of nephroureterectomy specimens. Keeley et al. demonstrated a biopsy grade to surgical specimen grade relation of 90% [29]. Grade at biopsy corresponded with eventual stage, with 87% of low-grade biopsies staged pTa or pT1 and 67% of high-grade biopsies staged as T2 or T3 at surgery. The diagnostic accuracy of tumor grade allows selection of patients either for future endoscopic treatment or nephroureterectomy for those who are at risk of progression [23].

Other studies have demonstrated under-staging and grading of tumors at biopsy. Guarnizo et al. [30] found that for tumors graded Ta at biopsy, 45% were upstaged based on the surgical specimen. In a review of 30 nephroureterectomies in Bristol, 75% of preoperative biopsies corresponded accurately with grade at surgery. Of the remaining cases, 90% were under-graded at biopsy. Of 18 lesions graded G2 at biopsy, 6 were surgically staged as pT2 or above [26].

Table 6.1 TNM 7 (2009) Classification Renal Pelvis and Ureter

T—Primary tumor			
TX	Primary tumor cannot be assessed		
T0	No evidence of primary tumor		
Ta	Noninvasive papillary carcinoma		
Tis	Carcinoma in situ		
T1	Tumor invades subepithelial connective tissue		
T2	Tumor invades muscularis		
T3	(Renal pelvis) Tumor invades beyond muscularis into peripelvic fat or renal parenchyma		
	(Ureter) Tumor invades beyond muscularis into periureteral fat		
T4	Tumor invades adjacent organs or through the kidney into perinephric fat		
N—Regional lymph nodes			
NX	Regional lymph nodes cannot be assessed		
N0	No regional lymph node metastasis		
N1	Metastasis in a single lymph node 2 cm or less in greatest dimension		
N2	Metastasis in a single lymph node more than 2 cm but not more than 5 cm in greatest dimension, or multiple lymph nodes, none more than 5 cm in greatest dimension		
N3	Metastasis in a lymph node more than 5 cm in greatest dimension		
M—Distant metastasis			
M0	No distant metastasis		
M1	Distant metastasis		
Histopathological grading			
GX	Grade of differentiation cannot be assessed		
G1	Well differentiated		
G2	Moderately differentiated		
G3–4	Poorly differentiated/undifferentiated		
Stage grouping			
Stage 0a	Ta	N0	M0
Stage 0is	Tis	N0	M0
Stage I	T1	N0	M0
Stage II	T2	N0	M0
Stage III	T3	N0	M0
Stage IV	T4	N0	M0
	Any T	N1, N2, N3	M0
	Any T	Any N	M1

The regional lymph nodes are the hilar, abdominal para-aortic, and paracaval nodes and, for ureter, intrapelvic nodes. Laterality does not affect the N classification

Table 6.2 WHO (2004 and 1973) histological grading of non-muscle-invasive bladder tumors

WHO (2004) grading
Urothelial papilloma
Papillary urothelial neoplasm of low malignant potential (PUNLMP)
Low-grade papillary urothelial carcinoma
High-grade papillary urothelial carcinoma
WHO (1973) grading
Urothelial papilloma
Grade 1: well differentiated
Grade 2: moderately differentiated
Grade 3: poorly differentiated

In contrast to 15% of bladder cancers, a significant 60% of UUT-TCC are invasive [31]. This is the reason nephroureterectomy has become the standard of treatment. It is an important consideration that any patient undergoing endoscopic treatment for UUT-TCC may potentially be denied a curative nephroureterectomy [28]. UUT-TCC is commonly multicentric, and unilateral upper tract multifocal tumors may account for up to 27% of all UUT-TCC [32]. Bilateral UUT-TCC occurs in 0.01–4% of cases.

Prognostic Factors

Staging is closely correlated with prognosis in UUT-TCC, with the stage and grade of tumor being the most important factors with regard to survival. Tumors that invade the muscle wall carry a very poor prognosis. The 5-year survival for a pTa tumor is >80% [10] compared to <50% of pT2/3 tumors and <10% for pT4 tumors [33, 34].

Lymphovascular invasion and extensive tumor necrosis (>10% tumor area) is associated with poorer outcomes [35–39]. The presence of CIS is associated with higher risk of recurrence and cancer-specific mortality [40].

Tumor location within the renal pelvis or ureter is no longer a prognostic factor according to recent data [41–43], even when adjusted for tumor stage [41, 44]. In addition, age and gender no longer accepted as adequate independent prognostic indicators [45–48]. Hydronephrosis on preoperative imaging is associated with more advanced disease and poorer outcomes [49].

Molecular markers such as E-cadherin, hypoxia-inducible factor (HIF), and telomerase RNA component have been heralded as prognostic markers [50] but have not yet been externally validated.

Management of Localized Disease

For patients with localized disease, the options for management include radical surgery (open/laparoscopic radical nephroureterectomy) or renal-sparing surgery (open/laparoscopic segmental resection or endoscopic treatment with or without adjuvant topical therapy).

Radical Surgery

Open Radical Nephroureterectomy

Le Dentu and Albarran performed the first nephroureterectomy with excision of the bladder cuff in 1891. Over the past 100 years, this has been the gold standard for treating UUT-TCC-allowing for complete tumor excision, good surgical margins, and assessment of disease spread and progression. UUT-TCC commonly presents multifocally within the urinary tract involved, therefore if there is a healthy contralateral tract it is the logical therapy. Recurrence rates in the contralateral tract are 6.5% at 15 years [51], whereas if only a simple nephrectomy is performed, the recurrence rate of UUT-TCC can be as high as 40% in the remaining ipsilateral stump [52]. Nephroureterectomy is therefore a safe curative therapy, and one should be aware of this when considering more conservative management options for patients.

Laparoscopic Radical Nephrectomy

This has become an accepted alternative to the open operation [32]. Laparoscopy offers reduced postoperative morbidity with no significant difference in disease-specific survival rates at 7 years in a study of laparoscopic versus open nephroureterectomy [53]. Specific concerns related to the laparoscopic approach are local seeding and port-site metastases.

Renal-Sparing Surgery

Segmental Resection

Segmental resection preserves the ipsilateral kidney whilst providing pathological information for staging and grading. Segmental distal ureteral resection is possible for low- and high-risk tumors [54, 55]. *Complete distal ureterectomy* is recommended for distal ureteral tumors that cannot be completely treated endoscopically. When the entire distal ureter is removed, a bladder psoas muscle hitch, a Boari flap, or both techniques may be required.

Open segmental ureterectomy and ureteroureterostomy is suitable for noninvasive grade 1 and grade 2 tumors of the proximal ureter or midureter too large for endoscopic treatment and for grade 3 or invasive tumors when nephron-sparing is required. In patients where renal-sparing is required but who have ureteral tumors that are numerous, multifocal but with low grade and stage, a *subtotal ureterectomy* which involves removal of long ureteral segments only may be appropriate [25]. *Open resection of renal pelvic or calyceal tumors* is now rare as it is technically challenging with higher recurrence rates compared to ureteral tumors [5]. Various techniques for *laparoscopic distal ureterectomy and reimplantation* have been reported [25] and early results are encouraging.

Endoscopic Treatment

Endoscopic management has gained acceptance in recent years. The aim is to ensure adequate cancer control while preserving renal function and the viability of the affected urinary tract. Approach to the tract can be made either antegradely in the same manner as a percutaneous nephrolithotomy or retrogradely via the ureter.

Percutaneous Approach

This approach allows tumor biopsy, resection, and/or cauterization. This is considered for low-grade noninvasive disease in the lower calyceal systems inaccessible or difficult to treat with ureteroscopy. There is a theoretical risk of tumor seeding in the tract and in perforations. Adjuvant therapy can be administered via a nephrostomy tube [5]. Recurrence rates following percutaneous therapy may be in the region of 30% for low-grade (1–2) tumors and 45% if low- and high-grade tumors are taken into account [56, 57]. This treatment modality is becoming less common due to advances in ureteroscopy [5].

Ureteroscopic Approach

Advances in ureteroscope technology have been vital in the progress of ureteroscopic management of UUT-TCC. With the development of smaller caliber rigid and flexible ureteroscopes, endoscopic management of ureteral and smaller renal collecting system tumors confers lower morbidity and also prevents tumor seeding in a closed system compared to the percutaneous approach [25]. Current flexible and semirigid ureteroscopes are small enough to allow accurate assessment of the ureter and collecting system. Flexible ureteroscopes are now produced with 180° upwards and downwards deflection allowing for accurate biopsy and ablation [58]. The Ho:YAG and Nd:YAG lasers in particular have allowed accurate treatment of larger tumors [23].

Ureteroscopic Management

Indications

Currently, there are three situations where ureteroscopic management is considered:

Existing or likely renal compromise. For patients with bilateral disease, solitary kidneys, or renal insufficiency, a renal-sparing approach is advocated. Ureteroscopic management can maintain

Table 6.3 Classification of indication for ureteroscopic treatment

Absolute	Patients who would not tolerate open surgery or would require dialysis
Relative	Those with severe medical problems or multifocal disease
Elective	Those with no contraindication to definitive surgery
Palliative	Those with large or bleeding tumors who would not tolerate open surgery

the kidney and also urinary tract integrity, thus avoiding rendering the patient dialysis-dependent.

Where a major operation would carry a high risk. For those patients who are unfit for major surgery, either open or laparoscopic, or for whom the risks associated with such an operation are high, endoscopic management can be considered as it is less invasive.

Low-grade, low-stage disease that can be managed conservatively. These cases can be managed endoscopically, given accurate preoperative tumor assessment and strict postoperative follow-up. A sound evidence base is essential for this group of patients as they are foregoing potentially curative nephroureterectomy.

A further classification of patients according to indication is shown in Table 6.3 [23].

Ureteroscopic Technique

Ureteroscopy for upper tract TCC involves inspection of the tract using rigid and flexible scopes, urine sampling, biopsy of suspicious lesions, and laser ablation of visible tumors [32, 33].

The procedure commences with an initial rigid cystoscopy as upper tract tumors are associated with bladder cancers [25]. The ureteral orifices are inspected for visible hematuria. Cannulation of the relevant ureteral orifice is performed to allow aspiration of urine or saline washings for cytological analysis followed by a retrograde study of the upper urinary tract. Rigid ureteroscopy of the ureter is performed with placement of a guidewire to the level of the ureteroscope, not beyond the immediate field of vision. If any suspicious area or lesion is encountered, cytology should be taken before biopsies or intervention.

On reaching the limit of the rigid ureteroscope, the rigid ureteroscope is replaced by a small caliber flexible ureteroscope which is advanced into the renal pelvis. At this point, further urine can be aspirated for cytological analysis. Contrast is injected to aid systematic ureteroscopic inspection of the calyces. Tumor biopsies are taken followed by tumor ablation. For tumors that protrude from the ureteral orifice, ureteroscopic ablation or transurethral resection of the most distal ureter is performed.

A retrograde ureteral stent or ureteral catheter is inserted at the end of the procedure. The former is left in situ for a variable period to allow healing and the latter to facilitate administration of adjuvant therapy in the postoperative period.

Tumor Ablation

Tumor ablation can be achieved by three methods [25].

Particularly suitable for low-grade papillary tumors on a narrow stalk, the first involves debulking the tumor with grasping forceps or flat wire basket. The base of the tumor is then ablated with electrocautery or laser.

The second method involves the use of a ureteroscopic resectoscope (12 Fr) where an intraluminal tumor is resected to the base. Resection beyond the lamina propria is not attempted, particularly in the upper and midureter where the wall is thin and the risk of perforation high. For higher volume disease of the distal ureter, resection with a long standard resectoscope after initial dilatation has been described. This technique has largely been replaced, as ureteral resectoscopes are of such a large caliber that access is problematic.

The final method involves taking an initial biopsy followed by ablation of the tumor bulk, including the base, with either electrocautery or laser. Electrocautery via a 2–3 Fr Bugbee electrode fulgurates tumors but variable depth of penetration is an issue in the ureter. There is a high risk of stricture formation with circumferential fulguration [25]. Laser ablation can be performed with a holmium:yttrium–aluminum–garnet (Ho:YAG) or neodynium:yttrium–aluminum–garnet (Nd:YAG) laser source via flexible, small diameter fibers (200–1,000 μm).

The Ho:YAG laser is used in the ureter as it has minimal depth of penetration of less than 0.5 mm which minimizes full-thickness ureteral injury during use. It ablates the tumor efficiently and provides precise cutting with excellent hemostasis. Laser settings are 0.6–1.2 J at 8–10 Hz. The Nd:YAG laser offers deep tissue penetration of up to 5–6 mm and is more suited to larger, renal pelvic tumors. It causes coagulation necrosis of the tumor with subsequent sloughing. Hemostasis is excellent. Its use in the ureter is limited due to increased risk of perforation. Settings employed are 15 W for 2 s for tumor ablation and 5–10 W for 2 s for coagulation [25].

Adjuvant Topical Therapy

Ureteroscopic treatment is associated with high recurrence rates and tumor progression. Reducing the rate of recurrence or progression is important in the management of these patients [59]. Postoperative topical immunotherapy and chemotherapy have been employed with success in the treatment of bladder TCC. These agents have also been administered as adjuvant treatment for UUT-TCC to decrease tumor recurrence and progression [60–65]. The agents available for use include bacillus Calmette-Guerin (BCG), mitomycin C (MMC), and doxorubicin. BCG is commonly used as adjuvant therapy and also when a tumor has been incompletely treated.

Administration. Adjuvant therapy can be administered by infusion via a retrograde ureteral catheter, reflux from the bladder via a ureteral stent, or percutaneously via a nephrostomy. Keeley and Bagley [59] described their technique of mitomycin C instillation in the treatment of UUT-TCC following endoscopic ablation. In their series, a 6 Fr open-ended ureteral catheter was placed in the renal pelvis under fluoroscopic guidance. The integrity of the collecting system and position of the ureteral catheter were confirmed by injection of contrast via the catheter. The ureteral catheter was secured to a urethral catheter under gravity drainage. Instillation was commenced after resolution of any visible hematuria to reduce the risk of systemic absorption. Three doses of 10 ml of mitomycin C (40 mg in 30 ml normal saline) were given at 2-hourly intervals. Each instillation was given over 2 min and the ureteral catheter clamped for 10 min following instillation. After the third instillation, both catheters were removed.

Safety. Concerns regarding the use topical therapies in the upper urinary tract include patient discomfort during instillation, local effects, systemic absorption and toxicity, and sepsis. Low pressure administration is required to prevent systemic absorption and sepsis. In the series by Keeley and Bagley [59], all 19 patients treated with MMC did not complain of discomfort during instillation with no cases of systemic toxicity. One patient had evidence of a local reaction with necrotic debris and overlying calcifications following extensive laser ablation of a renal pelvic tumor followed by MMC. This appearance persisted for at least 12 months. Eastham and Huffman [60] reported no systemic side effects or pyrexia in the seven patients treated with MMC.

However, out of 14 patients treated with MMC in the series by Martinez-Piero et al. [62], 1 patient died from aplastic anemia and sepsis secondary to extravasation. Their method of MMC delivery was not described.

With BCG therapy, the most common complication is sepsis but systemic BCG infection or granulomatous infection of the kidney can occur. Unfortunately, the upper urinary tract does not tolerate granulomas as easily as the bladder, as they can lead to obstruction and loss of function in our experience.

Efficacy. The medium term results of adjuvant topical therapy are similar to those for bladder cancer but have not been confirmed in long-term studies [14, 66, 67].

Ureteroscopic Complications

Ureteroscopic surveillance and treatment of upper tract tumors have a low rate of complications. The stricture rate following ureteroscopy is around 10% and the blood transfusion rate is very low.

Advantages of Ureteroscopic Management

Ureteroscopic treatment confers several advantages. A major advantage is the preservation of renal function which is important in patients where renal compromise would present a poor outcome. It is desirable in patients with low-stage and low-grade disease for whom endoscopic management would avoid radical surgery. For those with major co-morbidities, ureteroscopy is less invasive than radical surgery and confers a decreased risk of morbidity and mortalilty. A further benefit is that the integrity urinary tract is maintained thus limiting tumor spread.

There are few studies comparing outcomes for nephroureterectomy and ureteroscopic management of UUT-TCC [32]. Endoscopic management has a similar prognosis to nephroureterectomy if patients are well-selected, which is in turn dependent on accurate preoperative assessment [32]. In one study, Keeley et al. looked at 38 patients (41 kidneys) with UUT-TCC treated ureteroscopically. Complications during surgery were related to existing cardiopulmonary disease. Two patients subsequently developed urethral strictures but no patients required blood transfusions or emergency surgery for bleeding [23].

Disadvantages of Ureteroscopic Management

Ureteroscopic equipment is obviously small, and there are limits both to the extent to which biopsies can be performed and the amount of tumor that can be resected. Failure of ureteroscopic treatment is related to tumor size [23], hence the importance of accurate diagnostic assessment prior to ureteroscopy.

It has been noted that patients with grade 2 tumors are at particular risk of being understaged at biopsy [10]. However, the concurrent use of ureteroscopic biopsy is more accurate than using cytology, imaging, and retrograde studies alone. Thus clinicians should be cautious in interpreting biopsy results, especially for the *elective* group of patients with biopsy suggestive of middle-grade disease.

A chief concern is accurate preoperative staging and grading of tumors. This is especially pertinent for patients with suspected low-grade/stage disease for whom the option to undergo endoscopic therapy would be at the expense of potentially curative nephroureterectomy. Given that preoperative staging and grading is currently not 100% accurate, this is a point of contention that should be heavily weighed for any patient opting out of nephroureterectomy.

Maintaining the urinary tract comes at the price of higher recurrence rates. Thus it is essential that patients attend regular ureteroscopic follow-ups to assess disease progression. In the series by Keeley et al., recurrence rates were 27% for low-grade tumors and 45% for grade 2 tumors. A recurrence of 20% was noted for those patients classified as *elective*. These patients were followed up for a mean period of 50 months. No patient had local or metastatic progression or bulky recurrence while on surveillance [23]. Thus compared to nephroureterectomy, there is a higher rate of disease recurrence for patients treated ureteroscopically. However, if patients are followed up stringently, these recurrences can be picked up early with no increased rate of metastatic or local disease progression.

Outcomes

Endoscopic management of UUT-TCC preserves the urinary tract and controls local disease. However, the risk of disease recurrence necessitates long-term follow-up and good patient compliance.

Recurrence Rates

Retrospective studies have shown recurrence rates ranging from 31 to 86% [56]. While these figures are high, one must appreciate that UUT-TCC is a disease that tends to recur and it is fundamental to endoscopic management that recurrences are detected during follow-up. In essence, a high recurrence rate is not necessarily detrimental unless there is disease progression which affects patient survival and morbidity.

In a study involving 38 patients, there were 18 disease recurrences in 8 patients. Three of these recurrences were reported after 38 months from initial treatment, suggesting that long-term surveillance is necessary in patients treated endoscopically [23]. In the same study, looking at a select group of 11 low-grade, low-stage patients in whom treatment was solely elective (i.e., the decision for treatment was based on avoiding nephroureterectomy and not because of co-morbidities or inoperability), 10 patients became tumor free. There were only 3 recurrences in 2 patients in this group, who were followed up for a total of 53 months. These findings support managing low-grade, low-stage disease in a carefully selected group of patients [23].

The risk of recurrence is increased with initial multifocal disease. Studies concur that recurrence rates are lowest in low-grade, low-stage tumors and that these cases are more likely to become disease-free. Size of tumor is also related to recurrence, and tumors less than 1.5 cm in diameter are more likely to be treated successfully. The location of a tumor—be it intrarenal or ureteral—was less important to outcome and recurrence compared with multifocality, size, and grade [23].

Tumor Progression

Endoscopic treatment does not appear to increase the risk of tumor progression. Of the patients followed by Keeley et al., none developed local or metastatic progression of disease during the follow-up period of 53 months [23]. This suggests that a rigid surveillance program can adequately manage UUT-TCC endoscopically without increased risk of advanced disease.

However, clinicians should approach grade 2 tumors with a degree of caution, as these have a tendency to be under-graded at the time of initial biopsy and diagnosis. In the case of suspicious grade 2 tumors, it may be better to "over-treat" with nephroureterectomy than run the risk of under-treating a potentially life-threatening malignancy. As mentioned, it is tumor grade at biopsy which is the best indicator of overall patient survival. Of 38 patients, Keeley et al. found that 8 subsequently needed nephroureterectomy. These patients tended to have tumors larger than 1.5 cm and/or were grade 2 [23].

Survival Rates

The survival rates are similar to open nephroureterectomy [68]. In the long run, if patients continue to be carefully selected for ureteroscopy, one might expect the survival rates for endoscopic treatment to increase, as there are far fewer complications from endoscopic surgery compared to open nephroureterectomy. Of the 38 patients treated ureteroscopically in the study by Keeley et al., none required blood transfusions or emergency surgery for bleeding [23]. Patients chosen for endoscopic treatment have typically been carefully selected for non-standard treatment on the basis of medical co-morbidities or low-risk disease, so retrospective comparisons are inherently biased. Clearly, one must first exclude from endoscopic treatment those patients found to have high-grade or invasive disease.

There appears to be no difference in the survival rates or prognosis of those patients undergoing immediate nephroureterectomy compared to those with a delayed nephroureterectomy due to initial attempted endoscopic management [32, 69]. In a retrospective study, the authors concluded that their patients came to no harm from attempting ureteroscopic management even if nephroureterectomy was subsequently decided as the best management [32].

Ureteroscopic Tumor Propagation

There is no significant increase in the rate of metastatic disease in patients treated with nephroureterectomy compared to those with initial ureteroscopy followed by nephroureterectomy [70]. Kulp and Bagley looked specifically at the possibility of migration of malignant cells during endoscopy [71]. Thirteen patients underwent one to four ureteroscopic treatments, as well as biopsy, prior to nephroureterectomy. Only one patient had lymphatic/vascular tumor invasion, and this had been expected prior to endoscopy due to the tumor characteristics. Therefore, ureteroscopic management does not appear to increase the risk of tumor propagation.

Bladder Cancer

The de novo bladder cancer risk in patients treated for UUT-TCC with no prior history of bladder cancer has been reported as being 33% [23]. This does not appear to be higher than the bladder cancer recurrence rate in patients treated with nephroureterectomy; indeed, the rate of subsequent de novo bladder cancer occurrence is high regardless of therapy. The recurrence rate of bladder tumors in patients treated endoscopically for UUT-TCC has been reported as being 39% [72]. This compares to bladder tumor recurrence rates of 23–30% in patients treated by nephroureterectomy or distal ureterectomy.

Follow-Up

Follow-up of conservatively treated patients with UUT-TCC has to be rigorous in order to detect metachronous bladder cancers, upper tract recurrences, and disease progression. Given the high recurrence rate of UUT-TCC following excision of the affected tract and an even higher rate if the affected side is left in situ, the decision to treat ureteroscopically must take into account the high probability of subsequent disease [23].

Patients must be aware of these issues so that they can make an informed decision whether or not to pursue radical treatment and be more likely to comply with follow-up. Is the patient aware that although they are avoiding major surgery, they will, in all probability, face more future surgeries? Social issues should be taken into account in decision-making: is the patient frail or limited in terms of mobility and thus unlikely to attend follow-up?

Ureteroscopic surveillance is the safest way to follow patients up and should be carried out at 3, 6, 12, and 18 months. Thereafter, patients should attend annually. As with initial diagnosis, ureteroscopy should be complemented by urine cytology and upper tract imaging. Imaging alone is not sufficient as up to 75% of tumor recurrences are not visualized [23]. Regular check cystoscopies are mandatory.

Ureteroscopic management may subsequently become inappropriate due to tumor progression, when ureteroscopic surgery can no longer safely and completely treat tumor margins. At this point, it may be preferable for a patient to have radical surgery.

Conclusions

Ureteroscopic management of UUT-TCC has become an accepted alternative to nephroureterectomy in selected groups of patients. Ureteroscopy is a renal-sparing therapy for patients with renal compromise and confers a lesser risk of morbidity and mortality in patients who have significant medical co-morbidities. Moreover, ureteroscopy has a definite role in the conservative management of low-grade and low-stage disease in otherwise healthy individuals where a radical nephroureterectomy would be considered overtreatment, providing grading and staging is accurate. Patients who are treated ureteroscopically should expect to undergo long-term follow-up.

References

1. Munoz JJ, Ellison LM. Upper tract urothelial neoplasms: incidence and survival during the last 2 decades. J Urol. 2000;164(5):1523–5.
2. Hall MC, Womack S, Sagalowsky AI, Carmody T, Erickstad MD, Roehrborn CG. Prognostic factors,

recurrence, and survival in transitional cell carcinoma of the upper urinary tract: a 30-year experience in 252 patients. Urology. 1998;52(4):594–601.
3. Margulis V, Shariat SF, Matin SF, Kamat AM, Zigeuner R, Kikuchi E, Lotan Y, Weizer A, Raman JD, Wood CG. Upper Tract Urothelial Carcinoma Collaboration. Outcomes of radical nephroureterectomy: a series from the Upper Tract Urothelial Carcinoma Collaboration. Cancer. 2009;115(6):1224–33.
4. Olgac S, Mazumdar M, Dalbagni G, Reuter VE. Urothelial carcinoma of the renal pelvis: a clinicopathologic study of 130 cases. Am J Surg Pathol. 2004;28(12):1545–52.
5. Rouprêt M, Zigeuner R, Palou J, Boehle A, Kaasinen E, Sylvester R, Babjuk M, Oosterlinck W. Members of the European Association of Urology (EAU) Guidelines office. Guidelines on upper urinary tract urothelial cell carcinomas. In: EAU Guidelines edition presented at the 25th EAU Anaual Congress, Barcelona 2010. ISBN 978-90-79754-70-0.
6. Azémar MD, Comperat E, Richard F, Cussenot O, Rouprêt M. Bladder recurrence after surgery for upper urinary tract urothelial cell carcinoma: frequency, risk factors, and surveillance. Urol Oncol. 2011;29(2): 130–6.
7. Colin P, Koenig P, Ouzzane A, Berthon N, Villers A, Biserte J, Rouprêt M. Environmental factors involved in carcinogenesis of urothelial cell carcinomas of the upper urinary tract. BJU Int. 2009;104(10):1436–40.
8. Pommer W, Bronder E, Klimpel A, Helmert U, Greiser E, Molzahn M. Urothelial cancer at different tumour sites: role of smoking and habitual intake of analgesics and laxatives. Results of the Berlin Urothelial Cancer Study. Nephrol Dial Transplant. 1999;14(12):2892–7.
9. Shinka T, Miyai M, Sawada Y, Inagaki T, Okawa T. Factors affecting the occurrence of urothelial tumors in dye workers exposed to aromatic amines. Int J Urol. 1995;2(4):243–8.
10. Painter DJ, Timoney AG, Denton K, Alken P, Keeley Jr FX. The modern management of upper tract urothelial cancer: tumour diagnosis, grading and staging. BJU Int. 2007;99:973–7.
11. Acher P, Kiela G, Thomas K, O'Brien T. Towards a rational strategy for the surveillance of patients with Lynch syndrome (hereditary non-polyposis colon cancer) for upper tract transitional cell carcinoma. BJU Int. 2010;106(3):300–2.
12. Rouprêt M, Yates DR, Comperat E, Cussenot O. Upper urinary tract urothelial cell carcinomas and other urological malignancies involved in the hereditary nonpolyposis colorectal cancer (lynch syndrome) tumor spectrum. Eur Urol. 2008;54(6):1226–36.
13. Keeley FX, Bibbo M, McCue PA, Bagley DH. The use of p53 in the diagnosis of upper tract transitional cell carcinoma. Urology. 1997;49(2):181–6.
14. Oosterlinck W, Solsona E, van der Meijden AP, Sylvester R, Böhle A, Rintala E, Lobel B, European Association of Urology. EAU guidelines on diagnosis and treatment of upper urinary tract transitional cell carcinoma. Eur Urol. 2004;46(2):147–54.
15. Dillman JR, Caoili EM, Cohan RH, Ellis JH, Francis IR, Schipper MJ. Detection of upper tract urothelial neoplasms: sensitivity of axial, coronal reformatted, and curved-planar reformatted image-types utilizing 16-row multi-detector CT urography. Abdom Imaging. 2008;33(6):707–16.
16. Van Der Molen AJ, Cowan NC, Mueller-Lisse UG, Nolte-Ernsting CC, Takahashi S, Cohan RH. CT Urography Working Group of the European Society of Urogenital Radiology (ESUR). CT urography: definition, indications and techniques. A guideline for clinical practice. Eur Radiol. 2008;18(1):4–17.
17. Wang LJ, Wong YC, Chuang CK, Huang CC, Pang ST. Diagnostic accuracy of transitional cell carcinoma on multidetector computerized tomography urography in patients with gross hematuria. J Urol. 2009;181(2):524–31.
18. Wang LJ, Wong YC, Huang CC, Wu CH, Hung SC, Chen HW. Multidetector computerized tomography urography is more accurate than excretory urography for diagnosing transitional cell carcinoma of the upper urinary tract in adults with hematuria. J Urol. 2010;183(1):48–55.
19. Lang EK, Macchia RJ, Thomas R, Watson RA, Marberger M, Lechner G, Gayle B, Richter F. Improved detection of renal pathologic features on multiphasic helical CT compared with IVU in patients presenting with microscopic hematuria. Urology. 2003;61(3):528–32.
20. Buckley JA, Urban BA, Soyer P, Scherrer A, Fishmann EK. Transitional cell carcinoma of the renal pelvis: a retrospective look at CT staging with pathological correlation. Radiology. 1996;201:194–8.
21. Takahashi N, Glockner JF, Hartman RP, King BF, Leibovich BC, Stanley DW, Fitz-Gibbon PD, Kawashima A. Gadolinium enhanced magnetic resonance urography for upper urinary tract malignancy. J Urol. 2010;183(4):1330–65
22. Takahashi N, Kawashima A, Glockner JF, Hartman RP, Leibovich BC, Brau AC, Beatty PJ, King BF. Small (<2 cm) upper tract urothelial carcinoma: evaluation with gadolinium-enhanced three-dimensional spoiled gradient-recalled echo MR urography. Radiology. 2008;247(2):451–7.
23. Keeley FX, Bibbo M, Bagley DH. Ureteroscopic treatment and surveillance of upper tract transitional cell carcinoma. J Urol. 1997;157(5):1560–5.
24. Tavora F, Fajardo DA, Lee TK, Lotan T, Miller JS, Miyamoto H, Epstein JI. Small endoscopic biopsies of the ureter and renal pelvis: pathologic pitfalls. Am J Surg Pathol. 2009;33(10):1540–6.
25. Flanigan RC. Urothelial tumors of the upper urinary tract. In: Wein AJ, editor. Campbell-Walsh urology. 9th ed. Philadelphia: Saunders Elsevier; 2007. p. 1638–52.
26. Williams SK, Denton KJ, Minervini A, Oxley J, Khastigir J, Timoney AG, Keeley Jr FX. Correlation

of upper-tract cytology, retrograde pyelography, ureteroscopic appearance, and ureteroscopic biopsy with histologic examination of upper-tract transitional cell carcinoma. J Endourol. 2008;22(1):71–6.
27. Perez-Montiel D, Wakely PE, Hes O, Michal M, Suster S. High-grade urothelial carcinoma of the renal pelvis: clinicopathologic study of 108 cases with emphasis on unusual morphologic variants. Mod Pathol. 2006;19(4):494–503.
28. Stewart GD, Bariol SV, Grigor KM, Tolley DA, McNeill SA. A comparison of the pathology of transitional cell carcinoma of the bladder and upper urinary tract. BJU Int. 2005;95(6):791–3.
29. Keeley FX, Kulp DA, Bibbo M, McCue PA, Bagley DH. Diagnostic accuracy of ureteroscopic biopsy in upper tract transitional cell carcinoma. J Urol. 1997;157:33–7.
30. Guarnizo E, Pavlovich CP, Seiba M, Carlson DL, Vaughan Jr ED, Sosa RE. Ureteroscopic biopsy of upper tract urothelial carcinoma: improved diagnostic accuracy and histopathological considerations using a multi-biopsy approach. J Urol. 2000;163:52–5.
31. Papatsoris AG, Chrisofos M, Skolarikos A, Varkarakis I, Lekas A, Dellis A, Koritsiadis S, Deliveliotis C. Upper urinary tract transitional cell carcinoma. A 10-year experience. Tumori. 2008;94(1):75–8.
32. Arancibia MF, Bolenz C, Michel M-S, Keeley Jr FX, Alken P. The modern management of upper urinary tract urothelial cancer: surgical treatment. BJU Int. 2007;99:978–81.
33. Abouassaly R, Alibhai SM, Shah N, Timilshina N, Fleshner N, Finelli A. Troubling outcomes from population-level analysis of surgery for upper tract urothelial carcinoma. Urology. 2010;76(4):895–901.
34. Jeldres C, Sun M, Isbarn H, Lughezzani G, Budäus L, Alasker A, Shariat SF, Lattouf JB, Widmer H, Pharand D, Arjane P, Graefen M, Montorsi F, Perrotte P, Karakiewicz PI. A population-based assessment of perioperative mortality after nephroureterectomy for upper tract urothelial carcinoma. Urology. 2010;75(2):315–20.
35. Kikuchi E, Margulis V, Karakiewicz PI, Roscigno M, Mikami S, Lotan Y, Remzi M, Bolenz C, Langner C, Weizer A, Montorsi F, Bensalah K, Koppie TM, Fernández MI, Raman JD, Kassouf W, Wood CG, Suardi N, Oya M, Shariat SF. Lymphovascular invasion predicts clinical outcomes in patients with node-negative upper tract urothelial carcinoma. J Clin Oncol. 2009;27(4):612–8.
36. Kim DS, Lee YH, Cho KS, Cho NH, Chung BH, Hong SJ. Lymphovascular invasion and pT stage are prognostic factors in patients treated with radical nephroureterectomy for localized upper urinary tract transitional cell carcinoma. Urology. 2010;75(2):328–32.
37. Novara G, Matsumoto K, Kassouf W, Walton TJ, Fritsche HM, Bastian PJ, Martínez-Salamanca JI, Seitz C, Lemberger RJ, Burger M, El-Hakim A, Baba S, Martignoni G, Gupta A, Karakiewicz PI, Ficarra V, Shariat SF. Prognostic role of lymphovascular invasion in patients with urothelial carcinoma of the upper urinary tract: an international validation study. Eur Urol. 2010;57(6):1064–71.
38. Zigeuner R, Shariat SF, Margulis V, Karakiewicz PI, Roscigno M, Weizer A, Kikuchi E, Remzi M, Raman JD, Bolenz C, Bensalah K, Capitanio U, Koppie TM, Kassouf W, Sircar K, Patard JJ, Fernández MI, Wood CG, Montorsi F, Ströbel P, Wheat JC, Haitel A, Oya M, Guo CC, Ng C, Chade DC, Sagalowsky A, Langner C. Tumour necrosis is an indicator of aggressive biology in patients with urothelial carcinoma of the upper urinary tract. Eur Urol. 2010;57(4):575–81.
39. Seitz C, Gupta A, Shariat SF, Matsumoto K, Kassouf W, Walton TJ, Fritsche HM, Otto W, Tritschler S, Bastian PJ, Carballido J, Ficarra V, Karakiewicz PI, Artibani W, Mazzoleni G, Novara G. Association of tumor necrosis with pathological features and clinical outcome in 754 patients undergoing radical nephroureterectomy for upper tract urothelial carcinoma: an international validation study. J Urol. 2010; 184(5):1895–900.
40. Wheat JC, Weizer AZ, Wolf Jr JS, Lotan Y, Remzi M, Margulis V, Wood CG, Montorsi F, Roscigno M, Kikuchi E, Zigeuner R, Langner C, Bolenz C, Koppie TM, Raman JD, Fernández M, Karakiewizc P, Capitanio U, Bensalah K, Patard JJ, Shariat SF. Concomitant carcinoma in situ is a feature of aggressive disease in patients with organ confined urothelial carcinoma following radical nephroureterectomy. Urol Oncol. 2010;30(3):252–8.
41. Raman JD, Ng CK, Scherr DS, Margulis V, Lotan Y, Bensalah K, Patard JJ, Kikuchi E, Montorsi F, Zigeuner R, Weizer A, Bolenz C, Koppie TM, Isbarn H, Jeldres C, Kabbani W, Remzi M, Waldert M, Wood CG, Roscigno M, Oya M, Langner C, Wolf JS, Ströbel P, Fernández M, Karakiewcz P, Shariat SF. Impact of tumour location on prognosis for patients with upper tract urothelial carcinoma managed by radical nephroureterectomy. Eur Urol. 2010;57(6):1072–9.
42. Favaretto RL, Shariat SF, Chade DC, Godoy G, Adamy A, Kaag M, Bochner BH, Coleman J, Dalbagni G. The effect of tumor location on prognosis in patients treated with radical nephroureterectomy at Memorial Sloan-Kettering Cancer Center. Eur Urol. 2010;58(4):574–80.
43. Isbarn H, Jeldres C, Shariat SF, Liberman D, Sun M, Lughezzani G, Widmer H, Arjane P, Pharand D, Fisch M, Graefen M, Montorsi F, Perrotte P, Karakiewicz PI. Location of the primary tumor is not an independent predictor of cancer specific mortality in patients with upper urinary tract urothelial carcinoma. J Urol. 2009;182(5):2177–81.
44. Margulis V, Youssef RF, Karakiewicz PI, Lotan Y, Wood CG, Zigeuner R, Kikuchi E, Weizer A, Raman JD, Remzi M, Roscigno M, Montorsi F, Bolenz C, Kassouf W, Shariat SF, Upper Tract Urothelial Carcinoma Collaborative Group. Preoperative multivariable prognostic model for prediction of nonorgan confined urothelial carcinoma of the upper urinary tract. J Urol. 2010;184(2):453–8.

45. Fernández MI, Shariat SF, Margulis V, Bolenz C, Montorsi F, Suardi N, Remzi M, Wood CG, Roscigno M, Kikuchi E, Oya M, Zigeuner R, Langner C, Weizer A, Lotan Y, Koppie TM, Raman JD, Karakiewicz P, Bensalah K, Schultz M, Bernier P. Evidence-based sex-related outcomes after radical nephroureterectomy for upper tract urothelial carcinoma: results of large multicenter study. Urology. 2009;73(1): 142–6.
46. Lughezzani G, Sun M, Perrotte P, Shariat SF, Jeldres C, Budäus L, Latour M, Widmer H, Duclos A, Bénard F, McCormack M, Montorsi F, Karakiewicz PI. Gender-related differences in patients with stage I to III upper tract urothelial carcinoma: results from the Surveillance, Epidemiology, and End Results database. Urology. 2010;75(2):321–7.
47. Shariat SF, Favaretto RL, Gupta A, Fritsche HM, Matsumoto K, Kassouf W, Walton TJ, Tritschler S, Baba S, Matsushita K, Bastian PJ, Martínez-Salamanca JI, Seitz C, Pycha A, Otto W, Karakiewicz PI, Ficarra V, Novara G. Gender differences in radical nephroureterectomy for upper tract urothelial carcinoma. World J Urol. 2011;29(4):481–6.
48. Shariat SF, Godoy G, Lotan Y, Droller M, Karakiewicz PI, Raman JD, Isbarn H, Weizer A, Remzi M, Roscigno M, Kikuchi E, Bolenz C, Bensalah K, Koppie TM, Kassouf W, Wheat JC, Zigeuner R, Langner C, Wood CG, Margulis V. Advanced patient age is associated with inferior cancer-specific survival after radical nephroureterectomy. BJU Int. 2010; 105(12):1672–7.
49. Ng CK, Shariat SF, Lucas SM, Bagrodia A, Lotan Y, Scherr DS, Raman JD. Does the presence of hydronephrosis on preoperative axial CT imaging predict worse outcomes for patients undergoing nephroureterectomy for upper-tract urothelial carcinoma? Urol Oncol. 2011;29(1):27–32.
50. Eltz S, Comperat E, Cussenot O, Rouprêt M. Molecular and histological markers in urothelial carcinomas of the upper urinary tract. BJU Int. 2008;102(5):532–5.
51. Holmäng S, Johansson SL. Bilateral metachronous ureteral and renal pelvic carcinomas: incidence, clinical presentation, histopathology, treatment and outcome. J Urol. 2006;175(1):69–72.
52. Huben RP, Mounzer AM, Murphy GP. Tumor grade and stage as prognostic variables in upper tract urothelial tumors. Cancer. 1988;62(9):2016–20.
53. Bariol SV, Stewart GD, McNeill SA, Tolley DA. Oncological control following laparoscopic nephroureterectomy: 7-year outcome. J Urol. 2004;172: 1805–8.
54. Jeldres C, Lughezzani G, Sun M, Isbarn H, Shariat SF, Budaus L, Lattouf JB, Widmer H, Graefen M, Montorsi F, Perrotte P, Karakiewicz PI. Segmental ureterectomy can safely be performed in patients with transitional cell carcinoma of the ureter. J Urol. 2010;183(4):1324–9.
55. Thompson RH, Krambeck AE, Lohse CM, Elliott DS, Patterson DE, Blute ML. Elective endoscopic management of transitional cell carcinoma first diagnosed in the upper urinary tract. BJU Int. 2008;102(9): 1107–10.
56. Soderdahl DW, Fabrizio MD, Rahman NU, Jarrett TW, Bagley DH. Endoscopic treatment of upper tract transitional cell carcinoma. Urol Oncol. 2005;23: 114–22.
57. Palou J, Piovesan LF, Huguet J, Salvador J, Vicente J, Villavicencio H. Percutaneous nephroscopic management of upper urinary tract transitional cell carcinoma: recurrence and long-term follow-up. J Urol. 2004;172:66–9.
58. Grasso M, Bagley D. A 7.5/8.2F actively deflectable, flexible ureteroscope: a new device for both diagnostic and therapeutic upper urinary tract endoscopy. Urology. 1994;43:435–41.
59. Keeley FX, Bagley DH. Adjuvant mitomycin C following endoscopic treatment of upper tract transitional cell carcinoma. J Urol. 1997;158:2074–7.
60. Eastham JA, Huffman JL. Technique of mitomycin C instillation in the treatment of upper urinary tract urothelial tumors. J Urol. 1993;150(2):324–5.
61. Elliott DS, Blute ML, Patterson DE, Bergstralh EJ, Segura JW. Long-term follow-up of endoscopically treated upper tract transitional cell carcinoma. Urology. 1996;47(6):819–25.
62. Martínez-Piñeiro JA, García Matres MJ, Martínez-Piñeiro L. Endourological treatment of upper tract urothelial carcinoma: analysis of a series of 59 tumors. J Urol. 1996;156(2):377–85.
63. Schnapp DS, Weiss GH, Smith AD. Fever following intracavitary bacillus Calmette-Guerin therapy for upper tract transitional cell carcinoma. J Urol. 1996;156(2):386–8.
64. Sharpe JR, Duffy G, Chin JL. Intrarenal bacillus Calmette-Guerin therapy for upper urinary tract carcinoma in situ. J Urol. 1993;149:457–60.
65. Schoenberg MP, Van Arsdalen KN, Wein AJ. The management of transitional cell carcinoma in solitary renal units. J Urol. 1991;146(3):700–2.
66. Nonomura N, Ono Y, Nozawa M, Fukui T, Harada Y, Nishimura K, Takaha N, Takahara S, Okuyama A. Bacillus Calmette-Guerin perfusion therapy for the treatment of transitional cell carcinoma in situ of the upper urinary tract. Eur Urol. 2000;38(6): 701–4.
67. Thalmann GN, Markwalder R, Walter B, Studer UE. Long-term experience with bacillus Calmette-Guerin therapy of upper urinary tract transitional cell carcinoma in patients not eligible for surgery. J Urol. 2002;168(4):1381–5.
68. Rouprêt M, Hupertan V, Traxer O, Loison G, Chartier-Kastler E, Conort P, Bitker MO, Gattegno B, Richard F, Cussenot O. Comparison of open nephroureterectomy and ureteroscopic and percutaneous management of upper urinary tract transitional cell carcinoma. Urology. 2006;67:1181–7.
69. Boorjian S, Ng C, Munver R, Palese MA, Vaughan Jr ED, Sosa RE, Del Pizzo JJ, Scherr DS. Impact of delay to nephroureterectomy for patients undergoing

ureteroscopic biopsy and laser tumor ablation in upper tract transitional cell carcinoma. Urology. 2005;66(2):283–7.
70. Hendin BN, Streem SB, Levin HS, Klein EA, Novick AC. Impact of diagnostic ureteroscopy on long-term survival in patients with upper tract transitional cell carcinoma. J Urol. 1999;161(3):783–5.
71. Kulp DA, Bagley DH. Does flexible ureteropyeloscopy promote local recurrence of transitional cell carcinoma? J Endourol. 1994;8(2):111–3.
72. Fernández M, Bolenz C, Michel M-S, Alken P. Upper tract urothelial carcinoma: prognostic factors in 139 patients with a maximum follow-up of 16 years. Aktuelle Urol. 2006;37(S1):32.

Ureteral Calculi

7

Sri Sivalingam and Stephen Y. Nakada

Introduction

The prevalence of urolithiasis has increased from 3.8% in the 1970s to 5.2% in the 1990s, reflecting a 37% increase in lifetime risk in the USA [1]. Similar trends have been observed in other regions of the world [2–4]. Recent literature further indicates that the incidence of stone disease may be increasing faster in women than in men [5, 6]. Such gender trends have clinical implications for urologists in surgical management. As reviewed by Skolarikos and colleagues, less than 20% of these patients will actually become symptomatic from a new stone each year and only about half of these patients ultimately require surgical intervention [7]. Ureteral calculi create different diagnostic and therapeutic challenges in comparison to renal calculi. Ureteral stones present with renal colic with relatively smaller stones compared to renal calculi. Such symptoms arise during the passage of stones formed in the kidney; and if found incidentally, they are associated with some degree of hydronephrosis in patients with a prior diagnosis of nephrolithiasis [8]. This chapter carefully reviews the evidence and makes recommendations for the use of ureteroscopy (URS) in the treatment of ureteral stones.

The first reported URS was performed by Young in 1929, who used a pediatric cystoscope in the dilated ureter of an infant with posterior urethral valves [9]. Raney was the first to report on the use of an electrohydraulic lithotripter to fragment a ureteral stone in 1978 [10], followed by Das, who reported the first ureteral stone removal with a basket under direct vision using a pediatric cystoscope in 1981 [11]. The initial clinical use of URS with laser lithotripsy (pulsed dye laser) was reported by Dretler et al. in 1987, who successfully fragmented and cleared ureteral stones in 16 of 17 patients [12]. The introduction of the modern-day semirigid ureteroscope was reported, again by Dretler and Cho, in 1989 [13]. Table 7.1 shows this evolution of URS. Since the 1990s, ongoing advancement in both endoscopic and extracorporeal equipment has changed the indications, recommendations, and practice patterns for the treatment of ureteral calculi.

Natural History of Ureteral Calculi

Stone factors including size and location influence the rate of spontaneous passage, without any intervention. The majority of small ureteral calculi will pass spontaneously if given sufficient time. For stones less than 4 mm in diameter, two-thirds pass spontaneously within 4 weeks of symptom onset with an average time for passage being 1.6 weeks, compared with 2.8 weeks for

S. Sivalingam, M.D., M.Sc. (✉) • S.Y. Nakada, M.D., FACS
Department of Urology, University of Wisconsin,
1685 Highland Avenue, UW Medical Foundation
Centennial Building, RM 3267, Madison,
WI 53705, USA
e-mail: sivalingam@urology.wisc.edu

M. Monga (ed.), *Ureteroscopy: Indications, Instrumentation & Technique*, Current Clinical Urology,
DOI 10.1007/978-1-62703-206-3_7, © Springer Science+Business Media New York 2013

Table 7.1 Historical advances in ureteroscopy

Investigator	Year	Procedure	Instrument
Young	1929	Ureteroscopy for dilated ureter in infant with Puv	Pediatric cystoscope
Marshall	1964	Diagnostic ureteroscopy	
Goodman	1977	Therapeutic ureteroscopy—fulguration of ureteral tumor	Pediatric cystoscope
Raney	1978	Electrohydraulic ureterolithotripsy	
Das	1981	Ureteral basket stone removal under direct vision	Pediatric cystoscope + basket
Dretler, Watson, Parrish & Murray	1987	Ureteroscopy + laser lithotripsy	Pulsed dye laser
Dretler & Cho	1989	Modern-day ureteroscopy	Semirigid ureteroscope

stones 4–6 mm [14]. The current combined AUA/EAU guidelines on ureteral calculi report an estimated spontaneous passage rate of 68% (95% CI: 46–85%) for stones ≤5 mm [15]. For stones >5 mm and ≤10 mm, the estimated spontaneous passage is 47% (95% CI: 36–59%).

In the absence of ureteral disease, the width of the stone is the most significant measurement affecting the likelihood of stone passage [16]. As such, a linear association is seen between stone size and spontaneous passage rates, with rates of 87, 72, 47, and 27% for stones measuring 1, 4, 7, and 10 mm, respectively [17]. The systematic review by Hübner and colleagues showed a similar relationship between stone size and passage rates from a pooled analysis of 6 studies totaling 2,704 patients [14]. The rate of spontaneous passage for stones smaller than 4 mm was 38% compared to 1.2% for those larger than 6 mm within 4 weeks, irrespective of their position in the ureter at the time of presentation. Another systematic review of 37 pooled studies showed that in symptomatic ureteral calculi <4 mm, 38–71% will pass spontaneously and only 4.8% of stones <2 mm will need intervention during surveillance [7].

Stone location also influences clearance rates and has associated passage and impaction rates, i.e., proximal calculi pass less spontaneously than distal calculi, when controlled for size. Early studies showed a passage rate of 71% for distal calculi, and only 22% for proximal calculi, with an overall passage rate of 60% [18]. Other similar studies indicated less impressive results: calculi discovered in the distal third of the ureter had a spontaneous passage rate of 45%, compared with the mid third at 22%, and the proximal third at 12% [14]. Furthermore, the advent of medical expulsive therapy (MET) has improved the rate of spontaneous passage rates. Pooled results of high-quality randomized controlled trials in a contemporary meta-analysis showed a 65% greater likelihood of spontaneous stone passage with calcium channel blockers or alpha-blockers, compared to patients not receiving these drugs [19].

Some of the differences in reported stone passage rates can be attributed to measuring stone-free rates (SFRs). It should be kept in mind that the time needed for spontaneous clearance to occur can vary between patients and is not always apparent in the reporting criteria of studies; as such, an adequate period of observation is necessary if this is the chosen initial approach. The variability of observed spontaneous stone passage rates may be influenced by the duration of observation given before intervention is chosen, individual patient characteristics, and other confounding factors such as stone location or the use of MET. Furthermore, it has been shown that the criteria chosen to measure stone size can have interobserver differences [20]. However, cumulative results of studies indicate that 38–100% of stones <5 mm can be expected to pass spontaneously within 4 weeks. Thus, if spontaneous passage is chosen, the advantages of this approach must be weighed against the potential benefits of early definitive intervention. In general, literature supports that if significant progress has not occurred within 40 days of observation, intervention is necessary [18, 21].

Predictors of Spontaneous Passage

Interestingly, a recent study looking at the various factors influencing stone passage implicated serum WBC count as having a predictive potential for spontaneous passage. This study showed that its value, at the acute phase of a renal colic, is a significant predictor for stone spontaneous passage and should be considered [22]. The rationale for this observation is that a more mobile stone might cause more micro-trauma to the ureteral epithelium, causing a relatively more pronounced inflammatory response. However, the clinical utility of this is yet to be determined; even if a higher WBC count may suggest a greater likelihood for the stone to pass, it should be cautiously weighed against the possibility of an underlying infection or sepsis. Other potential predictors included stone sidedness, with a higher likelihood for left-sided stones to pass.

Ureteroscopic Treatment of Ureteral Stones

Ureteroscopy Versus Shock Wave Lithotripsy

The options for management of ureteral stones include conservative approaches such as active monitoring, and MET, minimally invasive procedures such as shock wave lithotripsy (SWL) and URS, and less often, laparoscopic ureterolithotomy. Taking together the observed rates of spontaneous stone passage, and variable time frame with which stones pass, the timing of when and modality with which to intervene can be challenging. Several factors, including patient preference, stone burden and location, resource availability, and surgeon skill, all contribute to the chosen treatment approach. Although conservative approaches such as observation or MET are acceptable options, passage of stones with such approaches may take several weeks to occur, during which period, patients may remain symptomatic, requiring ER visits, hospital admission, and analgesic use. Interestingly, despite its proven role in promoting stone passage, MET is still rarely used at the primary care level [19, 23]. In select cases, it might be prudent to offer early definitive therapy after a thorough discussion with the patient.

The indications and recommendations for URS have changed over the years, and is largely attributable to the refinement of flexible and rigid ureteroscopes, improved optics and ancillary instruments such as laser fibers and baskets, and to an extent evolution of surgical technique. Also, SWL has proven to be less effective than once thought. The updated ureteral stone guidelines reflect these changes, with an expansion for the indications of URS in treating ureteral stones [6]. While no differences in overall SFR were found between SWL and URS, the only instance in which SWL yielded slightly higher SFR was for proximal ureteral stones ≤10 mm. URS had significantly higher SFR for proximal stones >10 mm and for distal ureteral stones of all sizes. For all mid-ureteral stones, URS trended towards superior results but did not reach statistical significance. Such outcomes data would indicate that URS is perhaps less affected by stone burden than is SWL [24], and for obvious reasons, i.e., with SWL, the larger the stone burden, the more fragments that need to pass. URS is now deemed appropriate as first-line therapy for stones of any size in the proximal ureter, with clear benefits for stones >10 mm. Consistent with this is the updated Cochrane review comparing SWL to ureteroscopic management of ureteral calculi, which evaluated data from 7 randomized controlled trials. The authors report lower SFR (RR 0.84) and higher retreatment rates (RR 6.18) with SWL compared to URS, but with the benefit of shorter hospital stay and fewer complications (RR 0.43) [25]. This was further illustrated by Raman et al., where the number of primary procedures (i.e., the intended treatment modality) was fewer for URS compared to SWL at all ureteral locations, indicating a higher retreatment rate for SWL [24]. Scales and colleagues showed in a recent analysis that the odds of a second procedure following initial SWL were 1.54 times those of URS [26]. In their review, they showed that in beneficiaries undergoing initial SWL,

38% underwent an additional procedure within 120 days, versus 9% for URS and 18% for URS plus holmium laser.

Although the 1997 ureteral stone guidelines recommended SWL for stones <10 mm and either SWL or URS for stones >10 mm in the proximal ureter, the current guidelines, along with more recent data, reflect a change in this assertion. This shift in outcomes is largely due to improved endoscopic technology as discussed earlier, rendering URS easier and safer. Furthermore, newer devices such as the Stone Cone (Microvasive; Boston Scientific Corp., Spencer, IN) and N-Trap (Cook Urological, Spencer, IN) to prevent stone retropulsion during proximal URS may further contribute to the improved results [27, 28].

Unfortunately, it is very difficult to draw direct comparisons between available studies due to the variability in methodologies and criteria for determining SFRs; this continues to affect newer literature as well, as outlined in the Cochrane review discussed above. The limitations in assessing the currently available literature on SWL and URS stem from the lack of standardization in comparing stone size and burden, and more universal criteria in future study designs might permit a more accurate standard of comparison [20].

Current Trends in Treatment of Ureteral Calculi

In a recent review of over 9,000 beneficiaries in the USA who underwent an initial procedure for the treatment of ureteral stones, several patients, providers, and practice setting characteristics were associated with the selection of URS versus SWL [26]. As might be expected, the odds of undergoing URS was 44% higher when treated at a high-volume URS facility versus 68% lower odds when treated at a high-volume SWL facility. A significant and interesting finding in this review was that female patients were less likely than males to undergo URS. Such gender-based preferences for the treatment modality for ureteral stones may have subtle clinical implications, in light of the observed trend of higher rate of increase in the incidence of stone disease in women compared to men. Congruent with these findings was a study that showed more recently that trained urologists were more likely to use URS than SWL, based on an analysis of board certification logs [29]. Leijte et al. showed that surgeon experience was indeed a predictive factor for complications and success for ureteroscopic holmium laser lithotripsy for ureteric calculi. Experienced surgeons had fewer complications, and the success rate was higher [30]. Nonetheless, current practice patterns indicate a consistent trend among American urologists towards URS and away from SWL for the management of stones of all sizes throughout the ureter [31]. For example, even with an expansion of extracorporeal lithotripter ownership in the state of Michigan, an associated drop in the rate of URS was not seen [32].

A cost–benefit analysis showed that, after failed observation, URS is the most cost-effective treatment strategy for ureteral stones at all locations [33]. Although observation alone is purported to be more cost-effective than surgical treatment, costs of total observation are more difficult to ascertain as the observation regimen is less controlled due to variations in management, with variable hospital ER visits, loss of work secondary to pain, etc. Cumulative economic data suggest that URS is the most cost-effective treatment strategy for ureteral stones in all locations, after observation fails [34].

Stone Factors

Size and Location

The probability of spontaneous stone passage as discussed previously is directly correlated with the distance of ureter to be traversed and inversely with that of stone size. Greater ureteroscopic success is observed as the stone location is more distal, and as the stone burden is lower. It is known that ureteral stones are held up at predictable sites: the UPJ, crossing of the ureter over the iliac vessels, and at the UVJ, the narrowest portion of the ureter. However, recent clinical studies demonstrate the two most common sites of stones to lodge in patients presenting to the ER with renal colic: the UVJ (60.6% of cases), and the proximal ureter between the UPJ and the iliac vessels (23.4%) [35]. In this study, the proportion of stones lodged at the UPJ and crossing of the iliac were only 10.6 and 1.1%, respectively. These findings would indicate a greater role for URS over SWL, based on the previous outcomes discussion.

The technical challenge of treating proximal stones is greater than distal stones, potentially contributing to the lower SFRs at these locations. This is due to the instrumentation distance required to traverse and access the relatively more delicate upper ureter and added challenges due to stone migration during treatment. However, with the advent of newer and more sophisticated equipment, the gap in the SFRs between proximal and distal stones is decreasing [34]. Hollenbeck et al. showed that endoscopic management of proximal ureteral stones is highly successful, without an increase in complication rates, and that the differences in success rates between proximal and distal calculi have narrowed substantially [36].

The current ureteral stone guidelines report SFRs of 81, 86, and 94% for ureteroscopic management of proximal, mid, and distal ureteral calculi, respectively [15]. In comparing SWL versus URS in this report, the SFRs were 82 vs. 81%, respectively, for proximal ureteral calculi, 73 vs. 86% for middle ureteral calculi, and 74 vs. 94% for distal ureteral calculi [15]. Ureteroscopic SFRs showed less size dependence with comparable rates for proximal, middle, and distal stones ≤10 mm and >10 mm. Newer series report SFRs of 72, 95, and 99% [37] and 80, 94, and 91% [38], for proximal, mid, and distal calculi, respectively. It is important to note, however, that in some contemporary series, lower SFRs were observed for proximal stones, such as 69.4 [39] and 59% [40]. Another recent series showed SFRs of 77, 85, and 91%, but subgroup analysis for stones >10 mm showed that the SFRs were 54, 77, and 88%, respectively [41]. Table 7.2 highlights ureteroscopic outcomes from selected recent series since the 2007 guidelines for stones at various locations in the ureter.

In all, given the excellent overall results with URS, the guidelines on ureteral calculi now recommend URS to be appropriate for stones of any size and in any location in the ureter. This meta-analysis demonstrated that the URS yields significantly greater SFR for the majority of stone stratifications.

Stone Composition

Stone composition dramatically affects SWL efficacy, whereas URS is less affected by stone type. It is established that SWL is not as effective for cystine, brushite, or calcium oxalate monohydrate stones [42]. In contrast, studies evaluating the success rates of Holmium laser lithotripsy have shown equal efficacy for most stone types, including calcium oxalate monohydrate stones [43]. This study further demonstrated that radio-opacity of the stone has no bearing on laser lithotripsy. Teichman's review of his earlier studies showed that the holmium-YAG laser is effective for stones of all composition and sizes [42].

Very Large/Impacted Proximal Ureteral Stones

In cases with impacted stones in the proximal ureter, URS can be technically more challenging. As discussed above, URS yields better SFRs than SWL for proximal ureteral stones larger than 10 mm. Even in centers where flexible ureteroscopes are not available for example, semirigid URS is efficacious for proximal ureteral stones >10 mm, with excellent SFRs and safety profile [44]. This begs the question of a recommended maximum stone size for URS, i.e., in stones larger than 20 mm. Chen et al. showed that proximal ureteral stones >20 mm can be safely treated with semirigid URS and Holmium:YAG laser lithotripsy while achieving excellent SFR (84% at 4 weeks post treatment); here, no complications were reported [45]. In situations where traditional URS may not seem feasible or appropriate for proximal stones, i.e., for a stone that is too large or severely impacted, an antegrade approach may be suitable, which is discussed next.

Table 7.2 Ureterolithotripsy outcomes: Selected contemporary series (after 2007 guidelines review)

Investigators, year	Study type	Total # patients	Mean stone size (Mm)	Overall % SFR (# patients) Distal	Mid	Proximal	SFR (days, modality)	Instrument used
Al-Ghazo et al. 2011	Retrospective	244		96.6%	95.8%	69.4%	4 weeks, Kub	7.5, 8f Semirigid; Swiss Lithoclast
Best And Nakada 2011	Retrospective	43	9.1	N/A	N/A	86%		Flexible; Ho:Yag Laser
Ciftci et al. 2010	Retrospective	336	9.77	90.7%	85.5%	76.5%	4 weeks, Kub	9.5f Rigid; Pneumolithotripsy
Hong and Park 2009	Retrospective	341	8.8 (D) 8.7 (M) 10.9 (P)	96.9%	93.8%	80.3%	2 weeks, Kub	9.5f, 10f Rigid; Swiss Lithoclast
Yencilek et al. 2010	Retrospective	1,416	12.1	98.9%	94.8%	71.7%		Semirigid; Pneumatic Lithotripsy
Ather et al. 2010	Retrospective	265	>30 mm^2	92%	53%	59%	3 months	6.4, 7, or 8 F Semirigid; Swiss Lithoclast
Preminger et al. 2007	Systematic Review—2007 Aua Guidelines	8,194	N/A	94%	86%	81%	N/A	N/A

Antegrade Ureteroscopy for Proximal Impacted Stones

The treatment of larger or impacted proximal stones can be challenging, with the attendant risk of ureteral perforation and higher likelihood of stone migration during fragmentation. Antegrade URS has been described for impacted proximal and mid ureteral stones dating back to 1989 [46]. The AUA guidelines state that percutaneous antegrade URS is an acceptable first-line treatment in select cases [15]. As such, this, along with other studies, speaks to the feasibility and safety of this technique, in view of evolving technology [47, 48]. Retrospective series comparing antegrade with retrograde URS for impacted large upper ureteral calculi showed that better SFRs were achieved with the antegrade approach, and without complications [49]. A recent study prospectively looked at the utility of antegrade URS, where patients with large (>10 mm), impacted proximal ureteral calculi were randomized to either the standard retrograde URS or an antegrade approach [50]. This was based on a "mini-PCNL" technique for the antegrade group, with the access tract dilated to 16 F and utilization of a sheath that extended to the UPJ. Their results were in favor of the antegrade procedure, with SFR at discharge home being 95.3 vs. 79.5% for the retrograde group. It is to be noted, however, that the hospital stay was longer in the antegrade group (6.3 days vs. 2.1 days), although the complication rate was similar in both groups. Conversely, a randomized study comparing retrograde, antegrade, and laparoscopic approaches for proximal stones >15 mm failed to show any significant differences in stone clearance or an obvious benefit for one over the others [48].

The potential benefits of a higher SFR with antegrade URS need to be weighed against the added costs of a more prolonged operative time, longer hospital stay, and loss of work. Newer flexible and semirigid ureteroscopes in conjunction with stone migration devices may eventually obviate the need to consider alternatives to standard URS. The current literature, however, suggests that the antegrade approach can be performed safely and the approach to be taken must be based on the available resources, patient preference, and surgeon experience.

Bilateral Ureteral Calculi

In cases of bilateral ureteral calculi, various strategies can be utilized: observation, a combination of observation and staggered surgery with SWL and/or URS, or bilateral same-session URS. Modern-day URS permits safe and efficacious stone removal at all locations within the ureter. As briefly stated in the ureteral stones guidelines, URS can be used to safely treat bilateral ureteral stones simultaneously in select cases. In experienced hands, bilateral procedures may indeed be performed; however, the benefits of a single anesthetic induction and hospital admission must be weighed against the potentially increased complication rates.

A recent study assessed the outcomes of single-session bilateral URS and pneumatic lithotripsy for bilateral ureteral calculi, and showed that it was safe and effective, with a 6.2% overall complication rate, while the complication rate of unilateral procedure was 9.6% [51]. The authors suggest that although bilateral same-session URS is safe and effective, proximal ureteral calculi, or large/impacted calculi, carry the highest risk of unsuccessful results. Gunlusoy et al. obtained stone clearance rates of 72.7% for proximal ureteral calculi, 80.9% in the mid ureter, and 95.4% in the distal ureter after single, same-session bilateral URS, with no major complications [52]. For calculi <10 mm, the SFR was 94.1% and for stones greater than 10 mm, 76%. In Grossi and colleagues' comparative series of bilateral synchronous versus staged URS, they reported high SFR in both groups, although with a slight predominance of hematuria and urinary discomfort in the bilateral group, which did not reach statistical significance.

In contrast to these studies which endorse bilateral same-session procedures, other series suggest higher complication rates and advocate performing URS in a staged manner. For example, Hollenbeck et al. demonstrated a higher complication rate following bilateral same-session URS versus staged URS (29 vs. 14%), with a further increase in morbidity when a postoperative ureteral stent was not placed [53]. One case of anuric renal failure was also reported after bilateral URS, presumably because no stents were utilized after the procedure [54].

Given these data, the decision to pursue same-session versus staged URS should be based on a careful evaluation of several factors, including surgeon expertise, stone burden, renal function, and perhaps patient preference. It would be prudent, especially in bilateral proximal, large or impacted calculi to consider postoperative stent placement or staging the procedure.

Selected Patient Factors

Infection

Pain and infection secondary to ureteral obstruction are common indications for urgent decompression. URS, like SWL, should be avoided during active infection to avoid sepsis and other complications.

Obesity

Given the prevalence of obesity in stone patients, patient body habitus can influence the choice of optimal treatment modality. Studies have demonstrated the difficulty in targeting stones in the obese with SWL, and treatment with this modality will likely fail when skin-to-stone distance exceeds 10 cm [55]. However, ureteroscopic treatment of proximal ureteral stones has shown to be performed safely and with equal efficacy in both obese (BMI ≥ 30 kg/m^2) and non-obese patients [56]. Similar success rates were achieved between obese and non-obese patients, with SFRs of 91 and 81%, respectively. A more detailed review of URS in the obese patient will be discussed in a later chapter.

Anticoagulation

Stone disease in patients on oral anticoagulation poses a challenging management problem. In cases where anticoagulation medications cannot be stopped, SWL is absolutely contraindicated. The use of URS may be the only viable surgical option in such cases, providing a minimally invasive yet definitive treatment. In a study by Turna and colleagues, the use of flexible ureterorenoscopy with laser lithotripsy for the treatment of renal calculi was retrospectively reviewed in 37 patients on ongoing oral anticoagulation. Although the anticoagulated patients were older, and with higher ASA scores, all procedures were completed without complication and both groups had similar SFR [57]. Importantly, no procedure was terminated due to poor visibility from bleeding, and no transfusions or significant drop in hemoglobin were observed. Being the largest comparative study on the topic, this study attests to the safety of URS in these patients, in experienced hands.

Aberrant Anatomy

Aberrant anatomy poses obvious surgical challenges, and can affect treatment success. Small series have demonstrated successful URS for patients with stones within anomalous kidneys, i.e., pelvic or horseshoe kidney [58], albeit these studies were not exclusively for ureteral stones.

Other Considerations

Timing of Ureteroscopy

An initial management step for patients presenting to the emergency room with acute renal colic is to stabilize the patient and provide pain/emetic control. For the decompression of an obstructed and infected system, it is clear that urgent ureteral stents or nephrostomy tubes be placed and definitive treatment deferred. However, in the stable patient presenting with acute renal colic with pain refractory to medical management, the decision to perform immediate versus delayed URS or SWL needs to be made. Randomized control trials have shown that SWL can be safely and effectively performed in an emergent manner. However, there has been a relative paucity of data with respect to emergent URS for stone removal. Traditionally, URS is arranged as an elective procedure after initial management with medications or stenting.

In an effort to evaluate the feasibility of emergent URS, Guercio et al. conducted a prospective randomized control trial with 271 patients who presented to the ER with acute renal colic secondary to ureteral calculi. These patients were divided into two groups: immediate URS within

12 h of presentation, or medical treatment and delayed URS [59]. No differences in SFRs or complication rates were seen between the groups, and the results were consistent with other contemporary series. Sarica et al. showed retrospectively that equal SFRs were achieved in patients treated immediately with URS compared to those treated electively after 7 or more days of initial medical therapy [60]. SFRs in this study were 87.9 and 90.8% in the immediate and delayed groups, respectively. Further studies determined immediate URS to be safe and effective, with excellent SFRs [61]. Other retrospective data support this view, that emergent URS and laser lithotripsy can be performed safely in patients presenting with acute renal failure secondary to obstructive ureteral calculi [62]. These investigators achieved an overall SFR of 88.9%, and recovery of renal function in 96.3% of patients within 7 days, with no complications.

Taken together, these data suggest that immediate URS can be performed without an increased risk of complications and with similar efficacy compared to delayed URS. Immediate URS obviates the need for ongoing follow-up, prolonged analgesic requirements, and repeat ER visits, which can dampen some of the overall costs and morbidity of renal colic managed with medication or observation. As discussed by Guercio et al., immediate therapy also avoids complications such as urinary tract infection, worsening hydronephrosis, or renal function. It can be argued that deferred treatment can allow for spontaneous passage of stones and a complete avoidance of an invasive procedure and anesthesia altogether, and immediate URS decreases the opportunity for this. Without further prospective studies, it is difficult to generalize the currently available literature on this due to the relatively small number of studies and variability in study design.

The Role of Adjunctive Alpha-1 Blockers with Ureteroscopy

It is now well established that selective alpha-1 blockers enhance stone passage, especially in the distal ureter, and are routinely used for MET as primary conservative treatment and as an adjunct to SWL. Given these benefits, there has been growing interest in combining this strategy with URS to achieve better SFRs.

A recent prospective study showed a benefit in using alpha-1 blockers post ureteroscopic laser lithotripsy for relatively large ureteral stones (1–2 cm), with improved SFRs and decreased colic episodes [63]. Patients were randomized to receive tamsulosin with standard analgesia versus analgesia only following lithotripsy, and significant differences were demonstrated between the two groups: SFRs were 86.5 vs. 69.4%, and colic episodes were 5.4 vs. 22.2%, in the tamsulosin and control groups, respectively. Although it is difficult to know if some of these patients were already on tamsulosin following their initial episode of colic, the study was well designed, showing a benefit for adjunctive alpha-1 blockade post URS.

References

1. Stamatelou KK, Francis ME, Jones CA, Nyberg LM, Curhan GC. Time trends in reported prevalence of kidney stones in the United States: 1976–1994. Kidney Int. 2003;63(5):1817–23.
2. Yoshida O, Terai A, Ohkawa T, Okada Y. National trend of the incidence of urolithiasis in Japan from 1965 to 1995. Kidney Int. 1999;56(5):1899–904.
3. Hesse A, Brändle E, Wilbert D, Köhrmann KU, Alken P. Study on the prevalence and incidence of urolithiasis in Germany comparing the years 1979 vs. 2000. Eur Urol. 2003;44(6):709–13.
4. Trinchieri A, Coppi F, Montanari E, Del Nero A, Zanetti G, Pisani E. Increase in the prevalence of symptomatic upper urinary tract stones during the last ten years. Eur Urol. 2000;37(1):23–5.
5. Pearle MS, Calhoun EA, Curhan GC. Project UDoA. Urologic diseases in America project: urolithiasis. J Urol Mar. 2005;173(3):848–57.
6. Scales CD, Curtis LH, Norris RD, et al. Changing gender prevalence of stone disease. J Urol. 2007; 177(3):979–82.
7. Skolarikos A, Laguna MP, Alivizatos G, Kural AR, de la Rosette JJ. The role for active monitoring in urinary stones: a systematic review. J Endourol. 2010;24(6): 923–30.
8. Wimpissinger F, Türk C, Kheyfets O, Stackl W. The silence of the stones: asymptomatic ureteral calculi. J Urol. 2007;178(4 Pt 1):1341–4. discussion 1344.

9. Eisner BH, Kurtz MP, Dretler SP. Ureteroscopy for the management of stone disease. Nat Rev Urol. 2010;7(1):40–5.
10. Raney AM. Electrohydraulic ureterolithotripsy. Preliminary report. Urology. 1978;12(3):284–5.
11. Das S. Transurethral ureteroscopy and stone manipulation under direct vision. J Urol. 1981;125(1):112–3.
12. Dretler SP, Watson G, Parrish JA, Murray S. Pulsed dye laser fragmentation of ureteral calculi: initial clinical experience. J Urol. 1987;137(3):386–9.
13. Dretler SP, Cho G. Semirigid ureteroscopy: a new genre. J Urol. 1989;141(6):1314–6.
14. Hübner WA, Irby P, Stoller ML. Natural history and current concepts for the treatment of small ureteral calculi. Eur Urol. 1993;24(2):172–6.
15. Preminger GM, Tiselius HG, Assimos DG, et al. 2007 guideline for the management of ureteral calculi. J Urol. 2007;178(6):2418–34.
16. Ueno A, Kawamura T, Ogawa A, Takayasu H. Relation of spontaneous passage of ureteral calculi to size. Urology. 1977;10(6):544–6.
17. Coll DM, Varanelli MJ, Smith RC. Relationship of spontaneous passage of ureteral calculi to stone size and location as revealed by unenhanced helical CT. AJR Am J Roentgenol. 2002;178(1):101–3.
18. Morse RM, Resnick MI. Ureteral calculi: natural history and treatment in an era of advanced technology. J Urol. 1991;145(2):263–5.
19. Hollingsworth JM, Rogers MA, Kaufman SR, et al. Medical therapy to facilitate urinary stone passage: a meta-analysis. Lancet. 2006;368(9542):1171–9.
20. Patel SR, Nakada SY. Quantification of preoperative stone burden for ureteroscopy and shock wave lithotripsy: current state and future recommendations. Urology. 2011;78(2):282–5.
21. Miller OF, Kane CJ. Time to stone passage for observed ureteral calculi: a guide for patient education. J Urol. 1999;162(3 Pt 1):688–90. discussion 690–681.
22. Sfoungaristos S, Kavouras A, Perimenis P. Predictors for spontaneous stone passage in patients with renal colic secondary to ureteral calculi. Int Urol Nephrol. 2012;44(1):71–9.
23. Hollingsworth JM, Wolf JS, Faerber GJ, Roberts WW, Dunn RL, Hollenbeck BK. Understanding the barriers to the dissemination of medical expulsive therapy. J Urol. 2010;184(6):2368–72.
24. Raman JD, Pearle MS. Surgical management of ureteral stone disease. In: Dmochowski RR, Dahm P, editors. Evidence-based urology, vol. xiv. 2nd ed. Chichester, West Sussex, UK: Wiley-Blackwell; 2010. p. 417.
25. Aboumarzouk OM, Kata SG, Keeley FX, Nabi G. Extracorporeal shock wave lithotripsy (ESWL) versus ureteroscopic management for ureteric calculi. Cochrane Database Syst Rev. 2011;12:CD006029.
26. Scales CD, Krupski TL, Curtis LH, et al. Practice variation in the surgical management of urinary lithiasis. J Urol. 2011;186(1):146–50.
27. Lee HJ, Box GN, Abraham JB, et al. In vitro evaluation of nitinol urological retrieval coil and ureteral occlusion device: retropulsion and holmium laser fragmentation efficiency. J Urol. 2008;180(3):969–73.
28. Farahat YA, Elbahnasy AE, Elashry OM. A randomized prospective controlled study for assessment of different ureteral occlusion devices in prevention of stone migration during pneumatic lithotripsy. Urology. 2011;77(1):30–5.
29. Matlaga BR. Urology ABo. Contemporary surgical management of upper urinary tract calculi. J Urol May. 2009;181(5):2152–6.
30. Leijte JA, Oddens JR, Lock TM. Holmium laser lithotripsy for ureteral calculi: predictive factors for complications and success. J Endourol. 2008;22(2):257–60.
31. Gerber GS, Acharya SS. Management of ureteral calculi. J Endourol. 2010;24(6):953–4.
32. Tan HJ, Wolf JS, Hollenbeck BK, Ye Z, Hollingsworth JM. Use of ureteroscopy before and after expansion of lithotripter ownership in Michigan. Urology. 2011;78(6):1287–91.
33. Lotan Y, Gettman MT, Roehrborn CG, Cadeddu JA, Pearle MS. Management of ureteral calculi: a cost comparison and decision making analysis. J Urol. 2002;167(4):1621–9.
34. Matlaga BR, Lingeman JE. Surgical management of upper urinary tract calculi. In: Wein AJ, Kavoussi LR, Campbell MF, editors. Campbell-Walsh urology. 10th ed. Philadelphia, PA: lsevier Saunders; 2012.
35. Eisner BH, Reese A, Sheth S, Stoller ML. Ureteral stone location at emergency room presentation with colic. J Urol. 2009;182(1):165–8.
36. Hollenbeck BK, Schuster TG, Faerber GJ, Wolf JS. Comparison of outcomes of ureteroscopy for ureteral calculi located above and below the pelvic brim. Urology. 2001;58(3):351–6.
37. Yencilek F, Sarica K, Erturhan S, Yagci F, Erbagci A. Treatment of ureteral calculi with semirigid ureteroscopy: where should we stop? Urol Int. 2010;84(3):260–4.
38. Hong YK, Park DS. Ureteroscopic lithotripsy using Swiss Lithoclast for treatment of ureteral calculi: 12-years experience. J Korean Med Sci. 2009;24(4):690–4.
39. Al-Ghazo MA, Ghalayini IF, Al-Azab RS, et al. Emergency ureteroscopic lithotripsy in acute renal colic caused by ureteral calculi: a retrospective study. Urol Res. 2011;39(6):497–501.
40. Ather MH, Nazim SM, Sulaiman MN. Efficacy of semirigid ureteroscopy with pneumatic lithotripsy for ureteral stone surface area of greater than 30 mm2. J Endourol. 2009;23(4):619–22.
41. Ciftci H, Savas M, Altunkol A, Yeni E, Verit A, Celepkolu B. Influence of stone size, location and impaction on the success of ureteroscopic pneumolithotripsy. Georgian Med News Jun. 2010;183:7–12.
42. Teichman JM. Clinical practice. Acute renal colic from ureteral calculus. N Engl J Med Feb. 2004;350(7):684–93.

43. Seitz C, Tanovic E, Kikic Z, Fajkovic H. Impact of stone size, location, composition, impaction, and hydronephrosis on the efficacy of holmium:YAG-laser ureterolithotripsy. Eur Urol. 2007;52(6):1751–7.
44. Khairy-Salem H, el-Ghoneimy M, el-Atrebi M. Semirigid ureteroscopy in management of large proximal ureteral calculi: is there still a role in developing countries? Urology. 2011;77(5):1064–8.
45. Chen CS, Wu CF, Shee JJ, Lin WY. Holmium:YAG Lasertripsy with semirigid ureterorenoscope for upper-ureteral stones >2 cm. J Endourol. 2005;19(7):780–4.
46. Tan EC, Tung KH, Foo KT, Kwok R, Hoe J. Antegrade ureteroscopy and ultrasonic lithotripsy in the treatment of difficult upper and middle ureteric stones. Ann Acad Med Singapore. 1989;18(1):55–8.
47. Istanbulluoglu MO, Goren MR, Cicek T, Ozturk B, Ozkardes H. An alternative treatment for high-burden ureteral stones: percutaneous antegrade ureteroscopy. Urol Res. 2011;39(5):389–92.
48. Basiri A, Simforoosh N, Ziaee A, Shayaninasab H, Moghaddam SM, Zare S. Retrograde, antegrade, and laparoscopic approaches for the management of large, proximal ureteral stones: a randomized clinical trial. J Endourol. 2008;22(12):2677–80.
49. Maheshwari PN, Oswal AT, Andankar M, Nanjappa KM, Bansal M. Is antegrade ureteroscopy better than retrograde ureteroscopy for impacted large upper ureteral calculi? J Endourol. 1999;13(6):441–4.
50. Sun X, Xia S, Lu J, Liu H, Han B, Li W. Treatment of large impacted proximal ureteral stones: randomized comparison of percutaneous antegrade ureterolithotripsy versus retrograde ureterolithotripsy. J Endourol. 2008;22(5):913–7.
51. Chung SY, Chon CH, Ng CS, Fuchs GJ. Simultaneous bilateral retrograde intrarenal surgery for stone disease in patients with significant comorbidities. J Endourol. 2006;20(10):761–5.
52. Gunlusoy B, Degirmenci T, Arslan M, et al. Bilateral single-session ureteroscopy with pneumatic lithotripsy for bilateral ureter stones: feasible and safe. Urol Int. 2008;81(2):202–5.
53. Hollenbeck BK, Schuster TG, Faerber GJ, Wolf Jr JS. Safety and efficacy of same-session bilateral ureteroscopy. J Endourol/Endourol Soc. 2003;17(10):881–5.
54. Bandi G, Vicentini FC, Triest JA. Anuric renal failure after same-session bilateral atraumatic flexible ureteroscopy. Int Braz J Urol. 2007;33(2):193–4.
55. Pareek G, Hedican SP, Lee FT, Nakada SY. Shock wave lithotripsy success determined by skin-to-stone distance on computed tomography. Urology. 2005;66(5):941–4.
56. Best SL, Nakada SY. Flexible ureteroscopy is effective for proximal ureteral stones in both obese and nonobese patients: a two-year, single-surgeon experience. Urology. 2011;77(1):36–9.
57. Turna B, Stein RJ, Smaldone MC, et al. Safety and efficacy of flexible ureterorenoscopy and holmium:YAG lithotripsy for intrarenal stones in anticoagulated cases. J Urol. 2008;179(4):1415–9.
58. Raj GV, Auge BK, Weizer AZ, et al. Percutaneous management of calculi within horseshoe kidneys. J Urol. 2003;170(1):48–51.
59. Guercio S, Ambu A, Mangione F, Mari M, Vacca F, Bellina M. Randomized prospective trial comparing immediate versus delayed ureteroscopy for patients with ureteral calculi and normal renal function who present to the emergency department. J Endourol. 2011;25(7):1137–41.
60. Sarica K, Tanriverdi O, Aydin M, Koyuncu H, Miroglu C. Emergency ureteroscopic removal of ureteral calculi after first colic attack: is there any advantage? Urology. 2011;78(3):516–20.
61. Osorio L, Lima E, Autorino R, Marcelo F. Emergency management of ureteral stones: Recent advances. Indian J Urol. 2008;24(4):461–6.
62. Jiang H, Wu Z, Ding Q. Ureteroscopy and holmium:YAG laser lithotripsy as emergency treatment for acute renal failure caused by impacted ureteral calculi. Urology. 2008;72(3):504–7.
63. John TT, Razdan S. Adjunctive tamsulosin improves stone free rate after ureteroscopic lithotripsy of large renal and ureteric calculi: a prospective randomized study. Urology. 2010;75(5):1040–2.

Intrarenal Calculi

8

Ricardo D. Gonzalez and Benjamin K. Canales

Introduction

Flexible ureteroscopy (URS) has become an important tool for urologists who treat kidney stone patients. The popularity of this technique has grown due to improvements in ureteroscope design and rapid evolution and miniaturization of accessory instruments. Along with its increased prominence and use, flexible URS and its associated outcomes have been studied by a number of investigators with seemingly promising conclusions. Therefore, an evidence-based review of these outcomes should allow us to determine whether or not URS should be used as a sole treatment modality for kidney stones and what kind of stone-free outcomes our patients can expect.

The traditional factors determining the operative approach for nephrolithiasis are based on previous shock wave lithotripsy (SWL) studies and include renal anatomy, stone size, stone mineral composition, expected stone-free results, and patient body habitus/size. In 2000, the ureteral access sheath was introduced, facilitating multiple ureteral and renal reentries during flexible URS. Not only has the access sheath decreased operative time and cost, but it has also been shown to minimize patient morbidity and improve ureteroscopic success rates [1]. Ureteral access sheaths changed the paradigm of kidney stone surgery and brought retrograde flexible ureterorenoscopy with stone lithotripsy to mainstream urology operating rooms across the world. Now with modern URS, many of these "traditional factors" are no longer important—i.e., knowing the stone mineral composition is no longer an essential element in treatment decision-making as the holmium laser is capable of fragmenting all stone types. Patient body habitus is also less important, as obesity does little to change access to the patient's urethra or intrarenal anatomy. In light of these differences between URS and SWL, this chapter reviews the literature for ureteroscopic outcomes of intrarenal calculi and further emphasizes the most important factors that determine ureteroscopic outcomes: defining "stone-free" rates (SFRs), kidney stone size, lower pole (LP) kidney stone location, and URS "by default."

R.D. Gonzalez, B.A. • B.K. Canales, M.D., M.P.H. (✉)
Department of Urology, Center for the Study of Lithiasis and Pathological Calcification, University of Florida, 1600 SW Archer Rd, 00247, Gainesville, FL 32610, USA
e-mail: benjamin.canales@urology.ufl.edu

M. Monga (ed.), *Ureteroscopy: Indications, Instrumentation & Technique*, Current Clinical Urology,
DOI 10.1007/978-1-62703-206-3_8, © Springer Science+Business Media New York 2013

Evidence-Based Outcomes: Intrarenal Calculi

Materials and Methods

Relevant studies were identified from electronic databases, including Cochrane Central Register of Controlled Trials (*The Cochrane Library*), MEDLINE 1996–current, and EMBASE 1980–current. Reference lists were also made from urology and nephrology textbooks, review articles, and relevant studies. Search terms included all forms and abbreviations of URS, lithotripsy, lower pole, and nephrolithiasis. Studies were excluded if the language was not English, if published in a non-peer-reviewed journal, if sample size was less than 25 patients, if outcomes pertained solely to ureteral stones, if follow-up protocols were not reported, and/or if stone size data was not correlated to SFR. Ureteral access sheaths as an adjunct to increase SFRs became commonplace in studies published after 2002. Thus, studies prior to 2003 were titled "early series" while those published during or after 2003 were considered "contemporary." Mean stone size as well as SFR were taken directly from manuscript text or calculated from author results (if given). Imaging modality was recorded as well as the author's definition of "insignificant residual" fragments.

Results

We identified 29 published studies pertaining to URS for renal stones. Eleven studies were excluded due to failure to meet our inclusion criteria (see Table 8.1) [2–11]. Dasgupta et al. [4] were excluded due to reporting SFRs for patients with stone sizes <1.0 cm, 1–2 cm, and >2 cm without listing how many patients belonged to each group, thus making extrapolation unverifiable. Menezes et al. [3] were excluded due to limited number of patients in series ($N=22$) and because stone size and stone location (ureteric vs. renal) were not specified within the text. Chung et al. [6] compared percutaneous nephrolithotomy (PCNL) vs. URS for stones 1–2 cm but were excluded due to a very small intrarenal lithiasis cohort ($n=12$). The remaining studies were excluded due to small patient number (Table 8.1).

Table 8.1 Studies excluded from EBM review

Author	Reason for exclusion
Elbahnasy [2]	$N=13$
Menezes [3]	$N=22$
Dasgupta [4]	SFR for stone size not reported and unclear follow-up protocol
Breda [5]	$N=15$
Chung [6]	$N=12$
Ferrandino [7]	Not peer reviewed
Lahme [8]	Not peer reviewed
Riley [29]	$N=22$
Sejiny [9]	Stone series within calyceal diverticula
Desai [10]	$N=18$
Yili [11]	$N=13$

Key: *N* number of patients in study; *SFR* stone-free rate

A total of 18 studies with 1,362 patients met our inclusion criteria, including 566 patients in early series (Table 8.2) and 796 in contemporary series (Table 8.3). Of these, 90 patients were the result of "prospective" series with SFRs based on CT scan follow-up (see Table 8.3). Both of these (prospective randomized controlled trial Pearle et al. [12] and prospective trial Portis et al. [13]) are reviewed in greater detail in discussion section of this chapter. The remaining 16 studies were retrospective in nature and report a wide range of non-standardized follow-up protocols. It is important to note a significant lack of uniformity in outcome reporting among all trials. Therefore, SFRs from these studies were quite variable and have a high potential for bias and unreliability. Seven studies used more than one imaging modality to calculate SFR without stratifying patients per that modality, consequently making results unclear [14–20]. CT was the imaging modality of choice in 4/9 "modern" series (see Table 8.3), while kidneys–ureters–bladder films (KUB) the most common radiograph in the early series (7/9 studies, Table 8.2). Detection of residual stone burdens solely by CT scan was

Table 8.2 Results from early ureteroscopy series

Author	*N*	Mean size (cm)	Imaging modality	Median F/U	SFR	Notes
Fabrizio [20]	100	0.81	KUB, US, IVP	1 and 3 mos	77%	SFR includes 56 patients with concurrent ureteric calculi and includes fragments <3 mm
Grasso [19]	45	>2.0	KUB	3 mos	81%	45 stones (not patients) treated at 3 medical centers; SFR not stratified by center or by patient
Tawfiek [14]	59	0.68	KUB, US	Post-op to 3 mos	80%	Some patients had post-op KUB only as f/u data
El-Anany [16]	30	>2.0	KUB, US	1 mo	77%	Mean stone size NR; SFR includes residual calculi of <2 mm; 17/19 patients were stone free >6 mos
Sofer [30]	56	1.35	KUB	1–2 wks	84%	56/598 had renal stones only; unclear how SFR was calculated
Grasso [22]	90	NR	US	3 mos	82% (<1 cm) 71% (1–2 cm) 65% (>2 cm)	90 lower pole stones (not patients) treated at 3 medical centers; 70/90 stones had f/u data available
Kourambas [15]	34	NR	CT, IVP	3 mos	85%	30/34 patients had LP stones < 1.5 cm
Hollenbeck [23]	60	0.87	KUB	<1 mo	79%	Unclear number of ureteric stones and total follow-up; 21% of patients had stones >1 cm
Schuster [24]	78	0.86	KUB	1 mo	76%	16/72 pts had concomitant ureteral stones

Key: Bold—lower pole stone studies; *N* number of patients in study; *NR* not reported; *F/U* follow-up; *SFR* stone-free rate; *KUB* kidneys–ureters–bladder; *US* ultrasound; *IVP* intravenous pyelogram; *CT* computed tomography; *mo(s)* month(s); *wks* weeks

performed by three groups [12, 13, 21], while CT was combined with a variety of imaging modalities in two studies [15, 18]. Five studies have been published with a focus primarily on ureteroscopic treatment of lower pole stones (Tables 8.2 and 8.3) [12, 15, 22–24]. Four of these studies were published prior to widespread use of ureteral access sheaths in 2003, and two investigated patients who had previously failed SWL and/or had residual stones following PCNL [17, 25].

Using data from Tables 8.2 and 8.3, we created early and contemporary URS, Figs. 8.1 and 8.2. The number of patients was taken from each tabled study and multiplied by their reported SFR. These were summed and divided by total number of patients from all included studies, yielding an average. For example, five studies were reported before 2003 with a mean stone size <1 cm [14, 20, 22–24]. Total patient number multiplied by SFR and divided by total patient number resulted in the following: $[(47 \times 0.94) + (100 \times 0.77) + (59 \times 0.80) + (78 \times 0.76) + (60 \times 0.79)/(47 + 100 + 59 + 78 + 60)]$, equaling 79.9% which rounded to 80% (Fig. 8.1). All reported SFRs are termed "unadjusted" as they are pooled samples from a variety of studies and imaging modalities. Any use of imaging other than strict CT criteria (i.e., studies that combined CT and a variety of other imaging modalities) was termed "multiple imaging modality" or MIM.

Table 8.3 Results from contemporary ureteroscopy series

Author	*N*	Mean size (cm)	Imaging modality	Median F/U	SFR	Notes
Stav [25]	81	0.92	KUB and US	3 wks	46%	24/81 patients with ureteric and renal stones; all patients failed previous SWL
Pearle [12]	32	<1.0	CT	3 mos	50%	Randomized prospective trial comparing SWL and URS
Holland [17]	93	0.91	KUB and US	3 mos	73%	11/93 patients with ureteric and renal stones; 43 patients failed previous SWL; 8 patients failed previous PCNL
Johnson [31]	143	NR	US	3 mos	90% (<1.0 cm) 89 % (1–2 cm) 75% (>2 cm)	*n* = 10 for stones <1 cm, *n* = 100 for stones 1–2 cm, *n* = 33 for stones >2 cm
Portis [13]	33	0.94	CT	1 mo	54%	Prospective trial; 25/58 patients with ureteric and renal stones; SFR based solely on renal stones
Coccuza [21]	44	1.15	CT	2 mos	93%	15/44 patients had ureteric and renal stones; SFR based solely on renal stones
Alcaide [32]	100	1.5	IVP	3 mos	93%	95/128 stones treated were lower pole; 96% of patients had 3 mos follow-up
Hyams [18]	120	2.4	CT, KUB and US	2 mos	47%	Results from 3 different surgeons at 3 different centers; SFR not stratified by center nor imaging modality
Herrera-Gonzalez [27]	125	1.2	URS	Post-op and 1 day	74%	SFR calculated from direct visualization at case end; stone size ranged 2 mm–5 cm

Bold—lower pole stone study; *N* number of patients in study; *NR* not reported; *F/U* follow-up; *SFR* stone-free rate; *KUB* kidneys–ureter–bladder; *US* ultrasound; *IVP* intravenous pyelogram; *CT* computed tomography; *SWL* shock wave lithotripsy; *mo(s)* month(s); *wks* weeks; *URS* ureteroscopy

Outcomes in Ureteroscopy: SFR, Size, Location, and Default

Stone-Free Rate: CT Criteria

Since the advent of minimally invasive surgery, the definition of "success" in the management of kidney stones has undergone a series of transformations. Until the mid-1980s, open or percutaneous surgical series considered any residual stone an operative failure. With the widespread use of SWL in the late 1980s, small "clinically insignificant fragments" became an accepted term, as long as the residual stones were less than 4 or 5 mm in size, asymptomatic, and noninfected. Even today, there remains no consensus within the urologic community as to what constitutes a "clinically insignificant" fragment. Therefore, most urologists agree that attempts should be made to render a patient completely stone-free at the time of the first procedure, as any residual stone fragment may require continued radiological monitoring and may have the potential for future growth or symptoms.

Non-contrast, spiral computed tomography (CT) is the imaging modality of choice in the assessment of urinary stone disease, offering highly specific information such as renal anatomy and stone location, size, and density [26].

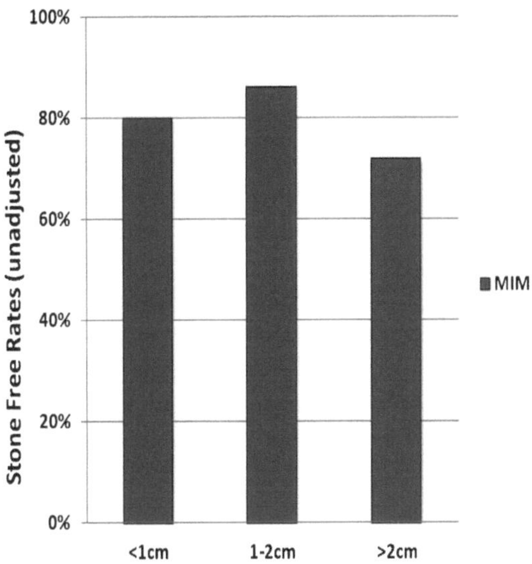

Fig. 8.1 Ureteroscopy stone-free rates, early studies. Average weighted stone-free rates reported by retrospective case series published prior to 2003 using multiple imaging modalities (MIM), including KUB, IVP, US, CT. Stone size <1 cm = 80%, 1–2 cm = 86%, and >2 cm = 72%. SFR includes all studies regardless of patient number in series

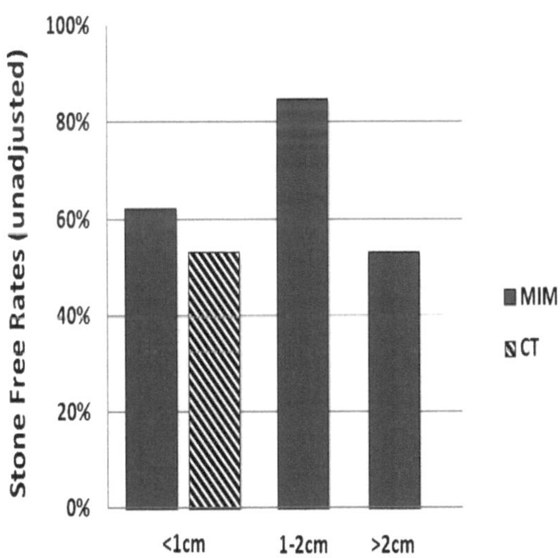

Fig. 8.2 Ureteroscopy stone-free rates, contemporary studies. Average weighted stone-free rates reported from both retrospective and prospective studies published during or after 2003 using either multiple imaging modalities (MIM—including KUB, IVP, US, CT) or strict CT criteria. Stone size <1 cm = 63% (MIM) and 53% (CT), 1–2 cm = 85%, and >2 cm = 53%. SFR includes all studies regardless of patient number in series

This increase in diagnostic accuracy has led to the detection of smaller residual fragments following URS than what was previously seen on intravenous pyelography (IVP), KUB, or renal ultrasound (RUS). One example of how CT can change reporting rates came from Portis et al. [13] (see Table 8.3). The authors of this study reported CT SFR 1 month after URS and stone lithotripsy in 35 patients with renal stones and 23 patients with proximal ureteral stones. They noted a 41% difference in CT SFR when patients were stratified into complete CT SFR (54%) versus residual fragments <4 mm (95%). Had the authors used KUB or RUS, these small fragments would likely have been missed, falsely elevating their reported stone-free success rates. These discrepancies are not trivial when comparing old and new outcomes and highlight the need to apply strict criteria for designing future studies in urologic stone disease.

Stone Size and Other SFR Criteria

Kidney stone size prior to surgery is one of the more reliable ways to stratify patient stone-free outcomes. Traditionally, renal stones are considered small if sized <1 cm, medium if 1–2 cm, and large if >2 cm. These stratifications are based more on cutoffs derived from the SWL literature than actual evidence-based results from URS studies. For URS in general, stone size is typically inversely correlated to success rate—i.e., the larger the stone, the lower the expected success rate. For studies reviewed in this chapter, eight included patients with ipsilateral ureteric stones in their analysis and calculation of SFR, potentially skewing results [13, 17, 19–21, 23–25]. Residual fragments, albeit small, were also occasionally used in the calculation of SFRs [16, 20, 21], and many studies published little as to follow-up protocols and mean/median follow-up range, as evidenced in Tables 8.2 and 8.3. Tawfiek et al. [14] particularly had unclear follow-up data. They used KUBs taken immediately post-op in their follow-up data and reported their success rates after only 1 month, even though "patients were followed postoperatively for a minimum of

3 months." Herrera-Gonzalez et al. [27] calculated their SFR from results of "after an ureteroscopic visualization" immediately post-op. As stated previously, we extrapolated the data from such studies that used a combination of imaging modalities or modalities that were not explicitly CT and represent the added results in Figs. 8.1 and 8.2 with the bars labeled "MIM," or "multiple imaging modalities."

Holland et al. studied URS as a second-line therapy for 51 of their 93 patients (8 having failed PCNL and 43 SWL) and thus are established difficult cases with a potentially negative effect on their SFR [17]. Some studies had to be excluded because of a failure to list adequate data for review. Cocuzza et al. were excluded from Fig. 8.1 and 8.2 because of unclear stratification of stone sizes per patient or SFRs; they reported SFRs of 93.1% but then reported "therapeutic success occurring in 70 and 66% of patients with stone size >15 mm and >20 mm, respectively," without adequate explanation [21]. Fabrizio et al. published SFRs for intrarenal calculi but 56% of their patients had concurrent ureteric stones; SFRs were not stratified to account for those with only renal calculi [20]. Stav et al. had 30% of their patients with concurrent ureteric stones and did not stratify SFR to location, making extrapolation of SFR for only intrarenal stones impossible [25]. Portis et al. studied ureteric, intrarenal, and combination stones and appropriately stratified SFRs for the 29% of patients with sole proximal ureteric stones, as well as the other 10% with combined ureteric and renal stones; their calculated SFR for intrarenal stones is 54% [13]. Grasso et al. did not specify how many patients had combined ureteric and intrarenal stones and instead stratified data by stone burden per location to calculate SFRs [19]. It is also unclear if the same patient database was used in Grasso et al. to study lower pole stone burdens [19, 22]. Because it is unclear, both published results are included here.

Lower Pole Location

Ureteroscopic management of lower pole stones is frequently more challenging than for stones located elsewhere in kidney. Not only can acute infundibular angles make deflection and maneuvering more difficult, but also the passage of accessory instruments through the ureteroscope working channel can reduce active ureteroscope deflection, creating a scenario where a lower pole stone can be visualized but not manipulated [22]. With the advent of newer, smaller flexible endoscopes as well as tipless nitinol stone baskets, many urologists basket and relocate lower pole stones into a more favorable location prior to fragmentation. Kourambas and colleagues describe the use of either a 3.2 F nitinol basket or 2.6 F nitinol grasper in ten cases where access to the lower pole was inhibited by decreased ureteroscopic deflection [15]. Fragmentation was achieved in all ten cases after stones were manipulated into a more favorable location. Schuster and associates reviewed their experience in 78 patients undergoing URS for lower pole stones [24]. Success rates were significantly better in cases where stones were displaced into a more favorable location than in those where lithotripsy was performed in situ. This was statistically significant for stones measuring 1–2 cm, as only 29% of cases in the in situ, lower pole group were successful compared to 100% success in the displacement group.

In perhaps one of the most important papers to date in the management of upper tract stones, Pearle and her associates in the Lower Pole Stone Study Group reported their results of a 19-center trial comparing SWL and flexible URS for the treatment of lower pole calculi less than or equal to 1 cm in diameter (the Lower Pole II study group) [12] (see Table 8.3). In this randomized, prospective trial, 78 patients were enrolled, and 67 remained on protocol with SFR being confirmed with CT scan at 3 months follow-up [12]. At trial end, 35 patients were randomized to URS group with very low attrition (32/35, see Table 8.2). Despite the study's early termination due to poor enrollment and lack of difference between the groups, several outcomes are notable. First, although a trend in higher success for URS cohort was seen, there was no significant difference in SFRs for SWL (35% at 4 months by

CT) vs. URS (50% at 4 months by CT, $p = 0.92$). SWL took significantly less time to complete than URS (66 vs. 90 min) and had fewer intra-operative complications (one non-visualized stone) compared to URS (14% failed lower pole access, 2% ureteral perforation rate). Postoperative complication rates were similar between the groups (23% SWL vs. 21% URS), and no differences were seen in the number of patients requiring retreatment or ancillary treatments. SWL was associated with greater patient acceptance (more rapid return to driving, return to work) and shorter convalescence (8.1 vs. 15.6 days for URS). In total, 90% of patients who underwent SWL would choose the procedure again as opposed to 63% in the URS group ($p < 0.05$). The results of this study would seem to support SWL treatment over URS for lower pole stones 1 cm or less in diameter due to superior patient acceptance and low morbidity although the required numbers calculated to show such a significant difference in stone-free outcomes were not reached. The authors do point out, however, that many of the symptoms encountered by the URS group could be attributed to the presence of a ureteral stent.

As a follow-up to the Lower Pole II study, the Lower Pole Stone Study Group compared URS to PCNL for medium-sized lower pole stones 11–25 mm [28]. This study, published in abstract form only, based outcomes on strict CT criteria. Significant differences were noted between CT SFRs for URS (31% at 4 months) versus PCNL (76% at 4 months) [28]. When "clinically insignificant" fragments were considered, success rates improve to 80% for URS and 100% for PCNL. The difficulties of URS are highlighted by these LP trials. The most obvious is the use of postoperative stents for small LP stones. Stents are responsible for irritative voiding symptoms and are almost always used following access sheath placement for manipulation of upper tract stones. Obviously, more prospective data using validated lower urinary tract questionnaires is needed in this area. Finally, ureteroscope size, flexibility, and design seem to change every 2–3 years. A prospective study that takes longer than this to implement falls well behind the technology curve and could be considered "outdated" before it is even published. However, when taken in context of scarcity of prospective randomized data, this "technology curve" should not deter urologists in the field to undertake solid prospective studies.

Ureteroscopy by Default

When counseling patients about expected outcomes for their specific kidney stone, comparisons are undoubtedly made to SWL and to PCNL. As demonstrated in this review, very little "head-to-head" evidence-based data exists to compare these modalities to URS. The previous section outlined the evidence-based data that does exist, namely, SFR based on CT criteria, stone size, and stone location. However, recall that a good deal of data (too broad to be discussed in this chapter) exists that precludes the use of SWL and PCNL in certain clinical situations. Thus, if SWL and PCNL are precluded or deemed to be less successful, URS becomes indicated "by default." Based on our clinical experience and data from SWL and PCNL studies, we created Table 8.4. The majority of this table includes topics not discussed in this evidence-based review. Nonetheless, we felt that this table was appropriate, as it summarized basic clinical and anatomical patient characteristics that are considered prior to ureteroscopic management of renal stones.

Ureteroscopic anatomic strengths (see Table 8.4) over SWL include access to the entire kidney regardless of stone location (lower pole) and similar success rates regardless of degree of hydronephrosis or distance of kidney from the skin (i.e., in setting of obesity). URS for renal stones during pregnancy or in patients with bleeding diathesis is unusual but would be considered the safest approach, if necessary. SWL success rates decrease in the presence of higher Hounsfield units, previously SWL failures, multiple stones (renal or ureteral), very dense stones (calcium oxalate monohydrate or cystine), and/or radiolucent stones. In these clinical situations, URS or

Table 8.4 Strengths and weaknesses for ureteroscopy in the treatment of kidney stones

	Renal anatomy	Patient/non-renal characteristics	Miscellaneous
Strengths			Radiolucent stone
	STSD >10 cm	Obesity	Failed previous SWL
	Lower pole access	Pregnancy	HU >1,000
	Hydronephrosis	Bleeding diathesis	Concurrent ureteral stone
			All stone compositions
Weaknesses	Inaccessible stone		
	Infundibular stenosis	Urethral stricture	Size >2 cm
	Tight tic ostium	BPH/median lobe	Stent-related urinary symptoms
	Inaccessible kidney		
	Horseshoe kidney	Tight ureter	Convalescence vs. SWL
	UPJO	Ureteral stricture	Complications vs. SWL

STSD skin-to-stone distance; *IP* infundibular pelvic, *IL* infundibular length; *IW* infundibular width, *tic* diverticulum; *UPJO* ureteropelvic junction obstruction; *BPH* benign prostatic hyperplasia; *SWL* shock wave lithotripsy; *HU* Hounsfield unit

PCNL would be considered first line, based on stone size and patient preference (see Table 8.4).

URS is not a panacea. The urologist must be able to access the stone in order to treat it, and a number of upper and lower urinary tract conditions can preclude this (see Table 8.4). These include infundibular stenosis, tight or inaccessible calcyeal diverticuli, ureteral or urethral strictures, or unusual congenital renal anatomy such as horseshoe kidney. Very large median prostate lobes or extremely small caliber ureters can present a clinical challenge to the urologist attempting to cannulate the ureter in the setting of primary URS. Based on our Figures 8.1 and 8.2, stones >2 cm in size have the lowest reported success rates (range 53–72%) and alternative therapies such as PCNL should be considered first-line for these stones, depending on the clinical situation. Last and perhaps most importantly, quality of life may be affected more by URS than other modalities, like SWL. Certainly, ureteral stents following ureteroscopy are associated with uncomfortable lower urinary tract symptoms. As discussed previously, Lower Pole II trial demonstrated longer recovery and convalescence (by 1 week) following URS. Although no significant difference was seen in complication rate, the postoperative complication profile between SWL and URS is certainly different [12]. All these must be taken into consideration when counseling patients on different stone treatment modalities.

Conclusion

While factors such as large stone size and unfavorable stone location lower the success rate of URS, the urologic endoscopist can bravely face these challenges with improved instrumentation and techniques. After reviewing the literature and noting URS' high reported success rates, it is not surprising that the annual number of ureteroscopic procedures for renal stones is rising. However, this evidence-based review has shown that defining ureteroscopic SFRs by MIM, compared to strict computed tomography, reduces the reliability of reported results and affects the urologist's ability to counsel patients on factual expectations compared to SWL or PCNL. Thus, it is important that future URS trials compare matched stone groups while measuring cost-effectiveness, validated postoperative quality of life scores, and SFR by strict CT criteria. Only by carefully designed studies can we increase patient satisfaction while optimizing patient outcomes.

References

1. Kourambas J, Byrne RR, Preminger GM. Does a ureteral access sheath facilitate ureteroscopy? J Urol. 2001;165:789–93.
2. Elbahnasy AM, Shalhav AL, Hoenig DM, et al. Lower caliceal stone clearance after shock wave lithotripsy or ureteroscopy: the impact of lower pole radiographic anatomy. J Urol. 1998;159:676–82.
3. Menezes P, Dickinson A, Timoney AG. Flexible ureterorenoscopy for the treatment of refractory upper urinary tract stones. BJU Int. 1999;84:257–60.
4. Dasgupta P, Cynk MS, Bultitude MF, et al. Flexible ureterorenoscopy: prospective analysis of the Guy's experience. Ann R Coll Surg Engl. 2004;86:367–70.
5. Breda A, Ogunyemi O, Leppert JT, et al. Flexible ureteroscopy and laser lithotripsy for single intrarenal stones 2 cm or greater—is this the new frontier? J Urol. 2008;179:981–4.
6. Chung BI, Aron M, Hegarty NJ, et al. Ureteroscopic versus percutaneous treatment for medium-size (1–2-cm) renal calculi. J Endourol. 2008;22:343–6.
7. Ferrandino MN, Preminger GM. Ureteroscopic management of stones in anomalous kidneys. Arch Ital Urol Androl. 2008;80:18–20.
8. Lahme S, Zimmermanns V, Hochmuth A, et al. Stones of the upper urinary tract. Update on minimal-invasive endourological treatment. Arch Ital Urol Androl. 2008;80:13–7.
9. Sejiny M, Al-Qahtani S, Elhaous A, et al. Efficacy of flexible ureterorenoscopy with holmium laser in the management of stone-bearing caliceal diverticula. J Endourol. 2010;24:961–7.
10. Desai MM, Grover R, Aron M, et al. Robotic flexible ureteroscopy for renal calculi: initial clinical experience. J Urol. 2011;186:563–8.
11. Yili L, Yongzhi L, Ning L, et al. Flexible ureteroscopy and holmium laser lithotripsy for treatment of upper urinary tract calculi in patients with autosomal dominant polycystic kidney disease. Urol Res. 2011;40(1):87–91.
12. Pearle MS, Lingeman JE, Leveillee R, et al. Prospective, randomized trial comparing shock wave lithotripsy and ureteroscopy for lower pole caliceal calculi 1 cm or less. J Urol. 2005;173:2005–9.
13. Portis AJ, Rygwall R, Holtz C, et al. Ureteroscopic laser lithotripsy for upper urinary tract calculi with active fragment extraction and computerized tomography followup. J Urol. 2006;175:2129–33.
14. Tawfiek ER, Bagley DH. Management of upper urinary tract calculi with ureteroscopic techniques. Urology. 1999;53:25–31.
15. Kourambas J, Delvecchio FC, Munver R, et al. Nitinol stone retrieval-assisted ureteroscopic management of lower pole renal calculi. Urology. 2000;56:935–9.
16. El-Anany FG, Hammouda HM, Maghraby HA, et al. Retrograde ureteropyeloscopic holmium laser lithotripsy for large renal calculi. BJU Int. 2001;88:850–3.
17. Holland R, Margel D, Livne PM, et al. Retrograde intrarenal surgery as second-line therapy yields a lower success rate. J Endourol. 2006;20:556–9.
18. Hyams ES, Munver R, Bird VG, et al. Flexible ureterorenoscopy and holmium laser lithotripsy for the management of renal stone burdens that measure 2 to 3 cm: a multi-institutional experience. J Endourol. 2010;24:1583–8.
19. Grasso M, Conlin M, Bagley D. Retrograde ureteropyeloscopic treatment of 2 cm or greater upper urinary tract and minor Staghorn calculi. J Urol. 1998;160:346–51.
20. Fabrizio MD, Behari A, Bagley DH. Ureteroscopic management of intrarenal calculi. J Urol. 1998;159:1139–43.
21. Cocuzza M, Colombo Jr JR, Cocuzza AL, et al. Outcomes of flexible ureteroscopic lithotripsy with holmium laser for upper urinary tract calculi. Int Braz J Urol. 2008;34:143–9. discussion 149–150.
22. Grasso M, Ficazzola M. Retrograde ureteropyeloscopy for lower pole caliceal calculi. J Urol. 1999;162:1904–8.
23. Hollenbeck BK, Schuster TG, Faerber GJ, et al. Flexible ureteroscopy in conjunction with in situ lithotripsy for lower pole calculi. Urology. 2001;58:859–63.
24. Schuster TG, Hollenbeck BK, Faerber GJ, et al. Ureteroscopic treatment of lower pole calculi: comparison of lithotripsy in situ and after displacement. J Urol. 2002;168:43–5.
25. Stav K, Cooper A, Zisman A, et al. Retrograde intrarenal lithotripsy outcome after failure of shock wave lithotripsy. J Urol. 2003;170:2198–201.
26. Smith RC, Rosenfield AT, Choe KA, et al. Acute flank pain: comparison of non-contrast-enhanced CT and intravenous urography. Radiology. 1995;194:789–94.
27. Herrera-Gonzalez G, Netsch C, Oberhagemann K, et al. Effectiveness of single flexible ureteroscopy for multiple renal calculi. J Endourol. 2011;25:431 5.
28. Kuo R, Lingeman J, Leveillee R, et al. A randomized clinical trial of ureteroscopy and percutaneous nephrolithotomy for lower pole stones between 11 and 25 mm. J Endourol. 2003;17:A31.
29. Riley JM, Stearman L, Troxel S. Retrograde ureteroscopy for renal stones larger than 2.5 cm. J Endourol. 2009;23:1395–8.
30. Sofer M, Watterson JD, Wollin TA, et al. Holmium:YAG laser lithotripsy for upper urinary tract calculi in 598 patients. J Urol. 2002;167:31–4.
31. Johnson GB, Portela D, Grasso M. Advanced ureteroscopy: wireless and sheathless. J Endourol. 2006;20:552–5.
32. Cansino Alcaide JR, Reinoso Elbers J, Lopez Sanchez D, et al. Flexible ureterorenoscopy (URS): technique and results. Arch Esp Urol. 2010;63:862–70.

Part III

Instrumentation for Ureteroscopy

Flexible Ureteroscopes: Fiberoptic and Digital

9

Vincent G. Bird

Introduction

In 1912 Young and McKay passed a rigid cystoscope into the ureter of a young boy with posterior urethral valves [1]. It is from this point that ureteroscopy began its long evolutionary course.

During this course both concept and design have changed a number of times to give us the flexible ureteroscopes we have today.

In time, with further refinements, rigid ureteroscopy opened up an entire new realm of possibility for approach to upper urinary tract pathologies. The rod lens optical systems that accompanied the rigid ureteroscope allowed for ever-improved visualization; however rigid ureteroscopes could not be torqued or deflected in any substantial way so as to allow reliable advancement of these ureteroscopes through tortuous anatomy and the renal calyceal system. Though the skilled ureteroscopist may optimize the use of semirigid ureteroscopes in cases of difficult anatomy, one must be careful that even in these cases, advancement of these ureteroscopes can result in inadvertent patient injury. Furthermore, in such cases, the semirigid ureteroscope can be bent and significantly damaged. As such, the semirigid scope cannot be practically used for treatment of pathologies in the renal pelvis and calyces. For these cases a ureteroscope with an articulating/deflecting nature would be required. Such ureteroscopes must also have reasonable "flexibility" and "give," so as not to cause undue damage to the kidney and ureter. For some time the construction of a flexible ureteroscope with such qualities eluded engineers. Nonetheless, Marshall first described the use of a flexible ureteroscope in 1964 [2]. The earliest flexible ureteroscopes were used only for diagnostic purposes. With subsequent addition of working channels, these ureteroscopes were used in a more active and therapeutic role [3]. Successive generations of engineering have produced ureteroscopes with narrower shaft diameters and greater distal tip active deflection. Later generation flexible ureteroscopes are also capable of secondary passive deflection, accomplished by creation of a second flexible segment of the shaft of the ureteroscope just proximal to the more distal active mechanism. The secondary point of deflection can serve as a new platform where then more distal deflection may be accomplished. One key purpose of the secondary mechanism is to allow the scope to be maneuvered in such that entry into the lower pole calyces is possible.

With smaller caliber and these combined deflective mechanisms, both factors that significantly facilitate passage of these scopes, currently

V.G. Bird, M.D. (✉)
Minimally Invasive Surgery Division, Urology Department, University of Florida College of Medicine, Gainesville, FL, USA

Minimally Invasive Surgery Division, Urology Department, Shand's Hospital, University of Florida, Gainesville, FL, USA
e-mail: vincent.bird@urology.ufl.edu

M. Monga (ed.), *Ureteroscopy: Indications, Instrumentation & Technique*, Current Clinical Urology, DOI 10.1007/978-1-62703-206-3_9, © Springer Science+Business Media New York 2013

available flexible ureteroscopes can now generally be advanced into all portions of the kidney and its associated calcyceal anatomy for treatment of a number of pathologies [4–6].

Required Components for Flexible Ureteroscope

The critical elements for successful construction of a modern-day working flexible ureteroscope include ability to acquire and transmit an image, ability to transmit or produce light sufficient for imaging, functional working channels for use of ancillary devices, adequate channel capacity for irrigation, ability to have active control maneuverability of the scope, and small shaft caliber. At first consideration of all of these elements, the task of design and construction certainly appears quite daunting. Early models of these ureteroscopes still had drawbacks, in terms of deflectability and caliber of working channels. Very tortuous and the well-known "lower pole" of the kidney would still oftentimes reveal the limitations of these ureteroscopes. Nonetheless, a number of technological innovations and improvements have made the realization of flexible ureteroscopes quite possible, with each successive generation of ureteroscope an improvement upon the last.

A thorough understanding of the construction of the flexible ureteroscope is critical in understanding how to properly use the instruments, in terms of understanding their capabilities, limitations, optimization of use, and their care, as these instruments, due to their small caliber and fragile nature, are prone to damage.

Fiberoptic Flexible Ureteroscopes

One of the largest hurdles to overcome with flexible ureteroscopy is provision of image and light transmission. This was first overcome with the advent and improvements in fiberoptic technology.

The evolution and nature of fiberoptic technology play a key role in the history and evolution of flexible ureteroscopy. Having an understanding of this technology is essential to the understanding of how fiberoptic flexible ureteroscopes are designed, used, degraded, and damaged.

Adequate transfer of light for proper visualization is critical to medical examination, as it is for a number of other related endeavors. The earliest forms of light transfer were in the form of head-mounted mirrors for reflection of sunlight, oil wick lamps, and incandescent light bulbs [7]. Application of continually evolving methods of illumination was employed in early rod lens rigid endoscopes. However, in the case of flexible endoscopes, light would need to follow a curve. The concepts key to the development of fiberoptics began 160 years ago, when Daniel Colladon, a professor of Physics at the University of Geneva, illuminated a fluid dynamics display for his class. As the lecture hall was poorly illuminated, he decided to focus sunlight through a lens into a tank of water that emptied into a cistern with holes in it. To great surprise, the light illuminated the water jets emanating through the holes of the tank. Essentially the light rays became trapped in the fluid by internal reflection and traveled through the arc of water [7, 8]. The critical observation here was that light, previously thought to only travel in a straight line, could be made to follow a curve [9]. Concurrently Jacque Babinet, who specialized in optics, also demonstrated that light could similarly be guided through bent glass rods [7, 10]. The British physicist John Tyndall replicated and further popularized these findings and is often credited development of theory relating to internal reflection and light guiding, likely due to limited communication and dissemination of ideas during the time period [11]. Thus, the foundation for fiberoptics was born. From this point, physicists continued development of this process by passing light through modified glass materials. Ultimately engineers developed arrays of flexible glass fibers that could guide light. These bare fibers were later covered with a transparent cladding of low refractive index to protect the reflection surface from light contamination and to reduce cross contamination between fibers. These refinements culminated in high-quality fibers capable of more powerful light transmission.

Use of fiberoptics for flexible endoscopy in the medical field began in the 1950s with development of the gastroscope by Basil Hirschowitz [12]. The feasibility of flexible ureteroscopes was demonstrated by Victor Marshall in the early 1960s [2]. Further miniaturization of these scopes has led to the most recent generation of fiberoptic scopes available today.

Working Paradigm

The common working paradigm for available fiberoptic flexible ureteroscopes is fairly similar, though different manufacturers may point out manufacturer-specific unique features and variations in basic construct. The ureteroscope consists of a handle with an eye piece and a long flexible shaft. The shaft contains both fibers for transmission of image and for transmission of light. The arrangement of bundles in ureteroscopes of different manufacture varies slightly in this respect. The fibers transmit the image to the more proximally located lens and eyepiece. Deflection is accomplished by means of a lever/pulley mechanism that may operate with either intuitive or counterintuitive deflection. The handle also includes ports of variable configuration that allow for working elements to be passed down a channel that travels through the shaft to the tip. This same mechanism allows for irrigant to pass in a similar manner. For this reason, as is well known to many users, irrigant flow may be decreased to variable degree depending on what working elements are being passed through the working channel.

Current Fiberoptic Flexible Ureteroscopes

A number of fiberoptic flexible ureteroscopes from a variety of manufacturers are now available for use. These ureteroscopes are summarized in Table 9.1, along with a number of commonly noted parameters, notably caliber along their shaft, degree and direction of deflection, working length, and diameter of working channels. Distal tip/proximal shaft diameter is variable along the working length of the scope, and is reported in a variable fashion to a degree. Ureteroscope specifications are given as stated by the manufacturer.

Many of the currently available fiberoptic flexible ureteroscopes are upgraded and enhanced version of prior models, and as such one must pay particular attention to the precise model in question. The most recent generation fiberoptic flexible ureteroscopes are described here. Though some

Table 9.1 Fiberoptic flexible ureteroscopes

Manufacture	Model	Working length (cm)	Tip diameter (Fr)	Proximal shaft diameter	Deflection up/down degrees	Channel diameter (Fr)
Gyrus ACMI	DUR 8E[a]	64	6.75	10.1	170/180	3.6
Gyrus ACMI	DUR-8 Ultra[a]	67.5	8.6	9.3 (avg)	270/270	3.6
Olympus	URF-P5[b]	70	8.4	8.4	180/275	3.6
Storz	Flex X2[c]	67.5	7.0	8.5	270/270	3.6
Stryker	Flex Vision U-500[d]	64	6.9	–	275/275	3.6
Wolf	Viper (7325. 076)[e]	68	6.0	8.8	270/270	3.6
Wolf	Cobra (7326.076)[e]	68	6.0	9.9	270/270	3.3/3.3

[a]Gyrus ACMI (Gyrus ACMI is now a business division of Olympus)
[b]Olympus Surgical, Orangeburg NY, USA
[c]Karl storz, Tuttlingen, Germany
[d]Stryker Endoscopy, San Jose CA, USA
[e]Richard Wolf Endoscopy, Vernon Hills, IL, USA

prior generation ureteroscopes are still in use, they are not described in detail here, as most are no longer produced, though they still may be serviced by the manufacturer. One must be mindful that active deflection will be affected to a variable degree by working elements placed through the working channel. Though newer generations of flexible ureteroscopes generally prove to have better irrigant flow [13], this parameter will also be affected to a variable degree by introduced working elements.

At the current time a large number of the most recent generation of fiberoptic-based flexible ureteroscopes are still in use, and a large portion of the data available regarding flexible ureteroscopes involves these ureteroscopes. Though these ureteroscopes are more commonly being replaced with their digital counterparts, a thorough understanding of these ureteroscopes is important in that studies of these ureteroscopes reveal a number of issues that impact the use and durability of ureteroscopes in a large number of ways. It is likely that a number of these findings will also facilitate improvements in digital flexible ureteroscopes. Though digital flexible ureteroscopes have a different operative paradigm in terms of optics and image production, many mechanical and structural features of these ureteroscopes remain quite similar to their fiberoptic counterparts.

There are also a number of other qualities and parameters that most manufactures generally allude to in description of these ureteroscopes. For example, the various manufacturers state that the working shaft of their flexible ureteroscope is coated with a type of proprietary coating or polymer that allows for expeditious and easy passage of the scope. They also all state that the efforts have been made to make the shaft crush resistant and torque stable during rotation of the scope. Nonetheless, some notable specific points about some of these flexible ureteroscopes are worthy of note.

The Gyrus ACMI (now a business division of Olympus) DUR 8 Elite ureteroscope has two points of active deflection, accomplished by use of a second lever that provides deflection of the scope more proximal on the shaft. The active secondary deflection adds 130° down. It has also been equipped with a moiré reduction filter. Moiré patterns are often an undesired artifact of images produced by various imaging techniques.

The Gyrus ACMI (now a business division of Olympus) DUR 8 Ultra has been created as a successor to the DUR 8 Elite. This ureteroscope is a hybrid of Olympus and ACMI technologies. The ureteroscope has been enhanced so that it has 270° up and down deflection. It has also been equipped with a moiré reduction filter. The manufacturer also claims that construction of this ureteroscope has also been improved such that it has improved endurance with commonly used sterilization methods.

The Olympus URF-P5 is also an enhanced version of prior Olympus fiberoptic flexible ureteroscopes. This ureteroscope has a 5.3 Fr beveled or bullet-shaped tip. This scope also has an incorporated moiré reduction filter to enhance image and provide a clearer picture. The deflective portion of the shaft is also covered with thicker rubber to resist potential puncturing (Fig. 9.1).

The Storz FLEX X2 ureteroscope is similar to its predecessor FLEX X scope in many aspects. Due to general concern regarding laser damage for all flexible ureteroscopes, this ureteroscope was enhanced with addition of a material laserite™ at its distal tip, in an attempt to make this portion of the ureteroscope more resistant to potential laser-induced damage.

Stryker offers the Flexvision U-500 fiberoptic flexible ureteroscope. Fiberoptic-based image quality relates in part to fiber number and density. This ureteroscope has been fitted with high-density fiber bundles in an effort to further improve image quality.

Richard Wolf produces the Wolf Viper and a more advanced flexible ureteroscope, the Wolf Cobra, which features dual channels for simultaneous use of two devices, such as a laser and a basket or a backstop. The dual 3.3 Fr. channels accommodate continuous irrigation capabilities with increased flow. The Cobra also includes an ergonomic laser dial with an integrated locking mechanism to advance the laser fiber and minimize laser damage, Figs. 9.2 and 9.3.

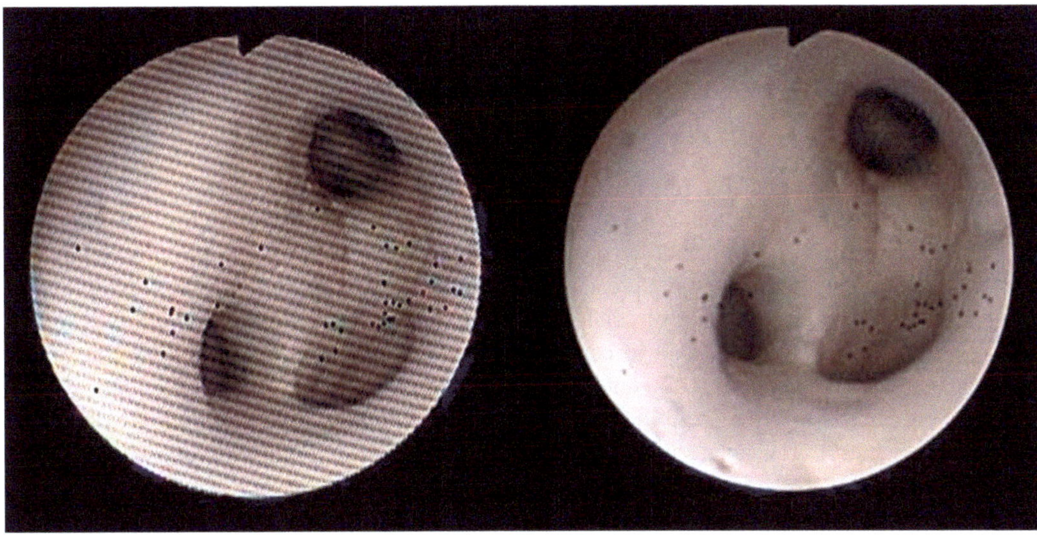

Fig. 9.1 Image through a fiberoptic ureteroscope showing moire effect and image after moire filtering. Also note that a number of fibers have been broken (courtesy of Olympus)

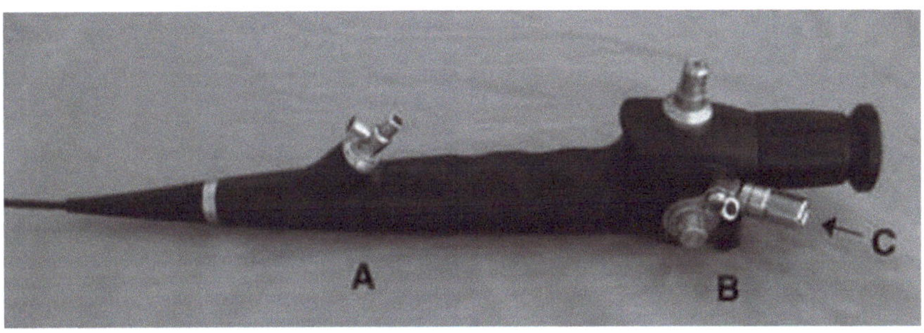

Fig. 9.2 Cobra dual-channel ureteroscope demonstrating two working channels (A, B) with laser advancement channel (B) being of longer length and optionally supported by thumb-operated laser advancement wheel (C) (thumb device not pictured). From [25], reprinted with permission from Mary Ann/Liebert Inc. Publishers

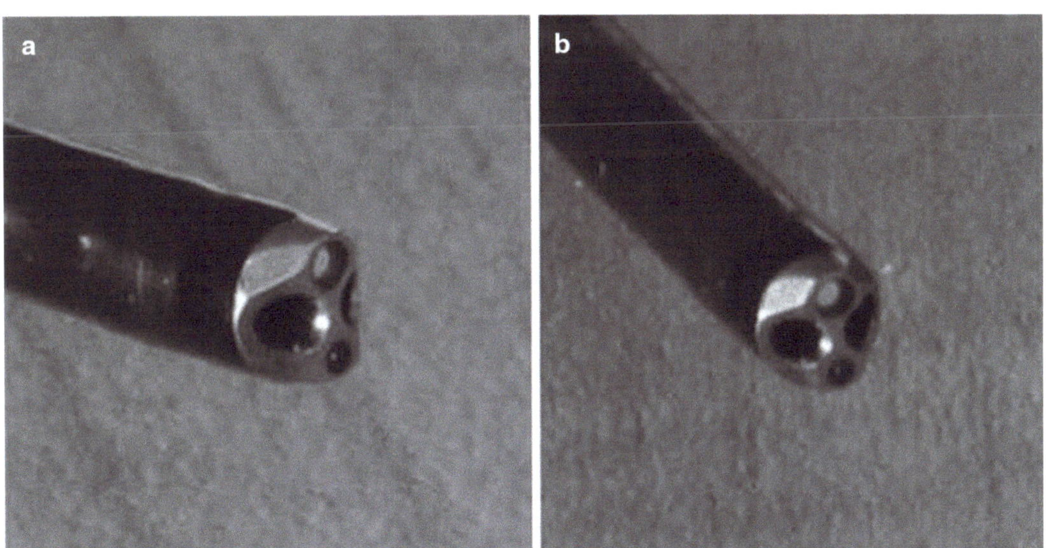

Fig. 9.3 Beveled tip of the dual-channel handle Cobra ureteroscope. From [25], reprinted with permission from Mary Ann/Liebert Inc. Publishers

Digital Ureteroscopes

Beyond doubt, the introduction of fiberoptic flexible ureteroscopes revolutionized urologic practice for management of upper urinary tract pathologies. Nonetheless, despite widespread use with these ureteroscopes, a number of concerns persist. Fiberoptic ureteroscopes tend to have a grainy image, water may leak into the lens, and fibers may burn out and fracture, resulting in loss of image quality [14]. The image produced by fiberoptic flexible ureteroscopes is not as sharp as that of a rod lens semirigid ureteroscope due to the smaller number of pixels in the flexible instrument's image, when compared to (a) rod/lens semirigid ureteroscopes [15]. Image quality may be improved by increasing the diameter of the flexible ureteroscope, but this is likely to increase the risk of failure of access to the upper urinary tract and decreased flexibility [16, 17]. Thus, strong impetus was present for improvement of available flexible ureteroscopes.

Digital Imaging

In order to avoid the operation-related weaknesses of film cameras, digital imaging was developed in the 1960s and 1970s. The impetus at that time was primarily for scientific and military use. In 1970, Boyle and Smith developed the charge-coupled device (CCD). This chip could store data in the form of electrical charges within a grid for subsequent retrieval [18, 19]. These grids could be stored as pixels [20]. The complementary metal oxide semiconductor (CMOS), a lower cost alternative to the CCD chip, was developed during the same time period. In addition to lower cost, the CMOS chip had the advantage of reduced device size and suitability for mass production [21]. Subsequent improvements and modifications of this technology resulted in real-time digital imaging. Evolution of this technology also suggests that successive generations of these chips will be further miniaturized.

Working Paradigm

The key paradigm change with digital flexible ureteroscopes is the "chip on tip" design, where an image is picked up, at times processed, then transmitted by a digital sensor, and sent to a proximal point via a single wire, where further processing and transmission take place. This arrangement bypasses the fragile optical fiber system of conventional fiberoptic flexible ureteroscopes. This arrangement may also include a distal more luminous light source built into the ureteroscope itself.

The specific configuration and operative paradigm of available digital ureteroscopes vary in certain aspects. The DUR D and Storz Flex XC flexible ureteroscopes have distally located light-emitting diode (LED) light source and a distally located CMOS chip that picks up and processes images. The Olympus URF V digital ureteroscope has a light source that is transmitted from a proximal source and a CCD chip that picks up images and transmits the data to a proximal source for processing. At the current time, it is of unknown significance what these different arrangements will mean for long-term scope operation, durability, and chance for malfunction/catastrophic failure.

Currently Available Digital Ureteroscopes

The aforementioned digital ureteroscopes are now available for use. Their general specifications can be seen in Table 9.2. Due to design changes these ureteroscopes are all lighter than their fiberoptic counterparts. They generally retain the non-optical related improvements in ureteroscope structure and composition available in their fiberoptic counterparts. All available digital ureteroscopes provide high-quality digital imaging, autofocusing capabilities, and digital magnification, which improve the user experience. The overall experience with digital ureteroscopes is growing, but is still somewhat limited.

Table 9.2 Currently available digital flexible ureteroscopes

Manufacture	Model	Working length (cm)	Tip diameter (Fr)	Proximal shaft diameter	Deflection up/down degrees	Channel diameter (Fr)	Light source/chip
Olympus-Gyrus ACMI	Invisio DUR D[b]	65	8.7	9.3	250/250	3.6	LED/CMOS chip
Olympus	URF-V[b]	67	8.5	9.9	180/275	3.6	Fiber/CCD chip
Storz	FLEX XC[a]	70	8.6	8.5	270/270	3.6	LED/CMOS chip

[a]Karl Storz, Tuttlingen, Germany
[b]Olympus Surgical, Orangeburg NY, USA

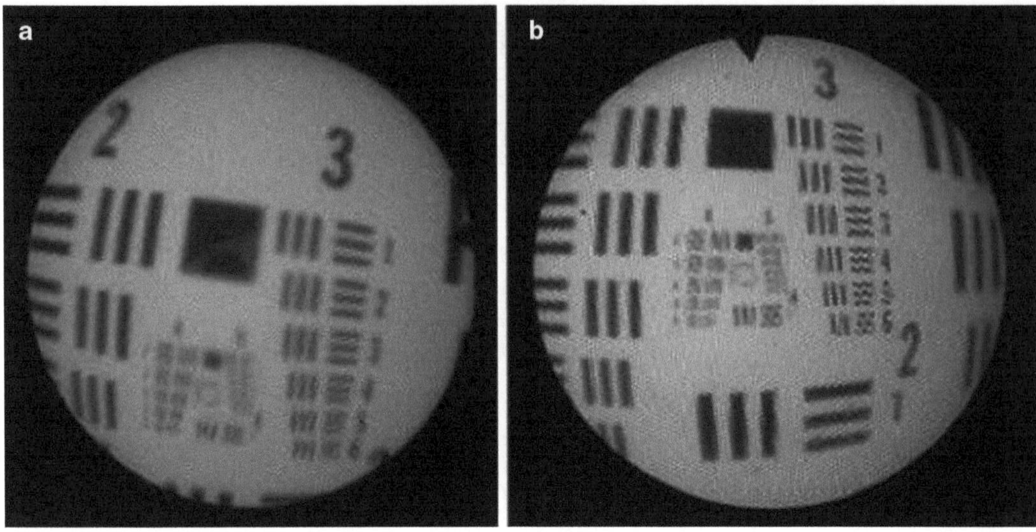

Fig. 9.4 (**a**) A photograph of the 1951 USAF test pattern card using the DUR-8 fiberoptic ureteroscope. (**b**) A photograph of the 1951 USAF test pattern card using the DUR-D digital ureteroscope. From [14], reprinted with permission from Mary Ann/Liebert Inc. Publishers

The Gyrus ACMI Invisio DUR D was the first digital flexible ureteroscope. The unique features of this ureteroscope are as aforementioned. The format of the hand piece, deflective mechanism, working port, and channels is relatively similar to its fiberoptic counterpart. The tip of the scope contains the dual LED light carriers and a 1-mm digital camera. The LED light can last for up to 10,000 h, which is significantly longer than more expensive xenon light sources. The ureteroscope has a configuration such that it is simply plugged in and ready for use. Of interest, the two aforementioned technological advances significantly reduce the weight of the scope (DUR D 505g, DUR 8E 1012g). Internalization of the light source also reduces risks of burning or fires. This ureteroscope also has a laser fiber detection system (IDC-1500-endoscope protection system) which can detect when the blue coating of a laser fiber is retracted within the ureteroscope and alert the operator. This option can be used to automatically disable (place on standby) the laser generator, with the goal of preventing laser-induced ureteroscope damage [14].

Though image quality is somewhat difficult to quantitate and qualify, the quality of the digital image that accompanies digital flexible ureteroscopy is notably improved. The DUR D allows digital magnification to 135%. Andonian et al. [14] compared the DUR 8 and DUR D ureteroscopes with test cards (USAF test pattern card), demonstrating a brighter image and higher resolution with the DUR D (Fig. 9.4).

The Olympus digital flexible ureteroscope, URF-V, is also available and currently in use. As aforementioned, this digital ureteroscope contains a CCD chip and has light transmitted from a proximal source. This scope also is fitted with moiré reduction capability. This ureteroscope also has narrow band imaging (NBI) capability, which operates by alteration of the white light source to specific wavelength bands, which is useful for observation of mucosal morphology. This modality is currently being used for identification of urothelial carcinoma in a number of settings.

The Storz FLEX XC has also recently become available for use. This digital ureteroscope has a similar design to that of the DUR D in that it contains LED and CMOS technology. A notable difference with this digital ureteroscope is that it retains a relatively low caliber shaft along its working length. The FLEX XC, like its most recent fiberoptic counterpart, is equipped with laserite™.

Comparison of Flexible Ureteroscopes

A number of different parameters of flexible ureteroscopes have been compared in a variety of fashions. However, comparison of these ureteroscopes must be viewed with caution. Individual investigators generally investigate only what is available to them. Most manufacturers, as previously stated, have also produced a number of successive models of their fiberoptic flexible ureteroscopes, and comparison of available models, available to investigators in a time staggered fashion, is also quite variable. The availability of digital ureteroscopes has only further confounded this issue, with both fiberoptic and digital ureteroscopes included in some studies that do not necessarily focus on optics. As such, both fiberoptic and digital scopes are assessed together in many respects. However, differentiation of these two types of scopes will be noted. Investigators may also have different degrees of experience with the ureteroscopes available for study. Variability in results may also occur due to investigative methods used. In summary there are few all-inclusive direct comparison studies. Nonetheless, a brief survey of these investigations is worthwhile in that it lends further understanding into the features and limitations of these ureteroscopes.

Studies involving flexible ureteroscopes themselves (not clinical outcomes associated with their use) are generally one of the two types: a comparison of working parameters (optical/mechanical) of the ureteroscopes and overall durability of the ureteroscopes. A large number of studies have been performed on successive generations of fiberoptic flexible ureteroscopes. Representative studies to point out key features and differences, and studies including a large number or representative types of available ureteroscopes at any given time, are summarized here to give the reader an overall picture of how these ureteroscopes generally compare with one another. Studies relating to ureteroscopes still in use were also used in selection. The key findings of these studies are noted. The detailed methodologies used are beyond the purview of this review.

Experience in flexible ureteroscopy has made evident that irrigation flow and related quality of vision certainly are a critical issue, and as such, this specific issue has received due attention. Bach et al. [17], in 2008, evaluated the effects of tools and probes on deflection angle and irrigation flow in five unloaded and instrument-loaded (273 μm laser fiber, 2.4–3.0 Fr biopsy forceps, and tipless nitinol baskets 1.5–2.4 Fr) flexible ureteroscopes, Wolf Viper, Storz FLEX X2, ACMI DUR 8 Elite, ACMI DUR D, and Olympus URF P5, and noted that deflection had no influence on unloaded scope flow rates and baskets had no influence on the maximum angle of deflection. Laser fibers and biopsy forceps lead to loss of deflection (laser fiber 4.44–10.21%; biopsy forceps 30.7–57.8%). Flow rates depended on the size of the working device introduced. Loss of irrigation volume ranged from 62.24 (1.5 Fr) to 99.1% (3.0 Fr). The laser fiber reduced irrigation volume by 53.7%. This study summarizes and outlines well that irrigation flow, loss of deflection, and intraoperative visualization are dependent on the working devices used. Another very important point here is that improvements in ancillary devices, such as smaller nitinol baskets, can help minimize the impact of these devices on ureteroscope function and performance. Indeed, other studies also corroborate that newer smaller caliber baskets have significantly less effects on deflection or irrigation [22]. One must also bear in mind that as smaller diameter ancillary devices are created, working channel caliber of successive generations of ureteroscopes has also been somewhat improved (Figs. 9.5 and 9.6).

Bach et al. [23] investigated the impact of working tools on light transmission, by measuring the time needed to irrigate clear an inked medium, as an objective measurement of visibility. Wolf Viper, Wolf Cobra, Storz FLEX X2, Olympus URF P5, and Olympus ACMI DUR 8 Elite unloaded and instrument-loaded (1.7 Fr basket, 2.2 Fr basket, and 273 μm laser fiber) ureteroscopes were compared. The dual-channel Wolf Cobra had the fastest restoration of light transmission. The authors also noted that the Olympus URF P5, with the longest working channel, needed the longest irrigation time to

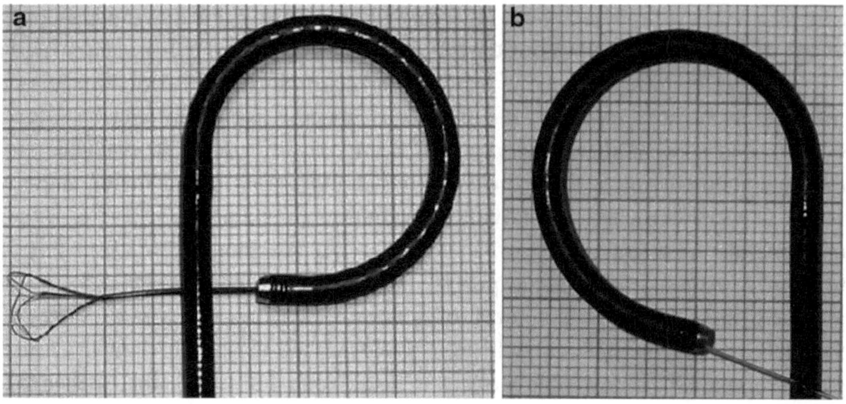

Fig. 9.5 (**a**) Viper (Richard Wolf) with 1.5-Fr NGage basket (Cook). (**b**) Viper (Richard Wolf) with 273-μm laser fiber (FlexiFib, Lisa Laser): loss of deflection (7.41%) and increased diameter (+1 mm) can be seen. From [17], reprinted with permission from Mary Ann/Liebert Inc. Publishers

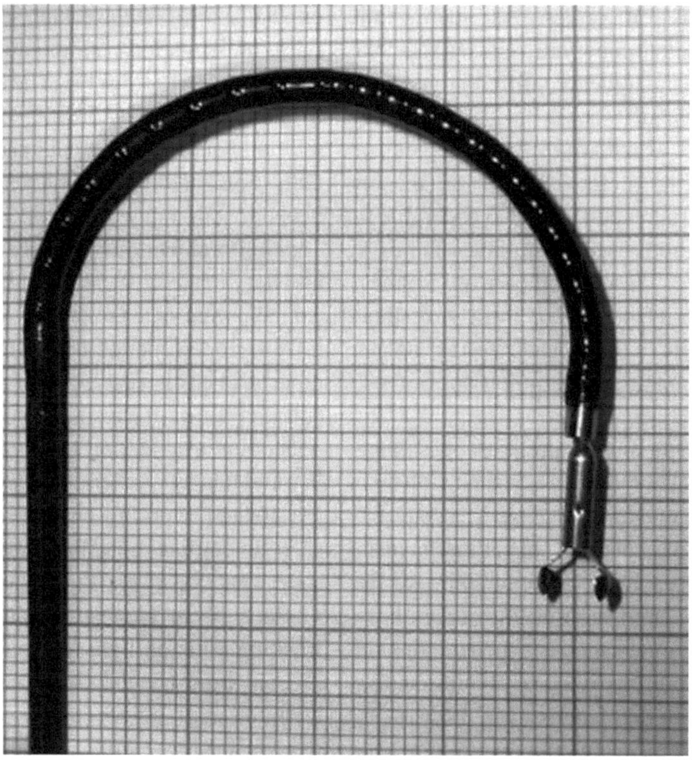

Fig. 9.6 Flex X2 (Karl Storz) with 2.4-Fr BIGopsy biopsy forceps (Cook): loss of deflection and increase of inner diameter can be seen. From [17], reprinted with permission from Mary Ann/Liebert Inc. Publishers

restore light transmission. These similar results were further corroborated with the inserted devices. The important observation in this study with a very sensitive methodology is that time needed to restore light transmission, i.e., to have good visualization, depends to a degree on working tool size and length of the working channel.

Kruck et al. [24] studied five ureteroscopes with 3.6 Fr working channels, the Wolf, Storz Flex X2 and Flex XC, and Olympus ACMI DUR

D and Olympus URF P5, in terms of irrigation flow in correlation to different deflection angles (0°, 90°, and 180°) and use of 1.9 Fr stone baskets. Mean flow rates without and with an inserted 1.9 Fr basket were noted. The authors noted that the 1.9 Fr basket significantly reduced flow in all five ureteroscopes. Mean flow rates without inserted baskets for all five scopes were fairly similar. With inserted baskets, the ACMI and Wolf ureteroscopes demonstrated the highest flow rate (12 ml/min) and the lowest reduction of flow rate. Measurements after deflection showed no further differences.

The Wolf Cobra ureteroscope is the only dual-channel ureteroscope. Haberman et al. [25] compared this scope to the Wolf Viper scope and noted that the deflection and related flow characteristics for the dual-channel scope were superior when larger or multiple working elements were used through the channels and suggested that such a new configuration may lead to development and implementation of novel endoscopic procedures.

Deflection and ability to manipulate flexible ureteroscopes is also an issue of particular concern. Manufacturers have addressed this concern with production of ureteroscopes with increasingly exaggerated deflection (see up/down deflection parameters in Table 9.1). Monga et al. [26] compared ease of manipulation of four flexible ureteroscopes, Stryker Flexvision U-500, ACMI DUR 8 Elite, Wolf Viper, and Olympus URF-P3, in the hands of eight experienced ureteroscopists, using a model. Operators maneuvered through a designated course. The Olympus URF P3 took the longest to reach the lower pole, of the kidney model and the Wolf Viper was the quickest to reach the mid kidney. Six of the eight endoscopists (all eight had more prior experience with Olympus URF P3 and randomized as to order of scope use during the study) said the Wolf Viper had better ease of manipulation, while 5/8 stated that the Olympus URF P3 was most difficult.

The DUR 8 Elite ureteroscope is the only ureteroscope with two points of active deflection. Ankem et al. [27] evaluated the clinical utility of a dual active deflection ACMI DUR-8 Elite ureteroscope in comparison to the DUR 8, and noted that the dual deflecting DUR-8 Elite ureteroscope may be helpful in cases in which the single deflection flexible instruments failed to access and treat upper urinary tract pathologic findings.

Durability of Flexible Ureteroscopes

The small caliber and deflectability of flexible ureteroscopes, core components to their success, are also of critical concern in regular use and durability of these instruments. Their very nature makes them quite fragile and prone to damage or "wear and tear" through repeated use. The implication here is that costs of damage and maintenance factor significantly into overall cost of ureteroscopy. A number of studies have investigated this issue.

Sung et al. [28] analyzed currently available manufacturer data regarding the character of ureteroscope damage from the four major ureteroscope manufacturers (ACMI, Olympus America, Karl Storz, and Richard Wolf) on the types, speculated causes, costs, and frequency of ureteroscope damage. Frequency of repair increased with decreasing ureteroscope diameter and increasing instrument length. Repair cost was greater for flexible ureteroscopes (mean $4,597versus $2,437 for semirigid ureteroscopes). The major causes of flexible ureteroscope damage were working channel damage from laser burn or instrument passage and extreme scope deflection with an indwelling instrument. Indeed most of the included studies mention laser damage, excessive torque, and damage to the deflection mechanism as common sources of damage.

Afani [29], in 2000, (r) compared early generation flexible ureteroscopes, Storz 11274AA, Circon ACMI AUR 7, Wolf model 7325.172, and Olympus URF-P3, for durability and function. They noted that although luminosity and irrigant flow remained relatively unchanged, active deflection deteriorated 2–28%, and the ureteroscopes were only used for 3–13 h, or 6–15 uses, prior to needing repair. The deflection mechanism was identified as fragile element. The information gained in this early study of these ureteroscopes is actually quite useful in that it served as a reference point for subsequent studies. In 2004 User et al. [30] compared six types of flexible ureteroscopes and found no statistically significant difference between them. In this investigation, 10–34 procedures were performed with the flexible ureteroscopes prior to their requiring major repair.

In 2006 Monga et al. [31] compared the Storz 11274AA and Flex X™, ACMI DUR 8 and DUR™ 8 Elite, Wolf™ models 7330.170 and 7325.172, and the Olympus URF-P3, all 9 Fr diameter and less flexible ureteroscopes, and noted that the DUR™ 8 Elite and Olympus URF-P3 appeared to be the most durable, assessed by average number of uses before repair, average ureteroscope operative time, minutes of use with an instrument in the working channel, average duration of lower pole use, and duration of use before repair.

In another large-scale study Carey et al. [32], studying the ACMI AUR 7, AUR 9, DUR 8 and DUR 8 Elite, and Storz model 11274AA and Flex X ureteroscopes, noted that one of the most important risk factors for predicting the number of uses of a ureteroscope was device age and prior repair of the ureteroscope. Newly acquired ureteroscopes had the best durability. Repeated damage occurred more frequently in ureteroscopes already having undergone repair and this factored into cost of maintenance. Future studies note whether ureteroscopes were newly acquired.

Traxer et al. [33] studied more specific damage that occurred to a Storz Flex X ureteroscope after being used in 50 ureteroscopies. Maximal ventral deflection deteriorated (270° to 208°), maximal dorsal deflection deteriorated (270° to 133°), irrigation flow (100 cm H_2O) decreased from 50 mL/min to 40 mL/min at last procedure, and number of broken mage fibers had reached 6 after 50 procedures. The authors concluded that the need for repair occurs less frequently with newer generation flexible ureteroscopes; however, no direct comparison was made. Nonetheless their findings correlate with those of Carey et al. [32] in that new ureteroscopes have fairly good durability.

Subsequently Knudsen et al. [34] studied (total time of use, number of scope insertions through an access sheath, working time in the lower pole, number of insertions and total time for accessory instrumentation in the working channel, and total laser energy used) newer generation flexible ureteroscopes, which included the Wolf viper, Olympus URF-P5, Gyrus ACMI DUR 8 Elite, and the Stryker FlexVision U-500, all received from the manufacturer and used until requiring major repair. Early catastrophic failure (less than 10 uses) occurred at three sites for the DUR 8 elite, and one site each for the Stryker and Wolf scopes. The Wolf Viper, Olympus URF-P5, and Stryker FlexVision U-500 ureteroscopes were deemed comparable in durability. Fragility of the DUR 8 Elite in this study contrasts to its being found to be most durable in the earlier study by Monga et al. [31] suggesting that other factors may have a role.

Most recently, Al-Qahtani et al. [35] also commented on the wear and tear noted with the use of the URF-V during 60 cases of use; active deflection deteriorated over time (up deflection, mean loss 10.5%, 180° to 161°; down deflection mean loss 21%, 275° to 217°). Subjective quality of the image remained the same throughout the 60 procedures. The authors finally noted that during the 60th procedure the digital flexible ureteroscope was ruptured in an attempt to enter a very narrow and angulated lower pole calyx, pointing to a similar fatigability and fragility of this new flexible ureteroscope.

In comparison of fiberoptic and digital flexible ureteroscopes Al-Qahtani et al. [35] offer three useful parameters for comparison: reliability of optical system, fatigability, and major malfunction that require major repair or replacement of the device. In terms of optical systems, it is already evident that the high-quality images given by digital flexible ureteroscopes are reliable and, for reasons relating to the technology, do not degrade. Crushed/broken fibers noted in the majority of durability studies relating to fiberoptic flexible ureteroscopes, that lead to decreased image brightness and poor image quality due to broken fibers, is simply not an issue.

The "chip on a tip" paradigm with wire transmission proximally has overcome this issue.

Ureteroscope fatigability, commonly noted as loss of deflection, is of great importance in that it may impact success in ureteropyeloscopic treatment of intrarenal/calyceal pathologies, where maneuverability and deflection are critical to the procedure. Pietrow et al. [36], in a study of fiberoptic flexible ureteroscopes, noted a mean of 50.3 passages before losing 25° of active deflection. Afane et al. [29], in their study of flexible fiberoptic ureteroscopes, noted that such scopes experienced 2–28% deterioration in active deflection per procedure. Busby et al. [37] postulated that loss of active deflection more specifically related to prolonged approach to lower calyx pathologies. Al-Qahtani et al. [35] 68 ureteroscope passages, noted a resultant loss of 58 and 19 degrees down and up deflection, respectively, with the Olympus URF-V. As documented in a number of the aforementioned studies, major malfunction generally is related to fractures, perforations, major deflection loss, and severe damage to the optical system. Al-Qahtani et al. [35] noted 60 uses with their newly acquired Olympus URF-V and considered this number to be significantly improved in comparison to previous results with fiberoptic flexible ureteroscopy. However, it is likely that this one finding is not enough to substantiate this claim. As noted by Carey et al. [32], newly acquired ureteroscopes in the hands of experienced ureteroscopists can have good durability. It is certainly reasonable to suspect that both fiberoptic and digital ureteroscope can sustain severe/catastrophic damage from improper advancement of the laser/ancillary devices, laser misfire, excessive torquing, and prolonged extreme deflection and maneuvering in the treatment of lower pole pathologies.

A number of issues relating to durability of flexible ureteroscopes are brought forth from these studies. Flexible ureteroscopes received new have potential for significant durability, though this in itself was variable and suggests that a number factors may be contributory. Ureteral access sheaths (UAS), now used more frequently, may reduce wear and tear on flexible ureteroscopes. Kourambas et al. noted that use of UAS may, in addition to decreasing operative time, extend durability [38].

Prevention of Damage

Laser misfiring is a common source of ureteroscope damage. Seto et al. [39] proposed introduction of the 200 μm laser fiber through a 2 Fr catheter to mitigate against this; however, this does result in diminished irrigant flow. Persistent deflection into the lower pole may result in loosening of the deflection tip cables, resulting in loss of deflection of the ureteroscope, which may be in part unavoidable. Cleaning and processing should be done with great care as flexible ureteroscope may sustain significant damage during the cleaning and handling process by hospital staff [40].

The issue of cleaning and handling of fiberoptic flexible ureteroscopes is difficult to assess in that none of the aforementioned comparative studies directly address this issue. These ureteroscopes may be sterilized in different fashions, and experience of ancillary personnel in cleaning them in association with this process is of unknown significance. Benito et al. [41] prospectively studied the effects of Steris 1™ sterilization and Cidex® ortho-phthalaldehyde high-level disinfection on durability of new-generation Storz Flex X Flexible ureteroscopes received new from the manufacturer. Substantial fiber damage and loss of resolution occurred in the ureteroscope first subjected to Steris 1 sterilization, which essentially rendered the scope in unusable condition. High-level disinfection with Cidex® ortho-phthalaldehyde had minimal impact on overall condition of the second ureteroscope. Despite these findings, most healthcare care institutions have very specific protocols and institutional requirements may influence the nature of sterilization of surgical instruments.

Though many fiberoptic flexible ureteroscopes are now being replaced by their digital counterparts, the information gained throughout the era of fiberoptic flexible ureteroscopes is likely to be quite useful in that will serve as a reference as to how durable digital ureteroscopes prove to be.

As digital ureteroscopes have only more relatively recently been introduced into more regular use, data regarding outcome with them, using a number of assessment parameters, will be forthcoming in the near future.

Future Directions and Considerations

In the evolution of both fiberoptic and digital flexible ureteroscopes much attention has been paid to many of the aforementioned parameters that include issues with the optical systems, functional mechanics, and durability. However, there are other factors, whose degree of impact is yet undetermined that may factor into successful development and use of flexible ureteroscopes.

One such area of interest concerns potential occupational hazards that may exist with performing endourologic procedures/flexible ureteroscopy. This has become more of a concern in that the diagnostic and therapeutic capabilities of flexible ureteroscopy have greatly expanded in recent times. New and advanced applications of flexible ureteroscopy may also be associated with increased operative times. Healy et al. [42] surveyed targeted urologists, who specialize in endourology, and psychiatrists, in both the academic and community settings. Physicians were queried regarding their practice settings and symptoms of hand pain, neuropathy, and/or discomfort. Hand/wrist problems were reported by 39% endourologists compared with 14% psychiatrists. Amongst endourologists, hand/wrist problems were much more prevalent amongst those who preferred counterintuitive ureteroscopic deflection as compared to intuitive deflection (56% versus 27%). The authors hypothesize that difficulty accessing lower pole calyces may explain this finding. Deflection is commonly accomplished with the use of the thumb. Studies show that the thumb naturally flexes, rather than hyperextends [43, 44]. In cases of intuitive deflection some deflection is need to reach the lower pole calyces; however counterintuitive instruments require extreme thumb extension, an ergonomically disadvantageous maneuver, to accomplish the same feat. The majority of respondents (85%) with hand/wrist problems needed either medical or surgical intervention. These findings suggest that the ergonomics involved with the performance of conventional ureteroscopy may have inherent problems and risks. The authors suggest that such findings give impetus to investigation and development of more ergonomic platforms for performance of flexible ureteroscopy. As will be discussed later, robot-assisted ureteroscopy has been promulgated as such an alternative paradigm. This study certainly has limitations that relate to response rate (20.3% endourologists and 12.8% psychiatrists) and other methodology-related issues [42]; nonetheless the study was designed to focus on an issue that specifically relates to flexible ureteroscopy. All major manufacturers offer flexible ureteroscopes with deflection of either design [42].

Though experience to date is limited, digital flexible ureteroscopes have been received quite favorably. They have notably improved image quality, a brighter image, are lightweight, and likely cause less operator-related fatigue.

Ongoing experience will likely reveal the durability and other possible limitations of digital flexible ureteroscopes. Observations to date do point to some areas where improvement and ongoing development may prove beneficial. Al-Qahtani et al. [35] noted in their use of the URF-V, which included both cases of urinary lithiasis and suspected urothelial carcinoma, and included the use of a ureteral access sheath (Cook Flexor 12/14 Fr ID/OD), that the scope had to be replaced in six cases by the thinner URF-P5 where the URF-V failed to access the entire collecting system, which was determined by the authors to be due to its larger diameter at the tip of the ureteroscope (8.4 Fr for URF-V versus 6.9 Fr for the URF-P5). The specific problem noted in all cases was inability to traverse a relatively narrow lower pole infundibulum/calyx. The authors also noted that in 7/60 procedures, balloon dilation of the distal ureter was necessary. Similarly, Humphreys et al. [45] reported that the DUR D digital flexible ureteroscope was unable to completely explore the renal collecting system in some patients due to ureteral narrowing/

stricture and inadequate deflection into lower pole calyces of the kidney, whereas conventional fiberoptic ureteroscopes were able to assess the entire collecting system. Thus, in the parameter of caliber, digital ureteroscopes to date take a step back to prior generations of flexible ureteroscopes where tip/shaft diameter may preclude ready passage of the ureteroscope, or limit its maneuverability in the pyelocalyceal system. The latest available digital flexible ureteroscope, the FLEX XC, however, appears to more closely resemble its latest fiberoptic counterpart, the FLE X2, in this respect.

Other new and innovative designs for ureteroscopes, focusing on mechanics rather than optics, are also under investigation. Castellanos [46] proposes SolidFlex™ endoscopic technology as one such design. The endoscope consists of a handle with rotor wheel (possibly adjustable to a robotic device) and a shaft with three or more elastic segments that include a rigid and semirigid segment, a passive flexible interface, and an active flexible section. The optical technology is not discussed in detail in the presentation. Bansal et al. [47] describe their early experience with "polyscope," an 8 Fr modular flexible ureteroscope that is assembled for use. Proposed advantages include easy replacement of damaged modular parts, and an optical fiber that does not come in contact with the patient, thus potentially precluding sterilization-related damage. Though these new designs are only in early phases of testing, they may influence subsequent design of flexible ureteroscopes, which are still fragile and costly.

Summary

Fiberoptic flexible ureteroscopes have undergone a substantial evolution and have pioneered modern-day ureteroscopy. Shortcomings of these ureteroscopes, in terms of fragility, mechanics, and optics, have greatly aided endoscopists and manufacturers in suggesting and making improvements in successive generations of flexible ureteroscopes. The next generation of flexible ureteroscopes, digital flexible ureteroscopes, has arrived. These ureteroscopes carry the immediate promise of better optics and visualization, but only further experience will dictate to what degree they address other shortcomings that exist beyond those of optics, namely, in terms of working channel parameters, reliable/user-friendly deflective mechanisms, and durability.

References

1. Young HH, Mckay RW. Congenital valvular obstruction of the prostatic urethra. Surg Gynecol Obstet. 1929;48:509.
2. Marshall VF. Fiberoptics in urology. J Urol. 1964;91:110–4.
3. Aso Y, Takayasu H, Ohta N, Tajima A. Flexible ureterorenoscopy. Urol Clin North Am. 1988;15:329–38.
4. Parkin J, Keeley Jr FX, Timoney AG. Flexible ureteroscope: a user's guide. BJU Int. 2002;90:640–3.
5. El-Hakim A, Tan BJ, Smith AD. Ureteroscopy: technical aspects. In: Stoller ML, Meng MV, editors. Urinary stone disease. Totowa: Humana press; 2007. p. 589–607.
6. Grasso M, Bagley D. Small diameter, actively deflectable, flexible ureteropyleoscopy. J Urol. 1998;160(5):1648–53.
7. Johnston WK. Epochs in endourology: the birth of fiber optics from "light guiding". J Endourol. 2004;18(5):425–6.
8. Hecht J. City of lights: the story of fiberoptics. New York: Oxford University Press; 1999. p. 13–27. 60–75.
9. Colladon D. On the reflections of a ray of light inside a parabolic liquid stream. Compt Rend. 1842;15:800.
10. Babinet J. Note on the transmission of light by sinous channels. Compt Rend. 1842;15:802.
11. Tyndall J. On some phenomena connected with the motion of liquids. Proc R Inst Great Britain. 1854;1:446.
12. Hirschowitz BI, Curtiss LE, Peters CW, et al. Demonstration of a new gastroscope, the fiberscope. Gastroenterology. 1958;35:50.
13. Chiu KY, Cai Y, Marcovich R, et al. Comparison of the mechanical, flow, and optical properties of contemporary flexible ureteroscopes. Urology. 2003;62(5):800–4.
14. Andonian S, Okeke Z, Smith AD. Digital ureteroscopy: the next step. J Endourol. 2008;22(4):603–5.
15. Sidorov DN, Kokaram AC. Suppression of moiré patterns via spectral analysis. In: Jay Kuo C-C, editors. Visual communications and image processing. Proceedings of the society of Photographic Instrumentation Engineers. vol. 4671; 2002. p. 895.
16. Hudson RG, Conlin MJ, Bagley DH. Ureteric access with flexible ureteroscopes: effect of the size of the ureteroscope. BJU Int. 2005;95:1043–4.

17. Bach T, Geavlete B, Hermann TRW, et al. Working tools in flexible ureterorenoscopy-influence on flow and deflection: what does matter? J Endourol. 2008;22(8):1639–43.
18. Natalin RA, Landman J. Where next for the endoscope? Nat Rev Urol. 2009;6:622–8.
19. Boyle WS, Smith GS. Charge coupled semiconductor devices. Bell Syst Tech J. 1970;49:587–93.
20. Damerell CJS, Farley FJM, Gillman AR, et al. Charge-coupled devices or particle detection with high spatial resolution. Nucl Instrum Methods. 1981;185:33–42.
21. Golden JP, Ligler FS. A comparison of imaging methods for use in an array biosensor. Biosens Bioelectron. 2002;17:719–25.
22. Nagele U, Horstmann M, Hennenlotter J, et al. Size does matter: 1.5 Fr stone baskets almost double irrigation flow during flexible ureteroscopy compared to 1.9 Fr stone baskets. Urol Res. 2006;34:389–92.
23. Bach T, Netsch C, Herrmann TRW, et al. Objective assessment of working tool impact on irrigation flow and visibility in flexible ureterorenoscopes. J Endourol. 2011;25(7):1125–9.
24. Kruck S, Anastasiadis AG, Gakis G, et al. Flow matters: irrigation flow differs in flexible ureteroscopes of the newest generation. Urol Res. 2011;39(6):483–6.
25. Haberman KH, Ortiz-Alvarado O, Chotikawanich E, et al. A dual-channel flexible ureteroscope: evaluation of deflection, flow, illumination, and optics. J Endourol. 2011;25(9):1411–4.
26. Monga M, Weiland D, Pedro RN, et al. Intrarenal manipulation of flexible ureteroscopes: a comparative study. BJU Int. 2007;100:157–9.
27. Ankem MK, Lowry PS, Slovick RW, et al. Clinical utility of dual active deflection flexible ureteroscope during upper tract ureteropyeloscopy. Urology. 2004;64:430–4.
28. Sung JC, Springhart WP, Marguet CG, et al. Location and etiology of flexible and semirigid ureteroscope damage. Urology. 2005;66(5):958–63.
29. Afane JS, Olweny EO, Bercowsky E, et al. Flexible ureteroscopes: a single center evaluation of the durability and function of the new ureteroscopes smaller than 9Fr. J Urol. 2000;164:1164–8.
30. User HM, Hua V, Blunt LW, et al. Performance and durability of leading flexible ureteroscopes. J Endourol. 2004;18:735–8.
31. Monga M, Best S, Venkatesh R, Ame C, et al. Durability of flexible ureteroscopes: a randomized prospective study. J Urol. 2006;176:137–41.
32. Carey RI, Gomez CS, Maurici G, et al. Frequency of ureteroscope damage at a tertiary care center. J Urol. 2006;176:607–10.
33. Traxer O, Dubosq F, Jamali K, et al. New-generation flexible ureteroscopes are more durable than previous ones. Urology. 2006;68(2):276–9.
34. Knudsen B, Miyaoka R, Shah K, et al. Durability of the next-generation flexible fiberoptic ureteroscopes: a randomized prospective multi-institutional trial. Urology. 2010;75(3):534–8.
35. Al-Qahtani SM, Geavlette BP, de Medina GS, et al. The new Olympus digital flexible ureteroscope (URF-V): initial experience. Urol Ann. 2011;3(3):133–7.
36. Pietrow PK, Auge BK, Delvecchio FC, et al. Techniques to maximize flexible ureteroscopy longetevity. Urology. 2002;60(5):784–8.
37. Busby JE, Low RK. Ureteroscopic treatment of renal calculi. Urol Clin North Am. 2004;31:89–98.
38. Kourambas J, Byrne RR, Preminger GM. Does a ureteral access sheath facilitate ureteroscopy? J Urol. 2001;165:789–93.
39. Seto C, Ishiura Y, Egawa M. Durability of working channel in flexible ureteroscopes when inserting ureteroscopic devices. J Endourol. 2006;20:223–6.
40. Chew BH. Durability of the next-generation flexible fiberoptic ureteroscopes: a randomized prospective multi-institutional trial. Editorial reply. Urology. 2010;75(3):538.
41. Benito J, Abraham A, Corollas S, et al. Effects of Steris 1TM sterilization and Cidex® ortho-phthalaldehyde high-level disinfection on durability of new generation Flexible ureteroscopes. J Endourol. 2007;21(9):985–92.
42. Healy KA, Pak RW, Cleary RC, et al. Hand problems among endourologists. J Endourol. 2011;25:1915–20.
43. Ingram JN, Kording KP, Howard IS, et al. The statistics of natural hand movements. Exp Brain Res. 2008;188:223–36.
44. Pearlman JL, Roach SS, Valero-Cuevas FJ, et al. The fundamental thumb-tip force vectors produced by the muscle of the thumb. J Orthop Res. 2004;22:306–12.
45. Humphreys M, Miller NL, Williams JC, et al. A new world revealed: early experience with digital ureteroscopy. J Urol. 2008;179:970–5.
46. Castellanos JAC. SolidFlex™ — the fourth generation in endoscopy. Arch Esp Urol. 2009;62(7):573–9.
47. Bansal H, Swain S, Sharma GK, et al. Polyscope: a new era in flexible ureteroscopy. J Endourol. 2011;25(2):317–21.

Guidewires and Angled Catheters 10

Nikhil Waingankar, Zeph Okeke,
and Arthur D. Smith

The field of endourology has undergone major transformations in the past three decades. These advances are largely due to improvements in fiberoptic visualization which has allowed for flexible instrumentation [1], development of smaller telescopes, and improvements in visual display [2, 3]. Equally important to the progression of urologic endoscopy has been the development and technological advances in ancillary equipment. The evolving use of wires and ureteral catheters has allowed for the evaluation and treatment of urinary tract pathology in areas that have previously been deemed inaccessible by minimally invasive means. This chapter describes the various types of guidewires and angled catheters, their mechanical characteristics, and their uses in clinical practice.

Guidewires

Guidewires were initially developed for vascular access and passage of intraluminal devices. In the technique attributed to Dr. Sven-Ivar Seldinger, the desired vessel is punctured with a hollow needle, a guidewire is passed through the needle, the needle is withdrawn, a blunt-tipped catheter (or other endovascular instrument) is passed into the vessel lumen over the wire, and finally the wire is withdrawn once access is secured [4]. Similarly, guidewires were adopted into urologic practice in 1981 to address anatomical and situational difficulties that prevented retrograde ureteral intubation with contemporary standard catheters [5]. Guidewires have since become a standard tool in the endourologist's armamentarium for use in routine stent placement and flexible and semirigid ureteroscopy; moreover, they have become essential in the completion of complex cases involving tortuous ureters, heterotopic orifices, and impacted stones. A variety of guidewires exist, and knowledge of four basic properties is essential in choosing the correct wire for a particular clinical situation: size, tip design, rigidity, and surface coating [6].

Size

Standard urological guidewires are 150 cm in length, although 145 cm wires are also available (Amplatz Super Stiff PTFE Coated Guidewire, Boston Scientific, Natick, MA). Wires shorter than this may make it more difficult to pass a flexible ureteroscope, while longer wires are simply unnecessary and can risk becoming entangled or accidentally pulled from outside the patient, resulting in lost access.

Perhaps more variable than wire length, and thus more individualized to procedure type and

N. Waingankar, M.D. (✉) • Z. Okeke, M.D.
A.D. Smith, M.D.
The Arthur Smith Institute for Urology,
Hofstra North Shore-Long Island Jewish Health System,
New Hyde Park, NY, USA
e-mail: nikhilwaingankar@yahoo.com

M. Monga (ed.), *Ureteroscopy: Indications, Instrumentation & Technique*, Current Clinical Urology,
DOI 10.1007/978-1-62703-206-3_10,

Fig. 10.1 Various tip shapes of guidewires. From [6], reprinted with permission from Elsevier Limited

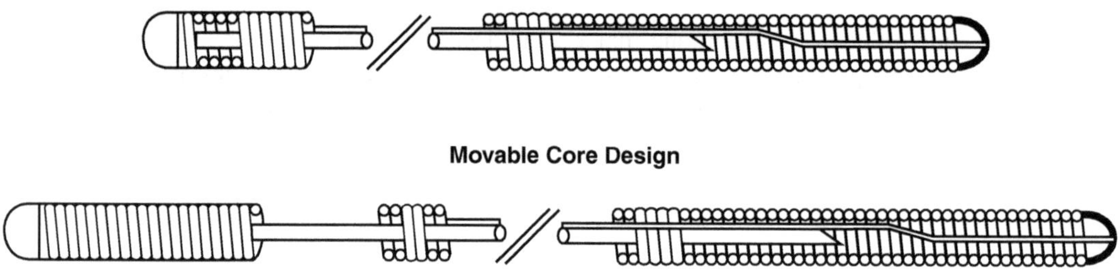

Fig. 10.2 Wire core design. From [6], reprinted with permission from Elsevier Limited

patient characteristics, is wire diameter. Standard diameters are 0.035 and 0.038 in.; however, wires as small as 0.018 in. are available.

Tip Design

Wire tips are available in straight, angled, and J-type (Fig. 10.1). Straight-tipped wires are most commonly used for routine ureteroscopy. Most wires in current practice lead with a soft, floppy tip designed to prevent iatrogenic ureteral or renal trauma. These flexible tips are available in various lengths, ranging from the standard 3 cm to the 15 cm Bentson-type, which is optimal for use as a safety wire as it allows for multiple coils within the renal pelvis. Angle-tipped wires are often utilized for accessing laterally displaced orifices or navigating beyond points of obstruction or tortuosity. J-wires are most commonly used to establish access within a calyx during percutaneous nephrolithotomy. In order to facilitate passage into an infundibulum or the UPJ, the J-tip can be straightened by applying increased tension on the outer core of the wire. Use of J-tip wires has also been described in cases of impacted stones and tortuous ureters [6].

Wire Rigidity

Urological guidewire shafts are composed of a solid metal core surrounded by a steel outer coil (Fig. 10.2). The core is made of either steel or nitinol, a metal alloy made of nickel and titanium that allows for shape memory and superelasticity while providing columnar strength to resist kinking. The core diameter determines the stiffness of the wire. Increased shaft stiffness is useful for straightening tortuous anatomy and serving as a working wire in cases where a routine guidewire is inadequate. The wire core is tapered as it approaches the tip, and the length and degree of tapering determine the tip flexibility; moveable core wires are available, where the length of the flexible tip can be adjusted simply by advancing or withdrawing the mandrel. The outer coil can either be flat or round; flat coils allow for a smoother outer surface and can accommodate in a larger diameter inner core. Among the stiffest guidewires in urological use, the Amplatz Super Stiff Guidewire (Boston Scientific, Natick, MA) features a flat outer coil for increased stiffness, thus providing stability within the urinary tract without compromising tip flexibility.

Surface Coating

Guidewires are coated with various substances that serve to decrease friction when passing instruments over them and/or to facilitate access into tortuous or obstructed ureters. Surface coatings include polytetrafluoroethylene (PTFE) or hydrophilic polymers. Most guidewires, including the Amplatz Super Stiff, Sensor, and Zebra hybrid wire (nitinol wire with striped PTFE jacket for increased torqueability; all Boston Scientific, Natick, MA), utilize a PTFE coating. The Roadrunner (Cook Urological, Spencer, IN) and Glidewire (Terumo Medical, Tokyo, Japan) feature a malleable nitinol core with hydrophilic coating and soft, floppy tip that provides a negligible coefficient of friction, thus making them useful for navigation beyond areas of impaction, stricture, or tortuosity. These wires can become quite slippery due to their hydrophilic nature, and thus should not be utilized as a safety wire. If access is achieved with a hydrophilic wire, it should be exchanged, if possible, for a PTFE-coated wire in order to prevent loss of access. A torque device can be used with hydrophilic wires for added control and assistance with maneuvering the wire into its desired position; if a torque device is not readily available, a loop can be made in the distal portion of the wire for better grasping and torque. Finally, dry gauze can be wrapped around the wire and manipulated by the surgeon to achieve the same result.

Comparison of Guidewires

Given the number of options available, intimate knowledge of the above properties becomes essential in selecting the appropriate wire for a given situation. The ideal guidewire should be flexible enough to bypass any point of obstruction, firm enough to secure access in the desired kidney, rigid enough to permit passage of instruments, and soft enough to do all of the above without traumatizing the urinary tract.

In attempt to predict their clinical performance, Sarkissian et al. analyzed the physical and mechanical properties of five commonly used guidewires: U-Nite (Bard Urological, Convington, GA), Sensor (Boston Scientific), Amplatz Superstiff (Boston Scientific), NiCore (Bard Urological), and RadiFocus glidewire (Boston Scientific). The primary aim was to compare their stiffness to a reference standard, the Amplatz SuperStiff wire. Secondarily, they compared the hydrophilic tips against the NiCore and the RadiFocus glidewires. Tests performed included measurement of coefficient of friction, shaft buckling force, tip bending force, and tip puncture force.

The Sensor wire was found to have the greatest coefficient of friction, while the U-Nite wire was found to have the lowest, with a maximum extraction force up to 0.1 N less than the reference standard. Shaft buckling measurements demonstrated that the Amplatz SuperStiff, as expected, had at least a 34.3% greater shaft buckling force compared to all other wires. The NiCore guidewire was found to have a significantly stronger tip than all of the other guidewires tested, with a 62% greater force than the RadiFocus, Sensor, and Amplatz SuperStiff, and up to a 47.6% greater force than the U-Nite guidewire. Finally, the Sensor wire required the least amount of force to puncture a standard 0.016 mm sheet of tin foil, while the RadiFocus required a minimum of 14.9%, 19.0%, 33.9%, and 47.9% greater force than the Amplatz SuperStiff, NiCore, U-Nite, and Sensor wires, respectively. The authors conclude from this work that these in vitro studies can be used to guide decision making in the operating room. The Amplatz SuperStiff wire remained the stiffest wire and was determined to be the best suited for placement of access sheaths and large stents, while all of the Boston Scientific Wires required less force than the Bard wires to bend around a point of obstruction [7].

In a similar in vitro trial, Clayman et al. compared tip bending force, shaft bending force, pull force, and tip puncture force of the UroWire XF,

Amplatz, and Bentson PTFE wires (All Applied Medical, Rancho Santa Margarita, CA); PTFE Guidewire (Bard); Glidewire, Amplatz Super Stiff, and Bentson guidewire (Boston Scientific); and PTFE Wire Guide, and Roadrunner (Cook urological). Featuring a 15 cm floppy tip, the Boston Scientific PTFE guidewire required the least amount of force to bend the tip. Of the wires with a 3 cm tip, the Applied Bentson wire was the most flexible, and there was no difference in tip flexibility between the Applied Medical or Boston Scientific brands of Amplatz wires, and there was no difference in tip flexibility among the hydrophilic wires. With regard to lubricity, the Boston Scientific glidewire required the lowest withdrawal force of all wires, and was found to have significantly less withdrawal force than the Applied Urowire ($p = 0.002$) but not significantly less than the Cook Roadrunner ($p = 0.155$). The Boston Scientific Amplatz wire required the greatest shaft bending force compared to all other wires ($p < 0.05$), while all of the nitinol hydrophilic wires appeared to be equally flexible. Finally, with regard to tip safety, the Boston Scientific glidewire required four times more force to puncture a sheet of aluminum foil than all of the other wires ($p < 0.001$), making it the safest wire in use [8].

A third comparative trial was performed by Liguori et al., who measured in vitro tip buckling, resistance to bending, and force at which permanent plastic deformation occurred. Fresh human cadaveric ureters were then used to determine force required to perforate a ureter and frictional coeffecient while traversing the ureter. Wires tested included the Boston Scientific PTFE guidewire, Radiofocus Guidewire M (Terumo Europe N.V., Leuven, Belgium), Medtronic PTFE guidewire (Medtronic, Danvers, MA), Emerald Guidewire (Cordis, Miami, FL), and Sensor Dual Flex wire (Boston Scientific). As expected, the wires with hydrophilic tips (Sensor Dual Flex and Radiofocus) required the least amount of bending force, while the Medtronic PTFE wire had the stiffest wire tip. The Boston Scientific PTFE wire was the most resistant to bending while the Terumo Radiofocus wire had the most flexible shaft. The Cordis Emerald and Medtronic PTFE wires were most easily deformed, while the Boston Scientific PTFE guidewire required the greatest force applied before undergoing plastic deformation. Both hydrophilic wires could not be deformed. The Medtronic PTFE wire required the least force to perforate the cadaveric ureter (less than 2.5 N), followed by the Boston Scientific PTFE and Cordis PTFE wires; both hydrophilic wires did not perforate the ureter during testing. This use of cadaveric ureter was validated in the same study as all five wires were tested for their ability to perforate paraffin film. The same results were seen, with the Medtronic wire requiring the least force, followed by the Boston Scientific and Cordis wires; in this test, the Terumo wire was able to puncture the paraffin wax, albeit at a much greater force. Finally, in the test of lubricity, the hydrophilic wires required the least withdrawal force, while the Cordis PTFE wire demonstrated the greatest force of friction [9].

Patriciu and colleagues, in an attempt to more closely estimate the forces applied by wires to anatomic structures, created a biomedical model composed of thermoplastic rubber, motion sensors, charge-coupled-device camera, computer, pneumatic grippers for wire control, and linear/torsional/axial force detectors (Fig. 10.3). Wires were tested on a model of a straight ureter, tortuous path, and a ureter obstructed with a 5.5 mm simulated stone. Calculations were made both for simple wire passage as well as for passage of a catheter over each wire. Wires tested included the Hydro-Glide (Bard); Glidewire, Lubriglide, and Sensor (all Boston Scientific); and Hiwire and PTFE guidewire (both Cook). Catheters tested were a 6 Fr Open-ended tapered tip catheter (Cook) and a prototype everting film catheter (Percutaneous Systems, Inc.) The authors found that the lowest forces recorded for passage along a straight path were with the Hydro-Glide. The Lubriglide wire demonstrated the lowest axial forces when placed on the tortuous and obstructed ureter models, while the Cook PTFE guidewire demonstrated the lowest transversal force applied to the ureteral walls. For all catheter placement tests, the everting film catheter demonstrated lower forces than the Cook catheter [10].

From all of these comparative studies on guidewire use in Urology, it is evident that the

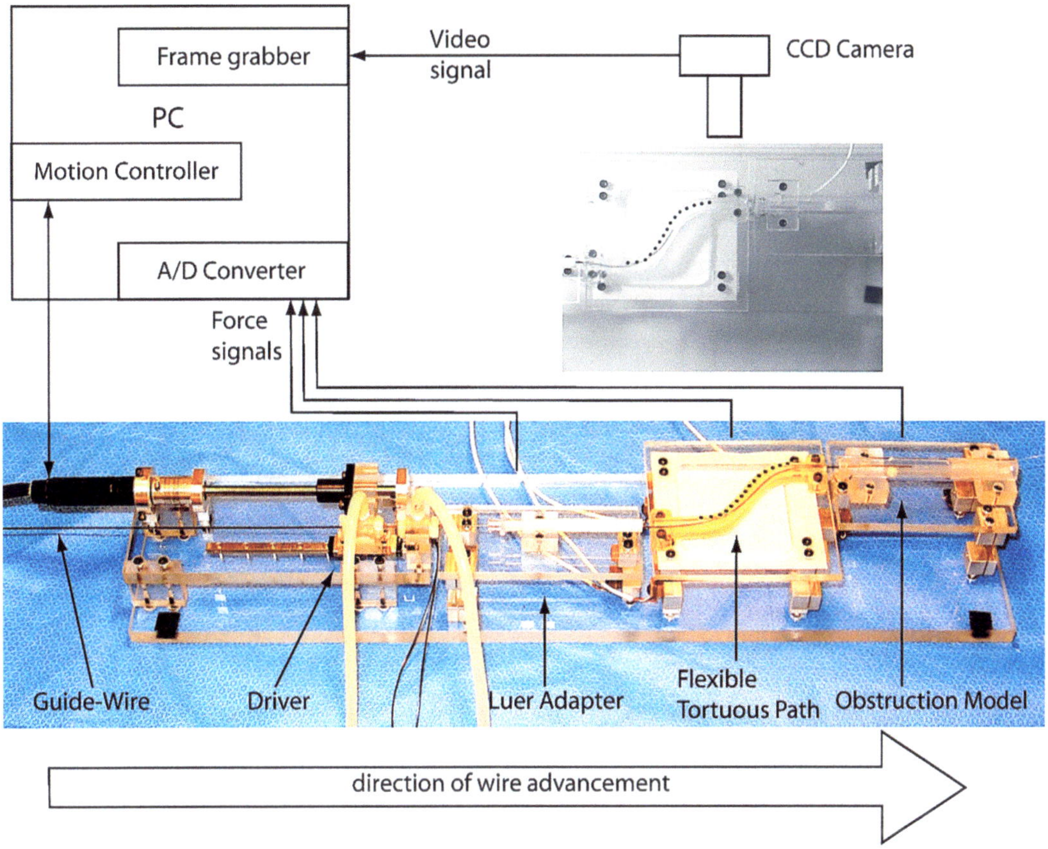

Fig. 10.3 Biomedical model for testing wires. From [10], reprinted with permission from Elsevier Limited

wire selected for a given procedure should provide the strength required to secure access, yet it should have a large "margin of error"—the difference between the force required to perforate a ureter and the force required to bend the tip [11]. As technology continues to evolve, it is imperative that continued product testing be performed to ensure that indications for use are current, safety standards are met, and techniques continue to evolve with novel product designs.

Angled Catheters

One of the earliest documented uses of angled catheters was by Smith and colleagues with their combined antegrade–retrograde placement of Gibbons ureteral stents in 1979. In this procedure, a nephrostomy tract was created, a 0.038 in. stiff wire was passed to the level of the ureteral obstruction, and then a 5- or 7-Fr angled tip catheter was advanced, and by manipulating the two instruments as a coaxial system, the obstruction was bypassed. An angiocath attached to a ureteral catheter was then passed antegrade and grasped cystoscopically and externalized through the urethra. A wire was then passed retrograde through the angiocath, and a Gibbons stent could then be passed retrograde over this wire (Fig. 10.4) [12].

This early avant-garde experience in endourology laid the foundation for the use of angled catheters and combined approaches in endourology today. While our most commonly used ureteral catheters in urology are 5- or 6-Fr open ended, straight-tipped catheters, situations arise where straight catheters are not sufficient—even when used in conjunction with angled wires—for establishing renal access. In such cases, angled ureteral catheters are an essential tool in the Endourologist's armamentarium. The most

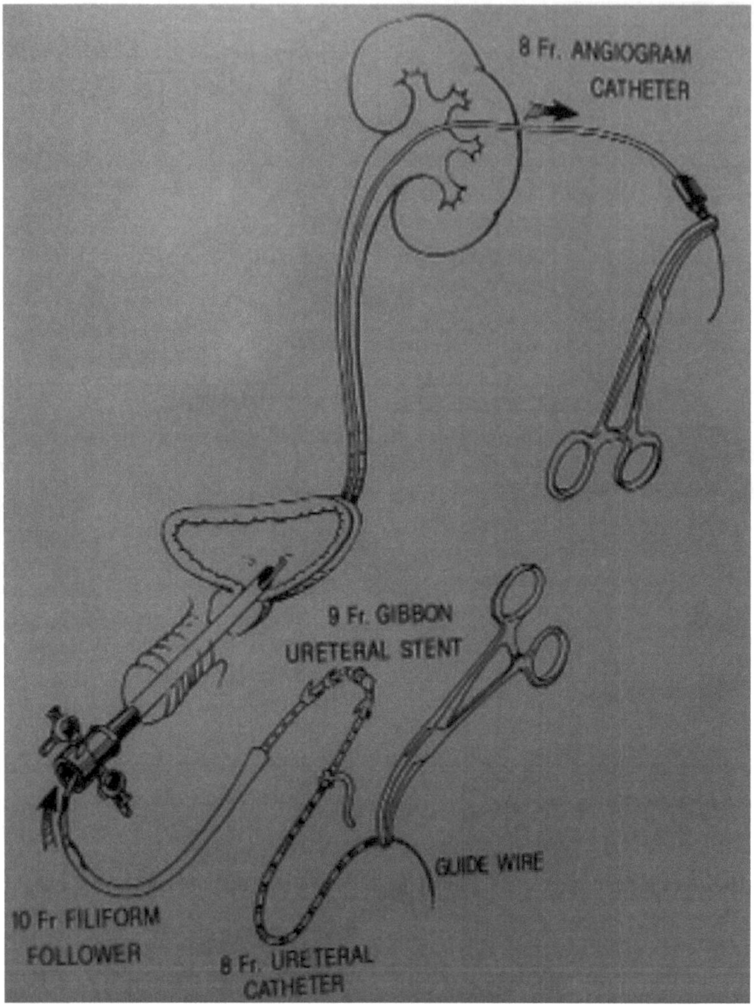

Fig. 10.4 Early use of angled catheter, rigid wire, and combined retrograde–antegrade endoscopy. From [12], reprinted with permission from Elsevier Limited

common cases where angled catheters are needed are for heterotopically displaced ureteral orifices (i.e., lateral openings, transplanted kidneys, and patients with a history of ureteral reimplant), J-hooked or otherwise tortuous ureters, and impacted stones. Angled catheters vary by length, diameter, tip angle, malleability, and tip shape.

Catheter Length

Standard angled catheter length is 70 cm, although sizes are available from 65 to 120 cm. Length should be chosen based on patient height and indication for using an angled catheter (e.g., gaining entry into the orifice vs. navigating around an impacted stone).

Catheter Diameter

Catheter diameter ranges from 3.0 to 8.0 Fr, and allows passage of instrumentation ranging from 0.028 to 0.038 in. in size. 3 Fr catheters are only available in closed-end models. Diameter should be chosen based on indication for using an angled catheter, and wire used with the ureteral catheter.

Tip Angle and Malleability

Flexible tip ureteral catheters are available in open- and closed-end models. Flexible catheters are primarily used for drainage and retrograde pyelogram. The flexible tip allows for atraumatic entry of the ureteral orifice and navigation of a tortuous ureter. Malleable tip ureteral catheters can be shaped to a desired configuration, thus facilitating navigation of partially obstructed systems. Nonmalleable angled ureteral catheters are available in 20° and 40° tips with either tapered or beveled ends. Angled catheters generally come prepackaged with flexible-tipped 145 cm guidewires, which can be directed through the angled tip into a ureteral orifice or around an area of obstruction.

Tip Shape

In addition to malleable and fixed 20–40° angled tips, alternative tip shapes exist to facilitate establishment of retrograde renal access in complex scenarios. Spiral tip catheters are available in 4–6 Fr diameter and 70 cm length, and are useful in very tortuous ureters with sharp-angled turns.

Kumpe catheters feature a hockey stick-shaped tip. Used in combination with a hydrophilic wire, Kumpe catheters are useful in gaining access in lateral ureteral orifices and transplant ureteral orifices, and reaching beyond a redundant or tortuous ureteral segment. Moreover, the angled tip can be used to dislodge a lightly impacted stone from the mucosal wall. The radiopaque tip makes them especially useful for identification of wire deployment under fluoroscopy.

Cobra catheters feature an S-shaped neck that can be utilized for accessing reimplanted ureters, J-hooked ureters, and tortuous segments. Cobra catheters have also been used for irrigation of lower pole calyceal stones to increase clearance during SWL [13]. An inner stainless steel braid traverses the shaft to provide torque, making direction of the tip much easier to control by the surgeon. Specific uses of the Cobra catheter are delineated below in the section "Clinical scenarios" (Fig. 10.5).

Given the variety in available catheter lengths, diameters, tip angles, and shapes, combined with the variety of previously discussed guidewires that can be utilized in concert with ureteral catheters, it is evident that Endourologists have a multitude of options in obtaining retrograde access. Knowledge of these ancillary equipment properties is imperative in order to treat patients with complex anatomical or disease characteristics. The following section delineates advanced scenarios where guidewires and angled catheters can be utilized in treating such patients.

Clinical Scenarios

Patients with transplanted kidneys often need retrograde access for stenting in cases of obstruction, or retrograde pyelogram to rule out urine leak. Cobra catheters are useful in such cases, especially in transplanted kidneys that indent into the lateral wall of the bladder. In these cases, the S-shaped neck can be used to maneuver around the indented wall, with the tip then being directed toward the ureteroneocystotomy site; angle-tipped wires can be used in conjunction with the Cobra catheter to assist with intubation of heterotopic orifices at acute angles from the orientation of the cystoscope (Fig. 10.6).

In patients with J-hooked ureters, the cobra catheter can be used initially to establish access with the tip of the S-shaped neck being directed inferiorly into the distal curve of the "J." An angled glidewire can then be passed through the Cobra catheter with the tip facing superiorly toward the proximal curve of the "J" and into the straightened ureter (Fig. 10.7).

Patients with a history of Cohen Cross-Trigonal reimplants present a particular challenge to obtaining retrograde access due to the acute angle formed by the direction of the orifice and the distal ureter as it traverses the trigonal tunnel. The Cohen Deflecting Wire Guide catheter (Cook Urological) features a deflecting tip that facilitates wire entry beyond this angle; moreover, it can also be used to negotiate a stenotic or tortuous ureter. Alternatively, ease of access has been demonstrated with a combination of an angle-tipped

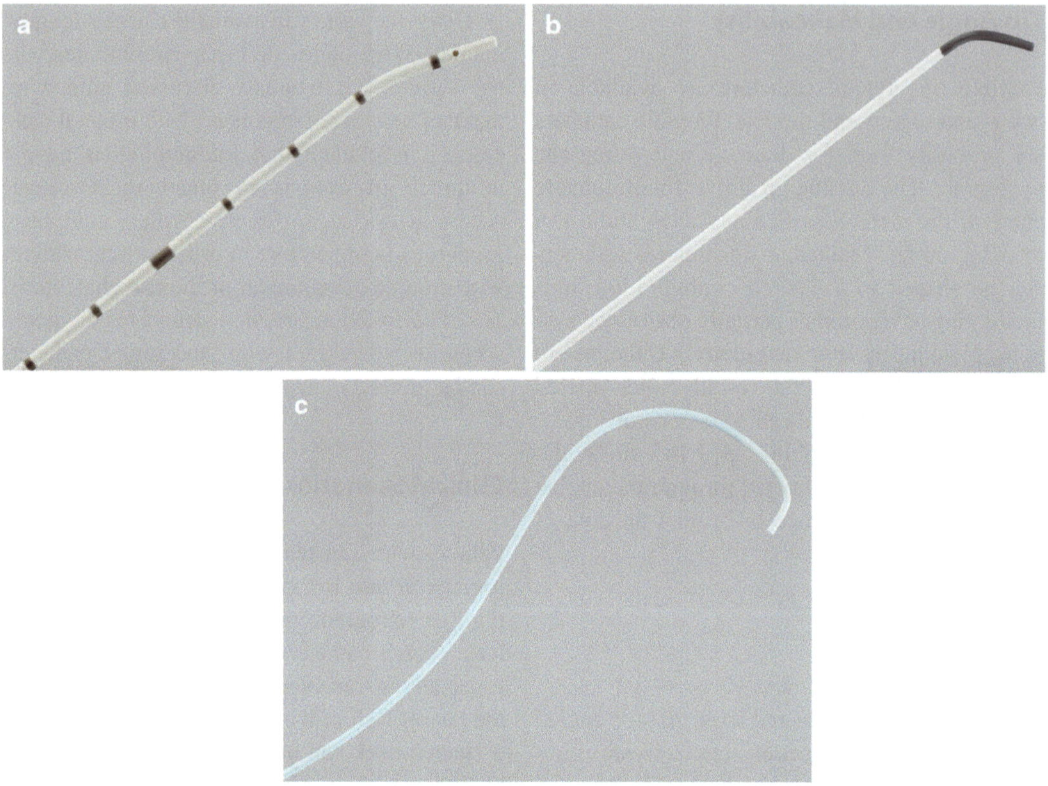

Fig. 10.5 *Left* to *right*: (**a**) Angled catheter, (**b**) Kumpe catheter, (**c**) Cobra catheter. Permission for use granted by Cook Medical Incorporated, Bloomington, IN

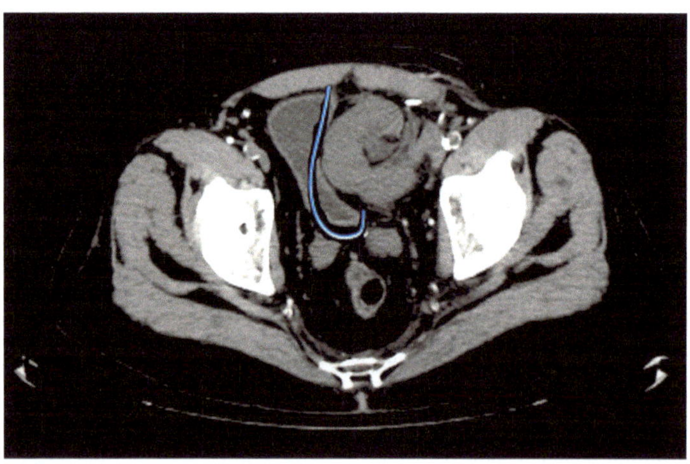

Fig. 10.6 Transplant kidney impinging on the left lateral wall of the bladder. Ureteroneocystotomy (left posterolateral wall near the dome)—previously inaccessible with a straight wire and ureteral catheter—was accessed with a Cobra catheter that arched around the transplanted kidney, and an angled glide wire

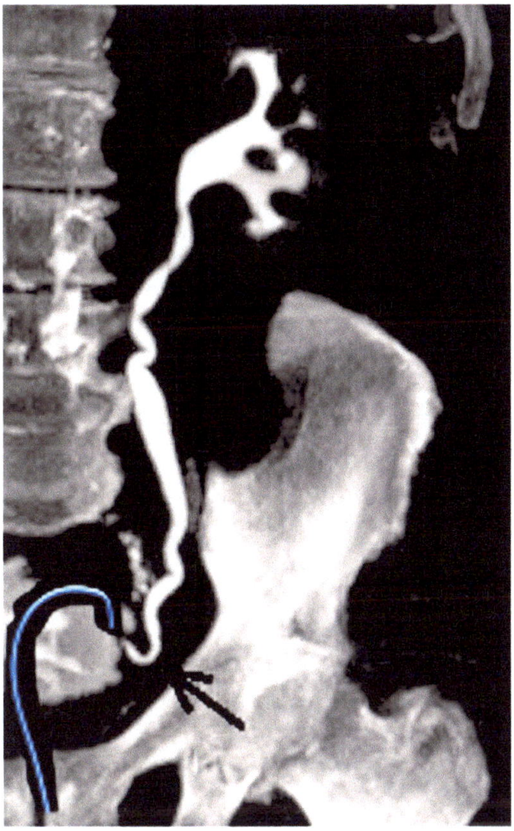

Fig. 10.7 Orientation of a Cobra catheter to access a J-hooked ureter. An angled glide wire can then be passed with the angle facing superiorly to navigate the curve of the J into the straightened portion of the ureter

catheter and angled glidewire with a torque device to permit wire passage in a direction perpendicular to the orientation of the cystoscope. With the glidewire in position, it could then be exchanged for a stiff guidewire, which could then be used as a working wire for stenting, catheter access for retrograde pyelogram, or ureteroscopy [14, 15].

Patients with ileal conduits often present with stone disease, cancer recurrence, benign stricture, or urine leak, all of which have traditionally been managed percutaneously. Drake and Cowan demonstrated success in placing new stents in 10/11 patients via a retrograde approach. Patients were placed supine on a fluoroscopy table and the conduit was opacified. An angled catheter was passed to the level of the ileoureteral anastomoses, and a glidewire was passed under fluoroscopic guidance into the ureter. A 5 Fr angiographic catheter was passed over the glidewire for retrograde pyelogram, and the glidewire was subsequently exchanged for an Amplatz stiff 0.035 in. guidewire, which facilitated stent passage. This procedure was successful in all ureters that demonstrated reflux from the conduit, and five of the nine ureters that did not. The authors concluded that this retrograde approach is feasible in patients with an ileal conduit as an alternative to the percutaneous antegrade approach [16]. Patel and Bellman recommended a percutaneous approach in patients with a smaller caliber stoma, such as a Mitrofanoff [17]. Nelson et al. demonstrated the feasibility of retrograde access in patients with neobladders. They performed cystograms to delineate the afferent limb and ureteral anastomoses. Access was achieved with a 0.035 in. Terumo stiff angled directional glidewire along with a 5 Fr open-ended ureteral catheter. The wire was advanced fluoroscopically, and a ureteroscope was subsequently passed over the wire. In this manner, 10/13 renal units were successfully accessed [18].

Conclusion

This chapter has described the physical and mechanical characteristics of guidewires and angled catheters commonly used in Urology today. The role of minimally invasive, endourological approaches can continue to expand with the growth of this ancillary equipment and modifications in technique.

References

1. Marshall VF. Fiberoptics in urology. J Urol. 1964;91:110.
2. Humphreys MR, Miller NL, Williams Jr JC, Evan AP, Munch LC, Lingeman JE. A new world revealed: early experience with digital ureteroscopy. J Urol. 2008;179(3):970–5.
3. Tan YH, Preminger GM. Advances in video and imaging in ureteroscopy. Urol Clin North Am. 2004;31(1): 33–42.
4. Seldinger SI. Catheter replacement of the needle in percutaneous arteriography; a new technique. Acta Radiol. 1953;39(5):368–76.

5. Fritzsche P, Moorhead JD, Axford PD, Torrey RR. Urologic applications of angiographic guide wire and catheter techniques. J Urol. 1981;125(6):774–80.
6. Rosenberg BH, Averch TD. Ancillary instrumentation for ureteroscopy. Urol Clin North Am. 2004;31: 49–59.
7. Sarkissian C, Korman E, Hendlin K, Monga M. Systematic evaluation of hybrid guidewires: shaft stiffness, lubricity, and tip configuration. Urology. 2012;79(3):513–7.
8. Clayman M, Uribe CA, Eichel L, Gordon Z, McDougal EM, Clayman RV. Comparison of guidewires in urology. Which, when, and why? J Urol. 2004;171(6):2146–50.
9. Liguori G, Antoniolli F, Trombetta C, Biasotto M, Amodeo A, Pomara G, Bucci S, Belgrano E. Comparative experimental evaluation of guidewire use in urology. Urology. 2008;72(2):286–9. discussion 289–90.
10. Patriciu A, Mazilu D, Bagga HS, Petrisor D, Kavoussi LR, Stoianovici D. An evaluation method for the mechanical performance of guide-wires and catheters in accessing the upper urinary tract. Med Eng Phys. 2007;29(8):918–22. Epub 2006 Oct 25.
11. Monga M. Re: comparison of guidewires in urology. Which, when and why? J Urol. 2005;173(5):1830.
12. Smith AD, Miller RP, Reinke DB, Lange PH, Fraley EE. Insertion of Gibbons ureteral stents using endourologic techniques. Urology. 1979;14(4): 330–6.
13. Nicely ER, Maggio MI, Kuhn EJ. The use of a cystoscopically placed cobra catheter for directed irrigation of lower pole caliceal stones during extracorporeal shock wave lithotripsy. J Urol. 1992;148(3 Pt 2): 1036–9.
14. Wallis MC, Brown DH, Jayanthi VR, Koff SA. A novel technique for ureteral catheterization and/or retrograde ureteroscopy after cross-trigonal ureteral reimplantation. J Urol. 2003;170(4 Pt 2):1664–6. discussion 1666.
15. Lusuardi L, Hruby S, Jeschke S, Zimmermann R, Sieberer M, Janetschek G. A new technique for retrograde flexible ureteroscopy after cohen cross-trigonal ureteral reimplantation. Urol Int. 2011;87(3):260–2. Epub 2011 Aug 26.
16. Drake MJ, Cowan NC. Fluoroscopy guided retrograde ureteral stent insertion in patients with a ureteroileal urinary conduit: method and results. J Urol. 2002;167(5):2049–51.
17. Patel H, Bellman GC. Special considerations in the endourologic management of stones in continent reservoirs. J Endourol. 1995;9:249–54.
18. Nelson CB, Wolf JS, Montie JE, Faerber GJ. Retrograde ureteroscopy in patients with orthotopic neobladder urinary diversion. J Urol. 2003;170: 107–10.

Ureteral Access Sheaths

11

Kendall J. Feia, Branden G. Duffey,
and J. Kyle Anderson

Introduction

Accompanying the development of more modern endoscopes in the 1970s and 1980s were technologies developed to further facilitate retrograde access to the upper urinary tract. The ureteral access sheath (UAS), first introduced by Takayaso and Aso in 1974, has proven to be a useful adjunct in ureteroscopy [1]. By simplifying repeated access to the upper urinary tract, the UAS has been shown to streamline ureteroscopy [2, 3] and decrease operative time and cost [2]. Furthermore, it has been associated with lower intrarenal pressures [4–6], decreased damage to operative equipment [7], and in a single study improved stone free rates following ureteroscopy [8]. The objective of this chapter is to provide a review of the current literature available regarding the UAS. This chapter will specifically address UAS construction and physical properties, purported benefits, potential complications, and uses in treating upper urinary tract pathology.

K.J. Feia, M.D. (✉) • J.K. Anderson, M.D.
Department of Urology, University of Minnesota, Minneapolis, MN, USA
e-mail: feia0003@umn.edu

B.G. Duffey, D.O.
Urology Division, Surgery Department, San Antonio Military Medical Center, San Antonio, TX, USA

Physical Properties and Deployment

Current ureteral access sheaths consist of an outer sheath and a tapered dilating obturator. They are frequently coated with hydrophilic polymers designed to decrease friction during passage, allowing for easier insertion. More recent models have been improved by incorporating a reinforced wall construction that provides more strength while minimizing wall thickness. They range in outer diameter from 9 to 18 Fr, and length from 20 to 55 cm, and are now available from several manufacturers (Table 11.1).

Prior to UAS deployment, two wires are placed into the upper tract under fluoroscopic guidance, one functioning as a safety wire and the other a working wire which is generally a stiff wire with a stainless steel core. The UAS is then moistened to ensure lubrication and advanced over the stiff wire under direct fluoroscopic guidance. It is important to ensure that the inner dilating cannula is securely engaged with the outer sheath during advancement to prevent ureteral injury from the exposed edge of the outer sheath. Once placed in satisfactory position, the inner dilating cannula and working wire are removed and the procedure performed.

While a UAS may be inserted without adjunctive maneuvers in the majority of endoscopic cases, it is not uncommon to encounter difficulty in passing the UAS. Harper et al. identified the following groups as at risk for conventional UAS insertion failure: young males with tight ureteral

M. Monga (ed.), *Ureteroscopy: Indications, Instrumentation & Technique*, Current Clinical Urology,
DOI 10.1007/978-1-62703-206-3_11, © Springer Science+Business Media New York 2013

Table 11.1 Commonly available ureteral access sheaths

Company	Product name	Size (Fr)	Length (cm)
Cook	Flexor	9.5, 12.0, 14.0	13, 20, 28, 35, 45, 55
BARD	Aqua Guide	10/12, 10/14, 11/13, 11/15	25,, 35, 45, 55
Boston Scientific	Navigator	11/13, 13/15	28, 36, 46
Gyrus-ACMI	Uropass	12/14	24, 38, 54
Applied Medical	Forté	10/12, 12/14, 14/16	20, 28, 35, 45, 55

orifices, duplicated collecting systems, and small caliber ureters [9]. If UAS placement is difficult the following manipulations may be attempted. Ensure the stiff working wire is correctly positioned with adequate coil in the intrarenal collecting system. Then eliminate slack in the guidewire by appropriately tensioning the wire while making sure it is not withdrawn. These two manipulations assist in straightening the ureter thereby facilitating UAS acceptance. If the aforementioned manipulations do not permit UAS passage, gentle coaxial dilation with the internal obturator of the UAS or specially designed ureteral dilators may prove useful, but care should be taken to avoid applying excess sheer force that could lead to ureteral injury or avulsion [10]. Should the preceding measures fail, balloon dilation of the ureter may be performed. However, this may increase the risk of ureteral perforation. Finally, placement of an indwelling ureteral stent allows for passive ureteral dilation and successful UAS or ureteroscope insertion in 10–14 days.

In vitro and clinical studies can be used to predict how specific UASs may perform with regard to kinking and buckling. In a randomized trial comparing the 12/15 F Applied Access Forte XE (Applied Medical, Rancho Santa Margarita, California) to the 12/14 F Cook Flexor (Cook Urological, Spencer, Indiana) access sheath, Monga et al. analyzed the ease of placement and rate of device failure [3]. While there were no statistical differences between the two groups with regard to preoperative stenting or use of rigid ureteroscopy before UAS placement, the device failure rates were 44% and 0% for the Applied Medical and Cook UASs, respectively ($p<0.001$). The device failures identified included buckling (25%), kinking (25%), and difficulty passing instruments (13%). The Cook sheath was also found to be superior with regard to ease of placement [3]. In a study evaluating the physical properties of next-generation UASs, Pedro and colleagues used an ex vivo model to better predict possible clinical failures [11]. Specifically, they evaluated the pressures at which buckling and kinking occurred, measured the coefficient of friction for each sheath during placement, and correlated that measurement to overall ease of placement. Testing included the Cook Flexor (Cook, 12/14 F×35 cm), Gyrus-ACMI UroPass (ACMI, 12/14 F×38 cm), Bard Aquaguide (Bard, 11/13 F×35 cm), and Boston Scientific Navigator (BSCI-11, 11/13 F×36 cm and BSCI-13, 13/15 F×36 cm) UASs. The authors found that the Cook UAS performed best with regard to buckling. The Bard catheter was the most likely to kink, while the ACMI was superior with regard to kinking. There was no significant difference between the tested sheaths with regard to the coefficient of friction upon placement [11].

Intrarenal Pressures

Increased intrarenal pressures have long been a concern during ureteroscopy. Attempts to maintain good visualization may inadvertently raise intrarenal pressure and over-distend the renal pelvis, resulting in pyelosinus/pyelovenous back flow. The adverse effect of increased renal pelvic pressure has been documented in animal studies [12, 13]. At pressures exceeding 150 mmHg many pathologic changes begin to occur. These include, but are not limited to, submucosal edema, vasculitis, tubular vacuolization, and focal renal scarring. As pressures rise above 330 mmHg, rupture of the collecting system can occur. These are all real risks in the modern era of ureteroscopy with hand irrigation where pressures can exceed 400 mmHg [13].

The ability of the UAS to lower renal pressure has been demonstrated in several well-designed studies. Functioning as an open conduit into the kidney, it allows fluid to enter through the endoscope, and flow out through the sheath around the scope thereby decreasing renal pelvis pressure [5].

Landman and colleagues demonstrated this relationship using the en bloc urinary tract from cadaveric donors. In their study, lower pole percutaneous access with a 30 F sheath was gained into the kidney and a nephroscope was then advanced into the renal pelvis. Irrigant was infused through the nephroscope at varying rates, while the intrarenal pressure and irrigant flow rates were measured in a variety of ureteral drainage conditions. Ureteral drainage included the native ureter, a 6 F ureteral catheter, a 10/12 F × 35 cm UAS, 12/14 F × 35 cm UAS, and a 7 F occlusion balloon catheter. Importantly, intrarenal pressures were significantly lower while using both the 10/12 F and the 12/14 F UASs compared to the other conditions [5].

Ureteral access sheaths have also been shown to decrease renal pelvis pressures during ureteroscopy in a cadaveric model [6]. Using a percutaneous pressure monitor, the authors were able to record renal pelvis pressures while performing ureteroscopy with a 7.5 F flexible ureteroscope. The ureteroscopes were then introduced into the collecting system using a 35 cm UAS with varying diameters (10/12 F, 12/14 F, and 14/16 F) or unsheathed (control). The authors then delivered irrigant through the ureteroscope at pressures of 50, 100, or 200 mmHg while measuring intrarenal pressure and irrigant flow. Irrigant flow was higher in all of the UASs tested compared to controls. In all experimental conditions with a UAS in place, intrarenal pressure was noted to stay below 30 cm H_2O. Notably, at low irrigant pressures (50 cmH_2O), flow through each sheath was similar, but at increasing pressures the 12/14 F and 14/16 F sheaths had better pressure and flow characteristics than the 10/12 F sheath. They also noted that the 12/14 F sheath performed equally to 14/16 F sheath, concluding that the 12/14 F UAS optimizes pressure and flow characteristics while limiting UAS diameter [6].

This same relationship has proven true with in vivo human studies. Auge et al. identified five patients who required placement of a percutaneous nephrostomy tube after presenting to the emergency department for obstructing ureteral calculi [4]. The patients then underwent interval treatment with flexible ureteroscopy. After clearance of all stone fragments, the flexible scope was then advanced and pressures were recorded through the percutaneous nephrostomy tube while hand irrigation was performed in the renal pelvis, proximal ureter, mid and distal ureter. This was initially performed with the ureteroscope alone, and then with the aid of a UAS. The authors found that collecting system pressures were significantly lower with the use of a UAS at all locations by 57–75% ($p < 0.05$) [4].

Operative Time and Cost

By simplifying repeated access to the upper urinary tract, the UAS has proven beneficial in reducing operative times and cost [2, 3]. To address these issues Kourambas and colleagues prospectively analyzed a cohort of 59 patients presenting for endoscopy above the level of the iliac vessels [2]. The patients were randomized to ureteroscopy with or without the aid of a UAS. The authors utilized a 12/14 F hydrophilic coated UAS ranging from 20 to 35 cm depending on patient size, sex, and stone location. They found that the operative time was significantly lower in patients randomized to the use of a UAS (43 min vs. 53 min, $p < 0.05$). Despite having a higher total stone burden in these patients (13.7 mm vs. 10.1 mm, respectively), the stone free rates between these two groups were similar. The overall calculated saving, based on operating room time saved, was $350 per procedure. They also found significant time saving when the UAS was used for ureteral dilation, and calculated an average saving of $700 per dilation when considering the cost of the balloon dilation system [2].

UAS use may further reduce overall costs by reducing wear and tear on endoscopic equipment.

Technologic advancement in materials science has permitted the miniaturization of ureteroscopes while concurrently increasing active range of motion and improving visualization. However, modern ureteroscopes are vulnerable to damage and the need for costly repairs, in previous studies requiring repair on average every 6–15 uses [14]. Not only is the monetary cost of these repairs high, but it can also lead to unnecessary delays in the operating room and possibly unexpected complications. The UAS decreases wear and tear on modern ureteroscopes by reducing axial forces on the ureteroscope as well as trauma to the working channel from repetitive backloading over a guidewire. With the use of a UAS, authors have shown that ureteroscopes could be used on average 27.5 times between repairs, thereby reducing the cost of ureteroscopy [15].

Stone Free Rates

Surgeons have postulated that UASs improve stone free rates following ureteroscopy by allowing for passive irrigation of stone fragments as well as quicker access to the upper collecting system. With this in mind, it is reasonable to consider the retrospective data available. Previously published reports have listed the stone free rates for ureteroscopy without the aid of a UAS ranging between 72 and 84% [16–20], and from 77 to 86% with the use of a UAS [2, 21].

To date, L'Esperance and colleagues have published the only study directly evaluating the effect of UAS utilization on stone free rates following ureteroscopy [8]. Following a retrospective review of their clinical database, they identified a total of 256 ureteroscopic procedures performed for renal calculi, 173 of which were performed with the use of a UAS. Demographic data, stone burden, and stone location were similar between groups. The authors found that overall stone free rates were significantly improved in those patients in whom a UAS was utilized 79% vs. 67%, $p=0.042$ [8]. It should be noted that while UAS use seems to facilitate ureteroscopy and possibly improve stone free rates, no level-one evidence exists to support or refute this claim.

Postoperative Course Following UAS Utilization

Ureteral stents are associated with symptoms such as frequency, dysuria, and flank pain [22], and for this reason efforts have been made to identify patients who do not require a ureteral stent post operatively. While symptoms are minimized with proper stent positioning [23, 24], they are still a significant cause of patient morbidity and their use has been discouraged following uncomplicated ureteroscopy [12, 25]. Post-operative pain, urinary symptoms, and narcotic use are lower in patients without ureteral stents, but these studies were performed on patients who did not require ureteral dilation [12, 25]. In a retrospective review, Rappaport and colleagues analyzed their data on 161 consecutive patients treated with ureteroscopy by evaluating the impact of stent vs. no stent on unplanned ER visits. In their cohort, 37% of patients treated with a UAS vs. 14% without a UAS returned to the ER for evaluation if a ureteral stent was not placed after the procedure ($p=0.04$). They concluded that use of a UAS precluded uncomplicated ureteroscopy and would therefore warrant placement of a ureteral stent [26].

In patients requiring dilation for ureteral narrowing, dilation with a UAS causes fewer symptoms compared to balloon dilation [2]. By using a comprehensive questionnaire, Kourambas and colleagues assessed the rates of flank pain, suprapubic pain, frequency, urgency, dysuria, and hematuria on post-operative days 0, 1, and 6. While the rate of hematuria was found to be similar between the two groups, there was a significant difference in all other symptoms favoring the patients who had dilation with the UAS [2].

Decreased Ureteral Blood Flow and Ureteral Strictures

Concerns have previously been raised regarding ureteral ischemia and eventual ureteral stricture formation following UAS utilization. Lallas and associates evaluated this question in a porcine model by measuring ureteral blood flow at 5-min intervals both with and without a UAS in place [20]. In all study groups, the ureteral blood flow decreased upon UAS insertion. Nadir blood flow was measured at 25% below baseline for the 10/12 F sheath, and at 65% below baseline with the 12/14 F and 14/16 F sheaths. However, this decrement in perfusion was only transient with ureteral blood flow trending toward normal by 70 min; to 88%, 70%, and 68% of baseline, respectively. It should, however, be noted that the 14/16 F sheath did reach the nadir level fastest, and also took the longest to normalize after removal of the UAS. The authors then performed histologic analysis on the ureters from the study. Ureteral specimens were collected at three time points: (1) immediate harvesting after the procedure, (2) 48 h post-procedure, and (3) 72 h post-procedure. In the longer time points, the access sheath group demonstrated nuclear changes, inflammation, and increased deposition of collagen leading to thickening of the ureteral wall, but importantly no overt signs of ischemic necrosis were evident [27]. While some may argue that these changes could lead to increased risk of ureteral stricture, this has not proven to be true in a well-designed study at this point.

Delvecchio and colleagues published a retrospective review of 150 patients who had undergone ureteroscopy aided by the use of a UAS and evaluated the rates of strictures among these patients [21]. The 12/14 F UAS was used in 79% of cases. They identified only a single ureteral stricture, and this occurred in a patient with a complex surgical history for recurrent struvite calculi. This study was, however, limited by a relatively short follow-up of 11 months on average, and included imaging in only 41% of these patients. Nevertheless their rate of stricture was similar to that published in large series for ureteroscopy without the use of a UAS at 1–2% [28–31].

UAS in Treating Upper Tract Urothelial Carcinoma

The UAS may prove to be particularly beneficial when diagnosing and treating upper tract urothelial carcinoma. While still unproven, some authors theorize that the sheath could protect the urinary tract from exposure to malignant cells, and the lower intrarenal pressures may help prevent the extravasation of malignant cells during ureteroscopy [32]. More recently authors have demonstrated benefits in diagnosing upper tract urothelial cell carcinoma with a UAS. Previously published reports have shown that biopsies obtained without the aid of a UAS are sufficient for analysis in only 75–82% of specimens [33, 34]. In a modern study of 235 procedures, the use of a UAS was shown to facilitate biopsy of upper tract lesions with over 90% of the specimens sufficient for analysis, and 88% concordance with final pathologic specimen [35]. More recently the benefits of easy passage of ureteroscopes utilizing a UAS have allowed the development of larger instruments that would otherwise not be safely passed through the ureter. In a study comparing the BIGopsy forceps (Cook Urological, Spencer, IN) to a more standard biopsy forceps ("Pirhana," Boston Scientific, Natick, MA), the BIGopsy performed better when comparing the average size of biopsy specimen and concordance with final pathologic result [36]. As this technology continues to improve, the success in diagnosing and treating pathology in the upper collecting system would be expected to improve as well, and it is with developments such as the UAS that this evolution continues to progress.

Conclusion

While evidence from randomized trials is generally lacking, multiple studies have suggested benefits of UAS use. Decreased operative time, reduction in ureteroscope damage, and improvement in stone free rates all appear to be benefits of the UAS. This tool will likely remain an important part of the urologist's armamentarium for some time to come.

References

1. Takayasu H, Aso Y. Recent development for pyeloureteroscopy: guide tube method for its introduction into the ureter. J Urol. 1974;112(2):176–8.
2. Kourambas J, Byrne RR, Preminger GM. Does a ureteral access sheath facilitate ureteroscopy? J Urol. 2001;165(3):789–93.

3. Monga M, Bhayani S, Landman J, Conradie M, Sundaram CP, Clayman RV. Ureteral access for upper urinary tract disease: the access sheath. J Endourol. 2001;15(8):831–4.
4. Auge BK, Pietrow PK, Lallas CD, Raj GV, Santa-Cruz RW, Preminger GM. Ureteral access sheath provides protection against elevated renal pressures during routine flexible ureteroscopic stone manipulation. J Endourol. 2004;18(1):33–6.
5. Landman J, Venkatesh R, Ragab M, Rehman J, Lee DI, Morrissey KG, Monga M, Sundaram CP. Comparison of intrarenal pressure and irrigant flow during percutaneous nephroscopy with an indwelling ureteral catheter, ureteral occlusion balloon, and ureteral access sheath. Urology. 2002;60(4):584–7.
6. Rehman J, Monga M, Landman J, Lee DI, Felfela T, Conradie MC, Srinivas R, Sundaram CP, Clayman RV. Characterization of intrapelvic pressure during ureteropyeloscopy with ureteral access sheaths. Urology. 2003;61(4):713–8.
7. Monga M, Best S, Venkatesh R, Ames C, Lee C, Kuskowski M, Schwartz S, Vanlangendock R, Skenazy J, Landman J. Durability of flexible ureteroscopes: a randomized, prospective study. J Urol. 2006;176(1):137–41.
8. L'esperance JO, Ekeruo WO, Scales Jr CD, Marguet CG, Springhart WP, Maloney ME, Albala DM, Preminger GM. Effect of ureteral access sheath on stone-free rates in patients undergoing ureteroscopic management of renal calculi. Urology. 2005;66(2): 252–5.
9. Harper JD, Ebrahimi KY, Auge BK, Lamberton GR, Pham AK, Zuppan C, Albala DM, Preminger GM, Baldwin DD. Comparison of a novel radially dilating balloon ureteral access sheath to a conventional sheath in the porcine model. J Urol. 2008;179(5):2042–5.
10. Gaylis F, Bastuba M, Bidair M, Friedel W. Ureteral dilation using a tapered dilator: a cost-effective approach. J Endourol. 2000;14(5):447–9.
11. Pedro R, Hendlin K, Durfee W, Monga M. Physical characteristics of next-generation ureteral access sheaths: buckling and kinging. Urology. 2007;70(3): 440–2.
12. Borboroglu PG, Amling CL, Schenkman NS, Monga M, Ward JF, Piper NY, Bishoff JT, Kane CJ. Ureteral stenting after ureteroscopy for distal ureteral calculi: a multi-institutional prospective randomized controlled study assessing pain, outcomes and complications. J Urol. 2001;166(5):1651–7.
13. Schwalb DM, Eshghi M, Davidian M, Franco I. Morphological and physiological changes in the urinary tract associated with ureteral dilation and ureteropyeloscopy: an experimental study. J Urol. 1993;149(6):1576–85.
14. Afane JS, Olweny EO, Bercowsky E, Sundaram CP, Dunn MD, Shalhav AL, McDougall EM, Clayman RV. Flexible ureteroscopes: a single center evaluation of the durability and function of the new endoscopes smaller than 9Fr. J Urol. 2000;164(4):1164–8.
15. Pietrow PK, Auge BK, Delvecchio FC, Silverstein AD, Weizer AZ, Albala DM, Preminger GM. Techniques to maximize flexible ureteroscope longevity. Urology. 2002;60(5):784–8.
16. Bilgasem S, Pace KT, Dyer S, Honey RJ. Removal of asymptomatic ipsilateral renal stones following rigid ureteroscopy for ureteral stones. J Endourol. 2003;17(6):397–400.
17. Chow GK, Patterson DE, Blute ML, Segura JW. Ureteroscopy: effect of technology and technique on clinical practice. J Urol. 2003;170(1):99–102.
18. Harmon WJ, Sershon PD, Blute ML, Patterson DE, Segura JW. Ureteroscopy: current practice and long-term complications. J Urol. 1997;157(1):28–32.
19. Schuster TG, Hollenbeck BK, Faerber GJ, Wolf JS. Ureteroscopic treatment of lower pole calculi: comparison of lithotripsy in situ and after displacement. J Urol. 2002;168(1):43–5.
20. Sofer M, Watterson JD, Wollin TA, Nott L, Razvi H, Denstedt JD. Holmium:YAG laser lithotripsy for upper urinary tract calculi in 598 patients. J Urol. 2002;167(1):31–4.
21. Delvecchio FC, Auge BK, Brizuela RM, Weizer AZ, Silverstein AD, Lallas CD, Pietrow PK, Albala DM, Preminger GM. Assessment of stricture formation with the ureteral access sheath. Urology. 2003;61(3): 518–22. discussion 522.
22. Haleblian G, Kijvikia K, Rosetta J, Preminger G. Ureteral stenting and urinary stone management: a systematic review. J Urol. 2008;179(2):424–30.
23. El-Nahas AR, El-Assmy AM, Shoma AM, Eraky I, El-Kenawy MR, El-Kappany HA. Self-retaining ureteral stents: analysis of factors responsible for patients' discomfort. J Endourol. 2006;20(1): 33–7.
24. Rane A, Saleemi A, Cahill D, Sriprasad S, Shrotri N, Tiptaft R. Have stent-related symptoms anything to do with placement technique? J Endourol. 2001;15(7): 741–5.
25. Cheung MC, Lee F, Leung YL, Wong BB, Tam PC. A prospective randomized controlled trial on ureteral stenting after ureteroscopic holmium laser lithotripsy. J Urol. 2003;169(4):1257–60.
26. Rapoport D, Perks AE, Teichman JM. Ureteral access sheath use and stenting in ureteroscopy: effect on unplanned emergency room visits and cost. J Endourol. 2007;21(9):993–7.
27. Lallas CD, Auge BK, Raj GV, Santa-Cruz R, Madden JF, Preminger GM. Laser doppler flowmetric determination of ureteral blood flow after ureteral access sheath placement. J Endourol. 2002;16(8): 583–90.
28. Abdel-Razzak OM, Bagley DH. Clinical experience with flexible ureteropyeloscopy. J Urol. 1992;148(6): 1788–92.
29. Elashry OM, Elbahnasy AM, Rao GS, Nakada SY, Clayman RV. Flexible ureteroscopy: Washington University experience with the 9.3 F and 7.5 F flexible ureteroscopes. J Urol. 1997;157(6):2074–80.

30. Francesca F, Scattoni V, Nava L, Pompa P, Grasso M, Rigatti P. Failures and complications of transurethral ureteroscopy in 297 cases: conventional rigid instruments vs. small caliber semirigid ureteroscopes. Eur Urol. 1995;28(2):112–5.
31. Geavlete P, Georgescu D, Niţă G, Mirciulescu V, Cauni V. Complications of 2735 retrograde semirigid ureteroscopy procedures: a single-center experience. J Endourol. 2006;20(3):179–85.
32. Vanlangendonck R, Landman J. Ureteral access strategies: pro-access sheath. Urol Clin North Am. 2004;31(1):71–81.
33. Keeley FX, Kulp DA, Bibbo M, McCue PA, Bagley DH. Diagnostic accuracy of ureteroscopic biopsy in upper tract transitional cell carcinoma. J Urol. 1997;157(1):33–7.
34. Tavora F, Fajardo DA, Lee TK, Lotan T, Miller JS, Miyamoto H, Epstein JI. Small endoscopic biopsies of the ureter and renal pelvis: pathologic pitfalls. Am J Surg Pathol. 2009;33(10):1540–6.
35. Gorin MA, Santos Cortes JA, Kyle CC, Carey RI, Bird VG. Initial clinical experience with use of ureteral access sheaths in the diagnosis and treatment of upper tract urothelial carcinoma. Urology. 2011;78(3):523–7.
36. Wason S, Schned A, Seigne J, Pais V. Evaluation of adequacy of pathologic specimens using a novel backloading ureteroscopic biopsy forceps. J Urol. 2010;183(4):e354–5.

12 Irrigation Systems and Irrigation Fluids

Renato Nardi Pedro

The endoscopic approach for treating urinary tract diseases has been made possible by a remarkable technological evolution in endoscopic devices. The design of small, digital, flexible, and more durable endoscopes with thin optic fibers or with light emitting diode (LED) has provided the endourologist the means to access the entire collecting system without the invasive characteristics of previous open surgical approaches.

Nowadays, ureteroscopies and renoscopies have become the mainstay treatment for several urinary tract diseases, such as urolithiasis. However, all those technological advances, by themselves, do not automatically correspond to safe and effective surgeries; on the contrary, one must always keep in mind that the basic principles of urinary endoscopy are still essential for a successful procedure. One of these basic principles comprises the irrigation systems and fluids, representing an important feat in endoscopic evolution.

Our current technique of active endoscopic fluid irrigation through a channel in the endoscope, which not only allowed the passage of fluids for a better visualization but also instruments for therapeutic and/or diagnostic proposals, has been the mainstay of endoscopy for the last two decades [1].

Nevertheless, the fluid flow injected into the collecting system may elevate the pressure within the kidney, potentially resulting in detrimental effects due to pyelolymphatic and/or pyelovenous backflow [2, 3]. Animal studies have demonstrated that, in the presence of pressures >150 mmHg, immediate gross alterations were detected in the renal papilla, such as diffuse denudation, flattening and submucosal congestion, and edema [4, 5]. Additionally, the authors showed that 4–6 weeks post-procedure there was a higher incidence of pericalyceal vasculitis, degeneration, renal tubules vacuolization, and columnar metaplasia in those papillas subjected to high pressures as compared to those with low irrigant pressures (<90 mmHg). Those microscopic findings were translated into focal renal scarring in five of seven renal units exposed to high pressures, whereas no scarring was noted in all the renal units exposed to low irrigation pressures [4].

Hence, despite all the undeniable benefits provided by the use of fluid irrigation systems during urinary tract endoscopy, endourologists must be aware of: (a) the potential hazards of pressure elevation during retrograde ureterorenoscopy, (b) what favors it to happen, and also (c) the options to avoid its consequences.

R.N. Pedro, M.D., Ph.D. (✉)
Ambulatory Surgical Unit, Lithotripsy Center, State University of Campinas, Rua Maruba, 631, Alphaville, Campinas, Sao Paulo 13098 340, Brazil

Clinica Padre Almeida, Endourology and Kidney Stones Treatment, Rua Maruba, 631, Alphaville, Campinas 13098 340, Sao Paulo, Brazil
e-mail: rnpedro@gmail.com

M. Monga (ed.), *Ureteroscopy: Indications, Instrumentation & Technique*, Current Clinical Urology, DOI 10.1007/978-1-62703-206-3_12,

Irrigation System

Historically, natural antegrade urine flow was the primary source of irrigation for urinary endoscopy [6]. In process of time and with the development of the working channel of the endoscope, the active retrograde fluid irrigation drastically improved upper urinary collecting system endoscopy [7].

To date, irrigation systems vary from gravity dependence to those operated by repetitive hand or foot control. The later enables the endourologists to correlate the frequency and force of pumps with the need of clearing the visual field [8].

The gravity-based irrigation systems create the least amount of pressure (50 mmHg), but it cannot be controlled by the surgeon and occasionally, it may result in impaired visual field. Pressure bags can be placed around the irrigation fluid to augment flow, and this can be titrated by the surgeon using the stopcock on the endoscope. In contrast, hand and foot pump irrigation systems are actively controlled by the surgeon resulting in peaks of high flow and pressure (up to 410 mmHg) according to the energy dispended onto the pump [9].

Figure 12.1 shows some of the different types of irrigation systems. A recent "in vitro" study compared all types of irrigation systems available for retrograde urinary endoscopy with regards to visual field clearing efficiency and forces exerted on a phantom stone. The authors demonstrated that, at the minimum fluid flow needed to visualize the phantom stone, the gravity dependent devices exerted less force on the stone; whereas, out of the pump-based irrigation systems, the hand-held device, Single Action Pump—Boston Scientific™, exerted the least total maximum impulse on the stone [9].

It is recommended using a hand-held irrigation system device during a retrograde ureterorenoscopy for its capacity to clear the visual field and also for providing a meticulous manual regulation of flow intensity when demanded by the surgeon.

Moreover, it is worthy to note that important factors affect the success of irrigation techniques including the use of a ureteral access sheath, size of the working channel, tip deflection in flexible ureteroscopes; number, size, and composition of instruments placed in the working channel; and of course, the type of irrigation system and irrigation fluids.

Irrigation Fluids

The fluid must be transparent, thin, sterile, warm, without debris, and chemically innocuous to the human tissue to be eligible for urinary endoscopy. As mentioned before in this chapter, during a ureteroscopy, fluid flow not only clears away blood, urine, and debris from the optical field but also distends the collecting system, permitting a thorough inspection of endoluminal structures [2].

Physiological saline encompasses all of the above-mentioned requisites, and it prevents electrolyte imbalance (hyponatremia) in the presence of mild to moderate fluid absorption, as in case of occasional pyelolymphatic/pyelovenous backflow during a high-pressure ureteroscopy. However, fluid overload, congestive heart failure, hypothermia, and hemolysis are associated with high fluid absorption seen in long operative times, sustained high intrarenal pressures or in advent of serious urothelial rupture with retroperitoneal extravasation, jeopardizing not only the endoscopic treatment success but also the patient's well-being [10, 11]. Given the factual risks of clinically relevant adverse events related to the retrograde ureterorenoscopy, identifying adjunctive measures by which intrarenal pressure could be lowered may be protective for the patient.

For this reason, the use of pharmacological agents in the irrigation fluid has been postulated, based on the premise that the renal pelvis and ureter have adrenergic, cholinergic and muscarinic receptors that directly interact with endoluminal pressure [12–15]. It has been demonstrated in an "in vivo" study that the use of catecholamines relaxes the ureteral muscle. This relaxant effect was attributed to activation of beta 2 and 3 receptors in the ureteral segment immersed in a saline solution with catecholamines [13]. In another animal study, the endoluminal norepinephrine injection into the ureter inhibited peristalsis,

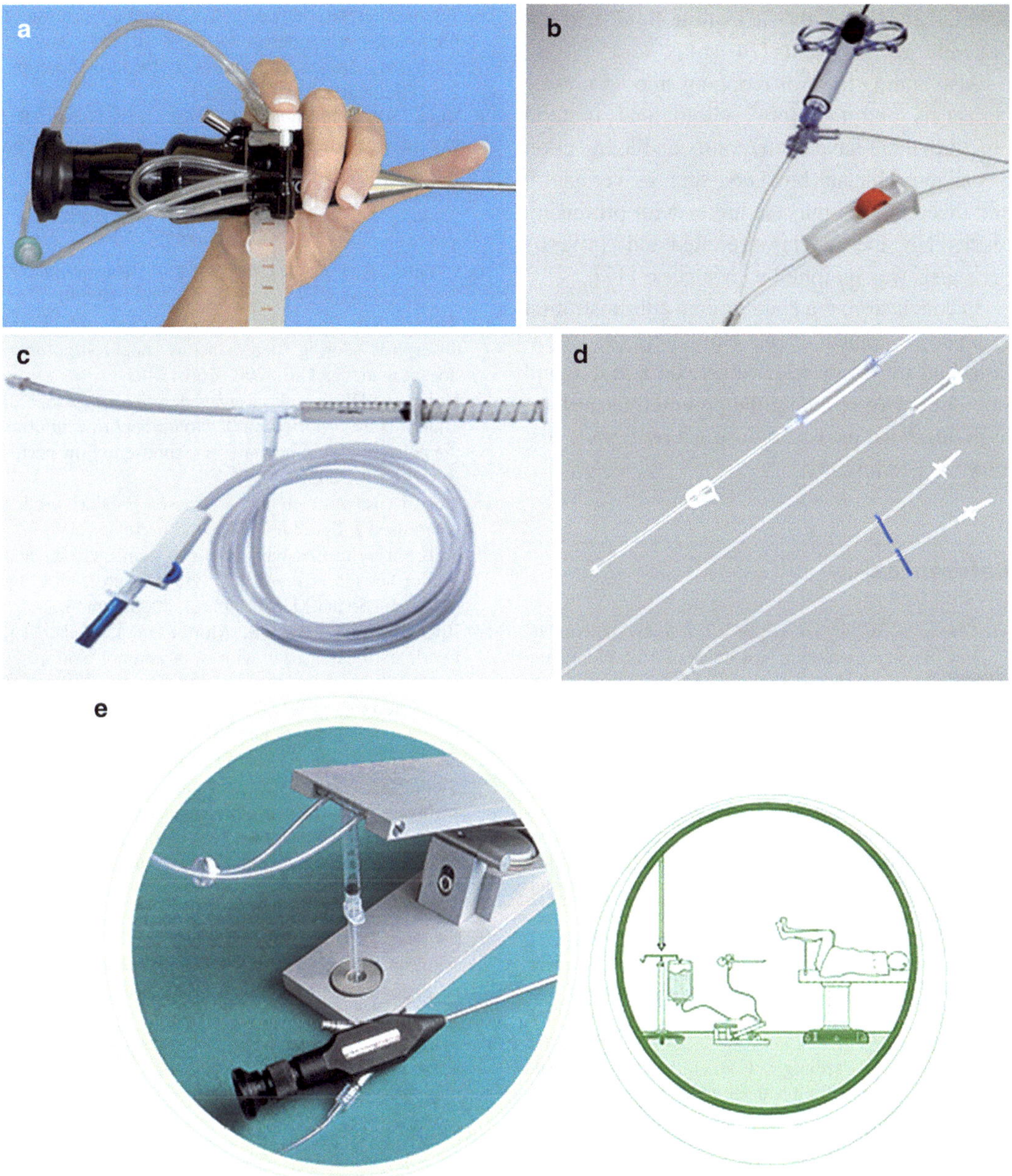

Fig. 12.1 Irrigation systems. (**a**) Kosin universal piggy-back irrigation system. Permission for use granted by Kosin Technologies. (**b**) Boston Scientific Single Action Pump (SAP). Permission for use granted by Boston Scientific. (**c**) Irri-flo irrigation delivery system, Gyrus ACMI. Permission for use granted by Gyrus ACMI and Olympus. (**d**) Ureteroscopy Irrigation System, Cook. Permission for use granted by Cook Medical Incorporated, Bloomington, Indiana. (**e**) Peditrol Foot Pump, Wismed. Permission for use granted by Wismed Medical Projects

resulting in a decrease of the smooth muscle tonus that in turn, eliminated the phasic pressure response to perfusion [12]. The most potent relaxing catecholamines were isoproterenol followed by epinephrine and norepinephrine subsequently [14]. These studies suggest it is possible to obtain a direct local response on endoluminal pressure by adding one of the above-mentioned catecholamines in the irrigation fluid without systemic adverse events [14–16].

Also aiming towards reducing smooth muscle peristalsis and therefore endoluminal ureteral pressure, there have been reports on the injection of calcium channel blockers, such as verapamil and theophylline, into the ureter with promising results. No side effects were cited and "in vivo" peristalsis was inhibited with success [17].

In conclusion, the endoluminal administration of pharmacological agents along with the irrigation fluid may, in a near future, be a viable and safe option for reducing the potential hazards of high intrarenal pressures during a retrograde urinary tract endoscopy.

References

1. Grasso M, Bagley D. A 7.5/8.2 F actively deflectable, flexible ureteroscope: a new device for both diagnostic and therapeutic upper urinary tract endoscopy. Urology. 1994;43(4):435–41.
2. Monga M, Hendlin K, Skenazy J, Ramani A. A novel dual-diameter ureteroscope working channel: impact on irrigant flow. Urology. 2004;64:892.
3. Auge BK, Pietrow PK, Lallas CD, Raj GV, Santa-Cruz RW, Preminger GM. Ureteral access sheath provides protection against elevated renal pressures during routine flexible ureteroscopic stone manipulation. J Endourol. 2004;18:33.
4. Schwalb DM, Eshghi M, Davidian M, Franco I. Morphological and physiological changes in the urinary tract associated with ureteral dilation and ureteropyeloscopy: an experimental study. J Urol. 1993;149:1576.
5. Wilson WT, Preminger GM. Intrarenal pressures generated during fexible defectable ureterorenoscopy. J Endourol. 1990;4:2.
6. Takayasu H, Aso Y, Takagi T. Clinical application of fiber optic pyeloureteroscope. Urol Int. 1971;26:97.
7. Bush IM, Guinan P, Lanners J. Ureterorenoscopy. Urol Clin North Am. 1982;9:131.
8. Blew BD, Dagnone AJ, Pace KT, Honey RJ. Comparison of peditrol irrigation device and common methods of irrigation. J Endourol. 2005;19:562.
9. Hendlin K, Weiland D, Monga M. Impact of irrigation systems on stone migration. J Endourol. 2008;22(3):453–8.
10. Cybulski P, Honey RJ, Pace K. Fluid absorption during ureterorenoscopy. J Endourol. 2004;18:739.
11. Kukreja RA, Desai MR, Sabnis RB, Patel SH. Fluid absorption during percutaneous nephrolithotomy: does it matter? J Urol. 2002;168:1348.
12. Holst U, Dissing T, Rawashdeh YF, Frokiaer J, Djurhuus JC, Mortensen J. Norepinephrine inhibits the pelvic pressure increase in response to flow perfusion. J Urol. 2003;170:268–71.
13. Holst U, Rawashdeh YF, Andreasen F, Djurhuus JC, Mortensen J. Endoluminal pelvic perfusion with norepinephrine causes only minor systemic effects and diminishes the increase in pelvic pressure caused by perfusion. Scand J Urol Nephrol. 2005;39:443.
14. Jung HU, Jakobsen JS, Mortensen J, Osther PJ, Djurhuus JC. Irrigation with isoproterenol diminishes increases in pelvic pressure without side-effects during ureterorenoscopy: a randomized controlled study in a porcine model. Scand J Urol Nephrol. 2007;6:1.
15. Danuser H, Weiss R, Abel D, Walter B, Scholtysik G, Mettler D, Studer UE. Systemic and topical drug administration in the pig ureter: effect of phosphodiesterase inhibitors alpha1, beta and beta2-adrenergic receptor agonists and antagonists on the frequency and amplitude of ureteral contractions. J Urol. 2001;166:714.
16. Jakobsen JS, Holst U, Jakobsen P, Steen W, Mortensen J. Local and systemic effects of endoluminal pelvic perfusion of isoproterenol: a dose response investigation in pigs. J Urol. 2007;177:1934.
17. Selmy GI, Hassouna MM, Khalafl M, Elhilali MM. Effects of verapamil, prostaglandin F2 alpha, phenylephrine, and noradrenaline on upper urinary tract dynamics. Urology. 1994;43:31.

Intracorporeal Lithotripsy: Electrohydraulic, Pneumatic, and Ultrasonic

13

Joe Miller and Marshall L. Stoller

Introduction

The terms lithotrite and lithotripsy derive from the Greek *lithos* for "stone" and the Latin *tritus*, a derivation of *terre,* meaning "to rub" [1]. Many lithotripsy energy sources were first used for lithalopaxy, the crushing of bladder stones. Electrohydraulic lithotripsy (EHL), pneumatic lithotripsy (PL), and ultrasonic lithotripsy (USL) for the treatment of ureteral stones also predated the development of the ureteroscope and the practice of ureteroscopy. These lithotripsy techniques were initially performed using a cystoscope for the blind placement of the lithotrite energy probe into the ureter, with intraoperative localization confirmed and monitored with fluoroscopy. Predictably, these blind techniques had poor success rates and an unacceptable incidence of complications, most commonly ureteral perforation [2, 3].

In the late 1970s ureteroscopy of the distal ureter was sporadically performed using short pediatric cystoscopes. The subsequent development of a dedicated 30 cm, 13–14.5 F rigid ureteroscope led to the routine performance of ureteroscopy and was an important step toward the practice of direct vision intracorporeal lithotripsy of ureteral stones. Due to the large diameter of the first ureteroscopes, early ureteroscopy was limited to the manipulation and extraction of stones in the distal ureter, but nonetheless ureteroscopy offered a much less invasive alternative to contemporary open ureterolithotomy, and a was major advancement for the fledgling field of endourology [4]. The rapid miniaturization of both ureteroscopes and lithotrite energy probes soon led to the widespread adoption of direct vision intracorporeal lithotripsy for the treatment for ureteral stones [5]. Just as ureteroscopy and the aforementioned methods of lithotripsy were maturing, shock wave lithotripsy (SWL) and laser lithotripsy (LL) systems became commercially available. SWL offered a less invasive means of treating some ureteral stones, but refractory cases due to stone composition or location were still common, and machine availability was initially limited to larger academic and urban centers. LL meanwhile offered a safer and often more effective means of stone fragmentation, but came at a greater financial cost that included initial equipment acquisition and high-priced disposable equipment. Combined with the required annual maintenance contract, the cost of early LL systems could reach $300,000 [6]. In the face of these competing techniques, and after 30 years and enumerable studies comparing the efficacy, safety and cost of the various methods of treatment for ureteral stones, ureteroscopy with intracorporeal lithotripsy remains a widely practiced and necessary tool in the urologist's armamentarium. Among the US population, the utilization

J. Miller, M.D. • M.L. Stoller, M.D. (✉)
Urology Department, University of California San Francisco, 400 Parnassus Avenue, A610, San Francisco, CA 94143-2200, USA
e-mail: mstoller@urol.ucsf.edu

M. Monga (ed.), *Ureteroscopy: Indications, Instrumentation & Technique*, Current Clinical Urology, DOI 10.1007/978-1-62703-206-3_13, © Springer Science+Business Media New York 2013

of ureteroscopy increased from 41.8 to 52.2/100,000 from 1998 to 2004, and the UK experienced a 131% increase in ureteroscopic stone procedures from 2000 to 2010 [7, 8].

In this chapter we review the history, mechanism, and performance of ureteroscopy with EHL, PL, USL, and the combination pneumatic-ultrasonic lithotripsy (PUL), for the treatment of ureteral stones. A survey of studies detailing safety, outcomes, complications, and costs of these techniques is also provided.

Electrohydraulic Lithotripsy

EHL, first described in the 1950s and initially called "electronic lithotripsy," was widely used to treat bladder stones prior to its adaptation for ureteroscopy. EHL is accomplished by the generation of an electrical spark at the distal end of a coaxial probe, which is placed in direct contact with the stone. Vaporization of the surrounding liquid medium by the spark produces a rapidly expanding plasma bubble [9]. Depending on the energy setting, the bubble expands to 4–11 mm in diameter and then persists for 400–500 μs before collapsing [10]. The dielectric irrigation medium transfers the resultant electrohydraulic shock wave from the rapidly expanding bubble to the surface of the stone to cause fragmentation [11].

The first commercially available EHL system was the Russian *Urat-1* (Medexport, Moscow, USSR). The system consisted of a pulse generator and a 10 F rigid probe that could be passed through the working channel of a standard 24 F rigid cystoscope. The *Urat-1* pulse generator stored electric energy in capacitors, which allowed electrical discharges to be delivered instantaneously to the end of the probe at variable power, rate, and duration [12]. An initial series of 304 patients undergoing lithalopaxy included bladder stones as large as 135 g and achieved a mean total operative time, including removal of fragments, of 26 (2–122) minutes. Complications were limited to 6 bladder perforations for a rate of 1.9%, including one extraperitoneal perforation that required laparotomy and repair [13]. Early experience in using EHL to treat bladder stones was transferred first to the ureters of dogs and cadavers before development of a smaller flexible probe that could be passed into the ureter and positioned with the aid of fluoroscopy [2]. Complications including ureteral perforation occurred in as many as 40% of early cases owing to the inaccuracy inherent in the blind radiological targeting and the rapid generation of heat at the distal tip of the probe [3]. Development of the 9.5 F ureteroscope with a 5 F-working channel to accommodate the new, smaller 5 F EHL probe allowed stone fragmentation in the ureter under direct vision, with markedly fewer complications and a higher success rate of approximately 90% [14, 15].

Further technical refinements resulted in miniaturization of the flexible EHL probes to 2–3 F and semirigid ureteroscopes to 7 F (Fig. 13.1). This allowed fragmentation of stones in the entire ureter and renal collecting system, utilizing a rigid or flexible ureteroscope, via retrograde ureteral access or antegrade percutaneous access. In a series of 94 ureteral stones 3–19 mm in diameter, ureteroscopy and direct vision EHL resulted in a complete fragmentation rate of 91.5%, with no major complications and a low incidence of minor complications including hematuria (2.2%), urinary tract infection (3.4%), and postoperative ureteral colic (2.2%) [16].

Due in part to the higher risk of ureteral perforation, the use of EHL for the treatment of ureteral stones was largely supplanted by the other modalities discussed within this section. EHL (as well as PL and USL) was further marginalized as the equipment for SWL and LL became more economically competitive and the techniques demonstrated high success rates and more favorable safety profiles [17, 18].

Pneumatic Lithotripsy

PL was introduced in the early 1990s with the development of the Swiss Lithoclast (Microvasive-Boston Scientific Corp., Boston, Massachusetts). This simplified means of stone fragmentation is accomplished via a rigid energy probe that is placed in direct contact with the stone (Fig. 13.2).

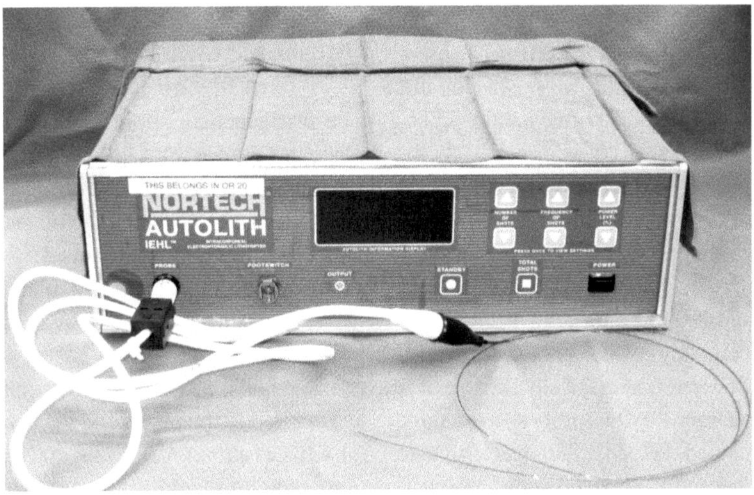

Fig. 13.1 Electrohydraulic lithotrite

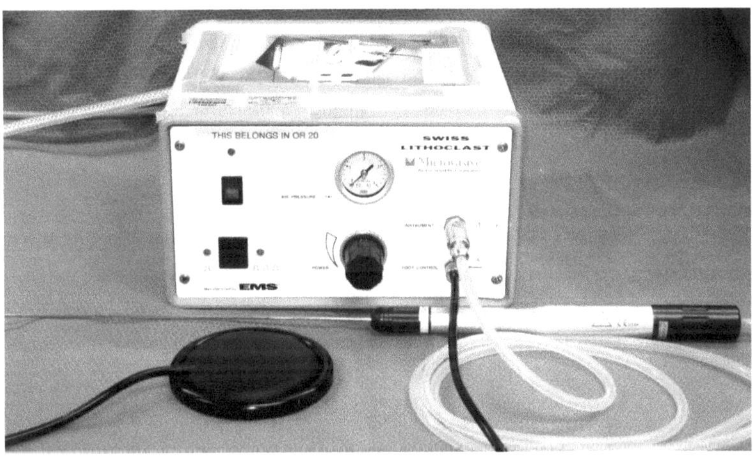

Fig. 13.2 Pneumatic lithotrite

The application of compressed air to a sliding metal projectile in the hand piece transmits energy to the probe and subsequently to the surface of the stone, facilitating stone fragmentation in a manner similar to that of a jackhammer [19]. Depending upon probe diameter and the air pressure setting, the rigid probe of the Lithoclast achieves a maximum velocity of 12.1–33.3 m/s with a maximum probe displacement of 2.53 mm [20]. The use of a readily available energy source (compressed air) as well as reusable probes and hand pieces made PL a practical and economical treatment option for ureteral stones upon its introduction [21].

The early rigid PL probes of the Lithoclast had to be used with a rigid ureteroscope or nephroscope, which initially restricted the application of the technique. To address this limitation, flexible pneumatic probes were developed for the Lithoclast. Although these new probes could be used through flexible ureteroscopes, a progressive loss of probe tip displacement, velocity, and energy, as well as stone fragmentation efficacy resulted, particularly with deflection angles greater than 24° [22, 23]. A rival PL system, the Browne Pneumatic Impactor (BPI; Browne Medical Systems, Minneapolis, MN), was the first lithotrite to come to market with flexible probes for PL. Utilizing the same basic principal as the Lithoclast, the BPI used compressed air to propel a 1.5–1.8 F nickel–titanium (Nitinol) wire through a polymer sheath that could be employed through a semirigid or actively deflectable flexible ureteroscope. Normal probe tip displacement and stone fragmentation efficacy was only maintained through 30 ° of deflection with the smallest flexible BPI probes, but larger flexible probes maintained tip displacement and velocity and were able to fragment even hard stones, at 90 ° of deflection [24]. In a small series of patients with stones as large as 20 mm, 7 of 8 ureteral stones were successfully fragmented using the BPI [25].

In addition to the maneuverability limitations imposed by PL probes, proximal stone fragment migration was a pervasive problem inherent to the nature of PL stone fragmentation. As many as 18% of patients undergoing PL for treatment of ureteral stones required secondary procedures due to proximal migration of large stone fragments [6, 26]. In an attempt to overcome this problem, as well as to provide an efficient means of small stone fragment evacuation, the Lithovac (Microvasive-Boston Scientific, Boston, Massachusetts) was developed. The Lithovac is a hollow suction probe through which the rigid Lithoclast energy probe projects. The device provides constant suction and is designed to facilitate the simultaneous evacuation of smaller fragments as the stone is destroyed, as well as helping to prevent proximal migration of larger fragments that would necessitate a secondary procedure. In a study performed shortly after its introduction, the Lithovac achieved a 100% ureteral stone fragmentation rate, with no proximal fragment migration and a stone-free rate of 95% [27].

As with EHL, the popularity of SWL and LL systems drastically decreased the utilization of PL. Some contemporary comparative studies suggest that PL remains an effective and economically treatment option for some ureteral stones [28, 29].

Ultrasonic Lithotripsy

The first practical application of ultrasound took place in France in 1916 when Chilowsky and Langevin patented the use of ultrasonic sonar for the underwater localization of submarines [30]. Ultrasonic energy is produced when alternating electrical current is applied to plates on the opposing sides of a crystal. The resultant mechanical vibrations of the crystal propagate waves of energy at a constant frequency, as determined by the voltage applied to the plates and the nature of the crystal. Observations of the disruptive effects of the first sonar on marine life led to the elucidation of the mechanism by which the ultrasonic vibrations affect objects within their path. The high frequency energy waves of ultrasound alternately compress and pull on particles within the radiation field. In transmission media such as water, this results in cavitation. When these cavities rapidly collapse instantaneous pressure is produced with magnitude and force capable of destroying solid objects [31]. Early attempts to fragment urinary and biliary stones by the direct application of ultrasound were unsuccessful due to the high electrical energy requirements and difficulties in conducting and focusing the ultrasonic energy [32–34]. In the early 1970s the ultrasonic lithotrite was developed. Rather than relying on the direct application of ultrasound energy and the resultant cavitation to disintegrate stones, the ultrasonic lithotrite uses an ultrasound transducer to rapidly vibrate a hollow probe and longitudinally transmit mechanical energy to the surface of stone, causing fragmentation in the same manner a drill (Fig. 13.3) [31]. The hollow USL probe facilitates simultaneous suction removal of stone fragments and constant-flow irrigation aids in fragment removal and cools the USL probe to reduce the risk of thermal damage to adjacent tissues [35].

Prior to its adoption for ureteroscopy, USL was widely employed in the transurethral treatment of bladder stones and in the percutaneous treatment of renal stones [36, 37]. Initially, USL in the ureter was performed in a blind fashion with fluoroscopic guidance. Results were more favorable than those seen with blind treatment of

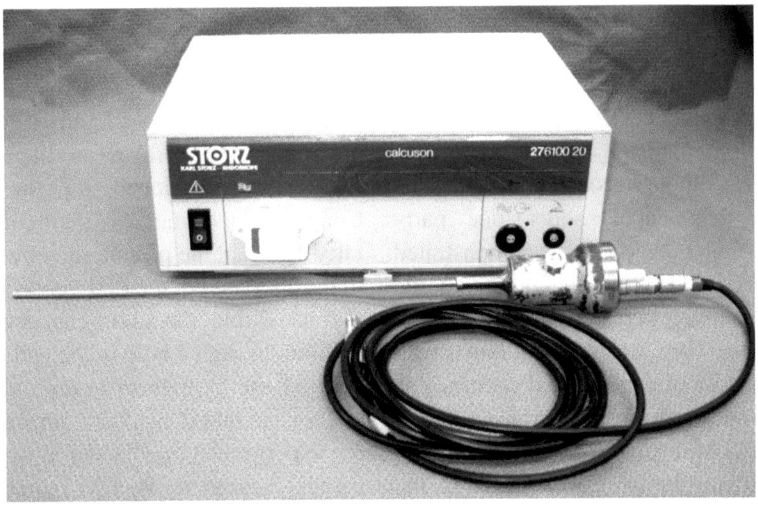

Fig. 13.3 Ultrasonic lithotrite

ureteral stones with EHL or PL, and complications rates were much lower [4]. Direct vision ureteroscopic USL was made possible by the miniaturization of ureteroscopes that could employ the first generation 4.5–6 F hollow probes. The development of a 2.5 F solid wire USL probe significantly increased the treatment range and efficiency of the technique [35]. The wire USL probe transmits the mechanical energy of the ultrasonic transducer to the stone in a transverse nature which, unlike the longitudinal energy transmission of a hollow probe, resulting in disintegration of the stone. A multi-institutional series of 118 upper, mid, and lower ureteral stones treated with USL demonstrated an overall success rate of 96.6% with a low rate of complications and secondary procedures [38].

As in the case of EHL and PL, SWL and LL systems have largely replaced USL in the treatment of ureteral stones, but they remain useful in some clinical situations such as patients with steinstrasse or a large ureteral stone burden [39].

Combination Ultrasonic and Pneumatic Lithotripsy

A combination intracorporeal lithotripter, the Lithoclast Ultra (Boston Scientific Corporation, Natick, MA) was introduced to take advantage of the rapid stone fragmentation of pneumatic lithotripsy and the efficient fragment evacuation ability of a hollow ultrasonic lithotripter. The pneumatic ultrasonic lithotripsy (PUL) allows the dual energy sources to be used individually or concomitantly depending on operator preference, stone composition, size, or location. Laboratory tests on stone phantoms found more efficient stone fragmentation and evacuation with the use of the combined energies at their highest settings, when compared to the highest setting operation of either mode alone [40, 41]. Early clinical experience verified the utility of PUL, but a randomized comparison revealed stone-free rates achieved with PUL were not significantly greater than those of USL alone [42].

The Safety of Intracorporeal Lithotrites

The emergence of each new lithotripsy technology prompted studies evaluating and comparing the risks associated with the use of their novel energy sources within the narrow confines of the ureter. The introduction of SWL and LL further highlighted the risks associated with all preceding methods of intracorporeal lithotripsy, and renewed concerns about the acute and long-term risks of their use. We provide a brief survey of the results of in vitro and in vivo analyses of the safety of each technique.

Electrohydraulic Lithotripsy

Among the methods of intracorporeal lithotripsy discussed in this chapter, EHL has the highest risk of acute tissue damage when used to treat ureteral stones. Although considered safe and effective for the treatment of bladder stones, early studies on the ureters of cadavers demonstrated the *Urat-1* was capable of rapidly inflicting tissue damage and ureteral perforation [11]. Direct application of the *Urat-1* to the abdominal wall and bladder mucosa of anesthetized canines was found to cause blistering and hemorrhage through the full thickness of the dermis and epidermis of the abdomen, and similar effects through the mucosa and detrussor muscle of the bladder [12]. High speed video of spark discharges at the tip of EHL probes revealed that the blast energy of the cavitation bubbles cause only small areas of trauma, limited in size to the diameter of the probe, even with the probe in direct contact with sections of opened human ureter. However, when confined within in the lumen of the ureter, the blast energy cannot be effectively dispersed and it causes rapid expansion of the ureteral wall and complete disruption of the ureter in a longitudinal fashion, as far as 1 cm from the tip of the probe [43]. To better characterize the immediate and potential long-term ureteral damage of EHL, the probe of a second generation EHL lithotrite was directly applied in a perpendicular fashion to the ureters of two anesthetized pigs. Histological samples were then analyzed at the time of injury, 1 day, and 6 days after injury. Within the ureter EHL produced an immediate partial abrasion of the urothelium and caused edema within the underlying lamina propria. By day one the urothelium was totally abraded and the edema in the lamina propria was increased and extended into the ureteric smooth muscle. Analysis of the ureteral sections 6 days after injury revealed worsening damage and reactive hyperplasia with excessive mucous secretion. This extensive damage can be partially attributed to the initial blast injury caused by the rapid expansion and collapse of the plasma bubble. To an even greater degree, full-thickness ureteral damage is due to the heat that is rapidly generated at the probe tip [44]. In an ex vivo model utilizing sections of pig ureter, application of EHL at the lowest power setting produced visible perforation of the ureter within approximately 25 pulses [45]. To reduce the risk of collateral tissue damage, a plasma shield was developed for the EHL probe. Composed of a stainless steel coil and a perforated end cap, the plasma shield was designed to fit the distal end of the EHL probe and confine the plasma within the coil. The energy was then focused through a hole in the end of the cap that reduced energy transfer to the tissue. In a study employing rabbit bladders, an unshielded EHL probe perforated the bladder in two pulses, compared to a mean of 35 pulses required to perforate with a shielded EHL probe [46].

While the EHL remains an efficient and economical tool for the treatment of some bladder stones, the propensity for tissue damage has limited its role for treatment of stones within the ureter.

Pneumatic Lithotripsy

In contrast to the early outcomes of EHL, PL the novel Swiss Lithoclast appeared to be effective and safe for use in the treatment of ureteral stones. Deliberate attempts to perforate the ureters of anesthetized female swine with 0.8 and 1.0 mm rigid Lithoclast probes resulted in perforation with the 0.8 mm probe, but not until after delivery of 250 consecutive shocks. Perforation of the ureter with the 1.0 mm probe was deemed impossible. Although no macroscopic lesions were visible on the ureteral epithelium, abrasion, and edema were seen on histologic analysis of treated sections of ureter [44]. Similar areas of transmural edema, abrasion, and hemorrhage were identified microscopically in sections of pig ureter subjected to direct firing of a 3.5 F Lithoclast probe for 5–7 s. In the same experiment, animals sacrificed 3 weeks later had no evidence of ureteral perforation on retrograde pyelography, and treated areas of ureteral tissue showed no microscopic evidence of damage. Animals sacrificed at 6 weeks posttreatment also had normal retrograde pyelograms and no direct evidence of microscopic tissue trauma to treated ureteral sections [47]. The safety of PL was further confirmed when the direct application of a 3 F rigid probe for 6 min of continuous activation failed to perforate ex vivo sections of pig ureter, even with "vigorous attempts to impale the ureter" [45].

An extensive study of the safety of PL, including its use to treat plaster-of-Paris stone phantoms in swine ureters and stones in the kidneys, ureters, and bladders of human patients, revealed that even direct and deliberate application to soft tissues results in minimal trauma. Among the 37 ureteral stones treated in the human portion of the study, one patient suffered a minor ureteral perforation attributed to "overenthusiastic ureteroscopy." Follow-up intravenous urograms of 25 patients obtained 1 month after PL demonstrated no ureteral injuries [48].

Ultrasonic Lithotripsy

Some of the earliest experiments to assess the effects of USL on the tissue of the ureter were performed in dogs. A 30-s application of the USL probe to human stones implanted in the canine ureter was followed by direct application of the probe to the ureteral mucosa for 5, 10, and 15-s intervals. Gross and histological examination of the ureteral tissue was performed after 48 and 72 h. No gross trauma to the ureteral wall was noted during applications of 10 s or less. Applications of the USL probe directly to the ureteral wall for 15 s caused visible and histologic changes consistent with thermal damage. The investigators theorized that this thermal damage could easily be prevented during routine use of the USL when pulses of 10 s or less are used and the buildup heat at the probe tip is avoided. Because this study was conducted prior to the introduction of ureteroscopy and direct vision intracorporeal lithotripsy, the main cause of most ureteral perforation was actually excessive force applied to the probe, and not ultrasound energy or the resultant heat [34]. A second study examining the effect of USL on the canine bladders revealed that direct contact application of the probe to the urothelium for 10 min produced only modest long-term histologic changes in sections examined 1 month after treatment [31]. A test of the ability of USL probe to cause perforation of swine ureter after 12 pulses of 3 s each resulted in no perforations and no macroscopic changes in the urothelium. Histologic examination of treated tissue on the day of treatment revealed no changes to the urothelium. Microscopic changes seen 1 and 6 days after treatment were moderate and less extensive than those seen in tissue samples of ureters treated with PL, EHL, or LL. The authors concluded that USL was among the safest of the lithotripsy technologies available at the time [44].

Because the energy of USL is produced by the generation of sound waves, its clinical use presented a unique safety concern regarding the effects of USL on the hearing of patients, physicians, and operating room personnel. In the US workplace noise exposure limits are established and monitored by the Occupational Safety and Health Administration (OSHA). The allowable continuous exposure is 8 h at 90 decibels (dBA), with a 50% decrease in duration mandated for each 5 dBA above 90 dBA. Measurements of the sound levels of the three commercially available USL units during actual cases of intracorporeal lithotripsy showed both decibel levels and exposure durations well below OSHA standards. Additionally, an audiogram performed on a urologist with a 3-year total of more than 40 cases of ultrasonic lithotripsy did not detect any hearing threshold sensitivity deficit [49]. An experimental model used to simulate the use of USL in the ureter during pregnancy concluded that the peak pressure of sound emitted during lithotripsy was unlikely to harm the hearing of the fetus [50].

Comparative Studies of Outcomes, Complications, and Cost

In addition to concerns regarding the safety of emerging lithotrite technologies, the introduction of each successive modality instigated comparisons to existing modes with special interest in the outcomes, complications, and costs. In this section we present summaries of a representative selection of these studies. Although LL is not

Table 13.1 Summary of comparative studies

Year author	n	Lithotrites (n)	Outcome measures and results
1991 Vicente J	100	USL (67) EHL (33)	• Successful fragmentation (USL vs. EHL): 93 vs. 73% • Three patients each group required secondary procedure • 1 EHL patient required ureteral reimplant
1994 Naqvi S	200	PL (152) LL (48)	• Non-fragmentation rate (PL vs. LL): 1 vs. 10% • Stone free ≤4 weeks (PL vs. LL) : 95 vs. 84%
1995 Hofbauer J	72	EHL (34) PL (38)	• Successful fragmentation (EHL vs. PL): 85 vs. 90% ($p=0.12$) • Need for secondary SWL (EHL vs. PL): 15 vs. 11% ($p=0.63$) • Ureteral perforation (EHL vs. PL): 18 vs. 3% ($p<0.01$)
1997 Teichman J	70	EHL (23) LL (47)	• Stone free at procedure (EHL vs. LL): 56 vs. 94% ($p=0.002$) • Stone free at 3 months (EHL vs. LL): 87 vs. 98% ($p=0.01$)
2001 Sun Y	286	PL (145) LL (140)	• Successful fragmentation (PL vs. LL): 70 vs. 96% ($p<0.01$) • Days to stone-free status (PL vs. LL): 31 vs. 18 ($p<0.01$) • Ureteral perforation (PL vs. LL): 5 vs. 0
2008 Maghsoudi R	82	PL (41) LL (41)	• Successful fragmentation (PL vs. LL): 73 vs. 90% ($p=0.46$) • Stone free at 1 month (PL vs. LL): 81 vs. 95% ($p=0.043$) • Proximal stone migration (PL vs. LL): 7.3 vs. 2.4% ($p=0.6$)
2008 Manohar T	50	PL (25) LL (25)	• Fragmentation time (PL vs. LL): 7.86 vs. 9.82 min ($p=0.12$) • Stone-free rate (PL vs. LL): 88 vs. 84% ($p=0.41$) • Proximal stone migration (PL vs. LL): 16 vs. 24% ($p=0.82$) • Secondary procedure (PL vs. LL): 12 vs. 16% ($p=0.99$) • Ureteral perforation (PL vs. LL): 12 vs. 8% ($p=0.34$)
2011 Binbay M	80	PL (40) LL (40)	• Operative time (PL vs. LL): 48 vs. 30 min. ($p=0.001$) • Stone-free rate (PL vs. LL): 80% vs. 98% ($p=0.03$) • Proximal stone migration (PL vs. LL): 4 vs. 1 ($p=0.29$) • Secondary procedure (PL vs. LL): 7 vs. 1 ($p=0.05$) • Ureteral perforation (PL vs. LL): 1 vs. 2
2012 Salvadó J	65	PL (22) PUL (20) LL (23)	• Operative time (PL vs. PUL vs. LL): 27 vs. 27 vs. 22 min ($p=0.97$) • Stone-free rate (PL vs. PUL vs. LL): 96% vs. 97% vs. 97% ($p=0.97$) • Proximal stone migration (PL vs. PUL vs. LL):14% vs. 20% vs. 17% ($p=0.87$) • Complications (PL vs. PUL vs. LL): 18% vs. 4.6% vs. 13% ($p=0.47$)

discussed in the chapter, studies comparing various types of lasers to EHL, PL, USL, and PUL are also included because the laser would eventually become the dominate energy source for intracorporeal ureteral lithotripsy. Table 13.1 summarizes the comparative studies detailed below.

USL vs. EHL

In a review of 100 consecutive cases of in situ lithotripsy of primary ureteral stones, Vicente and colleagues were among the first groups to compare the new USL and EHL systems. The study compared the outcomes and complications of 67 patients with 83 stones treated with USL to a group of 33 patients with 42 treated with EHL. Stone size, location, and composition between groups were similar. A favorable outcome was defined as successful stone fragmentation and extraction with preservation of the integrity of the urinary tract. Among the patients treated with USL, 92.5% of outcomes were considered favorable, compared to 72.7% of cases in which EHL was used. The need for secondary procedures was also documented and included open ureterolithotomy (EHL=2, USL=1), ureteral reimplant (EHL=1), percutaneous nephrolithotomy (EHL=1, USL=1), and SWL (USL=1) [51].

EHL vs. PL

A prospective, randomized study comparing the successful fragmentation rate and complications of EHL and PL included a total of 72 patients with ureteral stones not amenable to SWL. Among the patients in the EHL group, 29/34 (85.3%) of cases resulted in successful fragmentation of stone to ≤3 mm, as assessed by renal and bladder ultrasound or plain abdominal X-ray of the kidneys, ureters, and bladder (KUB). A similar rate of success of 89.5% ($p=0.12$) was achieved in the group treated with PL. The incidence of proximal fragment migration necessitating secondary SWL in each group was nearly identical. A notable difference between the two treatment groups was the rate of ureteral perforation; 6/34 (17.6%) patients treated with EHL, compared to 1/38 (2.6%, $p<0.01$) in the group treated with PL. This outcome is consistent with other reports of high risk of ureteral perforation with EHL, as well as the results of in vitro studies. A brief cost comparison included in the study noted the higher cost of the PL system, $17,000 compared to $11,000 for the EHL unit and was somewhat offset by the cost savings of the reusable PL probes [6].

EHL vs. LL

In a comparison of 70 consecutive patients with ureteral stones treated with either traditional EHL or the new Ho: YAG laser, LL resulted in a greater stone-free rate at completion of procedure (97 vs. 64%, $p<0.01$), but at 3 months the stone-free rates were similar (97 vs. 94%, $p=0.4$). In a direct comparison of operative times, EHL was faster for fragmentation of stones <15 mm, but LL was faster for stones ≥15 mm. Complications rates were similar between groups, but did not include three ureteral perforations in the EHL group that were treated at the time of occurrence with ureteral stenting. No direct cost comparison of EHL to LL was included in this study, but the authors noted that the laser system was shared with the departments of general surgery, orthopedics, and head and neck surgery to decrease the effective cost to any one department [52].

Although EHL was challenged by the development of LL in the early 1990s, EHL remained effective and widely used for many years largely because it was a far less costly alternative to the new lasers. The EHL system purchase price of $6,900 was considerably less than the cost of tunable dye laser that topped $187,500 and required an annual maintenance contract costing an additional $15,000 [5].

PL vs. LL

As LL became more widely available in the USA and other industrialized nations, the acquisition, maintenance, and operation costs began to decrease and the focus of comparative studies shifted to the efficacy and safety of the technologies. Some of the more contemporary studies at the end of this section highlight the important continuing consideration of the limited availability of modern laser systems in developing countries and document the efficacy of some the more traditional energy sources of EHL, PL, and USL.

A retrospective review of 200 ureteric stones treated with either the Swiss Lithoclast PL ($n=152$) or the Alexanderite Laser Impact (Dornier, Germany) ($n=48$) assessed the non-fragmentation rates, stone-free status <4 weeks and ≥4 weeks, treatment times, complications, and costs of each. Non-fragmentation rate of stones treated with LL was significantly higher (10.4 vs. 1.3%, $p=0.01$) and stone free status <4 weeks was lower (83.3 vs. 94.7%, $p<0.01$) when compared to PL. At ≥4 weeks stone-free status was similar, however. Treatment times were similar between the groups, though slightly shorter in the PL group. Cost per procedure comparison included the disposable laser fibers and favored PL that was accomplished at 1/8th the cost. Complications were not significantly different [53].

A study comparing the new Holmium:Yttrium-Aluminum-Garnet (Ho:YAG) to PL focused on the rates of successful fragmentation, mean operative times, time to stone-free status, and major complications. The state-of-the-art LL was superior in fragmentation (95.7 vs. 69.7%, $p<0.01$), mean operative time (25 vs. 35 min, $p<0.01$), and days until stone-free (18 vs. 31 days, $p<0.01$). The rate of major complications was greater in the PL patients with five ureteral perforations compared to none in the LL group. Stone-free status at 3 months was similar; however, 100% in the LL groups and 96% in the PL group, though 27 of those patients required a secondary SWL procedure. Although these results suggest the superiority of the LL system, a cost comparison was not provided [26].

A prospective randomized trial comparing 82 ureteral stones treated over a 1-year period included 41 stones each treated with PL or Ho:YAG. Successful fragmentation was accomplished in 37 (90.2%) cases of LL compared to 30 (73.2%) stones treated with PL. At 1-month stone-free status was assessed via KUB and ultrasound and was again superior in the LL group (95 vs. 80.5%). There were no major complications (ureteral perforation, urinoma, sepsis) in either group. Procedure costs were not assessed [18].

An assessment of the efficacy of PL and LL analyzed the fragmentation time, stone-free rate, complications, and secondary procedures among 50 randomized patients treated with the Swiss Lithoclast 2 ($n=25$) or Ho:YAG laser ($n=25$). Age, gender, and average stone size were similar. Stone-free rates were also similar, at 84% in the LL group and 88% ($p=0.41$) of patients treated with PL. Fragmentation times were not significantly different, neither was the need for secondary procedures. Instrument breakage and postoperative hematuria were more likely with PL, but ureteral perforation and proximal stone migration rates were the same [54].

The utility of PL and LL in the treatment of impacted ureteral stones was compared in a prospective randomized group of 80 patients. Stone size and location were similar. Among the 40 patients treated with LL, 97.5% were rendered stone-free after a single procedure, a rate significantly greater than the 80% achieved in the 40 PL patients ($p=0.03$). A secondary procedure was necessary in 7/40 patients treated with PL and 1/40 patients in the LL, after which 100% of patients in the study were stone-free. Complication rates after the procedure were similar, but 1 patient in the PL group developed a postoperative stricture, compared to none in the LL group [55].

PL vs. PUL vs. LL

There are few comparisons assessing the outcomes of more than two lithotripsy methods, but Salvadó and colleagues conducted a randomized controlled trial consisting of 69 patients with ureteral stones treated by PL, PUL, or LL. Stone-free rate was determined by computed tomography scan on postoperative day 15, and mean fragmentation time, proximal fragment migration rate, and complications were also assessed. In all metrics the lithotrites achieved statistically similar outcomes. A single case of ureteral perforation occurred in the PL group, but the study was not powered to detect a significant difference [29].

Conclusions

Beginning in the early 1970s modernization and miniaturization of endourologic equipment revolutionized the treatment of ureteral stones. Ureteroscopes and lithotrites would eventually render open ureterolithotomy obsolete, and each successive advancement in technology spurred development of the next.

As new energy sources became widely available, studies examining the safety, efficacy, and cost sought to determine the one best modality to treat all ureteral stones. EHL, while efficient and safe for treatment of bladder stones proved to be too powerful to use for the treatment of most stones within the ureter. USL and PL were safer and often times more efficient than EHL, but the breadth of their applicability was somewhat limited by the rigid nature of their probes. The advent of SWL and LL and their subsequent widespread affordability and availability eclipsed other energy sources as the first-line treatment for ureteral stones. Contemporaneous and modern clinical studies however prove that the traditional lithotrites, including EHL, PL, and USL, still have utility and can be especially effective when cost constraints dictate equipment choice.

References

1. Whitney WD, Smith BE. The century dictionary and cyclopedia, vol. 5. New York: The Century Co; 1911. p. 3483.
2. Raney AM. Electrohydraulic ureterolithotripsy. Urology. 1978 Sep;13(3):284–5.
3. Reuter HJ, Kern E. Electronic lithotripsy of ureteral calculi. J Urol. 1973;110:181–3.

4. Huffman JL, Bagley D, Schoenberg HW, Lyon ES. Transurethral removal of large ureteral and renal pelvic calculi using ureteroscopic ultrasonic lithotripsy. J Urol. 1983 Jul;130:31–4.
5. Denstedt JD, Clayman RV. Electrohydraulic lithotripsy of renal and ureteral calculi. J Urol. 1990 Jan;143:13–7.
6. Hofbauer J, Höbarth K, Marberger M. Electrohydraulic versus pneumatic disintergration in the treatment of ureteral stones: a randomized, prospective trial. J Urol. 1995 Mar;153:623–5.
7. Strope SA, Wolf JS, Faerber GJ, Roberts WW, Hollenbeck BK. Changing practice for upper urinary tract stone disease. J Urol. 2009 Sep;182:1005–11.
8. Turney BW, Reynard JM, Noble JG, Keoghane SR. Trends in urological stone disease. BJU Int. 2012; 109(7):1082–7.
9. Vorreuther R, Engelking R. Impact of voltage and capacity on the electrical and acoutstic output of intracorporeal electrohydraulic lithotripsy. Urol Res. 1992;20:355–9.
10. Corleis R, Vorreuther R, Engelmann U, Schaarschmidt U, Morgenstern B. First temporal and spatial quantification of single-shot electrohydraulic lithotripsy in vitro. Urol Res. 1996;24:167–70.
11. Rouvalis P. Electronic lithotripsy for vesical calculus with URAT-1. Br J Urol. 1970;42:486–91.
12. Eaton JM, Malin JM, Glenn JF. Electrohydraulic lithotripsy. J Urol. 1972 Dec;108:865–6.
13. Bülow H, Frohmuller HGW. Electrohydraulic lithotripsy with aspiration of the fragments under vision-304 consecutive cases. J Urol. 1981;126:454–6.
14. Green DF, Lytton B. Early experience with direct vision electrohydraulic lithotripsy of ureteral calculi. J Urol. 1985;133:767–70.
15. Green DF, Lytton B. Electrohydraulic lithotripsy in the ureter. Urol Clin North Am. 1988 Aug;15(3): 361–4.
16. See ACH, Ng FC, Ch'ng HC. Electrohydraulic lithotripsy: an effective and economical modality of endoscopic ureteric lithotripsy. ANZ J Surg. 1997;67: 551–3.
17. Leone NT, Garcia-Roig M, Bagley DH. Changing trends in the use of urteroscopic instruments from 1996 to 2008. J Endourol. 2010 Mar;24(3):361–5.
18. Maghsoudi R, Amjadi M, Norizadeh D, Hassanzadeh H. Treatment of ureteral stones: a prospective randomized controlled trial on comparison of Ho:YAG laser and pneumatic lithotripsy. Indian J Urol. 2008 Jul;24(3):352–4.
19. Schulze H, Haupt G, Piergiovnni M, Wisard M, von Niederhausern W, Senge T. The Swiss Lithoclast: a new device for endocscopic stone disitegration. J Urol. 1993 Jan;149:15–8.
20. Haupt G, van Ophoven A, Pannek J, Herde T, Senge T. In vitro comparison of two ballistic systems for stone disintegration. J Endourol. 1996 Oct;10(5):417–20.
21. Denstedt JD, Eberwein PM, Singh RR. The Swiss Lithoclast: a new device for intracorporeal lithotripsy. J Urol. 1992 Sep;148:1088–90.
22. Zhu S, Kourambas J, Munver R, Preminger GM, Zhong P. Quantification of the tip movement of lithotripsy flexible pneumatic probes. J Urol. 2000 Nov;164:1735–9.
23. Auge BK, Sekula JJ, Springhart WP, Zhu S, Zhong P, Preminger GM. In vitro comparison of fragmentation efficiency of flexible pneumatic lithotripsy using 2 flexible uteroscopes. J Urol. 2004 Sep;172:967–70.
24. Grasso M, Loisides P, Beaghler M, Bagley D. Treatment of urinary calculi in a porcine and canine model using the Browne Pneumatic Impactor. Urology. 1994 Dec;44(6):937–41.
25. Tawfiek ER, Grasso M, Bagley DH. Initial use of Browne Pneumatic Impactor. J Endourol. 1997 Apr;11(2):121–4.
26. Sun Y, Wang L, Liao G, et al. Pneumatic lithotripsy versus laser lithotripsy in the endoscoic treatment of ureteral calculi. J Endourol. 2001 Aug;15(5):587–90.
27. Delvecchio FC, Kuo RL, Preminger GM. Clinical efficacy of combined Lithoclast and Lithovac stone removal during ureteroscopy. J Urol. 2000 Jul;164:40–2.
28. Huang CY, Chen SS, Chen LK. Cost effectiveness of treating ureteral stones in a Taipei city hospital: shock wave lithotripsy versus ureteroscopy plus Lithoclast. Urol Int. 2009;83:410–5.
29. Salvadó JA, Mandujano R, Saez I, et al. Ureteroscopic lithotripsy for distal ureteral calculi: comparative evaluation of three different lithotripters. J Endourol. 2012;26(4):343–6.
30. Nelson PA, Herrick JF, Krusen FH. Ultrasonics in medicine. Arch Phys Med Rehabil. 1950 Jan; 31(1):6–19.
31. Howards SS, Merrill E, Harris S, Cohn J. Ultrasonic lithotripsy. Invest Urol. 1974;11(4):273–7.
32. Mulvaney WP. Attempted disintergration of calculi by ultrasonic vibrations. J Urol. 1953 Mar;70(5):704–7.
33. Suby H. The potential use of vibration for the disintergration of calculi. J Urol. 1957 Mar;77(3):364–71.
34. Goodfriend R. Disintergration of ureteral calculi by ultrasound. Urology. 1973 Mar;1(3):260–3.
35. Fuchs GJ. Ultrasonic lithotripsy in the ureter. Urol Clin North Am. 1988 Aug;15(3):347–59.
36. Marberger M, Stackl W, Hruby W. Percutaneous lithalopaxy of renal calculi with ultrasound. Eur Urol. 1982;8:236–42.
37. Çetin S, Özgür S, Yazicioglu A, Ünsal K, Ilker Y. Ultrasonic lithotripsy of bladder stones. Int Urol Nephrol. 1988;20(4):361–5.
38. Chaussy C, Fuchs G, Kahn R, Hunter P, Goodfriend R. Transurethral ultrasonic ureterolithotripsy using a solid-wire probe. Urology. 1987 May;29(5):531–2.
39. Gur U, Lifshitz D, Lask D, Livne PM. Utereral ultrasonic lithotripsy revisited: a neglected tool? J Endourol. 2004;18(2):137–40.
40. Auge BK, Lallas CD, Pietrow PK, Zhong P, Preminger GM. In vitro comparision of standard ultrasound and pneumatic lithotrites with a new combination intracorporeal lithotripsy device. Urology. 2002;60: 28–32.

41. Kuo RL, Paterson RF, Siqueira T, et al. In vitro comparision of Lithoclast Ultra intracorporial lithotripter. J Endourol. 2004 Mar;18(2):153–6.
42. Lehman DS, Hruby GW, Phillips C, et al. Prospective randomized comparision of a combined ultrasonic and pneumatic lithotrite with a standard ultrasonic lithotrite for percutaneous nephrolithotomy. J Endourol. 2008 Feb;22(2):285–9.
43. Vorreuther R, Corleis R, Klotz T, Bernards P, Engelmann U. Impact of shock wave pattern and cavitation bubble size on tissue damage during ureteroscopic electrohydraulic lithotripsy. J Urol. 1995 Mar;153:849–53.
44. Piergiovanni M, Desgrandchamps F, Cochand-Priollet B, et al. Ureteral and bladder lesions after ballistic, ultrasonic, electrohydraulic or laser lithotripsy. J Endourol. 1994;8(4):293–9.
45. Santa-Cruz RW, Leveillee RJ, Krongrad A. Ex vivo comparison of four lithotripters commonly used in the ureter: what does it take to perforate? J Endourol. 1998;12(5):417–22.
46. Bhatta KM, Rosen DI, Flotte TJ, Dretler SP, Nishioka NS. Effects of shielded or unshielded laser and electrohydraulic lithotripsy on rabbit bladder. J Urol. 1990 Apr;143:857–60.
47. Denstedt JD, Razvi HA, Rowe E, Grignon DJ, Eberwein PM. Investigation of the tissue effects of a new device for intracorporeal lithotripsy-the Swiss Lithoclast. J Urol. 1995 Feb;153:535–7.
48. Teh CL, Zhong P, Preminger GM. Laboratory and clinical assessment of pneumatically driven intracorporeal lithotripsy. J Endourol. 1998 Apr;12(2):163–9.
49. Teigland CM, Clayman RV, Winfield HN, Roeser RJ. Ultrasonic lithotripsy: the risk of hearing loss. J Urol. 1986 Apr;135:728–9.
50. Karlsen SJ, Bull-Njaa T, Krokstad A. Measurement of sound emission by endoscopic lithotripters: an in vitro study and theoretical estimation of risk of hearing loss in a fetus. J Endourol. 2001;15(8):821–6.
51. Vicente J, Caparrós J, Salvador J, Parra L, Rios G. Electrohydraulic and ultrasonic lithotripsy in 100 consecutive cases of primary ureteral stones. Urol Int. 1991;47:16–9.
52. Teichman JMH, Rao RD, Rogenes VJ, Harris JM. Ureteroscopic management of ureteral calculi: electrohydraulic versus holmium:YAG lithotripsy. J Urol. 1997 Oct;158:1357–61.
53. Naqvi SAA, Khaliq M, Zafar MN, Sizvi SAH. Treatmetn of ureteric stones. Comparision of laer and pneumatic lithotripsy. Br J Urol. 1994;74:694–8.
54. Manohar T, Ganpule A, Desai M. Comparative evaluation of Swiss Lithoclast 2 versus Holmum:YAG laser lithotripsy for impacted upper-ureteral stones. J Endourol. 2008 Mar;22(3):443–6.
55. Binbay M, Tepeler A, Singh A, et al. Evaluation of pneumatic versus holmium:YAG laser lithotripsy for impacted ureteral stones. Int Urol Nephrol. 2011; 43:989–95.

Flexible Ureteroscopy: Holmium:YAG Laser and Optical Fibers

14

Bodo E. Knudsen

This chapter contains video segments that can be found on the accompanying DVD

Introduction

After being used initially to treat biliary calculi, in 1995 the holmium:YAG laser was reported as a safe and effective method of intracorporeal urinary stone fragmentation [1]. Since the initial report, the holmium:YAG laser is now the "gold standard" for intracorporeal lithotripsy during ureteroscopic procedures [2]. Several properties of this laser have resulted in its widespread adoption.

Properties of the Holmium:YAG Laser

The 2,100 nm wavelength is highly absorbed in water making it ideal for the urologic environment. The laser energy is transmitted from the laser source efficiently via low OH-silica fibers that are relatively inexpensive and widely availability. Fibers may be constructed with small diameters that permit them to be passed through the working channel of both rigid and flexible endoscopes. Typical fiber core sizes used in urology range from 150 to 1,000 μm, but ≤365 μm are typically used for ureteroscopy.

The primary mechanism of action of the holmium:YAG laser for lithotripsy is photothermal ablation, although some weak photoacoustic effects likely also occur [3]. The tip of the laser fiber must be brought into direct contact with the stone when the laser in activated in order for fragmentation to take place [4]. Retropulsion during lithotripsy can be problematic leading to stone migration, but it is reduced with the holmium:YAG laser as compared to other types of lasers and pneumatic lithotripsy [5]. The holmium:YAG laser will fragment all types of urinary calculi including very hard stones such as cysteine, calcium oxalate monohydrate, and calcium phosphate brushite [6].

The holmium:YAG laser allows the user to select the fiber size, the pulse energy and frequency setting, and in some cases the pulse duration. Different laser manufacturers may offer lasers with different available settings, but most commercially available lasers will allow the user to select pulse energies between 0.4 and 1.0 J and pulse frequencies of 4–10 Hz, although some offer an expanded range depending on the total power rating of the laser. Fragmentation speed increases at higher pulse energies, but at the expense of larger fragment size and increased retropulsion [7, 8]. Increasing pulse energy above 1.0 J is rarely, if ever, needed for the treatment of ureteral and renal stones. Our practice is to routinely start with pulse energy and frequency settings of 0.6 J at 6 Hz. If the stone is very hard and not fragmenting efficiently the energy settings are slowly increased up to 1.0 J in 0.1 J increments.

B.E. Knudsen, M.D., F.R.C.S.C. (✉)
Department of Urology, Wexner Medical Center, The Ohio State University, Columbus, OH, USA
e-mail: bodo.knudsen@osumc.edu

M. Monga (ed.), *Ureteroscopy: Indications, Instrumentation & Technique*, Current Clinical Urology, DOI 10.1007/978-1-62703-206-3_14, © Springer Science+Business Media New York 2013

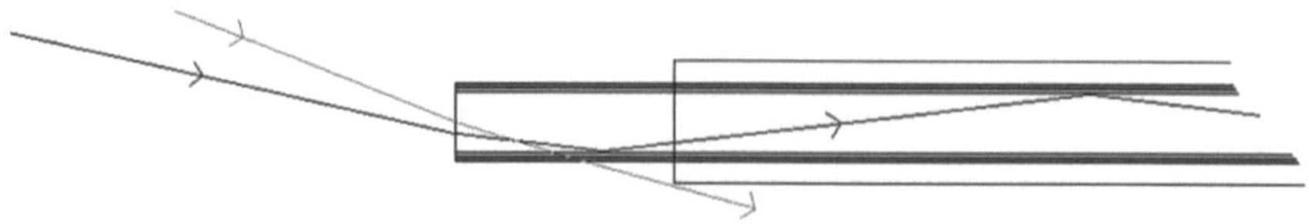

Fig. 14.1 High incidence angles cause by bending of the light

The pulse frequency may also slowly be increased to obtain the desired lasting effect. When working in the tight confines of the ureter it is best to keep the pulse frequency at ≤10 Hz to minimize potential injury to the ureter.

Most commercially available holmium:YAG lasers offer a fixed pulse duration of 350 μs, however the pulse width/duration is adjustable on the Odyssey 30 Holmium:YAG laser (Convergent Laser Technologies, Oakland, CA) with user selectable settings of 350 or 700 μs. In vitro study has demonstrated that the longer pulse duration results in decreased retropulsion of the stone while maintaining fragmentation efficiency [9].

Most commercially available holmium:YAG lasers used in urology are based on a single rod design, the Lumenis (Santa Clara, CA) VersaPulse 100 W laser is a four rod system that provides additional flexibility with additional pulse energy and frequency settings. This laser can be run at a pulse energy setting as low as 0.2 J and a pulse frequency settings as high as 50 Hz. While the lower pulse energy setting may be less efficient in regards to fragmentation speed, it creates smaller stone fragments and less retropulsion [7]. This, coupled with a high pulse frequency setting of 50 Hz, creates a "dusting" effect of the stone. This may be useful when the surgeon does not want to basket extract pieces or for larger stones where creating less fragments may be desirable.

Holmium:YAG Optical Fiber Design

A holmium:YAG optical laser fiber is constructed with a fiber core, a cladding surrounding the core, and an outer jacket. At the proximal end of the fiber is the connector that couples the optical fiber to the laser permitting the laser energy to launch into the fiber core. The components of the fiber need to work together to allow for the efficient transfer of the laser energy from the source to the target. If there are any breakdowns in this pathway there is, at best, reduced energy delivery to the target and, at worst, catastrophic damage to the fiber or laser.

Laser energy is normally transmitted through the core of the fiber by total internal reflection. When total internal reflection occurs, the laser energy reflected within the core of the fiber and it does not leak into the cladding or the jacket of the fiber. Energy transmission is most efficient in this scenario. When the fiber is bent, it increases the incidence angles of the laser light energy and the possibility of the energy entering the cladding or the jacket of the fiber increases (Fig. 14.1). Flaws in the design of the fiber can further contribute to this problem. The jacket of the fiber is not designed to transmit the laser energy and quickly heats up from laser energy entering into it. This leads to fiber failure and breakdown, a process that can happen with just several pulses of the laser.

Flexible Ureteroscope Design: Impact on Fiber Performance

Flexible ureteroscopes are capable of high degrees of both primary and secondary deflection. These small caliber flexible scopes are capable of reaching stones in the lower pole of the kidney where shockwave lithotripsy is less effective [10]. However lower pole access has correlated with the need for ureteroscope repair, which can be a very costly endeavor with repair costs as high as $10,000 per incident [11]. Laser fiber failure with the scope deflected in the lower pole may also be contributing to scope failure. Therefore it is critical that laser optical fibers used for laser lithotripsy are able to withstand

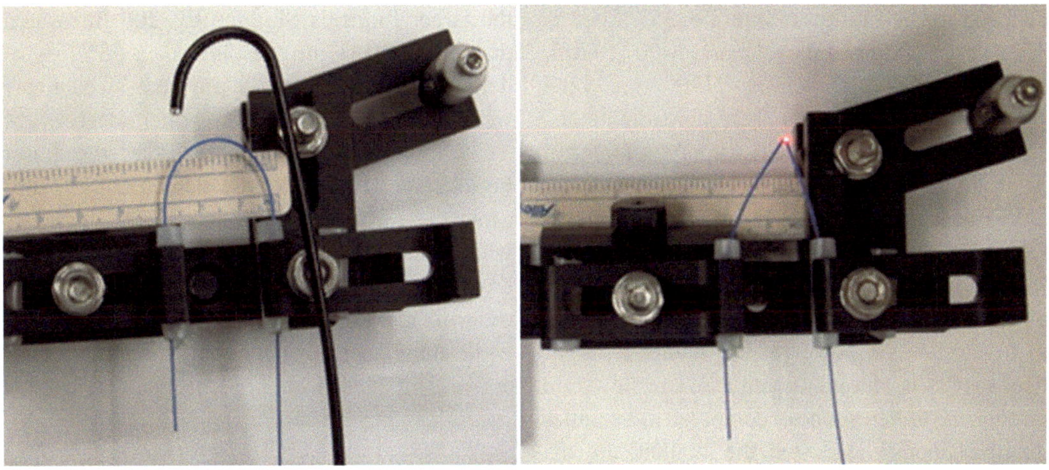

Fig. 14.2 Fiber failure during testing when the laser was activated

that sharp bends that are required to reach stones in difficult locations such as the lower pole of the kidney (Fig. 14.2).

Fiber Evaluation

During lower pole laser lithotripsy of renal stones it was identified by the author that fibers were periodically failing when highly deflected and the laser was activated. However the failure was sporadic and appeared to vary highly from fiber to fiber. What could be safely treated during one procedure may result in fiber fracture and ureteroscope damage in another procedure. Therefore a set of objective tests were created in an effort to safely test the performance characteristics of a series of commercially available holmium:YAG optical laser fibers.

Fiber Resistance to Fracture with Bending

A series of 24 commercially available holmium:YAG laser optical fibers were evaluated with core sizes ranging from 150 to 365 μm. Fibers were placed underwater in a testing apparatus that created 180° bends. The bend radius was set at 1.25 cm and the holmium:YAG laser was activated at a pulse energy setting of 1.2 J at a frequency of 10 Hz for 1 min or until fiber failure. If the fiber did not fail, the bend radius was decrease by 0.25 cm and the testing repeated. The continued until the bend radius reach 0.5 cm or until fiber failure. The results demonstrated that there was a wide range of failure thresholds for the fibers tested. The worst performing fiber was the AccuFlex 200 (Boston Scientific, Natick, MA), which failed at a bend diameter of 1.75 cm. The InnovaQuartz LLF273, Convergent OptiLITI SMH1020F, and Dornier Lightguide Super 270 had the best performance by not fracturing even at the tightest bend tested [12].

Fiber Diameter

Fibers used for laser lithotripsy can be broadly classified into four categories based on the core-size of the fiber: (i) ≤272 μm, (ii) 365 μm, (iii) 550 μm, and (iv) 1,000 μm. For flexible ureteroscopy, fibers with core sizes ≤365 μm are used. The fiber core size however does not accurately represent what the total diameter of the fiber is. The total diameter is the summation of all the components of the fiber, namely the core, cladding, and the jacket. The true diameter of the fiber is not always reported by the manufacturer but can be easily calculated using a hand held micrometer. For example, the measured total diameter of a Lumenis Slimline 365 fiber is 520 μm and the InnovaQuartz 400 (AMS, Minnetonka, MN) fiber is 718.5 μm, both significantly greater than their core diameters. The total fiber diameter is an important factor in determining the flow rate through the channel of a flexible ureteroscope, as most flexible ureteroscopes have only one working channel that is shared for both irrigation and instruments. Based on Poiseuille's Law that flow rate is proportional to four times the power of the radius, a larger fiber results is a dramatic reduction in flow rate through the ureteroscope as compared to a smaller diameter fiber. When tested, the smaller Lumenis Slimline 365 had a flow rate of 17.2 mL through a flexible ureteroscope channel whereas the larger InnovaQuartz 400 fiber had a greater than 50% reduction in flow measured at 7.7 mL/s [13]. Similarly, when fibers with ≤272 μm core sizes were measured, the fibers diameters varied greatly amongst those measured. For example, the Boston Scientific Accuflex 150 had a measured total diameter of 270 μm, while the Trimedyne FlexMAX 200 (Lake Forest, CA) had a true diameter of 445 μm [12].

Fiber Flexibility

An important aspect of fiber performance is the ability of the fiber to deflect easily so as to not limit the deflection of the ureteroscope. High fiber flexibility is essential when trying to reach stones located in the lower pole where high degrees of deflection are required [14, 15]. Furthermore, greater flexibility of the fiber will result in less strain on the deflection mechanism of delicate ureteroscopes potentially reducing costly failure.

The maximum deflection (primary and secondary active deflection) of a Stryker (Kalamazoo, MI) FlexVision U-500 ureteroscope without a laser fiber in the working channel is 275°. A series of laser fibers were placed in the working channel of the Styker ureteroscope and the loss of deflection from baseline was recorded. Fibers with the smallest diameters, such as the Boston Scientific AccuFlex 150 (measured diameter of 270 μm), resulted no loss of deflection, whereas the larger Lumenis Slimline EZ 200 (measured diameter of 423 μm) resulted in a 53° loss of deflection. When the 365 μm core sized fibers were tested, significantly greater degrees of deflection were lost. For example, the Laser Peripherals HBLF-365 (true diameter of 717 μm) a total of 97° of deflection were lost [12]. Therefore when selecting fibers to use with a flexible ureteroscope, a ≤272 μm fiber is recommended in order to maximize the flow rate and deflection, while simultaneously attempting to limit the wear and tear on the delicate ureteroscope.

Are Laser Optical Fibers Interchangeable with Different Holmium:YAG Lasers

A multitude of different holmium:YAG lasers and optical fibers are commercially available. Most laser manufacturers offer a product line of laser fibers to be used with their lasers. In addition, "fiber only" manufacturers may offer various optical fibers that are marketed to be used with various commercially available laser systems. Therefore innumerable combinations of different lasers and fibers can occur. While an exhaustive list of these combinations in beyond the scope of this chapter, it is important to note that not all combinations of holmium:YAG lasers and fibers are compatible and that incompatibilities can result in damage to both the fiber and to the laser energy source.

In an experiment where a series of laser optical fibers were tested, a catastrophic failure occurred when a Tridedyne 200 fiber was attempted to be coupled with a NewStar holmium:YAG laser. The laser energy from the NewStar laser was not effectively launched into the core of the fiber, resulting in heating and ultimately melting of the connector end of the fiber, requiring extensive repair. Similarly during clinical use, a 13% (4/30) rate of fiber failure occurred when the Trimedyne 200 fiber was coupled to a Lumenis VersaPulse 100 W laser [16]. Therefore, urologists should exercise caution when mixing and matching different brands of laser fibers with different lasers. One size does not fit all.

New Advances in Holmium:YAG Optical Laser Fibers

Both tapered and non-tapered connecters are used in commercially available sub-300 μm laser fibers. Fibers with core sizes ≤200 μm are usually tapered to more efficiently route the laser energy into the core of the fiber. Previous work has suggested that non-tapered holmium:YAG laser fibers have better overall performance and are less prone to failure that smaller tapered fibers, especially in regards to resistance to failure with bending (Fig. 14.3) [12]. The majority of non-tapered small core sized fibers used for flexible ureteroscopy and laser lithotripsy have been approximately 270 μm in diameter. More recently a new single-use 240 μm fiber has been introduced and represents a novel design. The fiber (Flexiva, Boston Scientific, Natick, MA) has a non-tapered connector and is rated to handle up to 50 W of power.

A recent study evaluated the performance of this fiber in both a bench setting and in clinical use [17]. A total of 100 fibers were used during 100 consecutive clinical procedures. None of the fibers fractured during the clinical procedures. There was an average of 1.664 mm of tip degradation per fiber, but this was highly variable as 33% of fibers demonstrated greater than 50% of the factory prepared tip to be degraded by the completion of the procedure. An analysis of the laser settings revealed that the degradation was independent of the laser pulse energy and rate settings. The same 100 fibers were then evaluated using the same bench testing described previously [12]. The results demonstrated no significant degradation in energy transmission with the fiber in the bent and 180 ° bend configuration. Fiber failure threshold testing established that 87/100 fibers did not fracture with energy transmission at the tightest bend radius tested (0.5 cm). Of the 13 fibers that did fail when bent, it was only at the tightest bend radius of 0.5 cm. This performance ranks amongst the best of all fibers previously tested [12]. However the variable degree of optical tip degradation during clinical use remains a weakness of this fiber, as needing to stop and strip the fiber during a procedure will lead to longer operative times and possibly poorer clinical outcomes if the target is lost.

The tips of holmium:YAG optical fibers are typically prepared and polished in the factory prior to packaging (Fig. 14.4). The tip is prepared

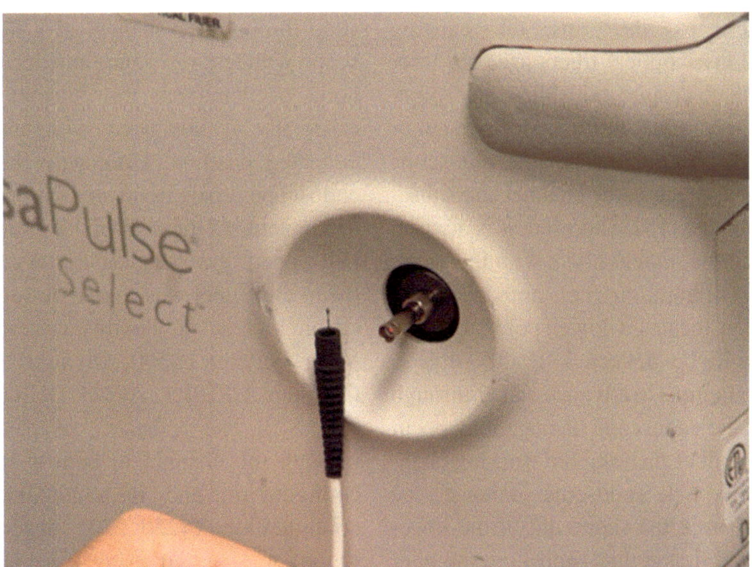

Fig. 14.3 Proximal connector failure

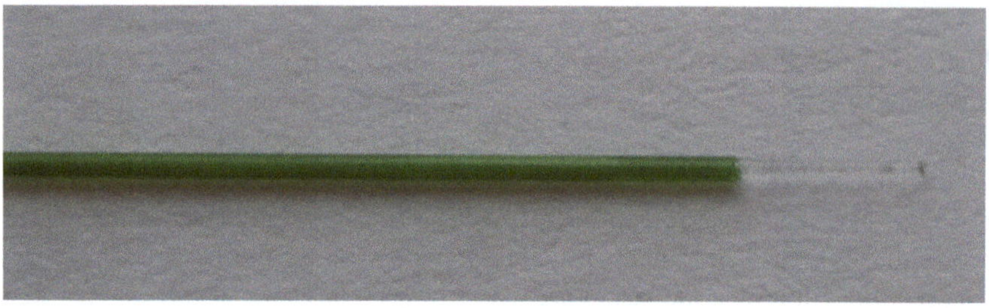

Fig. 14.4 Factory prepared fiber

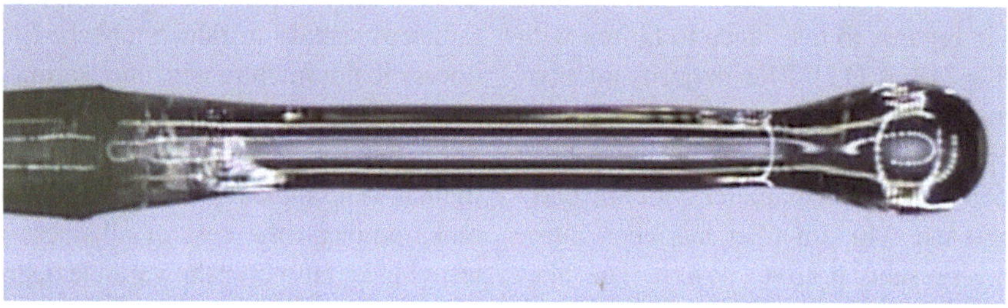

Fig. 14.5 Ball tipped laser fiber

by a combination of cutting the end of the fiber without cracking the glass core and then stripping off the overlying jacket. Variable degrees of polishing are used on the tip. During clinical use, the tip degrades and it may need to be recleaved and stripped when it burns back to the jacket. One drawback to the tips on existing holmium:YAG laser optical fibers used for laser lithotripsy is that, despite polishing, are somewhat sharp. It is possible for the fiber tip to cut or gouge the inside channel of a flexible endoscope which may cause a leak in the channel and subsequent scope damage [18]. Therefore it is advised to only advance the optical fibers with the scope in a straight configuration (i.e., not deflected). When a surgeon locates a lower pole stone the ureteroscope will be deflected. If the surgeon overzealously attempts to advance a fiber through the channel of the endoscope damage may occur for the tip of the fiber piercing the working channel. Rather than risk endoscope damage, the surgeon should back the scope out of the lower pole to straighten it, and then reposition the fiber at the tip of the scope before going back into the lower pole to lase the stone. If the stone is in a very difficult to reach position, it may be frustrating for the surgeon to have to relocate the stone.

A new prototype optical laser fiber with a novel ball tip design was evaluated. The tip of the fiber was melted to create a ball (Fig. 14.5). The purported advantage of this is to allow the fiber to slide through the channel of a flexible ureteroscope with less resistance and decrease the likelihood of damaging the channel of the scope especially if advanced with the scope in a deflected position. Ultimately this may reduce endoscope repair frequency. In order to evaluate the benefit of the ball-tip, a prototype 240 μm ball-tipped fiber was tested in a series of experiments. The fiber was passed through the working channel of seven flexible ureteroscopes (Wolf Viper, Stryker U-500, Olympus URF-V (two), Olympus URF-P5, ACMI DUR-8 Elite, Storz Flex-X2). The resistance of passing the fiber through the channel in both a 180 ° deflected configuration and in a maximally deflected configuration (≈250–270° depending on the scope) was scored using a subjective scale of 1–5. The fiber was passed successfully through the channels of all the endoscopes both in the

180° and in the maximally deflected configurations with no visible damage to the endoscope optics. Resistance to the fiber passage was score as either 1 (none) or 2 (minimal) for all scopes that had active primary deflection and passive secondary deflection. For the two scopes with active secondary deflection (Stryker U-500 and ACMI DUR-8 Elite) there was greater resistance to passage of the fiber scoring 3 (moderate) and 4 (large) on the resistance scale. This suggests that the tighter bend diameters that occur with the active secondary deflection create additional resistance to the passage of the fiber [19]. The results of the testing of this prototype fiber suggest that there is a benefit to the ball-tip especially with the first past through the endoscope. However optical tip degradation (burn back) is still likely to occur and the benefit of the ball-tip would likely be lost after laser lithotripsy is initiated. Further testing evaluating both energy transmission and efficiency of stone fragmentation are needed to validate the clinical performance of this fiber.

Conclusion

The holmium:YAG laser is the current gold standard for holmium:YAG laser lithotripsy during flexible ureteroscopy. Careful selection of the optical laser fiber coupled with appropriate pulse energy and frequency settings will result in safe and effective stone fragmentation. Future improvements in fiber design may lead to reduced damage and wear on fragile endoscopes.

References

1. Denstedt JD, et al. Preliminary experience with holmium:YAG laser lithotripsy. J Endourol. 1995;9(3):255–8.
2. Sofer M, Denstedt J. Flexible ureteroscopy and lithotripsy with the holmium:YAG laser. Can J Urol. 2000;7(1):952–6.
3. Vassar GJ, et al. Holmium:YAG lithotripsy: photothermal mechanism. J Endourol. 1999;13(3):181–90.
4. Pierre S, Preminger GM. Holmium laser for stone management. World J Urol. 2007;25(3):235–9.
5. Marguet CG, et al. In vitro comparison of stone retropulsion and fragmentation of the frequency doubled, double pulse Nd:YAG laser and the holmium:YAG laser. J Urol. 2005;173(5):1797–800.
6. Leveillee RJ, Lobik L. Intracorporeal lithotripsy: which modality is best? Curr Opin Urol. 2003;13(3):249–53.
7. Sea J, et al. Optimal power settings for holmium:YAG lithotripsy. J Urol. 2012;187(3):914–9.
8. Spore SS, et al. Holmium:YAG lithotripsy: optimal power settings. J Endourol. 1999;13(8):559–66.
9. Finley DS, et al. Effect of holmium:YAG laser pulse width on lithotripsy retropulsion in vitro. J Endourol. 2005;19(8):1041–4.
10. Albala DM, et al. Lower pole I: a prospective randomized trial of extracorporeal shock wave lithotripsy and percutaneous nephrostolithotomy for lower pole nephrolithiasis-initial results. J Urol. 2001;166(6):2072–80.
11. Afane JS, et al. Flexible ureteroscopes: a single center evaluation of the durability and function of the new endoscopes smaller than 9Fr. J Urol. 2000;164(4):1164–8.
12. Mues AC, Teichman JM, Knudsen BE. Evaluation of 24 holmium:YAG laser optical fibers for flexible ureteroscopy. J Urol. 2009;182(1):348–54.
13. Knudsen BE, et al. Performance and safety of holmium:YAG laser optical fibers. J Endourol. 2005;19(9):1092–7.
14. Traxer O. Flexible ureterorenoscopic management of lower-pole stone: does the scope make the difference? J Endourol. 2008;22(9):1847–50. discussion 1855.
15. Clayman RV. Flexible ureterorenoscopy for the treatment of lower pole calyx stones: influence of different lithotripsy probes and stone extraction tools on scope reflection and irrigation flow. J Urol. 2003;170(2 Pt 1):686–7.
16. Marks AJ, et al. Holmium:yttrium-aluminum-garnet lithotripsy proximal fiber failures from laser and fiber mismatch. Urology. 2008;71(6):1049–51.
17. Shore DM, Antiporda M, Teichman JM, Knudsen BE Evaluation of a new 240 μm single-use holmium:YAG optical fiber for flexible ureteroscopy. In: Engineering and Urology Society Annual Meeting. Washington, DC; 2011.
18. Sooriakumaran P, et al. Evaluation of the mechanisms of damage to flexible ureteroscopes and suggestions for ureteroscope preservation. Asian J Androl. 2005;7(4):433–8.
19. Knudsen BE Ball-tip holmium:YAG optical fiber. In: Engineering and Urology Society Annual Meeting. Washington, DC; 2011.

15 Stone Migration Devices

Evgeniy Kreydin and Brian Eisner

Introduction

Over the past two decades, the treatment of nephrolithiasis and endourological practices have changed dramatically—endourologic techniques such as ureteroscopy have become commonplace, and often the first-line treatment for renal and ureteral stones in many institutions [1]. Together with the increasing ureteroscopic experience of the urologic community as a whole, we have seen increasing stone-free rates, decreasing operative times, and decreasing complication rates for ureteroscopic stone treatment [1]. While the safety and efficacy of ureteroscopy have been established in multiple series and reports, the variation of stone characteristics, such as composition, size and location, has resulted in specific challenges pertaining to each. One such challenge is stone migration or retropulsion—the cephalad movement of kidney stone fragments towards to upper ureter or kidney as a result of ureteroscopic lithotripsy. Stone migration may lead to increased operative times secondary to the need to capture retropulsed fragments, increased costs when the urologist is required to switch from the semirigid to the flexible ureteroscope to find a retropulsed fragment in a more proximal location, and increased secondary procedures for retropulsed stone fragments left in the ureter or kidney which are of clinically significant size [2–5]. On the other hand, prevention of stone retropulsion has been shown in the laboratory setting to increase fragmentation efficiency and decrease the time required to fragment a stone [6, 7]. To this end, there are several commercially available devices which have been designed to prevent stone retropulsion. Herein we review the important aspects of stone retropulsion, prevention of migration, and the devices which are commonly used for this purpose.

Retropulsion: Risk Factors and Mechanisms

Retrograde stone migration has been shown to be a result of a combination of factors—some of which are modifiable while others are not. Among the "fixed" factors are surgeon experience, location, and size of the stone. Among the modifiable factors are the patient positioning, irrigation pressures, energy source (i.e., laser, pneumatic, electrohydraulic lithotrites), and the energy settings of the fragmentation device [2–4, 6, 8, 9]. The overall rates of stone retropulsion during ureteroscopic lithotripsy are reported to be between 5 and 15% [2, 7, 10]. The most important fixed risk factors are proximal stone location and the extent of ureteroscopic experience of the surgeon [6, 7, 9–11].

E. Kreydin, M.D. • B. Eisner, M.D. (✉)
Department of Urology, Massachusetts General Hospital, Harvard Medical School, 55 Fruit Street, GRB 1102, Boston, MA 02114, USA
e-mail: beisner@partners.org

M. Monga (ed.), *Ureteroscopy: Indications, Instrumentation & Technique*, Current Clinical Urology,
DOI 10.1007/978-1-62703-206-3_15,

Patient Positioning and Varying Irrigant Pressures

In the early days of ureteroscopy, adjusting patient positioning and decreasing irrigant pressure were two commonly applied techniques to prevent stone migration [2, 11, 12]. Placing the patient in the reverse Trendelenburg position was thought to decrease stone migration rates by using gravity to counteract the kinetic energy of a cephalad-migrating stone. However, as the force with which stones were propelled cephalad was stronger than partial gravitational pull, positioning was generally thought to be fairly ineffective at prevention of migration [10]. While minimizing pressure of irrigation fluid may be effective in decreasing cephalad stone migration, the urologist must balance this with the ability to effectively visualize and treat the stone. Various irrigation systems have been developed and studied—gravity-based systems have been shown to minimize retropulsion and also demonstrate poorer stone visualization compared to pressure-based systems (both automatic and hand-operated) [11].

Energy Source: Lithotrite Type

Currently the most common energy sources for ureteroscopic lithotripsy are pneumatic and laser, with electrohydraulic lithotripsy falling out of favor due to potential damage to the ureter [13, 14]. Studies comparing these lithotrites have demonstrated that retropulsion rates are significantly greater for pneumatic and electrohydraulic lithotrites than for the Holmium:YAG laser [14–16]. Recent studies have demonstrated a greater than twofold increase in clinically significant stone retropulsion for both pneumatic lithotripsy and electrohydraulic lithotripsy compared with laser lithotripsy, resulting in poorer stone-free rates [5, 8, 14, 17, 18]. These clinical findings are supported by laboratory studies, which have demonstrated significantly less stone migration with laser lithotripsy than pneumatic lithotripsy.

The Effect of Lithotrite Settings on Stone Retropulsion

The Holmium:YAG laser has proven to be the fragmentation device that is least likely to cause retrograde stone migration [4, 5, 14, 16, 17]. The physical properties that distinguish this laser from other lithotrites have been investigated and the critical difference appears to be the particularly long energy pulse generated by this laser [4, 5, 19, 20]. Due to this unique property, a different retropulsion pattern is produced by the Holmium:YAG laser than by other lithotrites, which produce short energy pulses.

Electrohydraulic lithotrites, pneumatic lithotrites, and short-pulse lasers, such as the frequency-doubled double-pulse neodymium laser (FREDDY), are thought to fragment stones by an "explosive ablation" process, in which the entire laser pulse energy is absorbed prior to the onset of ejection of a fragment from a stone. According to this model, a portion of the laser pulse provides the energy for fragmentation, and the remainder of the absorbed pulse is transformed to kinetic energy that determines the amplitude of recoil and the distance that the stone subsequently travels away from the energy source [18, 19]. On the other hand, a "continuous vaporization" model appears to be more appropriate to describe the action of a long-pulse laser, such as the Holmium:YAG. This means that during Holmium:YAG lithotripsy, most recoil is generated when a fragment is actually chipped off the stone, and the stone travels in the opposite direction of the ejected fragment in order to preserve the total momentum of the system [3–5, 19, 20]. Whereas for other devices the degree of retropulsion is primarily determined by the energy delivered by the fragmentation source, the shape and mass of an ejected particle appears to play a critical role in determining retropulsion in Holmium:YAG lithotripsy.

In turn, the size and shape of the ejected fragment is mainly determined by the energy of the delivered pulse and the size of the laser fiber used during the procedure. The largest fragments are chipped off by the largest fibers delivering pulses with the highest energy. Therefore stone retropulsion is diminished in cases, in which lower energy settings and smaller fibers are used. In vitro studies have also shown that varying the pulse width has an effect on stone retropulsion—in an experimental model which used 200 and 400 μm laser fibers and pulse widths of 350 and 700 μs, the 700 μs pulse width was associated with the least stone retropulsion, while the 700 μs pulse width and the 200 μm laser fiber was associated with the greatest stone fragmentation efficiency.

Anti-Retropulsion Devices

A number of effective antiretropulsion devices have been developed and studied. Early devices included the Parchute® (Boston Scientific, Natick, MA) and the Lithocatch® (MedSource, Norwell, MA). These were wire mesh devices placed above the ureteral stone to prevent migration. Both of these devices were quite small in the largest diameter (4 mm) and therefore often failed to occlude dilated ureters [2, 10]. Additionally, they suffered from poor ability to retrieve stone fragments.

In the twenty-first century, a new group of anti-retropulsion devices came to market. Currently available devices include the Stone Cone® (Boston Scientific, Natick, MA), NTrap® (Cook Medical, Bloomington, IN), and Accordion® (Percsys, Palo Alto, CA) which are devices positioned in the ureter alongside the stone and with retropulsion "elements" which are positioned cephalad to the stone to prevent the migration of fragments; and BackStop® (Boston Scientific, Natick, MA), which is a thermosensitive polymer injected cephalad to the stone to prevent migration.

Stone Cone®

The first of these devices to be commercially available was the Stone Cone® (Fig. 15.1) [2]. It is available in two sizes (7 and 10 mm outer diameters), to be used depending on the degree of dilation of the proximal ureter. This device consists of a strand of stainless steel wire wound with a strand of nitinol prebaked in a mold to produce a spiral form of varying sizes. This design allows the Stone Cone® to be collapsed inside an introducer sheath with a diameter of 0.038 mm (the diameter of a standard ureteral access wire) and delivered to the site of a ureteral stone. The wound portion of the device can then be expanded to a maximum diameter of 8–10 mm at a location proximal to the stone. Because the spaces between the rings of the cone are small, deployment of the device results in effective retention of stones larger than 2 mm. The polytetrafluoroethylene coating of the Stone Cone® is designed to protect the cone from damage by fragmentation sources. A safety-mechanism inherent in the design of the Stone Cone® is that the nitinol coils is to unwind to a diameter of less than 4 mm when sufficient tension is applied to the distal end of the Stone Cone® (0.127 pounds). This serves as a safety mechanism against avulsion of the ureter or entrapment of the device. The Stone Cone® is resistant to shocks delivered by pneumatic and electrohydraulic lithotrites. However, placement of the Holmium:YAG laser on and perpendicular to the wire caused wire melting and disruption after a number of pulses [2, 21–23].

Several studies have examined the efficacy of the Stone Cone® in prevention of stone migration. In the initial clinical experience, the Stone Cone® was used in 23 cases of pneumatic

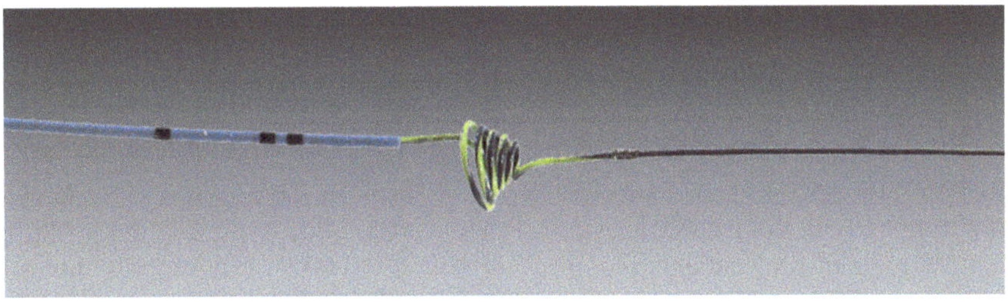

Fig. 15.1 Image of deployed Stone Cone (courtesy of Boston Scientific)

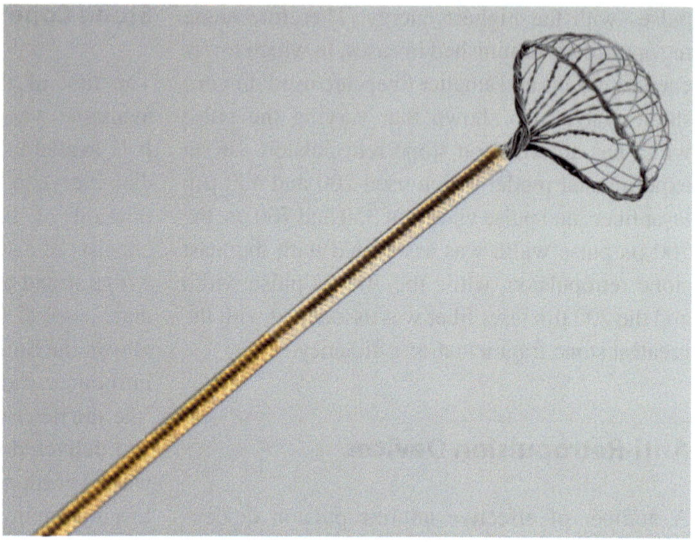

Fig. 15.2 Image of deployed NTrap (courtesy of Cook Urological)

lithotripsy for ureteral stones, compared with 27 control cases in which no migration device was used. When compared with controls, the Stone Cone® reduced the number of clinically significant residual fragments (0% vs. 30%, $p<0.001$) as well as the need for secondary procedures (0% vs. 20%, $p<0.01$) [23]. A second study compared electrohydraulic lithotripsy of ureteral stones with and without the Stone Cone® and noted significantly increased stone retropulsion (23% vs. 0%, $p<0.01$) and significantly increased residual fragments greater than 3 mm in diameter (31% vs. 0%, $p<0.001$) in cases without the Stone Cone® compared to those with the Stone Cone® [24].

Two noncontrolled series have been published using the Stone Cone® for ureteroscopic laser lithotripsy, with reported migration rates of 0–1.5%. Maislos et al. demonstrated that 19 consecutive patients with proximal ureteral stones underwent semirigid ureteroscopy with laser lithotripsy using the Stone Cone®. At the conclusion of the procedure, none of the patients had residual stone fragments larger than 2 mm and no auxiliary procedures were required [21]. An additional retrospective series of 133 consecutive cases of ureteroscopy with laser lithotripsy demonstrated a 1.5% incidence of patients requiring an additional procedure to treat migrated stone fragments [25].

NTrap®

The NTrap® is a device with a 3F shaft consisting of a wire mesh net composed of tightly woven Nitinol wires within a 115-cm sheath (Fig. 15.2). The net has central wires 1 mm apart and outer wires 2 mm apart. The original device had a mesh diameter of 8 mm and therefore had the ability to occlude a ureter dilated to that size. Because of the flexibility of its mesh fibers, the device is able to accommodate the ureter easily when it is deployed proximal to the stone. With the ureter occluded, the device can prevent proximal migration of stone fragments as small as 1.5 mm (in fact, fragments smaller than 1 mm are prevented from proximal migration by the central portion of the mesh, and only the peripheral wires allow passage of larger fragments) [9, 12, 26].

Wang et al. recently performed a prospective trial of 113 patients undergoing ureteroscopy with pneumatic lithotripsy for proximal ureteral stones [9]. In half of the patients, the NTrap® was used to prevent stone retropulsion. The authors noted a significantly lower incidence of stone migration in the NTrap® group (0% vs. 12%, $p=0.007$) as well as an improved stone-free rate in the NTrap® group (100% vs. 84%, $p=0.002$). There was no statistically significant difference in need for additional procedures. A second series compared 76

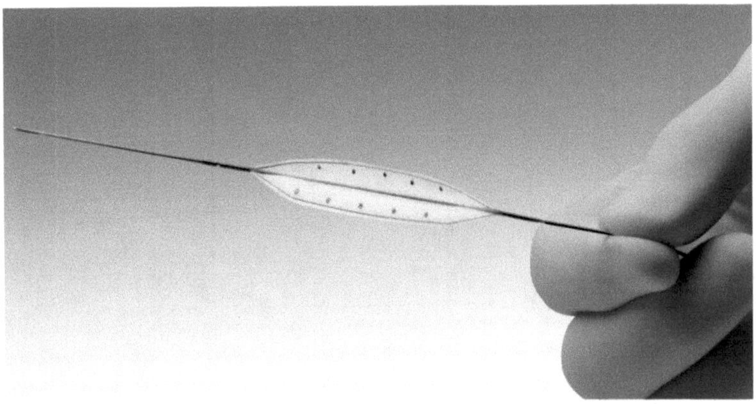

Fig. 15.3 Image of undeployed Accordion (courtesy of PercSys)

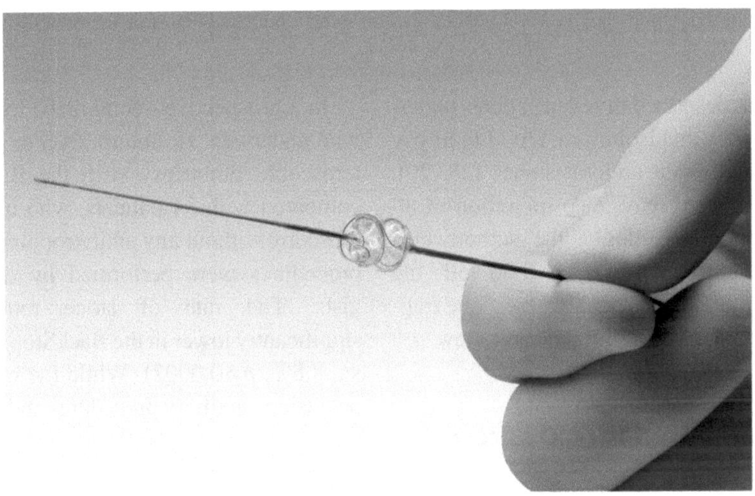

Fig. 15.4 Image of deployed Accordion (courtesy of PercSys)

patients who underwent ureteroscopic lithotripsy (81% with Holmium:YAG, 19% with Wolf pneumatic lithoclast) with the NTrap® with 68 patients who underwent standard ureteroscopy. Stone-free rate was significantly higher in the NTrap® group (98.7% vs. 89.7%, $p = 0.019$) [26].

Finally, a meta-analysis which includes the two aforementioned articles and a case series, totaling 456 cases noted that NTrap® was associated with a threefold increase in stone-free status, a fivefold reduction in stone retropulsion, and a threefold reduction in the need for auxiliary shock wave lithotripsy (SWL) treatment for migrated fragments [27].

Accordion®

The Accordion® is a sheath-wire system, 150 cm in length and with an outer shaft diameter of 0.038 in (Fig. 15.3). It has a floppy tip and a distal multifold film. When the device is deployed by coaxial retraction of the inner core of the coaxial wire, it "Accordions" to a 7 or 10-mm wide plug that blocks stone migration and provides the utility of a basket during stone fragment removal (Fig. 15.4). Because the Accordion® is the newest FDA-approved anti-retropulsion device, few clinical studies have evaluated its efficacy. In two abstracts published in 2007, the use of the

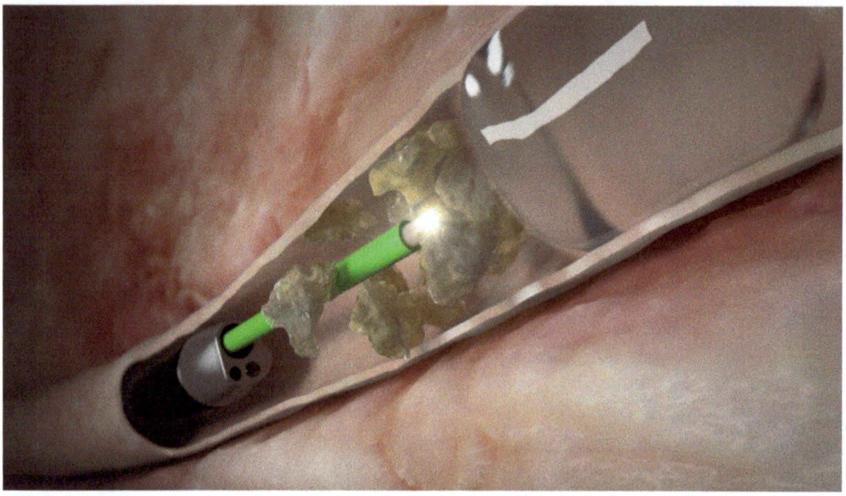

Fig. 15.5 Image of BackStop deployed proximal to ureteral stone (courtesy of Boston Scientific)

Accordion® was described in seven patients undergoing ureteroscopy and Holmium:YAG lithotripsy for proximal and distal ureteral stones [28, 29]. The device prevented retrograde migration of all stone fragments. Interestingly, the authors also noted rebounding of irrigation fluid off the deployed Accordion®, thus flushing the stone fragments distally and allowing for a clearer view.

Chemical Antiretropulsion Devices: BackStop® and Others

BackStop® is a unique biocompatible polymer with reverse thermosensitive properties (Fig. 15.5). It exists as a liquid at temperatures below 16 °C and as a soft but injectable gel at room temperature, and then transitions to a viscous gel at body temperature. BackStop® is dispensed with the accessory BackStop® injector and 3 or 5 Fr catheter. Before fragmentation the catheter is positioned 1–2 cm above the stone via the ureteroscope working channel or directly under fluoroscopy. BackStop® is dispensed above the stone, and forms a gel plug that conforms to the ureter and prevents the stone from migrating up the ureter and potentially into the kidney. After stone fragmentation is completed, the BackStop® plug is dissolved using saline irrigation; this process can be facilitated by using cold saline [30, 31].

In a prospective, randomized trial, 34 patients, who underwent Holmium:YAG or pneumatic ureteroscopic lithotripsy with the BackStop® were compared with 34 patients, who underwent ureteroscopy without any antiretropulsion device. The procedures were performed by different urologists. The rate of stone retropulsion was significantly lower in the BackStop® group (52.9% vs. 8.8%, $p=0.0002$). While the rates of ureteral occlusion, auxiliary procedures and adverse events were also lower in the BackStop® group, these differences did not reach statistical significance [30].

In addition to the BackStop®, other viscous materials have been tested to prevent stone retropulsion. In 2004, Ali et al. published a new technique, wherein 1–2 ml of lubricating jelly was injected proximal to a ureteral stone prior to electrokinetic lithotripsy [32]. Among seven patients treated in this manner, stone or fragment retropulsion was observed in none. A subsequent randomized control trial assessed the use of lidocaine jelly to prevent stone migration during pneumatic lithotripsy [33]. A stone retropulsion rate of 4% was observed among patients in whom the jelly was used, while the control group had a 28% rate of retrograde stone migration. Stone-free rates were also significantly different between the two groups (96% vs. 72%, $p=0.045$). In 2011, lidocaine jelly was compared with the Stone Cone® for its efficacy in preventing stone migration in a prospective randomized trial with 40 patients [34]. While both methods demonstrated effectiveness, the Stone Cone® was found to be superior to lidocaine jelly in stone retropulsion rates (0% vs. 15%, $p<0.05$) and operative time (41.8 vs. 51.4 min, $p<0.05$).

Other Issues: Device Deployment, Irrigation Characteristics, Damage, and Cost

In addition to the aforementioned clinical studies on the efficacy of using anti-retropulsion devices, there are number of characteristics common to each, which merit discussion. For any disposable device which is designed to improve outcomes in ureteroscopy, the ease of deployment and potential damage caused by deployment of the device is worth considering. A previously published study examined the dilation of the ureter proximal to obstructing calculi with an eye towards selection of the appropriate anti-retropulsion devices [35]. The authors analyzed 176 obstructing ureteral stones (nearly 1/3 proximal ureteral stones and 2/3 distal ureteral stones) and noted that the degree of dilation of the ureter just proximal to the stone was greater for proximal than for distal calculi, and that in total, 96% of all obstructed ureters could be occluded by a device of 7 or 10 mm diameter, while 4% of ureters demonstrated more dilation than 10 mm [35].

A subsequent study compared the insertion force and maneuverability as well as dilation and extraction forces for the Stone Cone®, Accordion®, and NTrap® in an ex vivo model. This study noted that the Stone Cone® demonstrated significantly higher insertion forces and required more attempts to bypass an experimental impacted stone than the Accordion® or the NTrap®. The Stone Cone® also demonstrated significantly greater radial dilation as well as required force of extraction than the Accordion® and the NTrap®. It remains to be seen how these differences observed in the laboratory setting may translate to differences in the clinical use of the devices [36]. In a related abstract, the pull-through forces of the Accordion®, Stone Cone®, and NTrap® devices were compared in a simulated ureter model and the Accordion® was found to have the lowest pull-through force [37].

The response of the Stone Cone®, NTrap®, and Accordion® to laser damage has also been tested in a laboratory model. Of note, the Accordion® was the most laser resistant device, able to be operated (i.e., deployed and un-deployed) after 100 direct contacts of the Holmium laser on the Accordion® film. The Stone Cone® was less laser resistant than the Accordion® but more resistant than the NTrap®. In a second experiment which tested the carrying catheters of the devices, the Stone Cone® and NTrap® catheters were more laser resistant than that of the Accordion® [22].

One study hypothesized that use of anti-retropulsion devices may decrease pressure transmitted to the upper tracts by decreasing the amount of irrigant which flows cephalad of the device. Using an ex vivo model, this report noted that the Accordion®, NTrap®, and Stone Cone® all significantly decreased renal pelvic pressures when compared to no device, and among them, the Accordion® demonstrated the greatest reduction [38].

A final issue to consider is the cost of the device. As mentioned briefly already anti-retropulsion devices have the potential to reduce costs by decreasing operative times, reducing the need to change from the semirigid to flexible ureteroscopy to chase migrated fragments cephalad, and also by preventing auxiliary procedures to treat clinically significant retropulsed fragments [8, 23, 39]. These cost benefits must be weighed, however, against the cost of the device. A single study examined the cost-effectiveness of use of the Accordion® to prevent stone retropulsion during pneumatic lithotripsy for ureteral stones. Using a decision analysis model which included the cost of additional ureteroscopy or shock wave lithotripsy for a clinically significant migrated stone fragment during the initial ureteroscopy, the authors noted that at a retropulsion rate of 14%, the device was cost-effective to use. It is noteworthy that this analysis model was strictly financial, and did not take into account other potential benefits, such as the potential for decreased operative times or decreased numbers of procedures for an individual [40] (Table 15.1).

Table 15.1 Published studies comparing ureteroscopic lithotripsy with and without anti-migration devices

Series	Device	Controls (*N*)	Device (*N*)	Lithotripsy type	Location in ureter	Control SFR[a] (%)	Device SFR[a] (%)	*P*-value
Lee et al. (2010)	NTrap®	68	76	Holmium:YAG/ pneumatic	Upper ureteral	89.7	98.7	0.019
Wang et al. (2009)	NTrap®	57	56	Pneumatic	Upper ureteral	84.2	100	0.002
Rane et al. (2010)	BackStop®	34	34	Holmium:YAG/ pneumatic	Upper ureteral	87.8	93.9	0.7[b]
Zehri et al. (2008)	Lidocaine jelly	25	25	Pneumatic	–	72	96	0.045
Desai et al. (2002)	Stone Cone®	20	23	Pneumatic	–	70[c]	100[c]	<0.001
Pardalidis et al. (2005)	Stone Cone®	30	26	Electrohydraulic	–	69.3[c]	100[c]	<0.001

[a] Stone-free rate
[b] The rate of stone retropulsion was significantly higher in the control group ($p=0.0002$)
[c] Residual stone size >3 mm

Summary

A variety of anti-retropulsion devices exist as adjunct tools for the urologist performing ureteroscopic lithotripsy. Each has been studied in several trials, and overall, results demonstrate that each device prevents stone migration when compared to controls (i.e., ureteroscopy performed without anti-retropulsion devices). It remains to be seen whether these devices become more commonplace as further studies are carried out and urologists' experience increases.

References

1. Preminger GM, et al. 2007 Guideline for the management of ureteral calculi. Eur Urol. 2007;52(6): 1610–31.
2. Dretler SP. The stone cone: a new generation of basketry. J Urol. 2001;165(5):1593–6.
3. Finley DS, et al. Effect of holmium:YAG laser pulse width on lithotripsy retropulsion in vitro. J Endourol. 2005;19(8):1041–4.
4. Lee H, et al. Stone retropulsion during holmium:YAG lithotripsy. J Urol. 2003;169(3):881–5.
5. Marguet CG, et al. In vitro comparison of stone retropulsion and fragmentation of the frequency doubled, double pulse nd:yag laser and the holmium:yag laser. J Urol. 2005;173(5):1797–800.
6. Eisner BH, Pengune W, Stoller ML. Use of an antiretropulsion device to prevent stone retropulsion significantly increases the efficiency of pneumatic lithotripsy: an in vitro study. BJU Int. 2009;104(6): 858–61.
7. Lee HJ, et al. In vitro evaluation of nitinol urological retrieval coil and ureteral occlusion device: retropulsion and holmium laser fragmentation efficiency. J Urol. 2008;180(3):969–73.
8. Chow GK, et al. Ureteroscopy: effect of technology and technique on clinical practice. J Urol. 2003;170(1): 99–102.
9. Wang CJ, Huang SW, Chang CH. Randomized trial of NTrap for proximal ureteral stones. Urology. 2011; 77(3):553–7.
10. Dretler SP. Ureteroscopy for proximal ureteral calculi: prevention of stone migration. J Endourol. 2000;14(7): 565–7.
11. Hendlin K, Weiland D, Monga M. Impact of irrigation systems on stone migration. J Endourol. 2008;22(3): 453–8.
12. Holley PG, et al. Assessment of novel ureteral occlusion device and comparison with stone cone in prevention of stone fragment migration during lithotripsy. J Endourol. 2005;19(2):200–3.
13. Elashry OM, et al. Intracorporeal electrohydraulic lithotripsy of ureteral and renal calculi using small caliber (1.9F) electrohydraulic lithotripsy probes. J Urol. 1996;156(5):1581–5.
14. Teichman JM, et al. Ureteroscopic management of ureteral calculi: electrohydraulic versus holmium:YAG lithotripsy. J Urol. 1997;158(4):1357–61.
15. Knispel HH, et al. Pneumatic lithotripsy applied through deflected working channel of miniureteroscope: results in 143 patients. J Endourol. 1998;12(6): 513–5.
16. Yang SS, Hong JS. Electrohydraulic lithotripsy of upper ureteral calculi with semirigid ureteroscope. J Endourol. 1996;10(1):27–30.
17. Bapat SS, et al. Comparison of holmium laser and pneumatic lithotripsy in managing upper-ureteral stones. J Endourol. 2007;21(12):1425–7.
18. Tipu SA, et al. Treatment of ureteric calculi—use of Holmium:YAG laser lithotripsy versus pneumatic lithoclast. J Pak Med Assoc. 2007;57(9):440–3.
19. Kang HW, et al. Dependence of calculus retropulsion on pulse duration during Ho:YAG laser lithotripsy. Lasers Surg Med. 2006;38(8):762–72.
20. White MD, et al. Evaluation of retropulsion caused by holmium:YAG laser with various power settings and fibers. J Endourol. 1998;12(2):183–6.
21. Maislos SD, et al. Efficacy of the Stone Cone for treatment of proximal ureteral stones. J Endourol. 2004;18(9):862–4.
22. Vejdani K, et al. Effect of laser insult on devices used to prevent stone retropulsion during ureteroscopic lithotripsy. J Endourol. 2009;23(2):249–51.
23. Desai MR, et al. The Dretler stone cone: a device to prevent ureteral stone migration-the initial clinical experience. J Urol. 2002;167(5):1985–8.
24. Pardalidis NP, Papatsoris AG, Kosmaoglou EV. Prevention of retrograde calculus migration with the Stone Cone. Urol Res. 2005;33(1):61–4.
25. Eisner BH, Dretler SP. Use of the Stone Cone for prevention of calculus retropulsion during holmium:YAG laser lithotripsy: case series and review of the literature. Urol Int. 2009;82(3):356–60.
26. Lee MJ, Lee ST, Min SK. Use of NTrap(R) during ureteroscopic lithotripsy for upper ureteral stones. Korean J Urol. 2010;51(10):719–23.
27. Ding H, et al. NTrap in prevention of stone migration during ureteroscopic lithotripsy for proximal ureteral stones: a meta-analysis. J Endourol. 2011;26(2): 130–4.
28. Chew BH, Gotto G, Teichman JM. The Accordion: a new device to prevent stone migration during ureteroscopic lithotripsy. J Endourol. 2007;21 Suppl 1:A108.
29. Ditrolio JV, Balla R. Limiting stone retropulsion during laser lithotripsy with a novel ureteral occluding device. J Endourol. 2007;21 Suppl 1:A285.
30. Rane A, et al. The use of a novel reverse thermosensitive polymer to prevent ureteral stone retropulsion during intracorporeal lithotripsy: a randomized, controlled trial. J Urol. 2010;183(4):1417–21.

31. Sacco D, McDougal WS, Schwarz A. Preventing migration of stones during fragmentation with thermosensitive polymer. J Endourol. 2007;21(5):504–7.
32. Ali AA, et al. A novel method to prevent retrograde displacement of ureteric calculi during intracorporeal lithotripsy. BJU Int. 2004;94(3):441–2.
33. Zehri AA, et al. A randomized clinical trial of lidocaine jelly for prevention of inadvertent retrograde stone migration during pneumatic lithotripsy of ureteral stone. J Urol. 2008;180(3):966–8.
34. Bastawisy M, et al. A comparison of Stone Cone versus lidocaine jelly in the prevention of ureteral stone migration during ureteroscopic lithotripsy. Ther Adv Urol. 2011;3(5):203–10.
35. Eisner BH, et al. Differences in stone size and ureteral dilation between obstructing proximal and distal ureteral calculi. Urology. 2008;72(3):517–20.
36. Ahmed M, et al. Systematic evaluation of ureteral occlusion devices: insertion, deployment, stone migration, and extraction. Urology. 2009;73(5):976–80.
37. Adam C. Maximum force generated to retract three stone-trapping devices around a stone in a ureter model with a stricture. J Endourol. 2007;21 Suppl 1:A3.
38. Tarin TV, Shinghal R. Ureteral anti-retropulsive devices decrease renal pelvic pressure. J Urol. 2009;181(4 Suppl):661–2.
39. Geavlete P, et al. Complications of 2735 retrograde semirigid ureteroscopy procedures: a single-center experience. J Endourol. 2006;20(3):179–85.
40. Olweny E, Eisner BH, Stoller ML. Cost-effectiveness of anti-retropulsion devices for ureteroscopic pneumatic lithotripsy. J Endourol. 2009;23 Suppl 1:A 121.

Stone Baskets and Forceps

16

Kirsten Foell, R. John D'A. Honey, and Kenneth T. Pace

Introduction

The field of endourology has made dramatic advancements largely due to the development of smaller flexible and semirigid ureteroscopes. However there have been equally dramatic improvements in ureteroscopic instrumentation that have allowed ureteroscopy to become a therapeutic and not merely diagnostic modality. In this chapter, the history of stone baskets will be briefly reviewed, and the currently available stone extraction devices for use in ureteroscopy will be described along with their strengths and limitations. Techniques and devices to prevent the proximal migration of fragments during ureteroscopy will be described. Complications associated with stone baskets and forceps will be discussed, and the chapter will conclude with a discussion of the role of stone extraction devices in endourology.

K. Foell, M.D., F.R.C.S.C.
R.J.D'A. Honey, M.D., F.R.C.S.C.
K.T. Pace, M.D., M.Sc., F.R.C.S.C. (✉)
Division of Urology, Department of Surgery, St. Michael's Hospital, University of Toronto, 61 Queen Street E., Suite 9-106, Toronto, ON, Canada M5C 2T2
e-mail: kenneth.pace@utoronto.ca

History of Ureteroscopic Stone Baskets

Early in the history of endourology, treatment of upper tract stones was accomplished by blind basketing of small lower ureteral stones followed by manual extraction. With the development of intraluminal ureteroscopes, the baskets were engaged under fluoroscopic guidance and direct vision. When the flexible ureteroscope was introduced in the early 1980s, flexible working instruments were developed with the goals of maintaining maximal scope deflection and irrigant flow, and optimizing the performance of the instruments.

The earliest stone baskets were of the Dormia design (Fig. 16.1): a classical helical structure that facilitated engagement of the stone and subsequent withdrawal [1]. The Dormia baskets were constructed with three or four wires, with or without a filiform tip that could be passed beyond the stone [1]. This helical design survived the transition to endoscopic stone removal, using the ureteroscope, and there are many urologists who still rely on modifications of this design during semirigid ureteroscopy.

With the introduction of percutaneous stone removal in the late 1970s, the helical design of the Dormia basket proved unsuitable for use in the kidney, especially for the removal of calyceal stones. Problems with the use of these baskets

M. Monga (ed.), *Ureteroscopy: Indications, Instrumentation & Technique*, Current Clinical Urology, DOI 10.1007/978-1-62703-206-3_16, © Springer Science+Business Media New York 2013

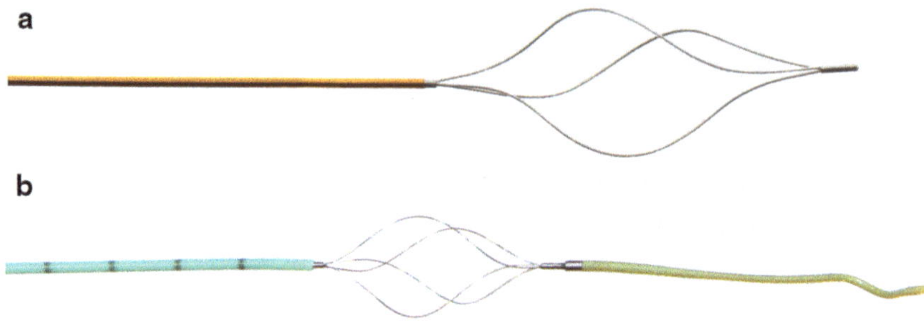

Fig. 16.1 Examples of Dormia helical stone baskets: (**a**) Bagley (Boston Scientific, Natick, MA, USA). Courtesy of Boston Scientific. (**b**) Dormia basket with filiform tip

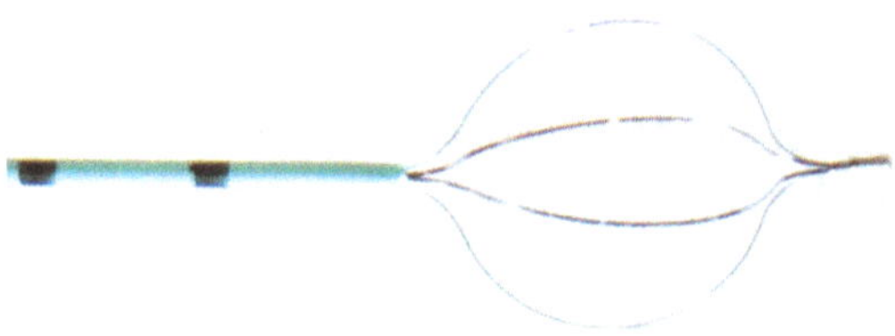

Fig. 16.2 Example of Segura flat-wire basket

included trauma to the collecting system from a rigid tip extending beyond the cage, particularly if the stone was in a calyx. Also, the long distance between the scope and the stone made engagement of the stone difficult.

The next generation of baskets was the Segura stainless steel four flat wire basket (Cook Urological, Bloomington, IN, USA), which was introduced in the early 1980s (Fig. 16.2). The basket could open widely in a relatively small space, which allowed capture of stones or stone fragments from the renal pelvis and calyces during PCNL (percutaneous nephrolithotomy). Although the Segura basket rapidly gained popularity, the rigid steel wires limited deflection of flexible nephroscopes and the protruding tip limited access to smaller calyces and tended to traumatize the papilla, causing bleeding.

The introduction of the nitinol tipless basket marks the transition to the modern era of endourology [2]. The N-Circle was the first nitinol basket introduced (Cook Urological) (Fig. 16.3). Nitinol is a combination of nickel and titanium, and the flexibility of the material allowed full deflection of nephroscopes and later flexible ureteroscopes. The tipless design and the flexibility of nitinol prevented trauma to the papilla during removal of calyceal stones. The combination of nitinol and the tipless design results in almost immediate opening of the basket on deployment, allowing the capture of stones in small, shallow calyces, or indeed anywhere in the collecting system.

Miniaturization of tipless nitinol baskets as small as 1.3 F in diameter allows improved irrigation when used with flexible ureteroscopes as small as 7.5 F. It was only with the introduction of nitinol baskets that it became possible to reliably access lower pole stones ureteroscopically, grasp and relocate them to the upper pole for fragmentation with the Holmium laser.

A number of companies have since modified the original Cook product, and at the latest count, there are 7 companies with 19 different nitinol baskets (Table 16.1). A variety of baskets with stainless steel construction and with tips remain commercially available (Table 16.2).

Some urologists have refrained from the use of stone baskets ureteroscopically for the fear of capturing a stone that could not be released. An unintentional benefit of the nitinol design is, however, the ability to flatten the loops of the open basket and release a stone; this was not possible with the flat wire baskets constructed of stainless steel. Since the 1990s, the use of nitinol baskets has increased dramatically, while the use of helical and Segura baskets has declined proportionally [3].

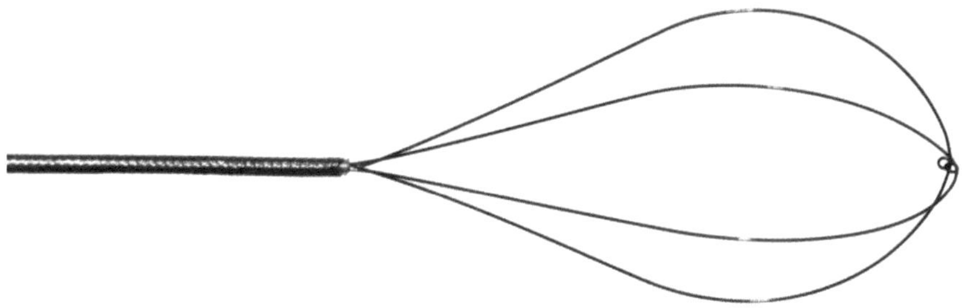

Fig. 16.3 NCircle (Cook Urological, 1.5 F): the earliest tipless nitinol basket. Permission for use granted by Cook Medical Incorporated, Bloomington, Indiana

Stone Extraction Devices

Stone Baskets: General Discussion

Though there are many different stone basket types available for use today (Tables 16.1 and 16.2), there are elements common to all. At the distal end, there are 3–16 wires forming a basket cage (most commonly four), composed of either stainless steel or nitinol (nickel/titanium). There are a variety of basket cage configurations, including spherical, helical, paired wire, or tipless. The cage diameter typically ranges from 10 to 20 mm. There may be a tip protruding beyond the basket cage. The sheath on the basket shaft is typically composed of either polyimide or PTFE (polytetrafluoroethylene) and ranges from 1.5 to 5.5 F. Baskets are typically available in two lengths: shorter for use through a semirigid ureteroscope (65–90 cm) and longer for flexible ureteroscopes (115–120 cm). At the proximal end of the basket is a handle that opens or closes the basket; some have locking or basket articulating mechanisms (Fig. 16.4). When the basket is closed, the basket wires retract into the sheath, and the basket appears to shorten. Most baskets can be disassembled for removal of the ureteroscope through which it is placed in the event that a stone becomes impacted or "stuck" in the basket [1]. All stone baskets are for use in a single patient, but multiple stone extractions can be performed with a single device, so basket durability is of utmost importance.

Key characteristics of a particular basket will affect its performance and its suitability for use in specific circumstances. These include

1. *Basket material.* The introduction of truly tipless nitinol baskets in the 1990s revolutionized the field of stone extraction devices. All previous baskets were composed of stainless steel which was strong, but these devices had several limitations (stiff tip, long excursion distances, etc.) related to the properties of the material and the basket designs of the time. Nitinol is flexible and resilient [2], and unlike stainless steel, it is kink resistant with excellent retention of shape in spite of repeated manipulations [4].
2. *Number and configuration of the wires.* Most baskets have at least three wires, and some even up to 16. Dormia helical baskets have classically been constructed of stainless steel and are most useful for the extraction of ureteric stones. Segura's flat wire baskets were strong, with high levels of radial force generated, but were more traumatic than round wires. Most baskets today are made of round wires, with configurations that include spherical, helical, paired wire, or tipless (Fig. 16.5). Some stainless steel baskets are shown in Figs. 16.1 and 16.2.
3. *Diameter of basket sheath.* Flow through the ureteroscope is inversely proportional to the cube of the sheath diameter, so the smallest possible sheath will help to optimize the flow of irrigant to maintain visibility. Flow will be further impaired if another instrument, such as

Table 16.1 Commercially available stone baskets for ureteroscopic use, constructed with nitinol

Configuration	Name	Company	Tip	Number of wires	Sizes (F)	Open diameters (mm)	Comments
Spherical	NCircle	Cook	Truly tipless	4	1.5, 2.2, 3.0, 4.5	10, 20	4.5 F is 20 mm
	NCircle MegaBasket	Cook	Truly tipless	4	2.2, 3.0	20	
	NCircle Delta Wire	Cook	Truly tipless	4	2.4	10, 20	Triangular Delta wire provides largest possible wire mass for strength
	Zerotip	Boston Scientific	Truly tipless	4	1.9, 2.4, 3.0	12, 16	16 mm for 3.0 F
	Escape	Boston Scientific	Truly tipless	4	1.9	11–15	2 long wires convert 11 mm basket to 15 mm
	Optiflex	Boston Scientific	Truly tipless	4	1.3	6–11	Wheel on handle provides 360° cage rotation
	Dormia No-Tip	Porges	Truly tipless	4	2.2, 3.0	11, 15	2.2 F with twisted wires. 3.0 F with straight ("flat") wires
	Halo	Sacred Heart	Truly tipless	4	1.5	12	Rotation control knob on handle
	Vantage	Sacred Heart	Truly tipless	4	2.4, 3.0	16	
	Apex Nitinol Flat Wire	Sacred Heart	Soft	4	2.4	15	Flat wire design
	Dimension	Bard	Truly tipless	4	2.4, 3.0	10, 13, 16	Articulating basket
	Nitinol Stone Basket	Applied Medical	Truly tipless	4	3.0	12–14	
Helical	Dormia NStone	Porges	Soft	4	2.5, 3.0, 4.0	12.5, 15	2.5 F: 12.5 mm. 3.0 and 4.0 F: 15 mm
	NCircle Helical	Cook	Truly tipless	4	3.0, 4.5	10, 20	4.5 F is 20 mm
	NForce	Cook	Soft or 5 or 7 cm filiform	3	2.2, 3.2	n/a	Soft tipped available in both sizes

Paired Wire	Surcatch NT	Gyrus ACMI	Truly tipless	6 (3 pairs)	1.9, 2.2, 3.0	16	Unique crossed paired wire design. Also available in stainless steel
	Paragon	Sacred Heart	Soft or 5 cm filiform	6	2.4, 3.0	10	3.0 F available with 5 cm tip
Other	NGage	Cook	Open (no tip)	3	1.7, 2.2	8, 11	
	NCompass	Cook	Truly tipless	16	1.7, 2.4	10,15	Partially opened, resembles three (or four wires). Tight weave of wires when fully opened

n/a information not available
Applied Medical, Rancho Santa Margarita, CA, USA
Bard, Covington, GA, USA
Boston Scientific, Natick, MA, USA
Cook Urological, Bloomington, IN, USA
Gyrus ACMI, Southborough, MA, USA
Porges Urology, Division of Coloplast, Minneapolis, MN, USA
Sacred Heart Medical, Minnetonka, MN, USA

Table 16.2 Commercially available stone baskets for ureteroscopic use, constructed with stainless steel

Configuration	Name	Company	Tip	Number of wires	Sizes (F)	Open diameters (mm)	Comments
Spherical	Segura Hemisphere	Boston Scientific	Short or 5 cm filiform	4	2.4, 3.0, 4.5	16, 20	Round wires. Filiform tip only on 4.5 F with 20 mm basket
	Atlas	Cook	Short or 5 cm filiform	4	1.7–4.5	17	
	Laser Flat-Wire	Cook	Short	4	2.5, 3.0	17	Hollow sheath for laser fiber; 150 μm fiber through 2.5 F and 273 μm fiber through 3.0 F
	Platinum Class Flat-Wire	Bard	Short	4	2.4	14	
	Summit	Sacred Heart	Short or 5 cm filiform	4	3	20	Flat wires
	Dormia with extractable basket	Porges	Short	4	2.5, 3.0, 4.0	n/a	Also in helical configuration
	Dormia with olive tip	Porges	Short	4	2.5, 3.0, 4.0	n/a	Also in helical configuration
	SurLok Flat-Wire	Gyrus ACMI	Short or 5 cm filiform	4	2.4, 3.0. 4.5	16, 20	With locking mechanism. Round wires
Helical	Platinum Class Helical	Bard	Short or 5 cm filiform	n/a	3	14	
	Expand 212	Bard	Short or 5 cm filiform	6	3	11	2-1-2-1 wire configuration. Nitinol drive wire
	Spira	Sacred Heart	Short or 5 cm filiform	4	3	n/a	
	Rutner	Cook	Balloon tip	3	5.0, 7.0	14	4 cm balloon proximal to basket for ureteral dilation
	Captura	Cook	Short or 5 cm filiform	3–6	1.7–4.5	10	
	Bagley	Boston Scientific	Short	3	1.9	10	
	Dormia with extractable basket	Porges	Short	3, 4, 6	1.9, 2.5, 3.0, 3.5, 4.0, 5.5	n/a	Also in spherical configuration
	Dormia with olive tip	Porges	Short	4	2.5, 3.0, 3.5, 4.0, 5.5	n/a	Also in spherical configuration
	Pickstone	Porges	Short	4	2.9, 4.0	n/a	No extractable basket
	Surlok Helical	Gyrus ACMI	Short or 5 cm filiform	3, 4, 6	1.9, 3.0, 4.5	n/a	With locking mechanism

Paired Wire	Hercules	Sacred Heart	Short or 5 cm filiform	6	3.0	11	2 pairs and 2 single wires
	Surcatch	Gyrus ACMI	Short or 5 cm filiform	3 pairs	2.4, 3.0	11	Unique crossed paired wire design. Also available in nitinol
	Gemini	Boston Scientific	Short or 5 cm filiform	3–5 pairs	2.4, 3.0	11, 14	Grouped pairs arranged in helix
Other	Lithocatch	Boston Scientific	Soft	12	2.2	7	Designed to immobilize and sweep small fragments from ureter
	Leslie Parachute	Boston Scientific	Short or 5 cm filiform	~ 8 (2 groups proximally)	3.1	11	2 proximal openings when open. When partially closed, multiple wires fan out to retain stone

n/a information not available

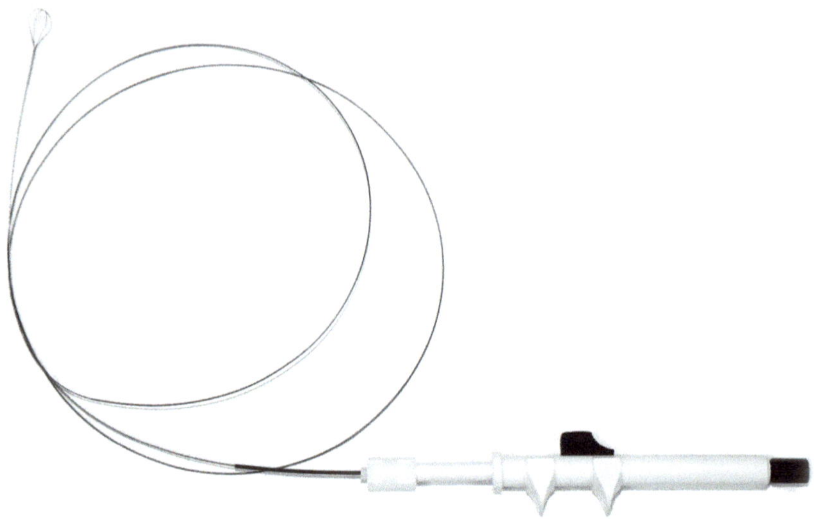

Fig. 16.4 Picture of Cook NCircle basket, showing distal basket cage, sheath (115 cm), and removable handle

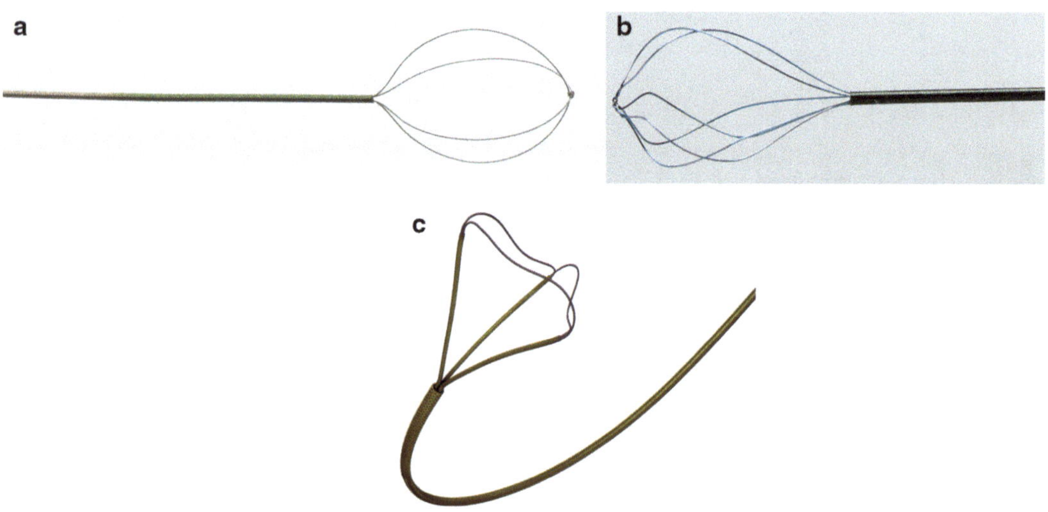

Fig. 16.5 Examples of nitinol basket configurations. (**a**) Spherical (Zerotip, Boston Scientific). Courtesy of Boston Scientific. (**b**) Paired wire (Surcatch, Gyrus ACMI). Courtesy of Gyrus ACMI. (**c**) Other (NGage, Cook Urological). Permission for use granted by Cook Medical Incorporated, Bloomington, Indiana

a laser fiber, is placed in the working channel. Smaller diameter baskets however are less kink-resistant and robust.

4. *The presence or absence of a basket tip.* The original Dormia and Segura stainless steel baskets all had tips protruding beyond the cage. The presence of a tip precluded the safe usage of the basket in the kidney, particularly for calyceal stones, due to the risk of collecting system or papillary trauma causing perforation or bleeding. Though most current nitinol baskets are tipless, baskets with 5–7 cm filiform tips remain available, intended specially for use in the ureter, particularly if it is

tortuous. However, the use of filiform tips has not, to our knowledge, been supported by any in vivo or in vitro studies. Even with a tortuous ureter, it is preferable to straighten it by the placement of a guidewire prior to ureteral stone basketing. The use of a filiform tip without a guidewire is equivalent to blind basketing which is not recommended [5].

Though various manufacturers have described some baskets as "tipless," there is still a definite tip remaining, with the potential to cause trauma to the collecting system. We have therefore classified baskets, through the remainder of this chapter and in Tables 16.1 and 16.2, into those that are "truly tipless," "soft-tipped" (nitinol baskets with a definite tip), "short-tipped" (stainless steel baskets without a filiform tip that could be potentially traumatic if used incorrectly or in the kidney).

5. *Degree of linear basket opening*. Linear basket opening is the 1:1 correlation of handle movement to basket opening. The more linear the basket movement, the easier it is to capture small stones. Some baskets open exponentially: that is, with handle movement, the basket opens little initially until it suddenly springs open. When 13 basket types were compared, the Cook N-Circle basket was the only one to exhibit linear opening [6]. With the nitinol baskets, linearity of opening is related to basket shape: "walnut shaped" baskets (e.g., Zero-tip, Boston Scientific, Natick, MA, USA) tend to have exponential opening, where "tear shaped" baskets (e.g., N-Circle) have linear opening [7].
6. *Radial dilation force*. The radial dilation force, or the radial force with which a basket will open, might be a factor in basket performance, particularly in more compact areas such as the ureter [8]. Though the radial dilation force varies between individual baskets, helical (stainless steel) baskets appear to exhibit much stronger radial strength than tipless nitinol baskets [8]. However, the radial dilation force appears to be of minimal importance clinically [7].

Stone baskets can be used during ureteroscopy for a number of indications, including

1. Stone extraction, either of intact stones or of stone fragments generated by intracorporeal lithotripsy.
2. To hold a stone in a stationary position while laser lithotripsy is being performed (i.e., as an anti-retropulsion device). This is typically feasible in semirigid ureteroscopy, with the basket through the same or a different working channel than the laser fiber. Some baskets are intended for this purpose, with a hollow central sheath that permits passage of the laser fiber (e.g., Laser Flat-Wire Stone Extractor, Cook Urological).
3. Repositioning of a stone to a more desirable location for laser lithotripsy to be performed. For example, a stone could be relocated with a basket from a lower calyx to an upper calyx, where it is released prior to laser lithotripsy. In the lower pole, laser fragmentation is more complex: the laser fiber cannot be advanced with the ureteroscope deflected, so the scope has to be deflected with the laser protruding. Movement of the stone with breathing can be across the line of the laser beam, whereas in the upper pole it is in line. Finally, stone-free rates for stones treated in the lower pole are inferior to those treated in other locations.
4. Grasping and extraction of a stent or foreign body.
5. Possible biopsy of a papillary urothelial tumor.

Regardless of the stone basket used, the principles of use include stone engagement, stone retention during manipulation or extraction, and stone release. The following factors influence the ability of a stone basket to successfully perform each of these steps.

1. Factors Affecting Engagement of the Stone by a Basket
   (a) *Stone size*. In vitro, baskets were capable of engaging beads of a variety of sizes, as long as the bead was smaller than the measured basket diameter [4]. In an in vitro model, braided nitinol wire baskets (such as Halo and Vantage by Sacred Heart Medical, Minnetonka, MN, USA) had the best retrieval characteristics for smaller (2 and 5 mm) stones.

This advantage may be related to increased deformability in the calyx or due to a smaller basket size [9].

(b) *Stone location*. For lower pole stones, engagement or retrieval with a stone basket may be challenging since adequate access to the stone may be limited by the degree of deflection that can be achieved by the flexible ureteroscope. Access may also be impeded by a narrow infundibulum. As will be discussed in a later section, the presence of a basket in the working channel may limit the degree of deflection attainable by the scope, though nitinol baskets of varying sheath sizes do not appear to affect scope deflection [10].

A basket with a high radial dilation force may make engagement of a ureteral stone more efficient [6], and the forces are higher for the helical baskets than the nitinol tipless [6]. In current practice, the best application for the helical baskets may be a ureteric stone, though the nitinol baskets are often appropriately used in this location. Baskets with a filiform tip (usually 5 cm) have been marketed for use if the ureter is tortuous proximal to the stone; the tip may help orient the basket. In practical terms, however, basketing should never be performed in the ureter without the presence of a safety guidewire. The wire should straighten the tortuous ureter, making a filiform tip unnecessary.

Lastly, before the advent of tipless stone baskets, stones in the kidney could not be safely retrieved, particularly calyceal stones. A truly tipless basket is required for stones in the calyceal location to avoid inadvertent papillary or urothelial injury caused by the tip, which could cause bleeding or perforation. It has been shown that tipless baskets are superior for calyceal stone extraction and cause less urothelial damage than a flat wire basket [2]. Apart from the safety considerations, it has also been shown that both helical and flatwire baskets are unsuitable for use in the calyces as they perform poorly in both engaging and releasing stones [4].

(c) *Degree of basket excursion*. The distance from the tip of the sheath to where the target basket width (TBW) is achieved is called the basket's excursion. In vitro, the 3.2 F nitinol N-Circle (Cook Urological) basket was shown to have excursion 12 mm shorter than the 3.0 flatwire Segura basket [2]. Another study showed that the tipless nitinol baskets opened more rapidly to TBW (9.4–14.8 mm) than did flat wire (17.5–22.7 mm) or helical (18.6–24.8 mm) baskets [6]. The implications are significant. If a basket (particularly with a tip that can perforate the collecting system) needs to extend over 2 cm to even engage the stone, the stone may not be visible if there is any degree of bleeding, and the ureter or calyx would be dangerous locations to basket the stone.

When a stone basket is used ureteroscopically, the TBW retracts towards the sheath as the basket is closed. Since the stone is stationary, the basket usually needs to be advanced slowly by an assistant in order to ensnare it.

(d) *Deformability of basket*. The wire should be deformable to minimize urothelial trauma. Deformable wires also permit basket opening in small locations, such as a calyx. Nitinol has all of these characteristics and, with the truly tipless basket designs currently available, a tipless nitinol basket should be the endourologist's first choice of stone basket.

2. Factors affecting Retention of the Stone during Manipulation

(a) *Basket size and configuration*. For a given stone, the larger the basket length, the greater likelihood the stone may escape after it is engaged [6]. Although many of the nitinol baskets are tipless, four-wire in configuration and safe for basically any stone, the helical and multiwire baskets are specifically marketed for the retention of small stone fragments. Several of the

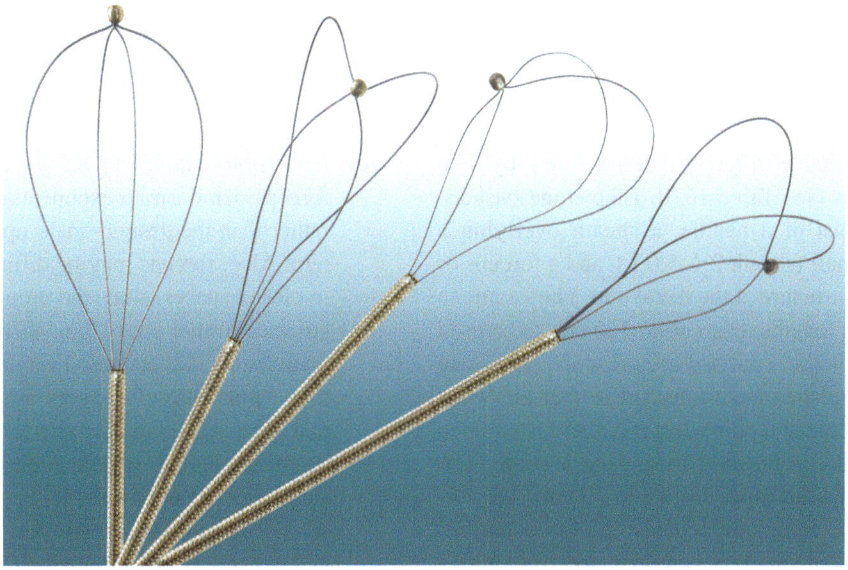

Fig. 16.6 The Dimension basket (Bard, Covington, GA, USA) with tipless nitinol construction. A wheel at the handle rotates one of the two pairs of wires to articulate, or deflect, the basket for improved stone release. Courtesy of Bard

multi-wire designs are grouped near the sheath (to allow wider spaces for stone engagement), then the wires fan out at the distal aspect to theoretically improve stone retention.

3. Factors Affecting Stone Release
   (a) *Lateral deflection of the ureteroscope.* This technique has been described for stone release, and is performed while opening and advancing the basket [11]. It is useful in both semirigid and flexible ureteroscopes and all basket types other than flat wire. In the four-wire configuration, the maneuver compresses two wires together, enlarging the opening between the other pair of wires to gently release the stone.
   (b) *Stone size.* Although stones can be easily engaged if they are slightly smaller than the size of the basket, the stone should be at least 4 mm smaller than the basket to ensure safe release [4].
   (c) *Deformability.* Similar to the engagement of the stone, for the release of a stone into a small space (e.g., relocation rather than extraction), the wires should be deformable in order to minimize trauma.
   (d) *Basket design.* The design or type of basket used appears to be important not only to engage the stone but also to release it. In vitro, nitinol tipless baskets could reliably release beads of all sizes, whereas flat-wire (Segura Hemisphere, Boston Scientific) and helical (Gemini, Boston Scientific) baskets were unable to reliably release beads 8–14 mm in both a ureteral and calyceal model [4]. Also, the Dimension nitinol basket (Bard Medical, Covington, GA, USA) has a unique articulating feature: with a wheel on the handle, one of the two pairs of basket wires can be rotated, to manipulate the basket into various positions (Fig. 16.6). In the same in vitro study, the articulating basket (Dimension) did have the best releasing capabilities of all the baskets, particularly for larger 10–12 mm beads [4] but is only available in 2.4 or 3.0 F sheaths.
   (e) *Inability to release a stone.* Occasionally, a stone can be engaged by the basket, but despite much effort the stone cannot be released. This is referred to as impaction and will be discussed in the complications section.

Stone Forceps: General Discussion

Stone forceps (or "graspers"), like baskets, are stone extraction devices that can be used ureteroscopically. There are approximately 12 commercially available forceps manufactured by five companies (see Table 16.3). Like stone baskets, they consist of a handle, a sheath overlying a flexible shaft (sheath 2.4–5.0 F), and a forceps or grasping structure at the distal end. They come in a range of lengths, from 40 to 120 cm, to be used in a flexible or semirigid ureteroscope. They can be distinguished from a basket in that the wires do not merge at a point. Instead, there is an open space that can be used to engage a stone. The grasping widths range from 8 to 20 mm. The forceps most commonly consist of three hooked prongs and are made of stainless steel, rather than nitinol, for sufficient closing or grasping strength (Fig. 16.7). The Boston Scientific Graspit has a unique design, with 2 nitinol loops that are serrated for additional grip (Fig. 16.8).

Stone forceps can be used for nearly the same indications as stone baskets. They can be used for stone extraction or manipulation and for the removal of foreign bodies. However, they are not used to mobilize a stone for facilitation of laser lithotripsy. Their grasping strength, in specific circumstances, may be greater than with that of a stone basket.

1. Factors affecting stone engagement by forceps
   (a) *Retracting or Non-Retracting Forceps.* Typically, when the forceps are opened the prongs are advanced forward toward the stone. When the prongs are closing to engage the stone, they retract back into the sheath and the whole device would need to be advanced toward the stone. This is similar to how baskets function when they are closing. Several forceps are available (e.g., Coaxial Sheath grasping forceps, Cook Urological) that have a separate inner sheath that advances to close the forceps while the prongs and outer sheath remain stationary.
   (b) *Grasping width of the forceps.* The widths range from 8 to 20 mm and need to be wider than the stone. Due to the open configuration of the forceps a stone may be easier to engage than with a basket, where the closed, distal portion of the basket must be maneuvered beyond the stone.
   (c) *Excursion distance of the forceps.* Many forceps demonstrate exponential opening, rather than the desired linear opening pattern. Also, forceps may be difficult to use in closed spaces, since the prongs need to advance further our of their sheath to fully open than a basket does. To improve upon this, "mini-throw" baskets are available that are designed to have shorter excursion distances, though specifications and measurements are not available. Examples are the Tricep Mini-Throw (Boston Scientific) and Captura (Cook Urological).
   (d) *Stone location.* Stainless steel prongs are not soft and deformable like a nitinol basket (with the exception of the Graspit) so the forceps should not be used unless the tips of the prongs are visible at all times. This may limit the use of forceps in the ureter, unless good visibility is achievable. Their use for calyceal stones may be limited due to the long excursion distance that may be greater than the depth of a calyx. Also, since forceps are composed of stainless steel and are typically somewhat wider than the sheaths of stone baskets, they tend to limit ureteroscope deflection more than nitinol baskets. The limitation of flexible ureteroscope deflection was shown with the Tricep grasping forcep (Boston Scientific) but not the Graspit (Boston Scientific, nitinol wires) [12]. With less maneuverability in the kidney, some lower pole stones will not be accessible.
2. Factors Affecting Stone Retention with Forceps
   (a) *Forceps Shape/Configuration.* With either the Graspit or the 3-prong forceps, the open configuration of the forceps may make stone retention more challenging than a basket if there is any resistance to stone manipulation. In all 3-prong

Table 16.3 Commercially available stone forceps for ureteroscopic use

Material	Name	Company	Sizes (F)	Open diameters (mm)	Comments
Nitinol	Graspit	Boston Scientific	2.6, 3.2	8, 10	2 serrated nitinol loops
Stainless steel	Tricep Retracting	Boston Scientific	2.4, 3.0	n/a	
	Tricep Mini-Throw	Boston Scientific	3.0	n/a	Permits close approximation to stone
	Tricep Extra-Strength	Boston Scientific	3.0	n/a	Heavier gauge wire
	Tricep Non-Retracting	Boston Scientific	3.0	n/a	No backward prong movement during closure
	Grasping	Cook	2.5, 3.5, 5.0	10, 14, 20	
	Platinum Class	Bard	3.0	n/a	Non-retracting (no backward prong movement during closure)
	Captura	Cook	2.8, 3.2	5, 15	Mini-throw (permits close approximation to stone)
	Coaxial Sheath	Cook	3.2, 4.5	10, 15	Forceps stay stationary as prongs are closed
	Delta Wire	Cook	3.2	10	Triangular delta wire allows largest possible mass for increased radial force
	Grasping	Bard	3.0	n/a	Retracting
	Grasper	Applied Medical	3.0	n/a	

n/a information not available

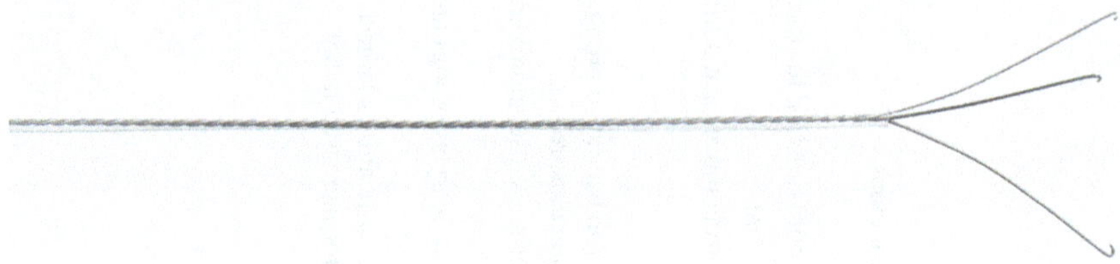

Fig. 16.7 Example of stone forceps with stainless steel construction and three hooked prongs (Tricep, Boston Scientific). Courtesy of Boston Scientific

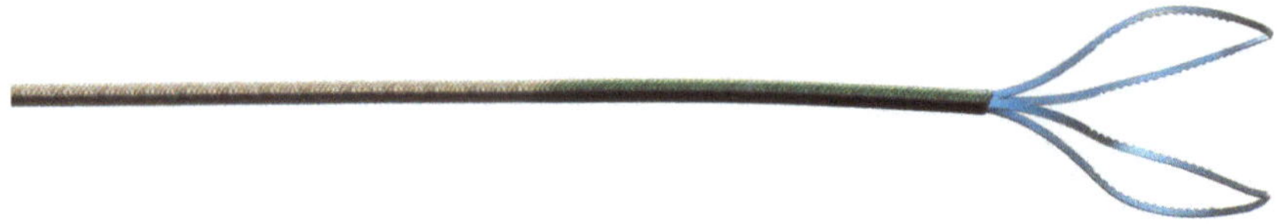

Fig. 16.8 Graspit forceps (Boston Scientific), constructed of serrated nitinol. Courtesy of Boston Scientific

designs, the distal portion of each prong has a hook to increase resistance to stone dislodgement.

3. Factors Affecting Stone Release with Forceps
   The most compelling reason for stone forceps instead of baskets is greater ease of disengaging stones; it should be much difficult to impact a stone with forceps than with a basket.

Anti-retropulsion Devices

There are a number of products and techniques that can limit retropulsion, or proximal migration, of stones during ureteroscopy and intracorporeal lithotripsy. Proximal migration of stone fragments during ureteroscopy and laser lithotripsy for a distal ureteral calculus can increase the length and cost of the procedure, and lead to additional procedures [13]. Three of the devices can also be used to "trawl" the ureter for small fragments after lithotripsy, so can also be considered stone extraction devices. These devices and techniques can be useful adjuncts to stone extraction devices, and some of the anti-migration devices have similar constructions to baskets.

1. NTrap (Cook Urological) (Fig. 16.9). This sieve-like device helps to catch stone fragments that may have migrated proximally due to the irrigation from the ureteroscope and also due to retropulsion from lithotripsy. When inside its sheath, it measures 2.8 F in diameter, and the nitinol umbrella measures 7 mm when deployed distal to the stone. Once fragmentation is complete, the device can be withdrawn carefully, under direct vision, to "trawl" the remaining fragments from the ureter. A retrospective case–control study of laser lithotripsy via semirigid ureteroscopy with or without the use of NTrap demonstrated its safety [14]. Intraoperative stone retropulsion into the renal collecting system occurred in 16.4% (25/152) in the no NTrap group and 0% (0/156) with NTrap.
2. Stone Cone (Boston Scientific). The stone cone is a nitinol retrieval device (Fig. 16.10). It is available with a coil of 3.0, 7.0, or 10.0 mm. It consists of an inner wire and an outer carrying catheter that is 0.038 in. There is a 10 cm hydrophilic tip of the inner wire that remains outside the radio-opaque carrying catheter. The coil shape is formed from a stainless steel wire wound with a strand of

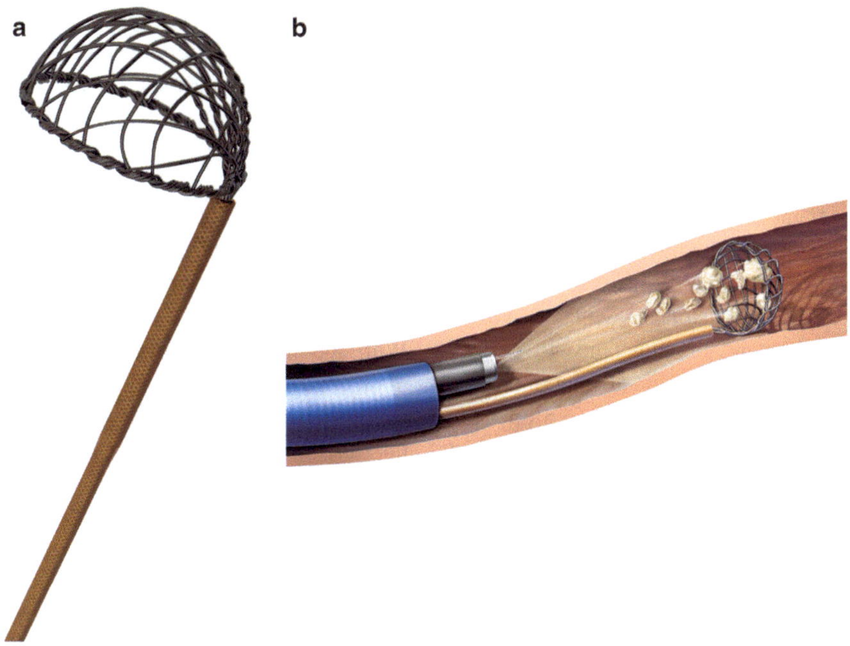

Fig. 16.9 (**a**) NTrap anti-retropulsion device (Cook Urological). (**b**) Illustration of NTrap alongside a flexible ureteroscope, within a ureteral access sheath. Permission for use granted by Cook Medical Incorporated, Bloomington, Indiana

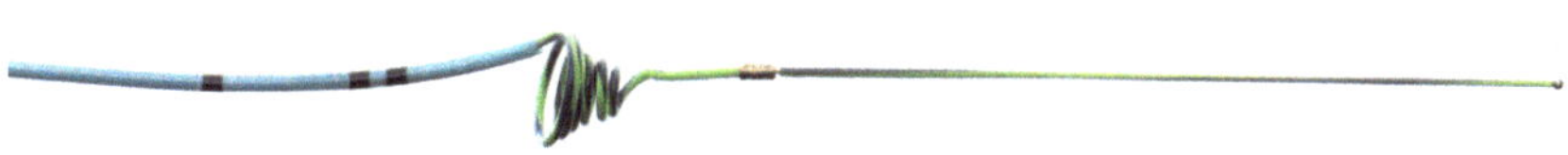

Fig. 16.10 The Stone Cone nitinol retrieval device (Boston Scientific), with hydrophilic tip on *right*. The coil shape is positioned outside the radio-opaque carrying catheter, seen on the *left*. Courtesy of Boston Scientific

nitinol, with memory such that it straightens within the carrying catheter and returns to its coiled position when in the ureter. The Stone Cone is passed just beyond the stone, and the carrying catheter is then removed. A guidewire is not used because it may distort the occlusive fit of the device to the ureteral wall. For proximal ureteral stones, a ureteral access sheath can be placed adjacent to the Stone Cone. The stone cone should not be used for stones at the UPJ or in ureters dilated more than 10.0 mm [13]. In 223 reported patients there was a retreatment rate of 1.5% for residual fragments, which is considered lower than the reported rates for retreatment after lithotripsy without the stone cone [13].

3. Accordion (Percsys, Palo Alto, CA, USA). The Accordion is a hydrophilic coated, microcatheter-based tool composed of a coaxial 0.038 in. guidewire with a floppy tip and a distal multifold film. When it is deployed by coaxial retraction of the inner core of the coaxial wire, the film "accordions" to a 7 or 10 mm wide device that blocks migration [15]. The safe use of the 7 mm accordion was described in six patients undergoing semirigid ureteroscopic laser lithotripsy, with the device inserted either through the ureteroscope, a ureteral access sheath or via a cystoscope with fluoroscopic guidance [16].
4. BackStop (Cook Urological). BackStop is a reverse thermosensitive water-soluble polymer

that is dispensed above the stone(s) and temporarily occludes the ureter to prevent retropulsion of stone fragments during intracorporeal lithotripsy. It exists as a liquid below 16°C and as a gel at room temperature. After lithotripsy is performed, the fragments are extracted, and irrigation with cool saline dissolves and flushes out the polymer. A randomized controlled trial of laser lithotripsy of proximal ureteral stones, with or without Backstop, showed the substance to be safe, with a patent ureter in all patients after flushing. Ureteroscopy with BackStop had a lower retropulsion rate (8.8%) than in patients without BackStop (52.9%), however it was not clear whether this difference was clinically significant as the stone-free rates and the need for additional procedures was not different between the groups [17].

5. Entrapment with nitinol basket during laser lithotripsy. During semirigid ureteroscopy, many nitinol baskets can be passed alongside the laser fiber in the working channel or in a separate channel. The stone can be engaged in the basket so the irrigation and retropulsion during lithotripsy do not cause migration of the stone. The nitinol wires are easily divided if the laser energy is directly applied, however the broken nitinol basket is safe clinically [18]: cut nitinol wires are not sharp and do not injure the urothelium. This strategy can be cost-saving since the same device used to prevent proximal migration can also be used to extract fragments.

Their safety has been described, though the clinical experience can be considered limited. When the Accordion, NTrap and Stone Cone were compared for efficiency of laser lithotripsy, at 20 and 80 W, all devices were more efficient than controls without a device [19]. No fragments larger than 2 mm migrated past any device. However, further experience and the cost of the disposable equipment or the substance need to be considered before their routine application. Furthermore, with the increasing availability of flexible ureteroscopes, the importance of stone retropulsion decreases: stones and fragments can be followed into the renal collecting system and treated even if they do migrate. As a group, anti-retropulsion devices or substances can be useful adjuncts to ureteroscopic laser lithotripsy in select cases.

The Effect of Stone Extraction Devices on the Functioning of the Ureteroscope

With the miniaturization of ureteroscopes, the main concerns regarding the use of stone baskets, or forceps, has been how these devices may affect the functioning of the ureteroscope and the ability to access all the calyces in the upper tracts. The main areas of concern are the effect they have on the flow of irrigation and the degree of deflection achievable by the flexible ureteroscope.

1. Effect on the Flow of Irrigant. Adequate irrigation is critical for visibility during ureteroscopy and laser lithotripsy. In a study of five different modern flexible ureteroscopes from four manufacturers, the flow of irrigant was not decreased by scope deflection. A 273 μm laser fiber caused a decrease in flow of 52.3–54.6%. A 1.5 F nitinol basket caused a decrease of 61.5–62.7% and a 2.2 F basket a decrease of 82.9–83.7% [10]. Another study confirmed that 1.5 F baskets caused less flow disruption than larger baskets [20]. A novel technique described to increase the flow of irrigant when using baskets is the use of a sheathless nitinol basket or "barenaked basket" [21, 22]. With the basket disassembled and the sheath removed, the barenaked basket allows a 2 to 30-fold increase in irrigant flow when larger baskets (2.2–3.2 F) were tested without the sheath in four different flexible ureteroscopes [22]. The unsheathed baskets were reduced to 0.8–1.2 F [23]. This technique has not been tested with smaller nitinol baskets.
2. Effect on Flexible Ureteroscope Deflection. Active single deflection up to 270° is possible with modern ureteroscopes, and some scopes offer secondary deflection (active or passive) [10], which can be useful particularly for lower pole stones. The presence of a 273 μm laser fiber in five different scopes results in a

4–25% loss in deflection, and an increase in the inner diameter of the arc formed by the maximally deflected scope of 1–4 mm. However, none of the 1.5–2.4 F nitinol tipless baskets disrupted the maximal deflection of the scopes or the inner diameter of the arc [10]. Another study showed minimal effect of nitinol baskets on ureteroscope deflection [12]. In contrast, Landman et al. [22] showed that sheathless baskets allowed an additional 15–20° of active deflection when using large baskets (2.2–3.2 F). While flexible ureteroscope deflection does not appear to be affected by the smaller nitinol instruments, stainless steel instruments, such as stone forceps, do restrict deflection [12]. The Tricep 3.0 F (Boston Scientific) decreased active deflection by 15–80° [12].

Current Stone Extraction Devices

Tables 16.1, 16.2, and 16.3 list currently available stone extraction devices. While it is not an exhaustive list, it attempts to list the available options and the manufacturer's specifications.

Complications

Despite improvements in endoscopes and their working instruments, complications still occur. Knowledge of device limitations and potential complications is essential for the endourologist. Ureteral avulsion is one of the most feared complications of ureteroscopy, and stone extraction devices are often involved. Blind basketing with the Dormia basket was associated with 2 of 3 ureteral avulsions reported in one series [24]. The reported rates of avulsion are variable (0.35% in one series [25]) but the risk can be reduced by adherence to good technique. Mostly importantly, stone baskets and forceps should *always* be used under direct ureteroscopic visualization. Adequate visualization of both the stone and the urothelium sliding over the stone as it is being extracted is essential. Blind basketing refers to basket manipulation of ureteral stones as practiced before the advent of ureteroscopy and fluoroscopy around 1981 and cannot be recommended [5]. Undue force should *never* be used [25]. Excessive force should also be avoided when advancing semirigid ureteroscopes. Modern semirigid ureteroscopes have a graduated increase in circumference over the length of the instrument, and forceful insertion can result in impaction of the proximal shaft of the instrument in the intramural ureter. Avulsion can occur with forceful removal of the scope [26].

Basket impaction refers to the inability to remove a basket or release a stone once it is engaged. It is important to avoid undue force if impaction is encountered. In one case of an impacted zero-tip nitinol basket with an engaged, 1.2 cm lower pole stone, the basket was eventually removed after three treatments with shockwave lithotripsy. A 6 F hydrogel ureteral dilator was then passed over the disassembled basket to force the wires closed [27].

All baskets are at risk for breakage if directly lasered with the holmium: YAG laser at energy levels used for lithotripsy, however nitinol baskets are divided with the least amount of energy (0.02–0.03 kJ), whereas the steel baskets broke at 0.06–0.78 kJ [18]. Stainless steel baskets tend to have wires that protrude outwards when broken, resembling fish hooks [18], whereas the nitinol baskets assume a safe configuration with soft pliable wires when broken. These qualities of the nitinol tipless baskets can be used if the basket becomes impacted: one or two adjacent wires of the nitinol basket can be divided with laser energy and then extracted under direct vision. Alternative methods of extraction have been described which include removal through a 7 F open-ended catheter, 8/10 coaxial dilator or a 20 F peel-away sheath. Broken baskets that are not nitinol cannot be extracted through any of these means [18] and may require more invasive measures.

A recent report detailed all of the adverse events associated with stone baskets and forceps from a search of the MAUDE database (Manufacturer and User Facility Device Experience) of the US FDA from 1996 to 2009 [28]. There were 556 adverse events reported, of which endoscopic management was undertaken in 79%, open surgery in 11% and no surgical management was required in 20%. Forty-eight percent of the complications were with tipped baskets, 36% with nitinol tipless, 8% with forceps, and 8% with the Stone Cone. The reported problems with baskets were breakage with detachment of a portion of basket in 49%, breakage without detachment in 39%, and an inability to withdraw the basket in 12%. The complications were considered serious in 42 patients who required major surgery: including ureteral reconstruction (7 patients), ureteral reimplantation (4 patients), and nephrectomy (7 patients). Specific diagnoses included ureteral stricture in three patients who required a repair, ureteral perforation or tear in 17 (59% were managed by stenting), avulsion in 5 and ureteral necrosis in 5. There was an increase in the rates of basket breakage during in 2008 and 2009, which was likely related to the miniaturization of baskets to less than 1.9 F; these very small baskets may be less durable for more complex procedures. There was a threefold increase in complications reported in 2005–2007 (relative to 2005–2007) and a sixfold increase in 2008–2009. These increases are likely due to the increased performance of ureteroscopy and the use of stone baskets in these more recent eras, but one limitation of the study is that the denominator, or total number of ureteroscopies performed, was unknown.

Stone extraction devices are crucial to the endourologist's armamentarium. The instruments have evolved significantly as more advanced and miniaturized flexible ureteroscopes have been developed. With proper technique and a good knowledge of the strengths and limitations of the stone extraction devices, they can be routinely used to improve stone-free rates.

Disclosures

Cook Urological partially funds the fellowship program at our institution. Dr. J. Honey is consultant with Cook Urological and Boston Scientific and has a royalty agreement with Cook Urological.

References

1. Honey RJD'A. Working instruments. In: Smith AD, Badlani GH, Bagley DH, Clayman RV, Docimo SG, Jordan GH, Kavoussi LR, Lee BR, Lingeman JE, Preminger GM, Segura JW. Smith's Textbook of Endourology. Hamilton, ON, Canada: BC Decker Inc.; 2007. p. 209–12.
2. Honey RJD'A. Assessment of a new tipless nitinol stone basket and comparison with an existing flat-wire basket. J Endourol. 1998;12(6):529–31.
3. Leone NT, Garcia-Roig M, Bagley DH. Changing trends in the use of ureteroscopic instruments from 1996 to 2008. J Endourol. 2010;24(3):361–5.
4. Chenven ES, Bagley DH. Retrieval and releasing capabilities of stone basket designs in-vitro. J Endourol. 2005;19(2):204–9.
5. Segura JW, Preminger GM, Assimos DG, Dretler SP, Kahn RI, Lingeman JE, Macaluso Jr JN. Ureteral stones clinical guidelines panel summary report on the management of ureteral calculi. J Urol. 1997;158:191501921.
6. Monga M, Hendlin K, Lee C, Anderson K. Systematic evaluation of stone basket dimensions. Urology. 2004;63:1042–4.
7. Blew BDM, Dagnone AJ, Fazio LM, Pace KT, Honey RJD'A. Practical comparison of four nitinol stone baskets. J Endourol. 2007;21(6):655–8.
8. Hendlin K, Lee C, Anderson JK, Monga M. Radial dilation force of tipless and helical stone baskets. J Endourol. 2004;18(10):946–7.
9. Lukasewycz S, Skenazy J, Hoffman N, Kuskowski M, Hendlin K, Monga M. Comparison of nitinol tipless stone baskets in an in vitro calyceal model. J Urol. 2004;172:562–4.
10. Bach T, Geavlete B, Herrmann TR, Gross AJ. Working tools in flexible ureterorenoscopy- influence on flow and deflection: What does matter? J Endourol. 2008; 22(8):1639–43.
11. Weiland D, Hendlin K, Canales BK, Lukasewycz S. Monga. Lateral deflection to release a stone: A simple method. J Endourol. 2007;21(10):1149–50.
12. Michel MS, Knoll T, Ptaschnyk T, Kohrmann KU, Alken P. Flexible ureterorenoscopy for the treatment of lower pole calyx stones: Influence of different lithotripsy probes and stone extraction tools on scope deflection and irrigation flow. Eur Urol. 2002;41(3):312–7.
13. Eisner BH, Dretler SP. Use of the stone cone for prevention of calculus retropulsion during holmium:YAG laser lithotripsy: Case series and review of the literature. Urol Int. 2009;82:356–60.
14. Feng C, Ding Q, Jiang H, Gao P, Wen H, Gu B. Use of ntrap during ureteroscopic holmium-yag laser lithotripsy of upper ureteral calculi. Minim Invasive Ther. 2012;21(2):78–82.
15. Wosnitzer M, Xavier K, Gupta M. Novel use of a ureteroscopic stone entrapment device to prevent antegrade stone migration during percutaneous nephrolithotomy. J Endourol. 2009;23(2):203–7.

16. Chew BH, Gotto G, Teichman J, Paterson RF. The accordion: A new device to prevent stone migration during ureteroscopic lithotripsy. J Endourol. 2007;21 Suppl 1:A108.
17. Rane A, Bradoo A, Rao P, Shivde S, Elhilali M, Anidjar M, et al. The use of a novel reverse thermosensitive polymer to prevent ureteral stone retropulsion during intracorporeal lithotripsy: A randomized, controlled trial. J Urol. 2010;183:1417–23.
18. Gallentine ML, Bishoff JT, Harmon WJ. The broken stone basket: Configuration and technique for removal. J Endourol. 2001;15(9):911–4.
19. Chew BH, Jonat L, Paterson R, Teichman J. Anti-Retropulsion devices increase stone fragmentation efficiency with holmium:YAG laser lithotripsy. J Endourol. 2009;23 Suppl 1:A345.
20. Nagele U, Horstmann M, Hennenlotter J, Walcher U, Kuczyk MA, Sievert KD, et al. Size does matter: 1.5 fr. Stone baskets almost double irrigation flow during flexible ureteroscopy compared to 1.9 fr. Stone baskets. Urol Res. 2006;34:389–92.
21. Watson G. The use of a sheathless basket via miniature ureteroscopes. Diagn Ther Endosc. 1995;1: 177–81.
22. Landman J, Monga M, El-Gabry EA, Rehman J, Lee DI, Bhayani S, et al. Bare naked baskets: Ureteroscope deflection and flow characteristics with intact and disassembled ureteroscopic nitinol stone baskets. J Urol. 2002;167:2377–9.
23. Bhayani SB, Monga M, Landman JL, Clayman RV. Bare naked baskets: Optimizing ureteroscopic stone extraction. Urology. 2002;60(1):147–8.
24. Alapont JM, Broseta E, Oliver F, Pontones JL, Boronat F, Jimenez-Cruz JF. Ureteral avulsion as a complication of ureteroscopy. Int Brazilian J Urol. 2003;29(1):18–23.
25. Elashry OM, Elgamasy AK, Sabaa MA, Abo-Elenien M, Eltatawy HH, El-Abd SA. Ureteroscopic management of lower ureteric calculi: A 15-year single-centre experience. Brit J Urol Int. 2008;102(8): 1010–7.
26. Ordon M, Schuler TD, Honey RJD'A. Ureteral avulsion during contemporary ureteroscopic stone management: "The scabbard avulsion". J Endourol. 2011;25(8):1259–62.
27. Allen D, Hindley RG, Glass JM. Baskets in the kidney: An old problem in a new situation. J Endourol. 2003;17(7):495–6.
28. Chotikawanich E, Korman E, Monga M. Complications of stone baskets: 14-Year review of the manufacturer and user facility device experience database. J Urol. 2011;185:179–83.

Ureteral Stents

17

Ben H. Chew, Ryan F. Paterson, and Dirk Lange

Introduction

Ureteral stents are commonly used in urology to provide urinary drainage of the kidney or to splint a ureteral anastomosis. Ureteral stents are commonly used to decompress acute obstruction from a kidney stone until definitive therapy can be utilized to treat the stone. This chapter discusses current stent materials including coatings and drug-elution, the methods used to improve stent symptoms including choosing the correct stent length and potential future technologies including new materials, coatings, and drug-elution.

Stents are commonly left indwelling after treatment for urolithiasis. The decision must be made at the end of stone surgery (e.g., ureteroscopy) as to whether or not a ureteral stent should be placed. The absolute indications to leave a ureteral stent are listed in Table 17.1 [1]. There are many randomized clinical trials with evidence that patients without ureteral stents have less postoperative pain and problems than those who receive a ureteral stent [2–7]. Patients without a ureteral stent tend to require less emergency room visits and have less postoperative pain. These studies show that patients who were randomized to not receive a stent after uncomplicated ureteroscopy did not have any more unexpected medical visits or requirements for stent insertion than patients who were stented postoperatively. However, there is also evidence to support the role for ureteral stenting following ureteroscopy—Borboroglu et al. report that the risk of admission for flank pain post-ureteroscopy was 7.4% in the unstented versus a 0% readmission rate in the stented group [8]. In this same study, however, the unstented patients did have significantly less flank pain. Although leaving a stent is justified to prevent ureteral strictures, a meta-analysis of randomized controlled trials by Nabi et al. indicated no difference in stricture rate between stented and unstented patients [9]. Although many studies have shown fewer symptoms and less pain in those patients without a stent, a meta-analysis found a trend towards fewer urologic complications in those patients who received a stent following ureteroscopy [10]. Some of the trials included in the analysis found no difference in complication rates between stented and unstented patients, but there was an overall 4.5% reduction in rate of complications in those patients who underwent placement of a stent following ureteroscopy (95% CI 1.8–7.3%, $P=0.001$). When a more stringent random effects model was applied, however, this difference was not statistically significant (4.1% risk difference, 95% CI 1.8–10.1%, $P=0.175$).

B.H. Chew, M.D., M.Sc., F.R.C.S.C. (✉)
R.F. Paterson, M.D., F.R.C.S.C.
D. Lange, M.Sc. (Hon)., Ph.D.
Department of Urologic Sciences, University of British Columbia, Level 6-2775 Laurel Street, Vancouver, BC, Canada V5Z 1M9
e-mail: ben.chew@ubc.ca

M. Monga (ed.), *Ureteroscopy: Indications, Instrumentation & Technique*, Current Clinical Urology, DOI 10.1007/978-1-62703-206-3_17, © Springer Science+Business Media New York 2013

Table 17.1 Indications to leave a ureteral stent following ureteroscopy

Absolute indications	Relative indications
Perforation of ureter or collecting system	Large stone burden fragmented during ureteroscopy
Infected system	Solitary kidney
Cannot achieve access and require passive ureteral dilation	Edematous ureter
	Severe hydronephrosis
	Bilateral ureteroscopy

Problems with Ureteral Stents: Infection

It is well known that ureteral stents can cause problems—namely irritative symptoms to the patient, infection, and encrustation. More than 80% of patients describe difficulties with an indwelling ureteral stent in place and are unable to work, carry out normal daily activities, or have sexual activity impaired by their stent [11]. Up to 35% of stents are colonized with bacteria following insertion and 24% of all stented patients are found to have bacteriuria [12]. Others report 24% of stents have adherent bacteria and of these patients, only 22.5% have bacteria in the urine [13]. Patients with more concomitant comorbidities have higher rates of bacteriuria following stent insertion: healthy patients had a bacteriuria rate of 28%, while patients with chronic renal insufficiency, diabetes, or diabetic nephropathy had bacteriuria rates of 57, 78, and 62%, respectively [14]. Furthermore, these authors also found that bacteria cultured from these stents were more likely to harbor antibiotic resistance, which is likely attributed to the fact that they are more likely to have been prescribed antibiotics for previous infections due to their immune compromised state. In fact, other authors have found immune compromised patients with diabetes, chronic renal insufficiency, or malignancy to be at higher risk for infection associated with ureteral stents [13].

This raises the question as to whether we should be continuously administered pre- and peri-operative antibiotics around ureteroscopy and stent insertion. In the latest best practice policy statement on antimicrobial prophylaxis in urologic surgery, analysis of four pooled studies with 345 patients covering a multitude of transurethral surgeries were summarized and oral fluoroquinolone prophylaxis had equivalent rates of bacteriuria to an intravenous cephalosporin [15]; there was a lower cost of patients taking ciprofloxacin, however, due to its oral administration. There is good level Ib evidence that one dose of oral ciprofloxacin prior to transurethral surgery is sufficient to reduce the postoperative infection rate when placing a stent. For ureteroscopy, the AUA recommends all patients be given prophylaxis with a quinolone or trimethoprim, or alternatively with an aminoglycoside, penicillin, or cephalosporin.

There is very little to no evidence that postoperative antibiotics are necessary in patients who had sterile urine preoperatively and receive a ureteral stent. Preoperative antibiotics do not prevent microbial colonization of the ureteral stent (EAU Guidelines on Urological Infections, 2009, http://www.uroweb.org/gls/pdf/15_Urological_Infections.pdf). In fact the European Association of Urology guidelines do not recommend antibiotic prophylaxis for healthy patients undergoing uncomplicated ureteroscopy for distal ureteral stones. Patients with a preoperative indwelling nephrostomy tube or ureteral stent or those that are immune compromised should receive antibiotic prophylaxis of second or third generation cephalosporin, trimethoprim–sulfamethoxazole, combination of penicillin and beta-lactamase inhibitor, or a fluoroquinolone. Similarly, patients with more proximal ureteral or renal stones, or impacted calculi, should receive antibiotic prophylaxis as mentioned above. Although the antibiotic treatment is recommended to be short term, the ideal length of time has yet to be determined.

Stent Biofilms

It has long been thought that stent encrustation and bacterial biofilm formation occur as a result of a urinary conditioning film that deposits on the stent surface. It has previously been shown that shortly after insertion of a ureteral device, components of the urine begin to deposit and cover its surface. Conditioning film components on the surface of ureteral stents with and without encrustation have been identified after stent removal from patients [16]. Immunoglobulins and Tamm–Horsfall protein were found to bind nonselectively to the stent surface immediately after insertion; it was hypothesized that their positively charged histones and nuclear DNA-condensing proteins promoted encrustation [16]. Similarly, our laboratory has compared urinary conditioning film components on stents between patients as well as between stents made of different materials (manuscript in progress). This study did not find any significant differences in the most common conditioning film components between stents and patients, suggesting that the major components of conditioning films are the same between patients. These conditioning film components included several cytokeratins associated with the urogenital tract, hemoglobin, Tamm–Horsfall protein, fibrinogen, apolipoprotein, serum albumin, and S100A9. Relating the identification of these conditioning film components back to stent-associated complications, bacteria have receptor molecules called adhesins on their surface that are able to interact with the majority of the components facilitating bacterial adhesion, colonization, and biofilm formation. In addition to this, calcium-binding proteins such as Tamm–Horsfall protein, serum albumin, and S100A9 may form a nidus for stent encrustation. Stent surface coatings and drug-eluting stents that are designed to prevent encrustation and infection are likely rendered ineffective by the formation of bacterial biofilms on the stent surface.

Infection can also lead to stent encrustation—particularly with organisms that possess the urea splitting enzyme urease (e.g., *Proteus mirabilis*) that forms an ammonium ion from ammonia in a process that utilizes free hydrogen atoms and results in the alkalization of urine (increasing pH) [17]. At a higher pH, magnesium, ammonium, and phosphate (i.e., struvite) crystals and calcium apatite crystals can form. Given the interaction of calcium and magnesium with proteins of the conditioning film, encrustation of the indwelling stent can occur. Aside from bacterial-induced urinary alkalization, other conditions that lead to an increase in urinary pH in the absence of bacteria can trigger precipitation of urinary ions that in the presence of the conditioning film will cause encrustation. Prevention of conditioning film deposition and bacterial adhesion are important points to consider for future research of ureteral stents. Although prevention of conditioning film formation will be a big step in preventing encrustation, it may not eliminate bacterial adhesion as they contain several factors on their surface that will allow them to interact with biomaterials in the absence of specific binding partners via ionic and hydrophobic interactions. Finding a biomaterial that resists both encrustation and bacterial adhesion is a great challenge.

Stent-Associated Discomfort

The most common complication of indwelling ureteral stents is pain experienced by the patient. Over 80% of patients with a ureteral stent experience pain and discomfort [11]. Much speculation has gone into the cause of the discomfort and the exact causes are unknown, but one theory is uroepithelial irritation during stent movement within the ureter as the patient goes about their day-to-day activities. A previous study showed that the ureteral stent moves within the ureter, kidney, and bladder when the patient moves and may cause discomfort [18]. This movement is likely attributed to the fact that ureteral JJ stents are not anchored in place: the pigtail curls in the bladder and kidney are designed to prevent migration of the stent, but allow the stent to slide and move. Using an in vitro stent-induced injury model, our laboratory has shown that the irritation of urothelial cells by a ureteral stent piece triggers the secretion of vast amounts of pro-inflammatory cytokines [19], which may be a cause of stent-associated pain.

Stent Length Relating to Discomfort

Even though there is no clear data to support the use of one type of stent over another, there is good data that longer stents that protrude into the bladder produce more symptoms. Choosing the correct length stent will significantly help reduce patient stent symptoms. Stents that cross the midline of the bladder result in significantly more dysuria, urgency and irritative voiding symptoms than patients with stents that do not cross the midline. Long stents are associated with excess material in the bladder—and, therefore, presumably with more bladder irritation—but do not result in excess stent length in the kidney [20]. Fluoroscopic studies of stented patients show that, with motion, the stent tends to bow in the mid and proximal ureter and the excess length slides in and out of the bladder at the ureterovesical junction, with relatively little motion seen in the kidney [18]. El Nahes and colleagues have identified additional factors that contribute to stent-associated symptoms that include crossing of the lower coil to the other side of the bladder, calyceal position of the upper coil, stent length, and larger stent diameter [21]. Certainly, stents that have a lot of excess material in the bladder may cause more mucosal irritation of the bladder and have been shown to result in more patient discomfort.

How is the correct stent length chosen? This question has baffled many urologists and many methods have been described including measuring patient height, torso length, intravenous urography, and direct ureteral measurement. One study found that direct intraoperative measurement of ureteral length was better than patient height at correlating with the correct stent length [22]. Another study evaluated several anthropometric factors, including patient height, BMI, and distances from the acromion process (shoulder) to the head of the ulna (wrist), olecranon process (elbow) to the head of the ulna, xiphoid process to pubis, umbilicus to pubis, and anterior iliac spine to anterior iliac spine [23]. They measured ureteral length intraoperatively with a 5 Fr ureteral catheter and found that height, xiphoid process to pubis distance, and the shoulder to wrist distance all correlated with ureteric length. Ho et al. recommend a 22 cm stent for patients 149.5–178.5 cm in height, but did not study patients outside this height range [24]. To date, there is no standard accepted method of determining the most appropriate length of ureteral stent.

Analgesics for Stent-Related Pain

Phenazopyridine and oxybutynin have been administered orally in an attempt to relieve stent-related symptoms. In a randomized trial involving 60 patients randomized to phenazopyridine, oxybutynin or placebo, the following measures were recorded: narcotic, use, flank pain, suprapubic pain, urinary frequency, urgency, dysuria, and hematuria [25]. There was a trend, although statistically insignificant due to the small group numbers, for a reduction in narcotic usage in the oxybutynin group. Phenazopyridine significantly reduced the amount of hematuria patients had on postoperative day 1 compared to placebo. Perhaps a larger study would discern if either of these medications would be helpful in relieving stent symptoms.

Alpha Blockers and Stent-Related Pain

Patients randomized to alfuzosin following ureteroscopy and stent insertion had significantly less narcotic use, less overall pain in the back and groin area, less flank pain during urination and less urinary frequency compared to patients given placebo [26]. Tamsulosin also produced similar significant results in other placebo-controlled prospective trials of patients undergoing ureteral stent placement following ureteroscopy [27, 28]. There is good data to suggest that alpha blockers are an excellent way to prevent and relieve ureteral stent symptoms [29].

Botulinum Toxin A and Stent-Related Symptoms

It is unknown exactly from where stent symptoms originate. There is evidence that the junction of the ureter and bladder play a role. In patients who had a ureteral stent post-ureteroscopy, a trial randomized patients to three injections of botulinum toxin A into the bladder around the ureteral orifice or no injection. Stented patients with botulinum toxin A experienced significantly less pain than controls and required less narcotic usage [30]. This lends evidence to the theory that detrusor muscle spasm around the intramural ureter is a cause of ureteral stent pain. Most interestingly, the stent used in this study was a multi-length ureteral stent [30]. There is a belief that more significant material in the bladder leads to more significant symptoms, but there is no randomized clinical data to support this anecdotal belief.

Which Stent is Most Comfortable?

This question is asked often, but there is no conclusive data as to which commercially available stent is the most comfortable for patients. There are a variety of factors that are taken into consideration including the softness (durometer) of the stent, its design, and its size both in length and in diameter. Intuitively, one would think that softer stents would be more comfortable than harder stents; however, randomized trials have shown no difference between soft and hard stents in terms of urinary symptoms, pain, time away from work or sexual dysfunction utilizing the Ureteral Stent Symptom Questionnaire (USSQ) [31]—the only validated tool for evaluating ureteral stent symptoms [32]. In one trial, patients randomized to a "stiffer" stent that was greater than 64A durometer in stiffness (Percuflex® stent; Boston Scientific, Natick, MA, USA) were compared to patients who received a softer stent (Contour™ stent, Boston Scientific; less than 64A) [32]. No differences between groups were seen at 1 and 4 weeks in terms of urinary symptoms, overall body pain, work performance, or general health index. Lennon et al. randomized patients to firm polyurethane stents or a softer Sof-Flex™ stent [33]. Patients with firmer stents did have a higher rate of dysuria, renal, and suprapubic pain; however, there was no significant difference in the degree of bladder inflammation, stent encrustation, urgency, frequency, nocturia or hematuria and patients in this study were not evaluated using the only validated stent symptom questionnaire, the USSQ. Dual durometer stents have a different firmness in the stent coil—typically the renal coil is firmer to maintain the curl and thus its position while the bladder curl is a softer durometer in an attempt to reduce bladder symptoms. The research group in Bristol, UK randomized 159 patients to receive a firm, single durometer stent (InLay stent, Bard) or a dual durometer stent (Polaris, Boston Scientific) [34]. There were no differences in stent symptoms between groups of patients: 91 and 94% of the Inlay and Polaris stented patients, respectively, still complained of stent symptoms. This study further outlines our poor understanding of why stents cause so much discomfort. Even with a softer bladder coil, patients still complained of symptoms.

In addition to irritating the uroepithelium, indwelling ureteral stents have been shown to affect the rate of ureteral *peristalsis*, which is the contraction of muscles surrounding the ureter that facilitate and drive urinary flow. This loss of ureteral peristalsis is also hypothesized to cause stent symptoms for patients. Several studies have shown that ureteral stents prevent ureteral peristalsis, which causes backpressure on the kidney due to decreased urinary flow down the ureter [35–37]. This backpressure may be an additional cause for patient discomfort. The decrease and disruption of ureteral peristalsis can also be attributed to the shape and location of the ureteral stent—the renal curl sits in the renal pelvis and may disrupt the pacemaker of ureteral peristalsis which are located in the renal pelvis [38–41]. Contact between the stent and the renal pelvis is believed to throw off the pacemaker, disrupting the rhythmic muscular contractions responsible for driving urinary flow into the bladder. Without these contractions, the renal pelvis becomes swollen or hydronephrotic and is thought to cause significant patient symptoms. Similarly, the diameter of the stent has also been shown to affect peristalsis, as smaller diameter stents have less contact with the ureteral wall compared to larger diameter stents [35, 42]. The prevention of stent symptoms needs to address the overall structure of the stent, minimize the degree of urothelial irritation and disruption of peristaltic activity.

Ureteral Stent Biomaterials

There are a variety of different biomaterials used in stent design with the most popular being a variation or combination involving polyurethane. Most are proprietary polymers based on this technology. Polyethylene stents originally used in stents are no longer used today due to their stiffness and brittleness which has a tendency to fracture when left indwelling for long periods of time. Newer blends of polyethylene and other polymers, such as polyurethane, have been developed to withstand the conditions of the urinary environment such as fracturing, encrusting, and causing infection [43]. Silicone is one of the most currently biocompatible materials used in the urinary tract today in terms of avoiding infection, encrustation, and biofilm production [44–46]. It is also very lubricious which makes insertion easier and may potentially help with patient comfort; however, silicone's flexibility and elasticity—two favorable properties—are also the cause of the problems with silicone. Namely, negotiating silicone ureteral stents through narrow or tortuous is very difficult since it is too flexible and elastic in these conditions and can often not be inserted under these situations. The development from brittle and firm polyethylene and soft silicone led to polyurethane—a compromise between these two extremes—and the most common biomaterial used in ureteral stents today. Although it is most commonly used, it is also fairly firm and is prone to causing significant discomfort in patients. Newer materials are constantly being developed and include many proprietary-based polymers from various companies.

The future of stent materials will likely include technologies to improve patient comfort while reducing encrustation, infection and maintaining its drainage characteristics. Newer coatings that will resist infection and encrustation will allow longer indwelling of ureteral stents without sequelae. Drug-eluting materials or coatings will be able to elute and deliver drugs locally to reduce symptoms or infection. The first drug-eluting ureteral stent was designed to elute the antimicrobial triclosan which has many mechanisms of action and is not classified as an antibiotic. It was shown to be very effective against susceptible bacteria in vitro [47] but not in patients who required long-term stents [48]. It is very effective to reduce bacterial adhesion to stents when tested in vitro [49] and there was no induction of antibiotic resistance when exposed to multiple low-dose antibiotics [50]. The second drug-eluting stent was designed to improve stent symptoms by eluting the nonsteroidal anti-inflammatory, ketorolac. In an animal study, the highest concentrations of ketorolac were found in the adjacent ureteral and bladder tissue without concomitant systemic side effects such as gastric ulceration which was found in the orally administered ketorolac group [51]. In a multicenter, randomized prospective trial, 276 patients received either a regular double J ureteral stent or a ketorolac-eluting ureteral stent [52]. There was a trend in the ketorolac eluting stent group to require less pain medication compared to controls ($P=0.057$) which was significant in younger males.

References

1. Wein AJ, Kavoussi LR, Novick AC, Partin AW, Peters CA. Campbell-Walsh urology. 10th ed. Philadelphia: Saunders; 2012.
2. Al-Ba'adani T, Ghilan A, El-Nono I, Alwan M, Bingadhi A. Whether post-ureteroscopy stenting is necessary or not? Saudi Med J. 2006;27(6):845–8 [Randomized Controlled Trial].
3. Chen YT, Chen J, Wong WY, Yang SS, Hsieh CH, Wang CC. Is ureteral stenting necessary after uncomplicated ureteroscopic lithotripsy? A prospective, randomized controlled trial. J Urol. 2002;167(5):1977–80 [Clinical Trial Comparative Study Randomized Controlled Trial].
4. Dominguez J, Clase CM, Mahalati K, MacDonald AS, McAlister VC, Belitsky P, et al. Is routine ureteric stenting needed in kidney transplantation? A randomized trial. Transplantation. 2000;70(4):597–601 [Clinical Trial Randomized Controlled Trial].
5. Hussein A, Rifaat E, Zaki A, Abol-Nasr M. Stenting versus non-stenting after non-complicated ureteroscopic manipulation of stones in bilharzial ureters. Int J Urol. 2006;13(7):886–90 [Randomized Controlled Trial].
6. Isen K, Bogatekin S, Em S, Ergin H, Kilic V. Is routine ureteral stenting necessary after uncomplicated ureteroscopic lithotripsy for lower ureteral stones larger than 1 cm? Urol Res. 2008;36(2):115–9 [Randomized Controlled Trial].

7. Mangus RS, Haag BW. Stented versus nonstented extravesical ureteroneocystostomy in renal transplantation: a metaanalysis. Am J Transplant. 2004;4(11):1889–96 [Comparative Study Meta-Analysis Review].
8. Borboroglu PG, Amling CL, Schenkman NS, Monga M, Ward JF, Piper NY, et al. Ureteral stenting after ureteroscopy for distal ureteral calculi: a multi-institutional prospective randomized controlled study assessing pain, outcomes and complications. J Urol. 2001;166(5):1651–7 [Clinical Trial Multicenter Study Randomized Controlled Trial Research Support, Non-U.S. Gov't Research Support, U.S. Gov't, Non-P.H.S.].
9. Nabi G, Cook J, N'Dow J, McClinton S. Outcomes of stenting after uncomplicated ureteroscopy: systematic review and meta-analysis. BMJ. 2007;334(7593):572 [Meta-Analysis Review].
10. Makarov DV, Trock BJ, Allaf ME, Matlaga BR. The effect of ureteral stent placement on post-ureteroscopy complications: a meta-analysis. Urology. 2008;71(5):796–800 [Meta-Analysis].
11. Joshi HB, Stainthorpe A, MacDonagh RP, Keeley Jr FX, Timoney AG, Barry MJ. Indwelling ureteral stents: evaluation of symptoms, quality of life and utility. J Urol. 2003;169(3):1065–9. discussion 9.
12. Akay AF, Aflay U, Gedik A, Sahin H, Bircan MK. Risk factors for lower urinary tract infection and bacterial stent colonization in patients with a double J ureteral stent. Int Urol Nephrol. 2007;39(1):95–8.
13. Al-Ghazo MA, Ghalayini IF, Matani YS, El-Radaideh KM, Haddad HI. The risk of bacteriuria and ureteric stent colonization in immune-compromised patients with double J stent insertion. Int Urol Nephrol. 2010;42(2):343–7.
14. Kehinde EO, Rotimi VO, Al-Hunayan A, Abdul-Halim H, Boland F, Al-Awadi KA. Bacteriology of urinary tract infection associated with indwelling J ureteral stents. J Endourol. 2004;18(9):891–6.
15. Wolf Jr JS, Bennett CJ, Dmochowski RR, Hollenbeck BK, Pearle MS, Schaeffer AJ. Best practice policy statement on urologic surgery antimicrobial prophylaxis. J Urol. 2008;179(4):1379–90 [Practice Guideline].
16. Canales BK, Higgins L, Markowski T, Anderson L, Li QA, Monga M. Presence of five conditioning film proteins are highly associated with early stent encrustation. J Endourol. 2009;23(9):1437–42 [Research Support, N.I.H., Extramural].
17. Sabbuba N, Hughes G, Stickler DJ. The migration of Proteus mirabilis and other urinary tract pathogens over Foley catheters. BJU Int. 2002;89(1):55–60 [Research Support, Non-U.S. Gov't].
18. Chew BH, Knudsen BE, Nott L, Pautler SE, Razvi H, Amann J, et al. Pilot study of ureteral movement in stented patients: first step in understanding dynamic ureteral anatomy to improve stent comfort. J Endourol. 2007;21(9):1069–75 [Research Support, Non-U.S. Gov't].
19. Elwood CN, Lange D, Nadeau R, Seney S, Summers K, Chew BH, et al. Novel in vitro model for studying ureteric stent-induced cell injury. BJU Int. 2010;105(9):1318–23 [Research Support, Non-U.S. Gov't].
20. Al-Kandari AM, Al-Shaiji TF, Shaaban H, Ibrahim HM, Elshebiny YH, Shokeir AA. Effects of proximal and distal ends of double-J ureteral stent position on postprocedural symptoms and quality of life: a randomized clinical trial. J Endourol. 2007;21(7):698–702 [Randomized Controlled Trial].
21. El-Nahas AR, El-Assmy AM, Shoma AM, Eraky I, El-Kenawy MR, El-Kappany HA. Self-retaining ureteral stents: analysis of factors responsible for patients' discomfort. J Endourol. 2006;20(1):33–7 [Comparative Study].
22. Jeon SS, Choi YS, Hong JH. Determination of ideal stent length for endourologic surgery. J Endourol. 2007;21(8):906–10 [Clinical Trial Research Support, Non-U.S. Gov't].
23. Hruby GW, Ames CD, Yan Y, Monga M, Landman J. Correlation of ureteric length with anthropometric variables of surface body habitus. BJU Int. 2007;99(5):1119–22.
24. Ho CH, Chen SC, Chung SD, Lee YJ, Chen J, Yu HJ, et al. Determining the appropriate length of a double-pigtail ureteral stent by both stent configurations and related symptoms. J Endourol. 2008;22(7):1427–31 [Evaluation Studies].
25. Norris RD, Sur RL, Springhart WP, Marguet CG, Mathias BJ, Pietrow PK, et al. A prospective, randomized, double-blinded placebo-controlled comparison of extended release oxybutynin versus phenazopyridine for the management of postoperative ureteral stent discomfort. Urology. 2008;71(5):792–5 [Comparative Study Randomized Controlled Trial].
26. Beddingfield R, Pedro RN, Hinck B, Kreidberg C, Feia K, Monga M. Alfuzosin to relieve ureteral stent discomfort: a prospective, randomized, placebo controlled study. J Urol. 2009;181(1):170–6 [Randomized Controlled Trial Research Support, Non-U.S. Gov't].
27. Damiano R, Autorino R, De Sio M, Giacobbe A, Palumbo IM, D'Armiento M. Effect of tamsulosin in preventing ureteral stent-related morbidity: a prospective study. J Endourol. 2008;22(4):651–6 [Randomized Controlled Trial].
28. Wang CJ, Huang SW, Chang CH. Effects of tamsulosin on lower urinary tract symptoms due to double-J stent: a prospective study. Urol Int. 2009;83(1):66–9 [Randomized Controlled Trial].
29. Yakoubi R, Lemdani M, Monga M, Villers A, Koenig P. Is there a role for alpha-blockers in ureteral stent-related symptoms? A systematic review and meta-analysis. J Urol. 2011;186(3):928–34 [Meta-Analysis Review].
30. Gupta M, Patel T, Xavier K, Maruffo F, Lehman D, Walsh R, et al. Prospective randomized evaluation of periureteral botulinum toxin type A injection for ureteral stent pain reduction. J Urol. 2010;183(2):598–602 [Randomized Controlled Trial].
31. Joshi HB, Newns N, Stainthorpe A, MacDonagh RP, Keeley Jr FX, Timoney AG. Ureteral stent symptom questionnaire: development and validation of a

multidimensional quality of life measure. J Urol. 2003;169(3):1060–4 [Validation Studies].
32. Joshi HB, Chitale SV, Nagarajan M, Irving SO, Browning AJ, Biyani CS, et al. A prospective randomized single-blind comparison of ureteral stents composed of firm and soft polymer. J Urol. 2005;174(6):2303–6 [Randomized Controlled Trial].
33. Lennon GM, Thornhill JA, Sweeney PA, Grainger R, McDermott TE, Butler MR. 'Firm' versus 'soft' double pigtail ureteric stents: a randomised blind comparative trial. Eur Urol. 1995;28(1):1–5 [Clinical Trial Comparative Study Randomized Controlled Trial].
34. Davenport K, Kumar V, Collins J, Melotti R, Timoney AG, Keeley Jr FX. New ureteral stent design does not improve patient quality of life: a randomized, controlled trial. J Urol. 2011;185(1):175–8 [Comparative Study Randomized Controlled Trial].
35. Venkatesh R, Landman J, Minor SD, Lee DI, Rehman J, Vanlangendonck R, et al. Impact of a double-pigtail stent on ureteral peristalsis in the porcine model: initial studies using a novel implantable magnetic sensor. J Endourol. 2005;19(2):170–6.
36. Kinn AC, Lykkeskov-Andersen H. Impact on ureteral peristalsis in a stented ureter. An experimental study in the pig. Urol Res. 2002;30(4):213–8.
37. Patel U, Kellett MJ. Ureteric drainage and peristalsis after stenting studied using colour Doppler ultrasound. Br J Urol. 1996;77(4):530–5.
38. Constantinou CE, Granato Jr JJ, Govan DE. Dynamics of the upper urinary tract: accommodations in the rate and stroke volume of ureteral peristalsis as a response to transient alteration in urine flow rate. Urol Int. 1974;29(4):249–64.
39. Constantinou CE, Djurhuus JC. Pyeloureteral dynamics in the intact and chronically obstructed multicalyceal kidney. Am J Physiol. 1981;241(5):R398–411 [Research Support, Non-U.S. Gov't Research Support, U.S. Gov't, P.H.S.].
40. Lang RJ, Davidson ME, Exintaris B. Pyeloureteral motility and ureteral peristalsis: essential role of sensory nerves and endogenous prostaglandins. Exp Physiol. 2002;87(2):129–46 [Research Support, Non-U.S. Gov't Review].
41. Mendelsohn C. Functional obstruction: the renal pelvis rules. J Clin Invest. 2004;113(7):957–9 [Comment].
42. Natalin RA, Hruby GW, Okhunov Z, Singh H, Phillips CK, Humphrey PA, et al. Pilot study evaluating ureteric physiological changes with a novel 'ribbon stent' design using electromyographic and giant magnetoresistive sensors. BJU Int. 2009;103(8):1128–31 [Evaluation Studies].
43. Mardis HK, Kroeger RM. Ureteral stents. Materials. Urol Clin North Am. 1988;15(3):471–9.
44. Tunney MM, Keane PF, Gorman SP. Assessment of urinary tract biomaterial encrustation using a modified Robbins device continuous flow model. J Biomed Mater Res. 1997;38(2):87–93 [Research Support, Non-U.S. Gov't].
45. Watterson JD, Cadieux PA, Stickler D, Reid G, Denstedt JD. Swarming of Proteus mirabilis over ureteral stents: a comparative assessment. J Endourol. 2003;17(7):523–7 [In Vitro].
46. Jones DS, Garvin CP, Gorman SP. Relationship between biomedical catheter surface properties and lubricity as determined using textural analysis and multiple regression analysis. Biomaterials. 2004;25(7–8):1421–8 [Comparative Study Evaluation Studies].
47. Chew BH, Cadieux PA, Reid G, Denstedt JD. In-vitro activity of triclosan-eluting ureteral stents against common bacterial uropathogens. J Endourol. 2006;20(11):949–58.
48. Cadieux PA, Chew BH, Nott L, Seney S, Elwood CN, Wignall GR, et al. Use of triclosan-eluting ureteral stents in patients with long-term stents. J Endourol. 2009;23(7):1187–94 [Clinical Trial Research Support, Non-U.S. Gov't].
49. Lange D, Elwood CN, Choi K, Hendlin K, Monga M, Chew BH. Uropathogen interaction with the surface of urological stents using different surface properties. J Urol. 2009;182(3):1194–200 [Research Support, Non-U.S. Gov't].
50. Wignall GR, Goneau LW, Chew BH, Denstedt JD, Cadieux PA. The effects of triclosan on uropathogen susceptibility to clinically relevant antibiotics. J Endourol. 2008;22(10):2349–56.
51. Chew BH, Davoudi H, Li J, Denstedt JD. An in vivo porcine evaluation of the safety, bioavailability, and tissue penetration of a ketorolac drug-eluting ureteral stent designed to improve comfort. J Endourol. 2010;24(6):1023–9 [Evaluation Studies].
52. Krambeck AE, Walsh RS, Denstedt JD, Preminger GM, Li J, Evans JC, et al. A novel drug eluting ureteral stent: a prospective, randomized, multicenter clinical trial to evaluate the safety and effectiveness of a ketorolac loaded ureteral stent. J Urol. 2010; 183(3):1037–42 [Multicenter Study Randomized Controlled Trial].

Part IV

Step-by-Step Technique

Informed Consent and Perioperative Antibiotics

18

Christopher L. Allam and J. Stuart Wolf Jr.

There is increasing use of ureteroscopy for a wide range of urological diseases [1, 2]. This results from technological advances, improved techniques and familiarity during training—all of which are associated with better outcomes and lower risks. Ureteroscopy is not a panacea, however. There are potential complications, most minor but some very serious, and outcomes can be less than optimal. In this chapter we review two issues pertinent to the balance of risks and benefits associated with ureteroscopy, informed consent and antimicrobial prophylaxis.

Informed Consent

It has long been established that physicians must obtain "permission" from their patients in order to perform treatments [3–5]. Specifically, in the case of *Schloendorff versus Society of New York Hospital*, Justice Benjamin Cardozo wrote in 1914, "Every human being of adult years and sound mind has the right to determine what shall be done with his body; and a surgeon who performs an operation without his patient's consent commits an assault, for which he is liable in damages [6]." This court ruling arguably is the foundation for the *consent* of a patient. The case law has evolved considerably since then [3]. The landmark case of *Salgo* versus *Leland Stanford Jr University Board of Trustees* in 1957 [7] added the notion of "informed" consent into the practice of medicine and surgery [5]. Over the next several decades, the courts and medical professional societies have defined and redefined the definition and interpretation of what constitutes *informed consent* of patients [3–5, 8]. This informed consent is essentially the concept that individuals have the right to make decisions affecting their bodies and health [4].

The physician–patient relationship and the associated fiduciary responsibilities form the ethical, moral, and legal basis of the patient's informed consent [4]. The American Medical Association's Code of Ethics [9] describes this relationship by stating "a physician is ethically required to use sound medical judgment, holding the best interests of the patient as paramount." This physician–patient relationship is based on thorough communication from the physician, not only about the best medical evidence and treatments available but also addressing the patient's questions about the benefits and risks of the procedures being considered [4].

The legal basis of informed consent starts with a discussion of the procedure including the expected benefits as well as the possible risks [3–5]. Initially, the patient should be informed of

C.L. Allam, D.O.
Endourology Division, Urology Department, University of Michigan, Ann Arbor, MI, USA

J.S. Wolf Jr., M.D. (✉)
Division of Endourology and Stone Disease, Department of Urology, University of Michigan Health System, 1500 East Medical Center Drive, TC 3875, Ann Arbor, MI 48109-5330, USA
e-mail: wolfs@umich.edu

M. Monga (ed.), *Ureteroscopy: Indications, Instrumentation & Technique*, Current Clinical Urology,
DOI 10.1007/978-1-62703-206-3_18,

the diagnosis and its potential consequences if left untreated. Next, for each of the available treatment options there should be discussion that includes a description of the treatments, their intended benefits, and the possible risks and/or consequences [3–5, 8]. This discussion includes framing the relative benefits and risks amongst the various alternatives, including non-treatment. The informed consent discussion between a physician and patient should be presented in terms that are easily understood by laypersons. In the case *Canterbury v. Spence* in 1972 the court stated the following topics are required for disclosure by a physician: (1) the inherent and potential hazards of the proposed treatment, (2) the alternatives to the treatment, if any, and (3) the results likely if the patient remains untreated [10]. In addition, the law has defined standards of disclosure as "professional" and "materiality" [3, 4]. The professional standard of disclosure is that the physician must disclose to the patient the same information that other physicians with similar skills would provide in the same circumstances [11]. The materiality standard of disclosure is that the physician must disclose all information that a reasonable person in the community would deem important in the decision-making process [3, 4]. Jurisdictions differ, with the professional standard of disclosure being using in some courts and the materiality standard of disclosure being used in others [3].

In order to obtain a valid consent, the patient must be competent and the consent given must be voluntary—"of free mind and free will [3, 4]." The ultimate decision of competency lies with the courts rather than the physician. The *capacity* of an individual specifically relates to processing of information and communication. Typically, capacity is assumed for any adult who has not previously been judged to be incompetent [3, 4]. This assumption may not be valid for the elderly population, where there is a greater incidence of dementia. According to the US Preventative Service Task Force on dementia in 2003, the aging population has had a dramatic increase in the prevalence of dementia, with up to 10% of people older than 65 and 50% older than 85 having some form of dementia [12]. Given the increasing age of our population, it is imperative that physicians not only provide excellent informed consent but also assess the *capacity* of our patients.

Endourology is held to the same standard of care with respect to informed consent as any surgical procedure. The jurisprudential rule of informed consent is for the Endourologist to discuss the procedure and associated risks (see Chap. 37 for specific complications of ureteroscopy) so that the patient can make an intelligent and informed decision of whether to consent to the procedure. All urologists are held to the same standard of care during endourology procedures regardless of experience or formal training. Certification to confirm "proficiency" is established by the American Board of Urology.

In the event of litigation regarding informed consent, a plaintiff has a two-part burden. First, it must be proven the physician did not meet the required standard for informed consents. Second, the plaintiff must prove a causal relationship between the physician's failure to disclose information and a direct damage to the patient [10]. The case LaCaze v. Collier in 1983 provided the basis for causation elements with regards to informed consent specifically in determining the objective standard whether a reasonable person in a patient's similar circumstances would have consented to a procedure if full disclosure was made. There are several factors that are considered in making this determination, which include the condition of patient and need for treatment, the seriousness of the risk and the likelihood of the occurrence [13].

Some relevant court cases pertaining to Endourology and *informed consent* include *Roussel v Sharp in 1990* in which a patient contested lack of informed consent with respect to possible risk of peritoneal extravasation for a bladder perforation following a transurethral resection of the prostate. The court ruled in favor of the physician as the plaintiff did not prove that a reasonable person in his position would have refused surgery if the risk was known [14]. However, in the case *Cross v. Trapp* in 1982, the verdict was in favor of the patient who suffered urinary incontinence and impotency after a transurethral resection of the prostate because the patient contested he never consented to the actual transurethral resection of the prostate [15]. Other cases have established that informed consent does not need to be obtained for every minor aspect of the endourologic procedure as long as the other standards of disclosure are met [16] and that unexpected findings during the course of the endourologic procedure can be addressed in the same setting without requiring the physician to obtain additional informed consent [17].

Antimicrobial Prophylaxis

"Infection of the operative wound is as old a problem as surgery is an art, and surely older than surgery is a science" [18]. (Described by Dr. Polk in the 1960s).

Antimicrobial prophylaxis has been shown to reduce the incidence of surgical wound infection, and as such is recommended for most operations [18–20]. In 2007, there were approximately 45 million procedures performed in the USA [21]. It is expected that almost 5% of all surgical procedures [21, 22] and up to 20% of intra-abdominal operations, will be complicated by surgical site infections (SSI) [22]. In addition, urinary tract infections (UTIs) and SSI are the first and third most common type of nosocomial infection, respectively [23]. These infections add significant morbidity to the surgical patient and contribute to rising health care expenditures. SSIs alone may add more than $10 billion in direct and indirect health care costs annually [24]. UTIs and SSIs can add several days of hospitalized care for the surgical patient [21–23].

The general risk of a procedure being complicated by SSI is related to the microbial density at the surgical site. Table 18.1 indicates a well-established system that classifies surgical wounds with regards to bacterial load [25]. The infection risk over the classification ranges from less than 2% for clean wounds to greater than 40% for dirty-infected wounds [25]. Antimicrobial prophylaxis is warranted in all procedures involving clean-contaminated, contaminated, and dirty-infected wounds. For clean surgical wounds, however, which carry less than 2% risk of SSI and account for more than 60% of all surgical procedures, the need for routine antimicrobial prophylaxis is uncertain [18, 26]. A large number of urological procedures, including all endourologic procedures, are classified "clean-contaminated" due to entering the urinary tract.

Table 18.1 Surgical wound classification

Clean	Uninfected operative site, with primary skin closure
Clean-contaminated	Entry into respiratory, alimentary, genital, or urinary tracts
Contaminated	Fresh accidental wounds, major break in sterile technique, gross spillage from gastrointestinal tract, or presence of acute but nonpurulent inflammation at the operative site
Dirty-infected	Old accidental wound with devitalized tissue or presence of clinical infection or perforated viscera at the operative site

Adapted from [25]

A necessary step in developing SSIs is microbial contamination of the surgical wound. The risk of developing an SSI is related to the amount of microbial contamination along with the virulence of the organism against the various host defenses. Surgical wounds contaminated with $>10^5$ microorganisms per gram of tissue increase the risk of developing an SSI [27]. The amount of microbial contamination needed to cause an infection is reduced with the presence of a foreign body in the wound [28]. Devitalized tissue likely has the same effect. Virulence factors contribute to microbial infection through a variety of mechanisms. Microorganisms may procedure substances, such as toxins, that contribute to its survival within a host or aid in the destruction of the host's environment [25]. For example, gram-negative bacteria produce endotoxins which stimulate cytokine production that initiate the systemic inflammatory response syndrome cascade [29]. Other bacteria have surface components that inhibit phagocytosis and facilitate microbial invasion. Gram-positive bacteria

Table 18.2 Patient and operation characteristics that may increase the risk pf surgical site infection

Factors that impair host defense
Very young or very old
Poor nutritional status
Diabetes mellitus
Smoking
Obesity
Immunosuppression, including corticosteroid use
Blood transfusion
Factors that increase amount and/or spectrum of microbes
Remote coexistent infection
Prolonged hospitalization
Foreign bodies
Inadequate sterile preparation (surgical scrub, skin antisepsis, preoperative shaving, sterilization of instruments)
Surgical factors
Type of operation and surgical wound
Prolonged operation
Insufficient antimicrobial prophylaxis
Inadequate operating room ventilation
Foreign material in the surgical site
Use of drains
Poor surgical technique
Poor hemostasis
Failure to obliterate dead space
Tissue trauma

Adapted from [18, 23, 25]

produce substances that interfere with a host's natural phagocytic defenses [30].

Most microbial invasion leading to SSIs involve endogenous flora from the patient's skin, mucous membranes, or hollow viscera. Skin and mucous membrane flora are typically aerobic gram-positive cocci (e.g., staphylococci), whereas anaerobic and gram-negative aerobes predominate in fecal flora [31]. Another source of pathogens can be exogenous from the operating room environment (e.g., personnel, instruments), and these microbes are typically gram-positive aerobes but can also include fungal elements [32, 33].

Host factors are also important in the pathogenesis of SSIs. Table 18.2 lists patient and operation factors that may increase the risk of SSI [18, 23, 25]. The patient factors weaken the host defenses or increase the amount and/or spectrum of microbes at the operative site. The surgical factors increase the likelihood that microbes can proliferate at the operative site. There are some additional factors that specifically increase risk of postoperative UTI, including anatomic anomalies of the urinary tract and externalized urinary catheters [34].

An antimicrobial prophylaxis program should ensure that the benefits of prophylaxis outweigh the risks. There are several ways in which antibiotic administration can harm. Allergic reactions can occur, which range from minor cutaneous events (e.g., rashes) to life-threatening reactions (e.g., anaphylaxis). Suppression of normal bacterial flora can lead to fungal infection, *Clostridium difficile* colitis, colonization, and other adverse events [35]. *C. difficile* infections (CDI) have typically been associated with clindamycin, third-generation cephalosporins, penicillins, and more recently, fluoroquinolones [36]. The incidence of CDI is rising and the economic cost annually is over $3 billion [37]. In addition, *C. difficile* is demonstrating increasing resistance to the typical treatment with oral metronidazole or vancomycin [36]. Finally, antibiotic administration can lead to selection of resistant microbes; the overuse and misuse of antibiotics is partially the cause of the worldwide increase in microbial resistance [38]. For example, the incidence of methicillin resistant *Staphylococcus aureus* in US hospitals is now greater than 55% [23]. A recent study that evaluated over 10,000 urine cultures noted resistance of *Escherichia coli* to fluoroquinolones in 25% and to trimethoprim/sulfamethoxazole in 30% [34]. Limiting and controlling the use of antibiotics should reduce the problem of resistance. Given these potentially very serious direct and indirect adverse effects of antimicrobial prophylaxis, it is clear that appropriate antimicrobial prophylaxis is indication-specific and of a limited duration [35].

Antibiotic regimens for prophylaxis entail administrating an antimicrobial agent before, and possibly for a limited time following, the procedure to prevent a postprocedural infection [34]. The agent should be targeted against disease-specific bacterial flora within the region of the operative field. It should be of a limited duration, to reduce cost, toxicity, and antimicrobial resistance [39]. The agent should obtain appropriate tissue and serum levels that exceed the minimum inhibitory concentration for organisms in the intended operative site. If possible, the drugs half-live should be such to maintain sufficient tissue concentration levels during the procedure without the need for additional doses [35]. Therefore the timing and dosing of antimicrobial prophylaxis are important for optimal drug-tissue concentrations during the procedure. Infusion of the first dose should be within 60 min of surgical incision, except for intravenous fluoroquinolones and vancomycin, which should be within 120 min [22]. The agent should be re-administered at one to two half-lives for prolonged procedures [18]. For the majority of procedures, the literature suggests a single dose prophylaxis or discontinuation within 24 h from the end of the procedure [25]. Some instances where antimicrobial prophylaxis may be extended include a preexisting infection, placement of prosthetic material or manipulation of an indwelling tube [35].

There are very few randomized controlled trials (RCTs) available to inform the specific antimicrobial prophylaxis regimen for genitourinary surgery. Currently, the best strategy is for urologists to familiarize themselves with the American Urological Association's (AUA) *Best Practice Policy Statement on Urologic Surgery Antimicrobial Prophylaxis*, in addition to consulting hospital antibiotic policies and local drug resistant patterns, to aid in the selection of a specific antimicrobial prophylaxis program [35].

Specifically for the genitourinary tract, fluoroquinolones, cephalosporins, and aminoglycosides have been advocated for prophylaxis due to their long half-lives, antimicrobial activity against the common encountered pathogens, minimal adverse reactions, and low cost [35, 39]. A review of the literature regarding antimicrobial prophylaxis typically involves trials within other surgical specialties outside of urology. While cephalosporins and aminoglycosides have been well established for SSI prophylaxis in general, fluoroquinolones are more particular to urological procedures. RCTs involving endourologic procedures have confirmed the efficacy and low cost of oral fluoroquinolones for antimicrobial prophylaxis for these procedures [40, 41].

The AUA recommendations cite level Ib evidence (evidence obtained from at least one RCT) as supporting antimicrobial prophylaxis during all types of ureteroscopic procedures [35]. The recommended agents include fluoroquinolone, trimethoprim–sulfamethoxazole (TMP-SMX), aminoglycoside ± ampicillin, first/second generation cephalosporin, or amoxicillin/clavulanate. Knopf et al. [42] in 2003 performed a RCT comparing perioperative single oral dose fluoroquinolone to placebo in patients undergoing ureteroscopic stone removal. The treatment arm had a bacteriuria rate of 2% versus 13% for the placebo group. Another RCT did not reveal any difference in bacteriuria rates between single dose oral fluoroquinolone or intravenous cephalosporins for ureteroscopic procedures or ureteral stenting [40]. A small RCT comparing a single intravenous dose of cefotaxime to placebo during upper tract ureteroscopy or percutaneous renal surgery revealed a treatment arm bacteriuria rate of 5% compared to 12% for placebo [43]. Aghamir and associates [44] performed an RCT in 114 patients, comparing semirigid ureteroscopy with pneumatic lithotripsy with and without perioperative administration of intravenous cefazolin, and found that the incidence of bacteriuria was significantly reduced in the group receiving antimicrobial prophylaxis, although the incidence of symptomatic UTI did not differ between groups. In a smaller retrospective review, use of antimicrobial prophylaxis was associated with a reduced admission rate following intended outpatient ureteroscopy [45]. Ureteroscopic procedures without antimicrobial prophylaxis have been associated with UTI rates as high as 25% [46].

The European Association of Urology (EAU) guidelines on urologic infections differentiate between various ureteroscopic procedures [47]. For diagnostic ureteroscopy or distal ureteral calculi manipulation, the EAU guidelines do not recommend prophylactic antibiotics. However, for proximal or impacted stones antimicrobial prophylaxis is recommended. The EAU guidelines also incorporate risk factors such as size of stone, length of procedure, bleeding, and surgeon experience into the consideration for an antibiotic regimen.

Adherence to either the AUA or the EAU recommendations is poor, however, with the primary infraction being excessively prolonged course of antibiotics after ureteroscopy. A survey of members of the Endourological Society revealed that only 30% complied with the AUA recommendations about antimicrobial prophylaxis for ureteroscopy [48]. In a follow-up study, the survey was repeated 1 month after an email notification that summarized the AUA recommendations; the compliance rate improved to only 40% [49].

As noted above, hospital antibiotic policies and local drug resistant patterns are an important adjunct to published recommendations for choosing an antimicrobial prophylaxis regimen. At the authors' institution, oral fluoroquinolones had been used for years as the perioperative antimicrobial prophylaxis for ureteroscopy, but in 2008 the preferred agent was changed to oral TMP-SMX owing to an increase in resistance of local *E. coli* urinary isolates to fluoroquinolones. In 2011, the preferred agent was changed again, to intravenous cefazolin, since sensitivity patterns had altered to the point that resistance to both fluoroquinolones and TMP-SMX was greater than to cefazolin.

An additional recommendation that urologists performed ureteroscopy should consider is the 2007 update by the American Heart Association (AHA) of their guidelines on prevention of infective endocarditis [50]. It is no longer recommended to administer antimicrobial prophylaxis during genitourinary procedures solely for the reason to prevent infectious endocarditis. Of course, antimicrobial prophylaxis may still be indicated to prevent postoperative UTI.

Urologists performing ureteroscopy also have to manage externalized and internalized catheters and ureteral stents. Antimicrobial prophylaxis for removal of externalized urethral catheters is not necessary if the urine is known to be sterile [35]. In addition, antibiotics are not of benefit in patients with long-term indwelling catheters or undergoing intermittent catheterization [51, 52]. However, since bacterial colonization rates with indwelling catheters or intermittent catheterization is about 5% per day [53], antimicrobial therapy at time of catheter removal may be warranted in select patients, especially following urinary tract surgery [35]. In an RCT by Duclos et al. [54], patients undergoing a transurethral resection procedure who were given a preoperative dose of cefotaxime and a second dose 1 h prior to urethral catheter removal were noted to have a decreased incidence of bacteriuria compared to patients only given a preoperative dose. The report of Ramaswamy et al. [55] regarding ureteral stent removal has been referenced earlier; prolonged antibiotics prior to stent removal were no more effective than a single antibiotic dose at the time of stent removal.

In summary, surgical site infections contribute not only to patient morbidity but also to the economic burden in health care. Antimicrobial prophylaxis, along with the surgical scrub and surgical suite sterile environment, are important components in decreasing the risk of infection in postoperative patients. Available published recommendations on antimicrobial prophylaxis, along with awareness of hospital antibiotic policies and local drug resistant pattern, can assist the urologist in optimal care of the ureteroscopy patient.

References

1. Pearle MS, Calhoun EA, Curhan GC. Urologic diseases of America project: urolithiasis. J Urol. 2005; 173(3):848–57.
2. Scales CD, Krupski TL, et al. Practice variation in the surgical management of urinary lithiasis. J Urol. 2011;186(1):146–50.
3. Metwalli AB, Metwalli AR, Donovan JF. Informed consent and related legal issues in laparoscopic surgery. In: Smith's textbook of endourology (2nd ed). Edited by Smith AD, Badlani GH, Bagley DH, Clayman RV, Jordan GH, Kavoussi, B. Lee LR, Lingeman JE, Preminger GM, and Segura JW. Hamilton, Canada: BC Decker, pp. 57–59, 2007.
4. Paterick TJ, Carson GV. Medical informed consent: general considerations for physicians. Mayo Clin Proc. 2008;83(3):313–9.
5. Beauchamp TL. Informed consent: its history, meaning and present challenges. Camb Q Healthc Ethics. 2011;20:515–23.
6. Schloendorff v. Society of New York Hospital. In: NE. vol 105. NY: 1914. P92 LEXIS 1028.
7. Salgo v. Leland Stanford Jr University Board of Trustess, 317 2d 170 (1957)

8. American Medical Association Code of Medical Ethics: Informed Consent. American Medical Association Web Site. http://www.ama-assn.org/ama/pub/physician-resources/legal-topics/patient-physician-relationship-topics/informed-consent.page. Accessed 16 Nov 2011.
9. The Patient-Physician Relationship: Report of the Council on Ethical and Judicial Affairs (1-A-01). American Medical Association Web Site. http://www.ama-assn.org/ama/pub/about-ama/our-people/ama-councils/council-ethical-judicial-affairs/ceja-reports.page? Accessed 16 Nov 2011.
10. Canterbury v Spence, 464F. 2d 772 (DC Cir 1972)
11. Rostolsky BM. Practice makes perfect: experience-related information should fall within the purview of Pennsylvania's doctrine of informed consent. Duquesne Law Rev. 2002;40:543–60.
12. Boustani M, Peterson B, Hanson L, et al. Screening for dementia in primary care: a summary of the evidence for the U.S. Preventative Services Task Force. Ann Intern Med. 2003;138:927–37.
13. LaCaze v. Collier, 434 So. 2d 1039, 1048 (La. 1983)
14. Roussel v. Sharp, 569 So. Ed 67 (1990)
15. Cross v. Trapp, 170W. Va 459 (1982)
16. Cheese v. U.S., Not Reported in F. Supp. 2d (2005)
17. Cistrunk v. Oakwoood Heritage Hosp., Not Reported in N.W. 2d (2010)
18. Woods RK, Dellinger EP. Current guidelines for antibiotic prophylaxis of surgical wounds. Am Fam Phyisician. 1998;57(11):2731–40.
19. Bratzler D, Houck PM, Richards C, et al. Use of antimicrobial prophylaxis for major surgery: baseline results from the National Surgical Infection Prevention Project. Arch Surg. 2005;140:174.
20. Platt R. Guidelines for perioperative antibiotic prophylaxis. In: Abrutyn E, Goldmann DA, Scheckler WE, editors. Saunders infection control reference service. Philadelphia: W.B. Saunders; 1997. p. 229–34.
21. Hall MJ, DeFrances CJ, et al. National hospital discharge survey: 2007, number 29. Hyattsville, MD: Centers for Disease and Prevention; 2010.
22. Bratzler DW, Houck PM. Surgical Infection Prevention Guideline Writers Workgroup: antimicrobial prophylaxis for surgery: an advisory statement from the National Surgical Infection Prevention Project. Am J Surg. 2005;189:395.
23. National Nosocomial Infections Surveillance (NNIS) System. National Nosocomial Infections Surveillance (NNIS) System Report, data summary from January 1992 through June 2004, issued October 2004. Am J Infect Control. 2004;32(8):470–85.
24. Urban JA. Cost analysis of surgical site infections. Surg Infect. 2006;7:S1–19.
25. Mangram AJ, Horan TC, Pearson ML, et al. Guideline for prevention of surgical site infection. Infect Control Hosp Epidemiol. 1999;20(4):250–80.
26. Culver DH, Horan TC, Gaynes RP, et al. Surgical wound infection rates by wound class, operative procedure and patient risk index. Am J Med. 1991; 91(3B):S152–7.
27. Krizek TJ, Robson MC. Evolution of quantitative bacteriology in wound management. Am J Surg. 1975;130:579–84.
28. James RC, MacLeod CJ. Induction of staphylococcal infections in mice with small inocula introduced on sutures. Br J Exp Pathol. 1961;42:266–77.
29. Morrison DC, Ryan JL. Endotoxins and disease mechanisms. Annu Rev Med. 1987;38:417–32.
30. Bergamini TM, Corpus Jr RA, Brittian KR, et al. The natural history of bacterial biofilm graft infection. J Surg Res. 1994;56:393–6.
31. Wiley AM, Ha'eri GB. Routes of infection: a study of using "tracer particles" in the orthopedic operating room. Clin Orthop. 1979;139:150–5.
32. Letts RM, Doermer E. Conversation in the operating theatre as a cause of airborne bacterial contamination. J Bone Joint Surg Am. 1983;65:357–62.
33. Giamarellou H, Antoniadou A. Epidemiology, diagnosis and therapy of fungal infections in surgery. Infect Control Hosp Epidemiol. 1996;17(8):558–64.
34. Schaeffer AJ, Schaeffer EM. Infections of the urinary tract. In: Wein AJ, Kavoussi LR, Novak AC, Partin AW, Peters CA, editors. Campbell-Walsh urology, vol. 1. 10th ed. Philadelphia: Saunders-Elsevier; 2011. p. 257–326.
35. Wolf Jr JS, Bennett CJ, Dmochowski RR, et al. Best practice policy statement on urologic surgery antimicrobial prophylaxis. J Urol. 2008;179:1379–90.
36. Owens Jr RC, Donskey CJ, Gaynes RP, Loo VG, Muto CA. Antimicrobial-associated risk factors for *Clostridium difficile* infection. Clin Infect Dis. 2008;46:S19–31.
37. Bobo LD, Dubberke ER, Kollef M. Clostridium difficile in the ICU: the struggle continues. Chest. 2011;140(6):1643–53.
38. Monroe S, Polk R. Antimicrobial use and bacterial resistance. Curr Opin Microbiol. 2000;3(5):496–501.
39. Enzler MJ, Berbari E, Osmon DR. Antimicrobial prophylaxis in adults. Mayo Clin Proc. 2011;86(7): 686–701.
40. Christiano AP, Hollowell CM, Kim H, Kim J, et al. Double-blind randomized comparison of single-dose ciprofloxacin versus intravenous cefazolin in patients undergoing endourologic surgery. Urology. 2000;55:182–5.
41. Lukkarinen O, Hellström P, Leppilahti M, Kontturi M, Tammela T. Antimicrobial prophylaxis in patients with urinary retention undergoing transurethral prostatectomy. Ann Chir Gynaecol. 1997;86:239.
42. Knopf HJ, Graff JH, Schulze H. Perioperative antibiotic prophylaxis in ureteroscopic stone removal. Eur Urol. 2003;44:115–8.
43. Fourcade RO. Antibiotic prophylaxis with cefotaxime in endoscopic extraction of upper urinary tract stones: a randomized study. The Cefotaxime Cooperative Group. J Antimicrob Chemother. 1990;26(Suppl A):77–83.
44. Aghamir SMK, Hamidi M, Salavati A, Mohammadi A, Farahmand H, Meysamie AP, Ghorbani B. Is antibiotic prophylaxis necessary in patients undergoing ureterolithotripsy? Acta Med Iran. 2011;49:513–6.

45. Taylor AL, Oakley N, Das S, Parys BT. Day-case ureteroscopy: an observational study. BJU Int. 2002;89:181–5.
46. Grabe M. Controversies in antimicrobial prophylaxis in urology. Int J Antimicrob Agents. 2004;23:S17–23.
47. European Association of Urology. Grabe M, Bishop MC, Bjerklund-Johansen TE, Botto H, et al. Guidelines on urological infections. European Guidelines online. Accessed 10 Jan 2012.
48. Kurtz M, Eisner B. Antibiotic use after routine ureteroscopic stone treatment (abstract 1448). J Urol. 2010;182(Suppl):e558.
49. Eisner B, Kurtz M, Wolf Jr JS. Antibiotic prescription and poor compliance with AUA Best Practice Statement (abstract 2154). J Urol. 2011; 185(Suppl):e862.
50. Wilson W, Taubert KA, Gewitz M, Lockhart PB, Baddour LM, Levison M, et al. Prevention of infective endocarditis. Guidelines form the American Heart Association. A Guideline From the American Heart Association Rheumatic Fever, Endocarditis and Kawasaki Disease Committee on Cardiovascular Disease in the Young and the Council on Clinical Cardiology, Council on Cardiovascular Surgery and Anesthesia, and the Quality of Care and Outcomes Research Interdisciplinary Working Group. Circulation. 2007;116:1736–54.
51. Niel-Weise BS, Van den Broek PJ. Urinary catheter policies for long-term bladder drainage. Cochrane Database Syst Rev 2005;(1):DC004201.
52. Clarke SA, Samuel M, Bobby SA. Are prophylatic antimicrobial necessary with clean intermittent catheterization? A randomized controlled trial. J Pediatr Surg. 2005;40:568.
53. Sedor J, Mulholland SG. Hospital-acquired urinary tract infections associated with the indwelling catheter. Urol Clin North Am. 1999;26:821.
54. Duclos JM, Larrouturou P, Sarkis P. Timing of antimicrobial prophylaxis with cefotaxime for prostatic resection: better in the operative period or at urethral catheter removal? Am J Surg. 1992;164:21S.
55. Ramaswamy K, Ojas S. Antibiotic prophylaxis after uncomplicated ureteroscopic stone treatment: is there a difference? J Endourol. 2011;26(2):122–5.

Ureteroscopy: Patient Positioning and Room Setup

19

Joseph A. Graversen, Debra Morrison, Jane Cho, Adam Kaplan, Corollos Abdelshehid, Achim Lusch, Michael A. Liss, and Jaime Landman

Introduction

Proper room setup is a key component to the successful outcome of any surgical procedure. This is especially true of ureteroscopic procedures as these procedures are technology intensive and space is at a premium. A poorly positioned back table or piece of equipment can not only extend operative times, but can also potentially endanger the patient, result in damage to expensive equipment, and can cause significant discomfort and inconvenience for the surgeon. Furthermore, due to the nature and size of the equipment utilized during ureteroscopy, it is important that the room is appropriately prepared prior to the patient entering the room. Even minor repositioning of the various elements involved can be difficult and time consuming once the patient is under anesthesia. Equally important, if not more so, is correct patient positioning. The ability for the surgeon to access structures of interest is solely dependent on patient positioning. Concomitantly, it is the surgeon's responsibility to reduce or eliminate the risk of position-related injuries. Any procedure that results in injury to the patient due to poor positioning should be deemed unsuccessful. In this chapter we discuss surgical suite ergonomics, room setup, X-ray positioning and safety, and choice of irrigant. We also discuss appropriate patient positioning in the dorsolithotomy and prone positions as well as associated complications.

J.A. Graversen, M.D. • J. Cho, M.D. • A. Kaplan, M.D.
C. Abdelshehid, M.D. • A. Lusch, M.D.
M.A. Liss, M.D. • J. Landman, M.D. (✉)
Department of Urology, University of California,
333 City Blvd West, Suite 2100, Irvine, CA 92868, USA
e-mail: landmanj@uci.edu

D. Morrison
Department of Anesthesiology, University of California,
Irvine, CA, USA

Room Setup

Endoscopic Suite Ergonomics

The goal of surgical ergonomics is to design the surgical suite and its instruments in such a manner as to optimize patient outcomes, to improve efficiency, to minimize the discomfort of the physicians and surgical staff, and to reduce their potential for injury [1]. While there is no question that newer endoscopic and surgical techniques are beneficial to the patient, the same techniques create technical and ergonomic challenges for the surgeon and operating room staff. Unfortunately, the cause and effect of poor ergonomics in the endoscopy suite are poorly characterized [2]. Several studies have demonstrated that the open surgeon suffers from less neck, back, and shoulder pain compared to the laparoscopic surgeon, but few have evaluated surgeon comfort in the endoscopic suite [2–5]. Certainly, surgeon experience and level of training affect comfort, but the very nature of minimally invasive and endoscopic

M. Monga (ed.), *Ureteroscopy: Indications, Instrumentation & Technique*, Current Clinical Urology,
DOI 10.1007/978-1-62703-206-3_19, © Springer Science+Business Media New York 2013

surgery along with the instruments utilized, patient positioning, and the equipment necessary to safely and efficiently complete the case are intrinsically detrimental to the surgeon and surgical staff [2–6].

The importance of maximizing endoscopic ergonomics is not only for the benefit of the surgeon but also for the patient. From minimally invasive surgery data it is known that surgeons and OR staff have reported such ill effects as neuropraxias, tremors, muscle and joint pain, eye fatigue, and generalized body fatigue [2–6]. Physical discomfort by the surgeon can potentially affect surgeon performance. In one report, surgeon fatigue was directly linked to surgical outcome [7]. Until recently, surgical suites were ill suited for endoscopic surgery with ergonomics largely ignored [1, 6, 8]. A recent boon in ergonomic awareness has led to intelligent room layouts and new innovations. For example, the use of ceiling hung monitors that can be easily positioned with interchangeable images has been introduced to great effect in both endoscopic and laparoscopic procedures. The routine use of large ceiling hung booms has facilitated the movement of commonly used equipment sets such as light sources and energy generators. More recently, the introduction of Gelmat floor pads to the endoscopic suite has been demonstrated to reduce surgeon discomfort and fatigue [9, 10]. When present, appropriate ergonomics in the endoscopy suite generally goes unnoticed; when absent, both the surgeon and the patient suffer. As such, it is paramount that ergonomics be considered for every case prior to the start of the case.

Room Setup

Setting up the operating room for optimal ureteroscopy is a team effort and should be an exercise in communication among surgeons and anesthesiologist, operating room staff, and the instrument processing team. It requires staff familiarity with the equipment, their functions and how to troubleshoot the basic problems encountered. This includes everything from handling the delicate ureteroscopic instruments to operating the often-complicated audiovisual equipment. Proper setup and attention to detail can help prevent complications and frustration during the procedure. Creation of a flawless and efficient routine for each type of case is a team-building exercise and sets the stage for a successful and satisfying operation. Similarly, the instrument processing staff has the equally important role of appropriately sterilizing, storing, and transporting equipment. A large part of endoscope durability and breakdown relies on their careful handling of the equipment. Furthermore, the efficient setup of the operating room prior to the start of the case largely depends on the appropriate storage of the various pieces of equipment. An open dialogue will ensure that all of the elements necessary to perform any given endoscopic case are readily accessible, properly sterilized, and appropriately stored, thereby obviating frustration and significant delays.

The room setup and positioning of each of the basic elements is shown in Fig. 19.1. For simplicity, the designation of laterality refers to the patient's right and left side. The operating table must be designed for GU imaging, with a springboard or removable footrest. The table must also be capable of supporting stirrups and, in the case of prone ureteroscopy, spreader bars.

The anesthesia setup is at the head of the bed. Our operating rooms all have a standard anesthesia setup. The anesthesia machine is typically on the patient's right side, with the left side of the machine near the head of the patient. There is a boom positioned just behind the anesthesia machine and all anesthesia power cords are plugged into the boom, as well as the power cord to the urology fluid warming device, which is positioned on a pole beside the anesthesia machine. There is a permanent cabinet on the wall behind the anesthesiologist, containing fluids, pumps, and special monitors. The anesthesia cart is to the right of the cabinet. There are IV poles at each side of the patient, at the level of the shoulders or as close to the anesthesia machine as possible. The Bair Hugger (Arizant Healthcare, Inc., Prairie, MN) warming device (an upper body Bair Hugger is used for ureteroscopy cases) is also at the right side of the patient near the head

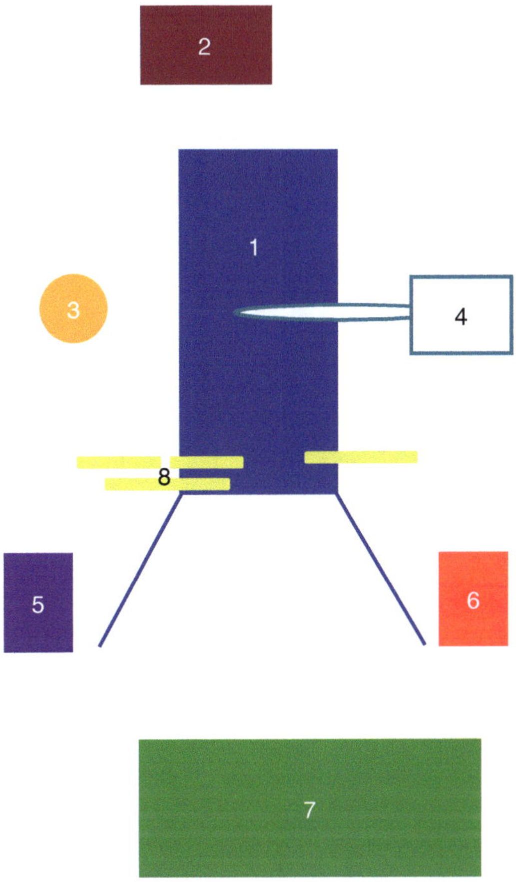

Fig. 19.1 Operating Room Setup Schematic: (1) GU imaging capable operating table with stirrups attached, (2) Anesthesia equipment, (3) IV pole with 4 hooks, (4) Fluoroscope, (5) Laser, (6) Endoscopy tower or boom, (7) Table with ureteroscopy and cystoscopy equipment, (8) Video screens

of the bed. There is room for a chair behind the drapes, but the anesthesiologist often stands to facilitate communication during critical periods of the case. The anesthesiologist can view at least one of the video monitors in order to be aware of the progress and challenges of the case. There is sufficient space on the left side of the patient to move a bed in and out of the room even with the C-arm fluoroscope in the room, although the endoscopic boom arm is moved into final position after the patient is asleep.

An endoscopic video cart or boom arm is positioned at the lower left of the table. The C-arm fluoroscope will enter often from the left side of the patient. An adjustable IV pole with 4 hooks and either a pressure bag or a pressure machine such as the Level 1® Rapid Infuser (SIMS Level 1®, Inc., Rockland, MA) should be at the upper right (Fig. 19.2). A laser setup (if used) is placed at the lower right. The laser fiber courses from the generator, over the patient's draped lower right leg, where a non-penetrating towel clamp is used to create a "canal" through which the fiber passes. In doing so, the fiber is secured to the drape without actually clamping the fiber itself (Fig. 19.3). When not in use, the fiber can be coiled, and placed onto the patient's right lower leg. A damp blue towel is placed on top of the coiled fiber to prevent the fiber from unraveling or falling to the floor. The laser generator is positioned near to the patient such that it is impossible to pass between the patient and the laser. In this way, we are able to avoid inadvertent internal avulsion of the laser into the ureteroscope by pulling of the fiber at this site.

Video screens must be positioned in clear view of the surgeon but not interfering with the fluoroscope (Figs. 19.2 and 19.4). Modern fluoroscope screens are generally of higher resolution than the typical flat screens utilized in minimally invasive suites. Occasionally when a higher resolution is necessary to complete a surgical task, we utilize the fluoroscope screen to provide an improved image. The use of booms or adjustable arms is suggested as they support the movement of a large number of energy generators, light sources, and camera hook-ups from one part of the room to another with relative ease. However, they are also a common source of "head bumping" by the operating room staff during the case, especially once the lights in the room are dimmed and the surgery is underway. The endoscopic suites are equipped with green lights. These lights are bright enough to provide adequate vision during the case, but the green color does not interfere with the surgeon's ability to clearly see the various monitors (Fig. 19.4).

A back table setup at the foot of the bed should include the ureteroscopy and cystoscopy tray. The table should be large enough to support a large array of endoscopes and supporting accessories while remaining uncluttered and well

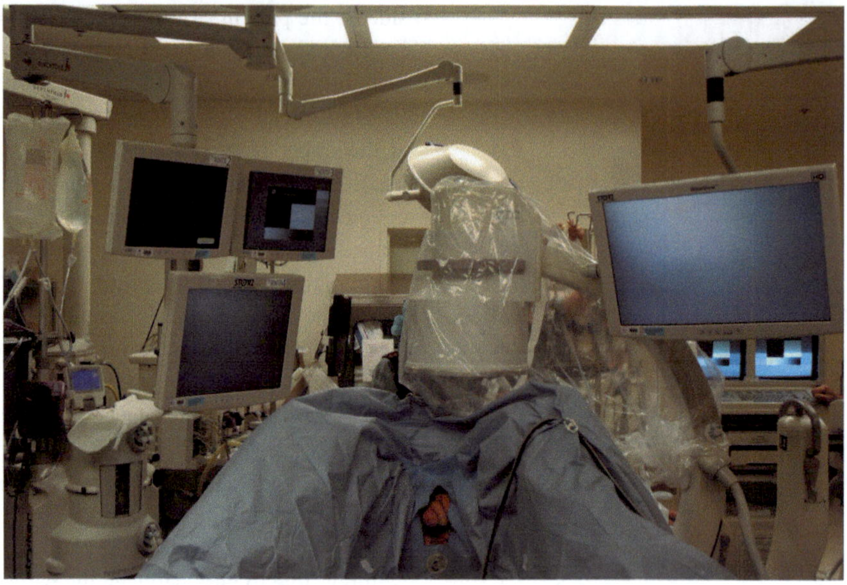

Fig. 19.2 Operating room setup. Video monitors are readily viewable and interchangeable, the C-arm is positioned from the lefts side of the patient, and the fluid and pressure bags are on the right

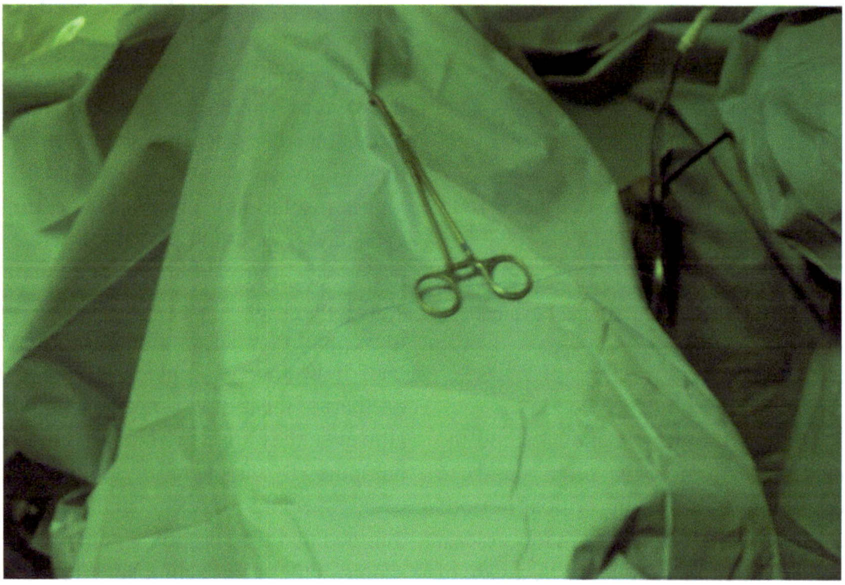

Fig. 19.3 The laser is positioned to the patient's right near the foot of the bed and the fiber is secured to the drapes by passing it through a "canal" created with a non-penetrating clamp

organized (Fig. 19.5). A large back table will also prevent sterile items from inadvertently falling or otherwise becoming contaminated as well as damage to the more sensitive pieces of equipment such as the flexible ureteroscope and cystoscope (Fig. 19.6). X-ray gowns with thyroid shields must be available for all personnel (Fig. 19.7).

Before beginning the procedure, a proper pre-check of the instruments should be performed. The lens and camera should be wiped dry,

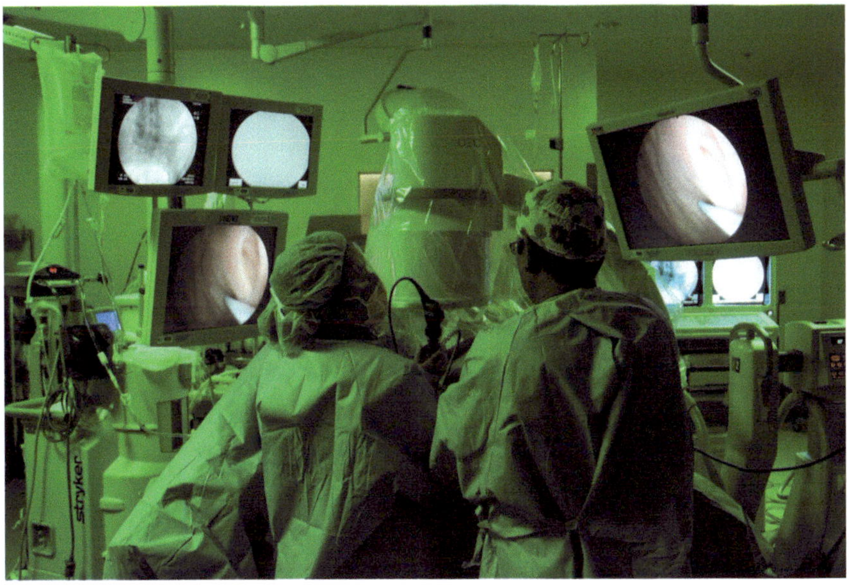

Fig. 19.4 The video screens are preferably ceiling hung so as to be easily adjustable. They are positioned in such a manner as to not interfere with the C-arm but are easily viewable by the surgeon and the surgical assistants

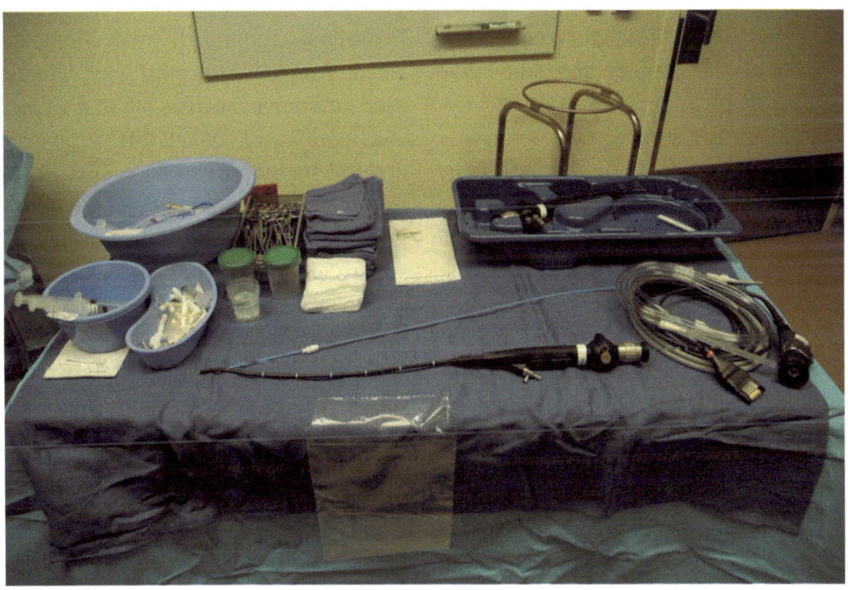

Fig. 19.5 A large, well-organized back table significantly improves efficiency and reduces the risk of inadvertent damage and contamination to the various pieces of equipment

focused, and appropriately white balanced (for fiberoptic systems). It is our preference that the zoom be adjusted so that the "ring" around the image is no longer visible. Zooming beyond this point can exacerbate the "screen door" effect commonly seen with fiber-optic ureteroscopes. Similarly, zooming in less typically creates an image that is too small. Digital ureteroscopes are different in that they do not require white balancing and there is a single hook-up that

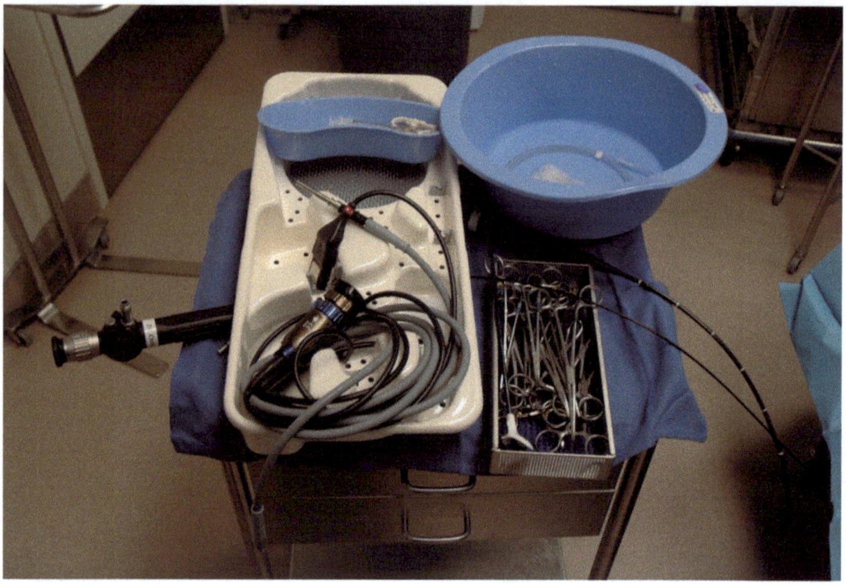

Fig. 19.6 Too small a back table not only risks contamination of the equipment but also places the expensive endoscopes, cameras, and light cords at risk for damage

provides the image and the light source. The proper function of the camera and adjunctive instruments (graspers, biopsy forceps, etc.) is essential. All instruments must be kept neatly arranged and readily available on the back table (Fig. 19.5).

The back table must be properly arranged with gowns and gloves for each surgeon, a ureteroscopy drape designed for stirrups with a collection bag for used irrigant, 12 foot suctioning tubing to be attached to the drape, Y-connecting tubing for irrigation, a camera with a cable and light cord, a sterile fluoroscopy drape, as well as gauze sponges, 2 towel clamps, 2 Kelly clamps, a Foley catheter, and a water based lubricant. A 16 Fr flexible and 22 Fr rigid cystoscope should be available, with an Albarran bridge and 2 gray nipples, and 2 Touey-Boursch or Sureseal adaptors. A large basin with sterile water (1 L) can be used to hold access wires and stents. A smaller basin should be arranged with 100 mL of a mix of 50% Hypaque (70 mL) with sterile water (30 mL), along with a 10 mL and a 20 mL syringe. Commonly used access wires can be opened, including (based on preference) a 0.035 hydrophilic Terumo glidewire, Bentson guidewire and an Amplatz Superstiff wire. Other commonly used equipment such as a 5 or 6 Fr ureteral catheter, a preferred coaxial dilator, an access sheath, ureteral balloon dilator, or dual lumen catheter should be in the room but remain unopened until just prior to use. The table should also include a semirigid ureteroscope or flexible ureteroscope of choice.

Prior to each case it is our practice to discuss with the operating room staff what equipment should be opened and placed on the back table and what equipment should be readily available in the room but unopened. The surgeon should be aware of the general cost of the equipment (capital and disposables) so as to minimize cost while optimizing outcome. While it is less expensive to having some equipment in the room but not "open," there is also a cost of manpower associated with pulling the equipment and putting it away. Each surgeon should thoughtfully review their equipment needs and work with their OR staff to assure the patient care is optimized with the least amount of surgical waste possible.

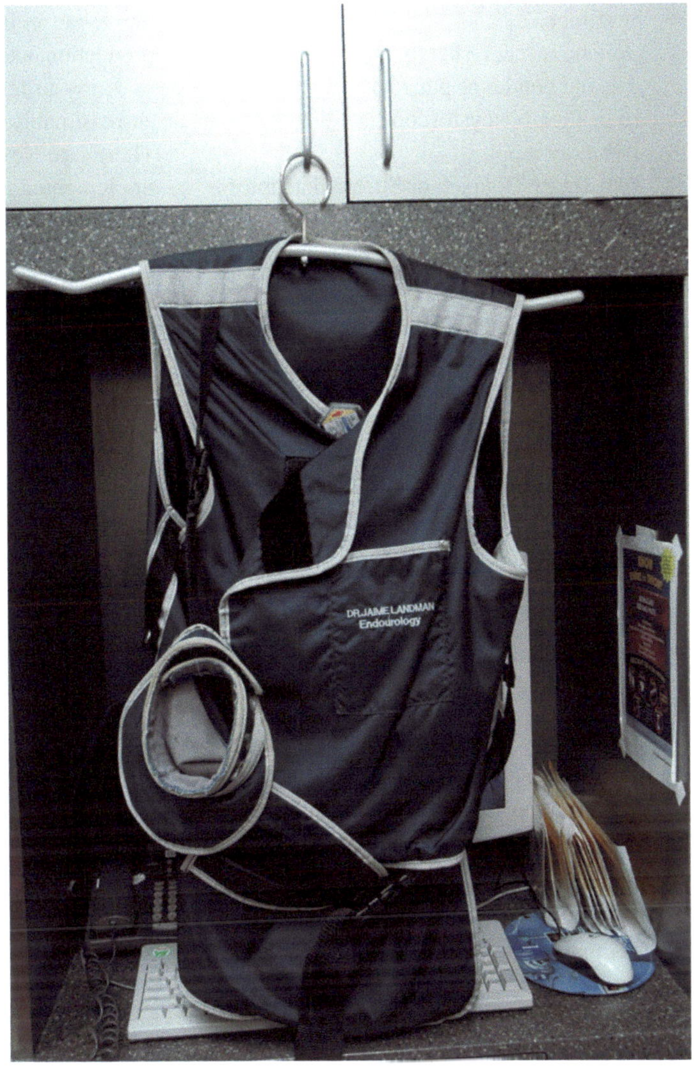

Fig. 19.7 Radiation protection, including thyroid shield should be made available for all staff in the surgical suite. Note that the equipment is stored on a hangar that is specifically designed to hold the lead apron. This is important as it reduces cracking and breaking which reduces the radiation blocking capability of the shield

Typically, the following pieces of equipment are routinely used in every case and should be opened and on the back table:

1. Gowns and gloves for all members of the surgical team.
2. Ureteroscopy drape with collection bag (i.e., Lingeman drape).
3. 12 ft suctioning tubing for drape.
4. Y irrigation tubing.
5. Light cable.
6. Camera.
7. Gauze sponges for white balance.
8. Large basin with sterile water (1 L).
9. Small basin containing 50% Hypaque (70 mL) + 30 mL sterile water (100 mL total).
10. Guidewires (0.035 Terumo glidewire, Bentson Guidewire, Amplatz Superstiff wire).
11. 10 and 20 mL syringes for contrast injection in the small basin.
12. 5 or 6 Fr open ended ureteral catheter with adaptor.
13. 12 Fr Foley catheter.
14. Two towel clamps.
15. Two Kelly clamps.

16. Surgilube.
17. Ureteral access sheeth (size dependant on size and gender of patient).
18. 16 Fr Flexible cystoscope.
19. Two gray nipples.
20. Two Touey-Boursch or Sureseal adaptors.
21. Semirigid or flexible ureteroscope (depending on case and surgeon preference).
22. Surgical towels ×4.
23. Sterile fluorscopy drape.

Equipment typically available in the room but not opened include:

1. 22 Fr Rigid cystoscope with 30° and 70° lenses.
2. Albarrans bridge.
3. Selection of ureteral stone baskets.
4. Selection of laser fibers 200–1,000 μm.
5. Ureteral balloon dilator.

The room itself should have the following basic pieces of equipment

1. GU imaging ready table (spring board vs. lowering foot).
2. Stirrups.
3. X-ray gowns.
4. Adjustable IV pole with 4 hooks and pressure bags.
5. Endoscopic video cart or arm.
6. Video camera.
7. C-arm fluoroscope.
8. Multiple 3 L bags warm saline.
9. Anesthesia machine.
10. Anesthesia cart.
11. Appropriate irrigant fluids plus any medications specific to the procedure, including antibiotics, mannitol, lasix, IV blue contrast of choice, glucagon, etc.
12. Laser.
13. One table setup (Cysto and Ureteroscopy instruments).

X-Ray Setup

Radiography in ureteroscopy is critically important for instrument guidance, stone or tumor localization, and positioning of guidewires and catheters. The endourologist must be well acquainted with the X-ray equipment, basic principles of X-ray production, and radiation safety.

X-ray usage should comply with the "as low as reasonably achievable" (ALARA) approach. There are several key principles that can be implemented to help achieve this: decrease usage time, maximize user distance from the source, and provide adequate shielding. Usage of spot fluoroscopy instead of continuous imaging for smaller steps of the procedure can dramatically decrease radiation exposure. Increasing operator distance from the radiation source decreases X-ray exposure exponentially (doubling distance from the fluoroscope decreases X-ray exposure by one-fourth). As a rule of thumb, at 12 ft, away, X-ray exposure is immeasurable. Effective shielding with lead aprons and thyroid collars should be required of all staff (Fig. 19.7). Lead aprons should have an equivalent lead thickness of 0.5 mm to adequately attenuate the radiation. The lead aprons should be checked regularly for cracks or breaks in the radiation barrier. Additionally, every staff member exposed to ionizing radiation should be provided with badges that are closely monitored to reduce the risk of excessive exposure.

The image intensifier of a fluoroscope is lead lined to minimize scatter. The preferred configuration to minimize leakage and scatter radiation from both the X-ray and the patient is to place the image intensifier *above the table.*

Use of modern digital fluoroscopy equipment can aid in radiation reduction. Images can be manipulated and enhanced, obviating the need for retakes. Pulsed fluoroscopy simply means that the output of the X-ray machine is coupled with the video screen refresh rate (30 times per second), allowing for radiation reduction without compromising resolution. Reducing the pulse rate even further, to frame rates as low as four frames per second have been associated with a further reduction in radiation exposure with no effect on stone-free rates [11]. To help minimize the radiation exposure, be sure to alert all members of the team when the X-ray is active. X-ray badges should be required by the hospital or surgical facility for monthly dosimetry reports.

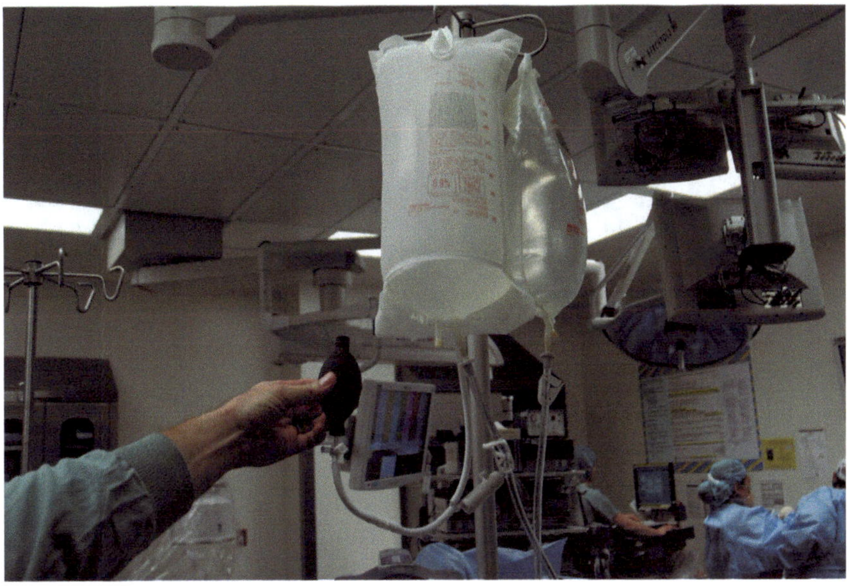

Fig. 19.8 A simple yet effective method of pressurizing the irrigant is with a 3 L pressure bag. The pressure bag provides consistent pressure throughout the case, however it requires careful vigilance by the surgeon and OR staff to ensure that the pressure is maintained

Choice of Irrigant

The choice of irrigant is dependent on the type of procedure to be performed [12]. For most stone and endopyelotomy procedures in which a laser or electrohydraulic lithotripter is to be used, normal saline (0.9% NaCl) is the preferred irrigant. For procedures in which monopolar current is used (resection of renal tumors, or fulguration of a renal cyst or calicyceal diverticulum) the irrigant must be changed to glycine or water. Use of saline with monopolar instruments will dissipate the current, rendering the instrument ineffective and creating the potential for thermal injury to surrounding structures.

It is important to warm the irrigant to body temperature to promote cardiovascular stability and prevent hypothermia and postoperative shivers. The ideal warming system maintains a consistent temperature as the irrigant leaves the bag via the Y-connecting tubing. Warming cabinets can be inconsistent in their temperature.

The irrigant should be hung on a height-adjustable pole with 4 hooks, with 2-way or 4-way Y-connecting tubing. During ureterscopic procedures, the irrigant can be pressurized to 100–250 mmHg. There are two primary mechanisms of pressurizing irrigant. The simplest and least expensive is application of a simple pressure bag. This simple device typically includes a pressure gauge and is designed to hold the 3 L bags typically utilized in ureteroscopy (Figs. 19.8 and 19.9). Contrarily, pressurized rapid transfusion systems such as the Level 1® not only provide excellent pressure production and accurate monitoring but also have the capability to warm the irrigant thereby minimizing the risk of hypothermia. Regardless of the system utilized by the surgeon, it is important that the surgeon optimize visualization by increasing the flow, and therefore the bag pressure, with the understanding that increasing the flow at the tip of the scope also increases the pressure that is generated. Passing an accessory device such as a laser fiber or a basket through the channel decreases the effective channel diameter with the resulting effect of a flow reduction. Often times, pulling the instrument back or removing it all together can significantly improve flow. It is the responsibility of the surgeon to ensure that the lowest pressure that provides optimal flow is utilized at all times.

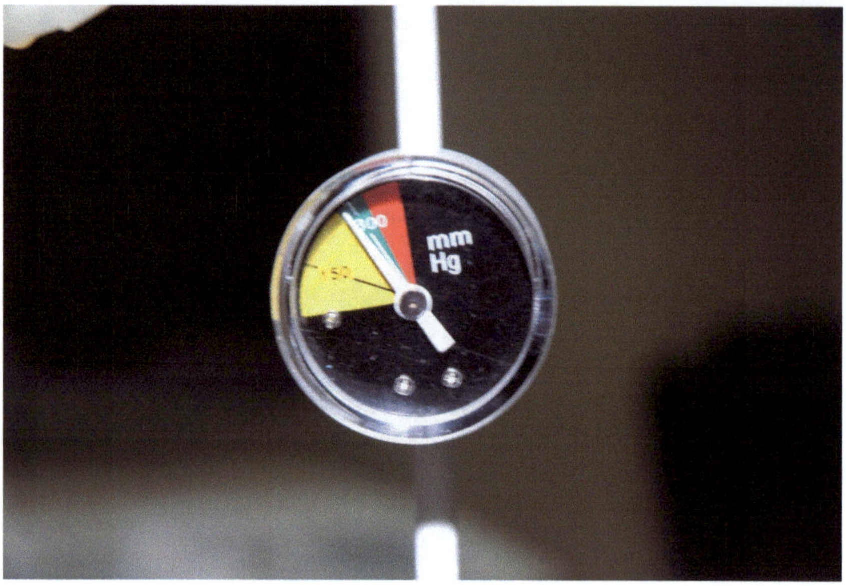

Fig. 19.9 Pressure bags typically come with a pressure gauge that allows accurate monitoring of the pressure throughout the surgery. Typically pressures are maintained between 100 and 250 mmHg

Patient Positioning

Goals of Positioning

There are currently two standard positions utilized during ureteroscopy: dorsolithotomy and prone. There are limitations and advantages to both positions, which will be covered in greater detail elsewhere in this chapter. Prior to discussing the individual positions it is important to consider the goal of surgical positioning. As in all surgery, patient positioning should optimize the ability to successfully complete the intended procedure while concomitantly minimizing the risk of positional injury. As it pertains to ureteroscopy, the important aspects of positioning include

1. Access to the urethra: In the rare case of urinary diversion this is not mandatory, but otherwise, retrograde ureteroscopy is performed per urethra.
2. Maintenance of mobility: Especially during rigid ureteroscopy or proximal ureteroscopy, the surgeon's ability to manipulate the endoscope extracorporeally is paramount to a swift and successful outcome.
3. Fluoroscopic Imaging: The details of fluoroscope use are discussed elsewhere, but the ability to completely visualize the bladder, and the kidneys and ureters bilaterally is important.
4. Access to instrumentation: Ureteroscopy often incorporates a multitude of small and often fragile devices that are passed on and off the back table in rapid succession. In routine and complex cases alike, the inability to easily give and receive these devices could result in surgical delay, loss of ureteral access, and dropped or damaged equipment.
5. Visualization: The ability to comfortable manipulate the endoscope while simultaneously viewing the monitors is key. Modern minimally invasive suites have often utilize multiple, high definition ceiling hung monitors that can be switched from the fluoroscopic view to views from 1 or more cameras. This is especially advantageous during endoscopic assisted percutaneous access where multiple cameras along with fluoroscopic imaging are used simultaneously.

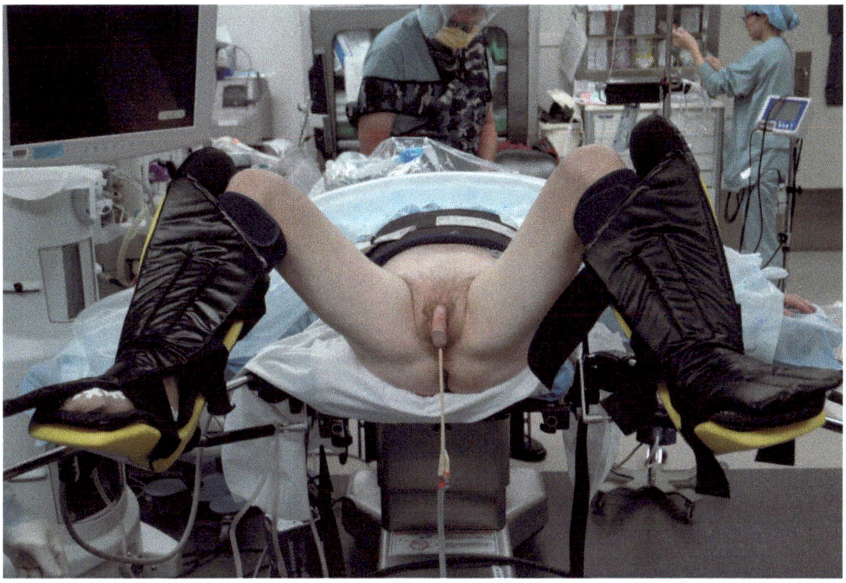

Fig. 19.10 When appropriately positioned, the hip and knee joints are flexed approximately 90 ° and the great toe and ipsilateral knee are aligned with the contralateral shoulder. The lower legs are well padded and secured snugly

Dorsolithotomy Position

The use of the dorsolithotomy position is considered standard for routine ureteroscopy. It is important that the operating room bed utilized in this position have a removable footrest. This allows the fluoroscope to freely move superiorly and inferiorly, thereby allowing complete visualization of the kidneys, ureters, and bladder. Beds that only break at the foot significantly limit the superior movement of the fluoroscope and should be reserved only for cystoscopy cases in which fluoroscopy is not utilized. If the bed is capable of sliding, then the table top should be positioned as inferiorly as safely possible. The bed itself must be radiolucent to allow for complete visualization above the level of the pelvis.

Once comfortably under anesthesia, the patient is brought down near the foot of the bed such that the patient's coccyx is at the edge of the springboard. Beds with a pelvic cutout are advantageous as they provide improved pelvic support laterally, allow for maximal genital exposure/mobility, and provide a space for the cystoscopic fluid collection pouch. The patient's legs are then simultaneously placed into padded stirrups. It is our preference to use Allen® Yellowfin® Stirrups (Acton, MA) since they are easy to use, provide well-padded support, secure the leg firmly, and provide a significant range of motion. When positioned appropriately, the hip and knee joints are flexed at approximately 90 ° and the great toe of each leg is in a straight line with the ipsilateral knee and the contralateral shoulder. The legs should be secured into place with additional padding placed as necessary (Fig. 19.10).

All of our patients, whether in the prone or dorsolithotomy position have sequential compression devices placed in the preoperative holding area. Sequential compression devices have been demonstrated to reduce the risk of both proximal and calf deep venous thrombosis, and in some series were equivocal or outperformed chemical prophylaxis [13–15]. Furthermore, the table upon which ureteroscopy is to be performed should be well padded, especially over the bony prominences, in order to prevent neural injury or prolonged muscle compression which can lead to rhabdomyolysis.

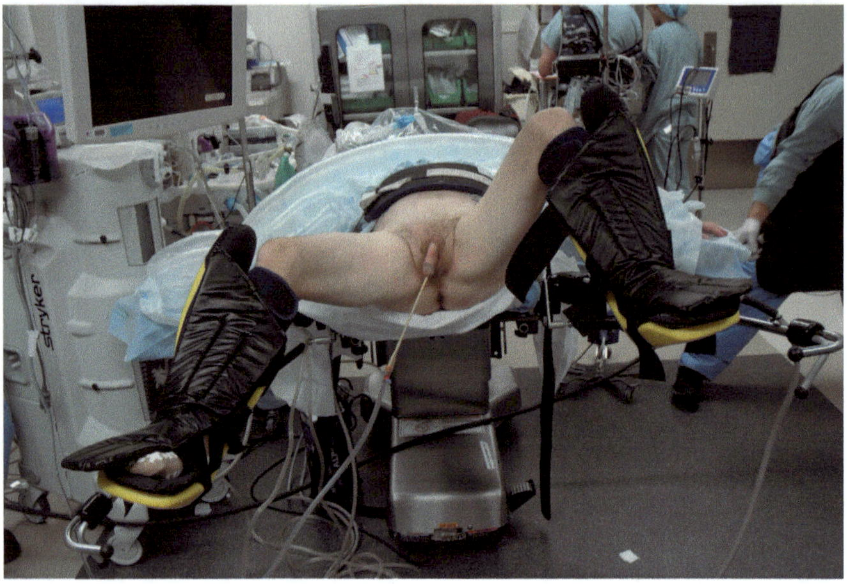

Fig. 19.11 In the extended leg dorsolithotomy position, the leg ipsilateral to the stone is straightened and slightly abducted compared to the contralateral leg. This puts the ipsilateral psoas on stretch and improves access to the mid and proximal ureter by a rigid ureteroscope

When contemplating semirigid ureteroscopy, a modified extended leg dorsolithotomy (ELDL) position should be considered. In the ELDL, the leg ipsilateral to the stone is extended, in line with the patient's body, and slightly abducted (Fig. 19.11). In this position, the psoas muscle is stretched making the distal and mid-ureter more accessible. When compared to rigid ureteroscopy in the standard dorsolithotomy, the ELDL has been associated with shorter operative times while maintaining equivalent stone-free rates [16].

Additional padding should be placed at the elbow and wrist, and the arms are then subsequently tucked into draw sheets. Leaving the arms on arm boards often restricts the fluoroscope superiorly and should be avoided. It is critical to maintain the arms in a position slightly anterior to the midline of the body in the coronal plane in order to avoid stretch on and consequent injury to the brachial plexus. This is potentially challenging in obese patients and attention should be paid to appropriately supporting the arms with additional padding. In some instances, arm boards may be necessary to widen the surface of the table to provide the appropriate support. When tucking the arms, it is important to exclude any intravenous lines from the draw sheet in order to maintain easy access by the anesthesia team and to make sure no lines are occluded. The patient's head should rest on a gel-foam donut and should be moved gently from side to side during the case to minimize prolonged compression and ischemia to the scalp.

The genitals are then prepped with either betadine- or chlorohexadine-based prep kits. Alcohol-based preps should be avoided as they cause significant irritation to the mucosal membranes of the uncircumcised penis, vagina, and urethra. The area of prep should include the genitals, including the introitus of the vagina, perineum, inner thigh, and anterior abdomen to just below the level of the umbilicus. It is our preference to drape the patient first with blue towels, followed by leggings, and finally with a Lingeman drape (or similar product). A sterile sleeve is then placed over the C-arm, and it is advanced into the desired position. The monitors are then over the patient's pelvis (ideal) or to the left or the right of the patient. Finally, irrigation tubing, lighting cords, and camera cables are draped over the patient's legs toward the boom that houses their respective generators. They are then tightly anchored to the drapes in a manner similar to that of the laser fiber. Doing so prevents the diminution of the surgeon's sense of touch caused by the weight of the cords pulling on the instruments (Fig. 19.2).

Prone Position

Ureteroscopy in the prone position is mainly utilized during retrograde percutaneous access, although it can certainly be used as the main approach for treatment. The use of retrograde percutaneous access was first introduced in the early 1980s by two independently published reports [17, 18]. The original technique of retrograde percutaneous access involved an inside-out puncture from the kidney to the skin surface which often resulted in long, serpiginous tracts. In 1995, Grasso and colleagues were the first to describe ureteroscopic guidance for percutaneous access when they utilized the method as a salvage technique [19]. The ability to use a flexible ureteroscope for access guidance was primarily a result of an evolution in flexible endoscope technology that allowed for reliable access to each calyx of the kidney [20]. In the early 2000s, studies began to emerge that the retrograde placement of ureteral access sheaths as an adjunct to PCNL significantly improved flow and lowered intra-renal pressure [21, 22]. In 2006, Khan and colleagues described their refinement of the endoscopic guided percutaneous access technique whereby a ureteral access sheath is deployed and ureteroscopy is utilized from the outset to guide percutaneous tract establishment [23]. Currently, this is the method by which the University of California, Irvine team gains access for PCNL procedures. In a retrospective review of our data there was a reduction in blood loss and blood transfusion rates, with no detrimental affect on stone-free rates compared to fluoroscopic access alone [20, 23].

As it pertains to the room setup, the various pieces of equipment are arranged in the same manner as in the dorsolithotomy position. Similarly, the table utilized is a radiolucent, slide-top table with a pelvic cutout and removable footrest. The only modification is that in lieu of stirrups, spreader bars are utilized to support the legs in an abducted position. The knees are padded with additional egg crate foam and secured to the upper part of the spreader bar with gauze wrapping. In order to reduce the risk of sciatic nerve over-extension, the lower legs are slightly flexed at the knees and the ankles supported with pillows. The lower legs are then similarly secured to the spreader bars with a gauze wrapping. The legs are abducted to allow free access to the vagina or penis. The patient is then prepped and draped in standard fashion as previously described.

The patient's upper body should be supported on chest rolls to allow excursion during respiration and the head should be in a neutral position. We use a Prone View device to support the head and minimize pressure to the eyes and face. The eyes are lubricated and taped with porous tape to prevent the skin from becoming damp and macerated and likely to tear with any traction during movement or tape removal. The endotracheal tube is tied rather than or in addition to being taped. No Opsite/Tegaderm is used on the face because it is occlusive, not porous, and can cause maceration. The Prone View device includes a mirror that allows the anesthesiologist to check the face. A short accordion connector is inserted between the endotracheal tube and the circuit to ease the transit of the circuit out the side of the prone view to prevent accidental disconnection. The arms are placed on arm boards at the level of the head, anterior to the midline of the body in the coronal plane, or slightly lower than the top of the table, with elbows slightly bent and wrists supported.

Complications of Positioning

Although injuries and complications associated with patient positioning are rare, they can have devastating consequences. Therefore, optimal positioning is a critical step in any urologic procedure as these complications are often preventable.

Dorsolithotomy

The risk of neuropraxia during lithotomy positioning is a well-documented complication. Thirty-eight percent of all urology claims during the past 20 years reported by the American Society of Anesthesiologists Closed Claims Project database were for nerve injuries [24]. The injury usually occurs when a peripheral nerve is stretched or compressed at the time of surgery. With these nerve injuries, varying degrees of compression lead to varying degrees of ischemia. The injury can be as mild as temporary conduction block lasting only a few minutes to as severe as Wallerian degeneration and complete axonal loss [25].

Specific nerves that may be affected during lithotomy positioning include the peroneal nerve and the saphenous nerve. The peroneal nerve is derived from the dorsal branches of the fourth and fifth lumbar spinal nerves and the first and second sacral nerves. It descends obliquely on the lateral aspect of the popliteal fossa before coursing around the lateral aspect of the head of the fibula. At this point it divides into superficial and deep branches. The superficial peroneal nerve innervates the muscles of the lateral compartment of the lower leg, while the deep peroneal nerve innervates the muscles of the anterior compartment. These muscles are largely responsible for dorsiflexion of the foot and injury to the peroneal nerve usually results in foot drop. The peroneal nerve is most susceptible to injury at the point where it winds laterally around the head of the fibula where it lies in a relatively exposed position. In this location, it can be easily compressed between the stirrup and the bony prominence of the fibula. A large retrospective review of 198,461 patients at the Mayo clinic who underwent surgical procedures in the lithotomy position reported 55 patients (1/3,608) with persistent neuropathy and of these, 78% of which involved the common peroneal nerve [26]. Significant risk factors were found to be low BMI, recent smoking history, and long duration of surgery (greater than 3 h). The risk of nerve injury increased 100-fold for each additional hour spent in lithotomy.

The saphenous nerve is the largest and longest branch of the femoral nerve. It originates in the upper thigh within the femoral triangle and terminates at the great toe. It initially courses in close relation to the femoral artery before turning laterally where it travels along the medial aspect of the knee behind the Sartorius muscle. It pierces the fascia lata and continues to descend along the medial aspect of the leg subcutaneously. The saphenous nerve supplies general sensory to the anteromedial aspect of the leg and foot. It is most vulnerable to compression as it courses against the medial tibial condyle. Injury at this point is secondary to medially placed stirrup holders while in lithotomy and can lead to pain and paresthesia along the anteromedial leg. Recovery after saphenous nerve injury is slow due to the long course of this nerve [25].

In any variation of the supine position, including lithotomy, the arms should be slightly anterior to the midline of the body in the coronal plane to minimize traction on the brachial plexus. An obese patient is at much higher risk of brachial plexus injury as the coronal plane in these patients is altered anteriorly compared to that of a non-obese patient. The arms should be elevated accordingly, whether tucked or on arm boards. Arm boards or lateral table extensions may be required to support the tucked arms of the obese patient.

In addition, especially during long cases, and especially in males whose arms may not fully extend, the elbows should be padded and slightly flexed to prevent the biceps tendons from being on prolonged stretch, causing postoperative pain and dysfunction. If arm boards are used, the position of the arms should be alternated between slight pronation and slight supination. Wrists should be supported and secured in neutral position.

Compartment syndrome is an even rarer complication than neuropraxia. It occurs in a closed fascial compartment when either interstitial pressure increases or capillary perfusion pressure decreases. The initial ischemia leads to local changes and subsequent reperfusion injury leads to further ischemia and damage [27]. Factors that affect incidence include preexisting peripheral vascular disease and duration of surgery. There are only 27 reported cases in urology and 26 of the cases reported were more than 4.5 h in duration [24]. An additional 65 cases were reported after a survey of 261 urologists [28]. Of these cases, 33 were low lithotomy, 29 were standard lithotomy, and 3 were exaggerated lithotomy. Of note, only 2 of the cases were less than 4 h in duration and none of the cases were endoscopic in nature.

Prone

Neuropraxia and compartment syndrome are potential complications associated with prone positioning of patients. However, there are additional potential complications that are unique to the prone position including pressure injuries and cardiovascular issues. Despite this, there is very minimal published data in urology. Most data regarding complications of the prone position are from our anesthesia and neurosurgery colleagues.

Cardiovascular changes in the prone position include decreased cardiac index, inferior vena caval obstruction, as well as potential arterial occlusion. Excessive neck movement should be avoided to allow adequate blood flow in carotid and vertebral arteries as stroke has been reported in at least six cases. Of note, none of these reported cases were from urology patients [29]. Pressure injuries can be a result of direct or indirect pressure. Direct pressure injuries include skin necrosis and sores in dependent body parts such as iliac crests, chin, nose, and eyelids. Tracheal compression has also been reported in four patients with history of scoliosis. Indirect pressure injuries are a result of pressure on vascular supply and include macroglossia, mediastinal compression, visceral ischemia as well as compartment syndrome [29].

Management of Complications

The management of neuropraxia is dependent on the degree of symptoms. Once the symptoms manifest after the dissipation of anesthesia, a complete history and physical should be conducted to determine the distribution of the nerve injury and neurology should be consulted. Electromyography of muscles along the distribution of the suspected nerve can be conducted. However, denervated muscles are usually not evident for 2–3 weeks. Earlier abnormalities on the electromyography may be a result of preexisting injury. The test is usually repeated 4 weeks postoperatively to document denervational changes. Treatment includes physical therapy to maintain range of motion and in extreme cases, repair with nerve graft. Neurogenic pain should be controlled with non-narcotic analgesics such as gabapentin [25].

The signs of compartment syndrome include the 5 "P"s—pain (disproportionate), paresthesia, pallor, paralysis, pulselessness. The last two signs are consider late symptoms [30]. Obesity, prior peripheral vascular disease, and prolonged surgery should prompt low threshold for orthopedic or vascular consult when symptoms are present. Useful laboratory values include creatinine kinase >2,000 IU and myoglobinuria. Intracompartmental pressure >45 mmHg is an indication for immediate fasciotomy. However, some do advocate lower thresholds [31]. The administration of mannitol has also been shown to reduce pressures as well as prevent the adverse effect of myoglobin [32].

Summary

Due to the overwhelming number of advantages that ureteroscopy has to offer, it has become a requisite addition to the urologist's armamentarium. In order to maximize efficacy and efficiency, it is paramount that the room is intelligently and ergonomically laid out. Furthermore, it is equally important to have all the appropriate instruments available during the surgery. When positioning the patient, it is important to consider the sources of injury so as to avoid them. Avoiding injury begins prior to draping the patient and is just as important a consideration as the position itself.

References

1. van Deet MJ, Meijerink WJHJ, Hoff C, et al. Optimal ergonomics for laparoscopic surgery suites: a review and guidelines. Surg Endosc. 2009;23:1279–85.
2. Kaya OI, Moran M, Ozkardes AB, et al. Ergonomic problems encountered by the surgical team during video endoscopic surgery. Surg Laparosc Endosc Percutan Tech. 2008;18:40–4.
3. Hemal AK, Srinivas M, Charles AR. Ergonomic problems associated with laparoscopy. J Endourol. 2001;15:499–503.
4. Berguer R, Chen J, Smith WD. A comparison of the physical effort required for laparoscopic and open surgical techniques. Arch Surg. 2003;138:967–70.
5. Johnston 3rd WK, Hollenbeck BK, Wolf Jr JS. Comparison of neuromuscular injuries to the surgeon during hand assisted and standard laparoscopic urologic surgey. J Endourol. 2005;19:377–81.
6. Beurger R. Surgery and ergonomics. Arch Surg. 1999; 134:1011–6.
7. Wong SW, Smith R, Crow P. Optimizing the operating theatre environment. ANZ J Surg. 2010;80:917–24.
8. McKenna JV. The case for motion and time study in surgery. Am J Surg. 1957;94:730–4.
9. Haramis G, Rosales JC, Palacios JM, et al. Prospective randomized trial of foot gel pads for operating room staff comfort during laparoscopic renal surgery. J Urol. 2010; doi:10.1016/j.urology.2010.01.018
10. Graversen JA, Korets R, Mues AC, et al. Prospective randomized evaluation of gel mat foot pads in the endoscopic suite. J Endourol. 2011;25:1793–6.
11. Elkoushy MA, Shahrour W, Andonian S. Pulsed fluoroscopy in ureteroscopy and percutaneous nephrolithotomy. Urology. 2012;79(6):1230–5.
12. Shultz RE, Hanno PM, Wein AJ, et al. Percutaneous ultrasonic lithotripsy: Choice of irrigant. J Urol. 1983; 130:858–60.
13. Hull RD, Raskob GE, Gent M, et al. Effectiveness of intermittent pneumatic leg compression devices for preventing deep vein thrombosis after total hip replacement. JAMA. 1990;263:2313–7.
14. Bailey JP, Kruger MP, Solano FX, et al. Prospective randomized trial of sequential compression devices vs low-dose warfarin for deep venous thrombosis prohylaxis in total hip arthroplasty. J Arthroplasty. 1991; 6(Suppl):S29–35.
15. Hansberry KL, Thompson Jr IM, Bauman J, et al. A prospective comparison of thromboembolic stockings, external sequential pneumatic compression stockings and heparin sodium/dihydroergotamine mesylate for the prevention of thromboembolic complications in urological surgery. J Urol. 1991;145:1205–8.
16. Korkes F, Lopes-Neto AC, Mattos MH, et al. Patient position and semi-rigid ureteroscopy outcomes. Int Braz J Urol. 2009;35:542–7.
17. Hunter PT, Hawkins IF, Finlayson B, et al. Hawkins-Hunter retrograde transcutaneous nephrostomy: a new technique. Urology. 1983;22:583–7.
18. Lawson RK, Murphy JB, Taylor AJ, et al. Retrograde method for percutaneous access to kidney. Urology. 1983;22:580–2.
19. Grasso M, Lang G, Taylor FC. Flexible ureteroscopically assisted percutaneous renal access. Tech Urol. 1995;1:39–43.
20. Sountoulides PG, Kauffman OG, Louie MK, et al. Endoscopy-guided percutaneous nephrostolithotomy: benefits of ureteroscopic access and therapy. J Endourol. 2009;23(10):1649–54.
21. Landman J, Venkatesh R, Ragab M, et al. Comparison of intrarenal pressure and irrigant flow during percutaneous nephroscopy with an indwelling ureteral catheter, ureteral occlusion balloon, and ureteral access sheath. Urology. 2002;60:584–7.
22. Landman J, Venkatesh R, Lee DI, et al. Combined percutaneous and retrograde approach to staghorn calculi with application of the ureteral access sheath to facilitate percutaneous nephrolithotomy. J Urol. 2003;169:64–7.
23. Khan F, Borin JF, Pearle MS, et al. Endoscopically guided percutaneous renal access: "Seeing is believing". J Endourol. 2006;20:451–5.
24. Akhavan A, Gainsburg DM, Stock JA. Complications associated with patient positioning in urologic surgery. Urology. 2010;76:1309–18.
25. Winfree CJ, Kline DG. Intraoperative positioning nerve injuries. Surg Neurol. 2005;63:5–18.
26. Warner MA, Martin JT, Schroeder DR, et al. Lower-extremity motor neuropathy associated with surgery performed in patients in a lithotomy position. Anesthesiology. 1994;81:6–12.
27. Ubee SS, Manikandan R, Athmanathan N, et al. Compartment syndrome in urological practice. BJU Int. 2009;104:577–8.
28. Simms MS, Terry TR. Well leg compartment syndrome after pelvic and perineal surgery in the lithotomy position. Postgrad Med J. 2005;81:534–6.
29. Edgecombe H, Carter K, Yarrow S. Anesthesia in the prone position. Br J Anaesth. 2008;100:165–83.
30. Matsen 3rd FA, Winquist RA, Krugmire Jr RB. Diagnosis and management of compartmental syndromes. J Bone Joint Surg Am. 1980;62:286–91.
31. Pearse MF, Harry L, Nanchahal J. Acute compartment syndrome of the leg. BMJ. 2002;325:557–8.
32. Hutton M, Rhodes RS, Chapman G. The lowering of postischmic compartment pressures with mannitol. J Surg Res. 1982;32:239–42.

20 Radiation Safety During Ureteroscopy

Don C. Arnold II and D. Duane Baldwin

Introduction

Since the first description by Hugh Hampton Young in 1912 [1], there have been major advances in ureteroscopy including miniaturization of ureteroscopes and instruments, the development of the holmium laser for stone fragmentation, and the creation of actively deflectable flexible ureteroscopes [2–4]. The imaging has also advanced from the use of plain films and intravenous pyelograms (IVP) with long acquisition times and the risk of dye administration to the use of noncontrast spiral CT imaging with rapid image acquisition, high sensitivity and specificity and no requirement for intravenous contrast. Although these advances in imaging have improved patient care, they have produced a moderate to significant increase in radiation exposure.

Since radiation cannot be seen, smelled, or felt, it is not surprising that its risks could be underestimated. In a survey of 45 emergency and 38 radiology physicians published in 2004, it was found that 91 and 53% believed that radiation did not increase the risk of malignancy, respectively. Furthermore, 51% of emergency and 24% of radiology physicians underestimated the radiation exposure by a factor greater than tenfold [5].

In 2009, a tragic set of circumstances at Cedars-Sinai Hospital in Southern California forever altered both patient and physician perceptions of the risks associated with medical imaging. More than 200 patients were exposed to radiation levels up to 8–10 × normal over an 18-month period while having CT brain scans during stroke evaluation. Hair loss and skin erythema developed in 40% of patients. Perhaps most concerning was the fact that this was not an isolated practice as several other hospitals in California and across the nation were employing similar practices [6]. The images of these patients portrayed in the media and the ensuing lawsuits forever changed both the physicians and patients' perspectives of radiation safety [7, 8]. Furthermore, the use of CT has grown exponentially from 3 million in 1980 to 62 million in 2007 [9], producing some public health concerns as it is estimated that 1.5–2.0% of all cancers diagnosed in the USA may be due to radiation from CT scans [10]. It is estimated that in 2007 alone, 29,000 cancers would develop, 14,000 due to CT of the abdomen and pelvis [10]. These public health concerns prompted the US Food and Drug Administration (FDA) to issue a white paper in February of 2010, describing the impact of the >60 million CT scans, 18 million nuclear medicine procedures, and 17 million interventional

D.C. Arnold II, M.D.
Department of Urology, Loma Linda University School of Medicine, Loma Linda, CA, USA

D.D. Baldwin, M.D. (✉)
Department of Urology, Loma Linda University Medical Center, Loma Linda University School of Medicine, 11234 Anderson Street, Room A560, Loma Linda, CA 92354, USA
e-mail: dbaldwin@llu.edu

M. Monga (ed.), *Ureteroscopy: Indications, Instrumentation & Technique*, Current Clinical Urology, DOI 10.1007/978-1-62703-206-3_20,

fluoroscopy procedures that were performed in the USA in 2006. This FDA campaign was designed to reduce the exponential growth rate in radiation exposure [11].

The primary dictum of the Hippocratic Oath is to "do no harm." Yet, as evidence mounts suggesting that the radiation associated with medical imaging is potentially harmful to the patient, it becomes essential for the physician to develop a clear understanding of the units of radiation exposure, the amount of radiation provided by different diagnostic and therapeutic interventions, the potential risks associated with this radiation exposure, and the reduced radiation alternatives currently available.

Historical Implications of Medical Radiation

X-rays were first discovered in 1895 by Wilhelm Conrad Roentgen [12]. Later, Henri Becquerel demonstrated that uranium salts caused fogging of an unexposed photographic plate and Marie Curie is credited with discovering that thorium and uranium gave off rays of energy and she coined the term "radioactivity" [13, 14]. Scientists eager to recreate Roentgen's discoveries exposed themselves to large amounts of radiation, and due to the latency noted no harmful effects initially. With time, however, the devastating effects of their large radiation exposure became evident. Clarence M. Dally, who assisted Thomas Edison in early X-ray experiments over 8 years, was one of the early victims of radiation toxicity and developed facial burns, degenerative skin changes in his hands, and extensive hair loss. He later required hand amputation for a non-healing wound and ultimately died of metastatic cancer at the age of 39 [15].

Despite the accepted risk of high radiation doses, there is still debate regarding the harmful potential of low and moderate doses of radiation exposure. One theory, called radiation hormesis, is that low doses of ionizing radiation stimulate the activation of repair mechanisms that not only cancel the detrimental effects of ionizing radiation but also inhibit disease that is not related to radiation exposure. This view is not widely accepted [16–19]. A second view of radiation biology is the threshold model which contends that small doses of radiation may not be damaging until a certain threshold is reached [20]. The predominantly held view is the linear no-threshold model. This theory suggests cancer risk will increase in direct proportion with an increase in radiation exposure and the risk of sequential radiation doses is equivalent to their sums. Furthermore, there is no safe radiation exposure and small amounts of radiation have the potential to result in future malignancy. This is the view supported by the US National Research Council and the National Council on Radiation Protection and Measurements and the United Nations Scientific Committee on the Effects of Atomic Radiation (UNSCEAR) [19].

Radiation Physics

The physical term radiation includes ionizing and nonionizing forms and describes a process in which energetic particles or energetic waves propagate through space. The lowest frequency of electromagnetic radiation is radio waves, followed in increasing frequency by microwaves, terahertz, infrared, visible light, ultraviolet, X-rays, and gamma rays [21]. Nonionizing forms of radiation may include radio waves, heat or visible light and are usually considered harmless to organisms at low levels that do not produce temperature rise [22]. In contrast, ionizing radiation contacts atoms and removes an electron, leaving the atom with a net positive charge. This ionization of individual atoms may result in DNA damage and subsequently the development of malignancy [21]. Just as the effects of low to moderate dose radiation exposure are poorly understood, the units used to express radiation exposure are also not well understood by many medical professionals. The absorbed dose is the energy absorbed per unit of mass and is measured in Gray (Gy). One Gray is equal to 1 J of radiation energy absorbed per kilogram of tissue (1 J/kg). The organ dose is the absorbed dose averaged over an organ. In other words, it is the

Table 20.1 Radiation equivalents

1 Gy	1,000 mGy
1 mGy	100 mrad
1 Sv	1,000 mSv
1 Sv	100 rem
1 mSv	100 mrem
10 mSv	1 rem
1 rad	1 rem
1 rem	1,000 mrem
1 Gy[a]	1 Sv[a]
1 Gy	100 Roentgen
10 mGy	1 Roentgen
1 mGy[a]	1 mSv[a]

[a]This only holds true when discussing X-rays, gamma rays, and beta-radiation
Data from [25, 123–126].

amount of energy absorbed by the organ divided by the mass of the organ and is expressed in Gray. The organ dose is the preferred entity to use when assessing the risk to the organ from radiation [9, 23]. The effective dose is expressed in Sieverts (Sv) and is used for dose distributions that are not homogenous like those which occur in CT imaging. It is designed to be a proportional estimate of the overall harm to a population caused by a defined radiation exposure [24]. When discussing X-rays, gamma radiation, and beta radiation, Grays and Sieverts are equivalent [25]. Dose is expressed in Gray for matter or Sieverts for biological tissue when using SI units. In this instance 1 Gy or 1 Sv is equal to 1 J/kg. Non-SI units are still often employed where dose is expressed in rads (1 Gy = 100 rad) and dose equivalent in rems (1 Sv = 100 rem). Table 20.1 provides radiation exposure conversions. Individuals living in the United States are routinely exposed to approximately 3.0 mSv annually due to environmental background exposure although significant regional differences do exist [26]. A lethal dose of radiation for a human is between 3 and 5 Sv over an hour [27]. The Nuclear Regulatory Commission has mandated that 50 mSv is the maximal permissible annual radiation dose for occupational exposure in adults [28], while exposure should not exceed 100 mSv over any 5-year period [29].

There are two types of side effects seen following radiation exposure; the immediate deterministic effects and delayed stochastic effects. Deterministic effects (like those seen in the Cedars-Sinai patients) have a short latency and are rarely seen in urologic applications but are seen more commonly after cardiology, interventional and neurointerventional procedures. They will not occur unless a threshold of 2–3 Gy are exceeded at one setting [30–35].

The second type of radiation side effect, known as stochastic effects, includes the development of secondary malignancies. Much of our understanding of stochastic effects of radiation exposure is inferred from the side effects seen in the atomic bomb survivors, although this may not be an ideal comparison since atomic bomb survivors also received neutrons, protons, and other radioactive materials for which the biological significance is less well-characterized [36, 37]. Brenner and colleagues reviewed a group of victims that were exposed to a mean of 200 mSv with 50% of that cohort being exposed to less than 50 mSv. The stochastic effects were usually not seen for many years following radiation exposure and increased as the relative radiation exposure and the period from exposure increased. Although variable, the average effective dose of a single noncontrast CT of the abdomen or pelvis has been estimated at 10 mSv [38]. Therefore, >3 single phase CT scans of the abdomen and pelvis or one 3-phase study in 1 year (60 mSv) would exceed the maximum permissible "occupational" exposure [28] and be similar to the exposure of a Japanese atomic bomb survivor within 3 km of detonation [39].

According to Preston and colleagues after exposure at age 30, it is estimated that at age 70 solid cancer rates will increase by 35% per Gy for men and 58% per Gy for women [40]. Individuals that have been exposed to 50–100 mSv over a protracted amount of time or 10–50 mSv during an acute exposure have a dose response relationship with regards to solid cancer related mortality [41]. The likelihood that ionizing radiation will result in cancer is dependent upon the absorbed dose of radiation, as adjusted for the damaging tendency of the type of radiation (equivalent dose) and the sensitivity of the organism and tissue to radiation which is the effective dose.

Preoperative Imaging for Patients Undergoing Ureteroscopy

Typically, the most common indication for ureteroscopy is in the management of urinary stone disease and flank pain. Imaging options in these patients include plain KUB, renal and bladder US, IVP, MRI, and CT imaging. The modality selected for imaging may have significant effects upon imaging time, study cost, and patient radiation exposure.

One of the oldest, simplest, and fastest imaging modalities for the evaluation of stone patients is the flat plate of the abdomen (KUB). The KUB is low cost (US national average $240) [42], rapid to acquire and easy to interpret. It provides a sensitivity of 44–77% and a specificity of 77–80% [43]. The radiation exposure provided by a KUB is modest at 0.7 mSv [44]. The disadvantage of a KUB is that it will not detect radiolucent stones (uric acid and cysteine), stones <4 mm and it may be difficult to distinguish small stones from phleboliths. Finally, KUB cannot determine if hydronephrosis is present, if the system is obstructed, or evaluate renal function [45].

Ultrasonography of the kidney and bladder represents another method to image patients with flank pain, or potential stones and results in no radiation exposure. Ultrasound has other advantages including a rapid performance time (20–30 min) and a high sensitivity for detection of large renal stones (96–100%) [46]. Ultrasound also can determine ureteral patency indirectly by identifying ureteral jets and absence of hydronephrosis. The disadvantages of ultrasound are that it is user dependent, it is difficult to image non-obstructing ureteral calculi, it may image poorly in obese individuals, and it is moderately costly ($400) [47].

Historically, IVP was considered the diagnostic test of choice for evaluating the upper urinary tract and had a mean exposure of 3.3 mSv [48]. Today this study is rarely performed in the USA as it has largely been replaced by CT imaging [49]. IVP would diagnose both radio-opaque and larger radiolucent stones (by their negative filling defect), and was excellent in providing information regarding the presence of function and obstruction. The sensitivity (87–90%) and specificity 94–100% were good [50]. Of concern the contrast causes adverse allergic reactions in up to 13% with ionic and 3% of people that receive nonionic contrast. Severe, life-threatening reactions can occur between 0.04 and 0.22% of the time [51]. Secondly, the use of contrast media may result in renal deterioration due to acute tubular necrosis in 3–26% of patients which is increased in patients with chronic renal insufficiency, diabetes mellitus, dehydration, multiple myeloma, and congestive heart failure [52]. Furthermore, IVP is potentially labor intensive sometimes requiring hours to perform [53]. The total cost of an IVP is typically between $150 and 200 [54].

Another imaging modality with no radiation exposure is the MRI. Although good at evaluating soft tissue lesions, it is not sensitive at diagnosing urinary calculi with a sensitivity and specificity of 78 and 96.1%, respectively [55]. Other limitations of MRI include slow acquisition time, limited availability during off hours, and high cost. The national average cost of an abdominal-pelvic MRI is approximately $5100.00 [56]. MRI is predominately used to determine the presence or absence of hydronephrosis and can also detect a filling defect if contrast is used [57, 58]. Until imaging times and costs are reduced it is not likely that MRI will replace CT imaging in the evaluation of flank pain and urinary stone patients.

The noncontrast CT scan of the abdomen and pelvis is currently the standard of care for the evaluation of patients with acute flank pain and potential urolithiasis due to its high sensitivity and specificity, rapid acquisition time, and universal availability. The sensitivity and specificity of CT scan has been noted to be 94–100% and 92–100%, respectively [46]. In addition noncontrast CT has no risk of dye allergy, or ATN, and requires very little technician time. Another advantage of CT imaging is its ability to establish alternative diagnoses other than urinary stones in the 14% of patients that present with flank pain that will require immediate or deferred treatment for other conditions [59]. The only

Table 20.2 Characteristics of imaging modalities employed prior to ureteroscopy

	Sensitivity	Specificity	Time to perform exam	Radiation exposure
IVP	87–90% [50]	94–100% [50]	Intermediate to long	3.3 mSv
KUB	44–77% [43]	77–80% [43]	Rapid	0.7 mSv
Ultrasound	74–96% [46]	100% [46]	Intermediate	0 mSv
unenhanced CT scan abd/pelvis	94–100% [46]	92–100% [46]	Rapid	20 mSv
MRI	69–78% [55]	89–96% [55]	Long	0 mSv

significant disadvantages of computed tomography are the amount of radiation exposure and relatively high cost. The radiation exposure with a single abdomen and pelvic CT is approximately 20 mSv but there can be tremendous range between protocols employed at different centers [60]. The cost of a CT in one study was approximately $2200.00 [47].

CT urogram, although not often employed, is a useful tool to assess the upper and lower urinary tract in patients that present with hematuria, strictures, or complicated anatomy [61]. Traditionally, a CT urogram has multiple phases including a noncontrast phase and delayed phase following opacification of the collecting system and has a relatively high radiation exposure at 25–35 mSv [62, 63]. It has a sensitivity for detecting upper tract neoplasms of 64% and a specificity of 98% in patients with asymptomatic hematuria. Furthermore, the sensitivity and specificity of a CT urogram to detect lower tract neoplasms was 79 and 94%, respectively. CT urography should be cautiously applied in high-risk patients with hematuria and complicated anatomy, but should probably not be routinely employed for evaluation of routine urinary stone patients due to its high radiation exposure.

Another imaging modality sometimes employed in the evaluation of patients prior to ureteroscopy is nuclear medicine renography which is associated with approximately 3.7 mSv per study [64]. This test is typically conducted when one is evaluating a patient for obstruction and in an attempt to determine the function of a renal unit. Technetium-99m-mercaptoacetyltriglycine (MAG3) is commonly used because 40–50% of it is extracted by the proximal tubules and then secreted into the tubular lumen. This radiotracer is a good diagnostic agent in neonates, patients with impaired renal function, patients with suspected obstruction, and can be used as a independent measure of renal function [65]. Technetium-99m-diethyenetriaminepentaacetic acid (DTPA) is also commonly used in renal nuclear renography and has the advantage that it is less expensive than MAG3. The extraction rate of DTPA is approximately 20%. Table 20.2 provides a summary of the characteristics of the imaging modalities employed prior to ureteroscopy along with other commonly employed studies.

Imaging Employed During Ureteroscopy

Fluoroscopy provides important information to the urologic surgeon that improves the safety and efficacy of this procedure and it is almost universally employed during ureteroscopy. It identifies stones, assists in the placement of guidewires, ureteral access sheaths, and stents and assists during renal mapping. Extensive use of fluoroscopy during ureteroscopy has the potential to provide a large radiation exposure.

The amount of radiation that the patient is exposed to during fluoroscopy is dependent upon fluoroscopy time, distance between the patient and the X-ray source, and the parameters on the fluoroscopy machine (kVp, mA). When the kVp is increased the penetration and exposure are increased and the contrast is decreased. Increasing the milliamperage (mA) increases the exposure which causes the film to darken [66]. During a typical fluoroscopic examination the X-ray tube is typically operated below 100 kVp and 3 mA current. Despite this, the radiation exposure from fluoroscopy is quite variable and it is estimated to produce a radiation dose between 10 and 500 mGy per minute, with spot films increasing this dose by a factor of 10–60 times [67].

In a study by Bagley and Cubler-Goodman published in 1990, it was determined that patients undergoing ureteroscopy received 100 mGy to the posterior skin at the level of the costovertebral angle. In this study fluoroscopy time ranged from 2 min for a simple diagnostic rigid ureteroscopy up to 4.7 min for a combined rigid and flexible ureteroscopy [68]. In a more recent study performed by Krupp and colleagues in 2010, all clinical ureteroscopy cases from 2006 to 2008 were reviewed. Simulating ureteroscopy, male and female cadavers were then exposed to 145 s of fluoroscopy. Dosages seen in this study were posterior skin 10.5 mGy, left kidney 3.5 mGy, and left ureter 2.7 mGy. Additionally, the left ovary received a higher radiation dosage (3.4 mGy) than the left testicle (0.36 mGy) which should be considered when performing ureteroscopy in younger females [69].

In addition to the patient, urologists, radiologic technicians, and nurses are also exposed to radiation primarily from patient scatter. Bagley and Cubler-Goodman performing 13 ureteroscopies during 1 month and found the urologist had a neck dose of 0.3 mSv and a hand dose of 12.7 mSv [68]. Giblin and colleagues measured the radiation exposure to the urologist positioned 6 in. from the perineum during direct vision endoscopy using a fluoroscopy table. The urologist's head and neck received 11 mSv per hour from radiation scatter [70]. Certainly, the use of video endoscopy has moved the surgeon further from the source and decreased exposure but the dosage received by patients and staff from fluoroscopy may be considerable.

Imaging During Follow-Up of Ureteroscopy Patients

Ureteroscopy patients receive ionizing radiation during the preoperative evaluation, intraoperatively during fluoroscopy, and also during imaging performed for follow-up with all exposures being cumulative. In the postoperative evaluation of stone patients a combination of a KUB for residual stones and a renal ultrasound to detect possible silent hydronephrosis are adequate for most uncomplicated patients and has minimal radiation exposure. In a study conducted by Ferrandino and colleagues, 108 patients received 4 radiographic examinations with a mean effective dose of 29.7 mSv (excluding fluoroscopy) during the year following stone presentation. Twenty percent of patients received >50 mSv [71]. The frequent young age of presentation and high recurrence rates in stone patients should encourage urologists to strongly consider alternative imaging strategies to decrease the radiation exposure whenever possible. Table 20.3 provides a summary of the different amounts of radiation exposure from various imaging modalities and environmental exposure.

Alternative Imaging Strategies for Ureteroscopy Patients

As discussed previously, there is no ideal imaging modality for the evaluation of ureteroscopy patients. The sensitivity of ultrasound, MRI, and KUB are too low. In addition the acquisition time is too long for MRI and the risks associated with contrast are too high to justify use of IVP. As a result, noncontrast CT has become the diagnostic test of choice for patients with flank pain and renal colic despite its high radiation exposure. There are several potential ways to reduce radiation exposure in ureteroscopy patients including avoiding medical imaging whenever possible, spacing out the interval of ionizing radiation and finally reducing the radiation associated with conventional imaging studies.

In today's litigious medical environment physicians have become accustomed to routine CT imaging in a high proportion of patients presenting to the emergency room. Between 1996 and 2007, CT utilization increased by 330%, despite only a 30% increase in ER visits. The utilization of CT for abdominal pain increased 10× and the use of CT for flank pain increased from 3.5 to >40% over the same time period [72]. Physicians

Table 20.3 Radiation dose comparison[a]

Diagnostic procedure	Average effective dose (mSv)	PA chest X-rays (equivalent effective dose)	Ranges reported in the literature (mSv)
Chest X-ray (PA film)	0.02	1	0.007–0.050
Chest X-ray (PA and lat)	0.1	5	0.05–0.24
Mammography	0.4	20	0.10–0.60
Lumbar spine X-ray	1.5	75	0.5–1.8
Abdominal X-ray (KUB)	0.7	35	0.04–1.1
Intravenous urogram	3.0	150	0.7–3.7
Renal scan DTPA	1.8	90	n/a
Renal scan MAG3	2.6	130	n/a
Renal scan DSMA	3.3	165	n/a
Bone scan	6.3	315	n/a
Upper G.I. (with fluoroscopy)	6.0	300	1.5–12.0
Barium enema (with fluoroscopy)	8.0	400	2.0–18.0
CT head	2.0	100	0.9–4.0
CT chest	7.0	350	4.0–18.0
CT chest (PE protocol)	15.0	750	13.0–40.0
Ventilation/perfusion scan	0.5	25	n/a
CT abdomen	10.0	500	3.5–25.0
CT pelvis	10.0	500	3.3–10.0
Thallium cardiac stress test	40.7	2,035	n/a
PET scan	14.1	705	n/a
Chernobyl containment workers (mean)	165 mSv	8,250	n/a
Organ-specific radiation dose (kidneys) during 1 min of fluoroscopy	1.8 mSv/min	n/a	n/a
Fluoroscopy exposure 1 min	10 mGy/min	n/a	10–500 mGy

[a]Actual exposures received may vary widely based upon patient and imaging parameters
Data from [26, 43, 44, 46, 123, 127–130]

fearing a missed diagnosis must also now contend with the threat of lawsuit for malignancy resulting from unnecessary conventional CT imaging. It is imperative that physicians use sound medical judgment and consider the risks and benefits of each imaging modality prior to its use.

Ureteral stones 2–4 mm in size have a 95% spontaneous passage rate [73]. Therefore, in a known stone patient with signs and symptoms compatible with ureteral colic, adequate pain control and no infection, imaging is not mandatory. Furthermore, in patients with recent imaging it is not mandatory to repeat imaging with each subsequent presentation.

In patients presenting with flank pain, another option to reduce radiation exposure is to use imaging that does not employ ionizing radiation. Renal ultrasound has excellent sensitivity for the detection of renal stones and hydronephrosis and may be a reasonable alterative to CT in uninfected, minimally symptomatic patients. The combination of renal ultrasound and a KUB has been shown to increase the sensitivity and specificity as high as 97 and 67%, respectively, with a negative predictive value of 95% while providing minimal ionizing radiation [50].

Perhaps one of the most promising means to decrease radiation exposure in ureteroscopy patients is the use of reduced radiation CT imaging. A variety of studies have consistently shown that low-dose CT provides a sensitivity and specificity that is greater than 90% and similar to conventional CT [74]. Zilberman and colleagues added noise to a 160 mA CT simulating a 70, 100 and 130 mA CT. There was no difference in interobserver and intra-observer variability for stone detection or radiographic signs of obstruction between settings [75]. Similarly, Poletti and colleagues performed low-dose CT (30 mAs) and conventional CT (180 mAs) for 125 stone patients and found that when BMI was <30, the low-dose CT had a sensitivity of 95%, a specificity of 97%, and detected all ureteral calculi >3 mm [76]. Hamm and colleagues performed a study utilizing a low-dose 70 mA (1.5 mSv) CT scan in 109 patients and discovered that low-dose CT scan had a sensitivity and specificity of 96 and 97%, respectively [74]. In a cadaveric study, Jellison and colleagues compared mAs settings ranging from 7.5 to 140 and found no difference in sensitivity or specificity at any setting despite a 95% reduction in radiation (the radiation dose similar to a KUB). All stones >3 mm were detected [38]. Similarly, Jin and colleagues used a cadaver model to compare renal stone detection at 100, 60, and 30 mAs equivalent to a CT dose index volume of 6.7, 4.0, and 2.0 mGy, respectively. The blinded radiologists determined that there was similar detection for stones >3 mm despite a 70% reduction in radiation exposure [77].

However, there are still some factors that have not been fully characterized with low-dose CT. Low-dose CT works well in patients with normal BMI but detection of calculi may be decreased when using ultra-low-dose CT (5–7.5 mAs) in very thin and obese patients [78, 79]. Additionally, it may be harder to determine an accurate size of the stone with low-dose computed tomography when the stone is less than 3 mm [76]. Finally, the ability of low-dose CT to detect other pathology will need to be further characterized, although early reports show that low-dose studies are capable of diagnosing bowel disease and metastatic testicular cancer [59, 80]. In the clinical study by Poletti and colleagues, low-dose CT was 100% sensitive and specific for establishing alternative non-urinary tract diagnoses in six patients [76]. Although some questions remain, low-dose CT appears to be a safe, effective, and easily implemented technique to reduce radiation exposure in ureteroscopy patients that does not affect stone detection.

One technique applicable to the CT urogram is use of a split bolus technique where an initial noncontrast CT is performed. Eight to ten minutes after injection of 30–50 cc of contrast, another injection of 80–100 cc of contrast is given. The nephrogram and delayed urogram views can then be consolidated into a second phase avoiding a three phase study. The sensitivity (100% for upper tract and 99% for lower tract) and specificity (74% for upper tract and 99% for lower tract) remain high [81]. Also similar to noncontrast CT, reducing the mAs and employing the use of tube current modulation can be implemented with the CT urogram resulting in a radiation reduction from 26 to 10 mSv [82].

Intraoperative Strategies for Reduction of Radiation to Patients and Staff

Intraoperative fluoroscopy is a fundamental and integral portion of ureteroscopy. Appropriate utilization of fluoroscopy provides important anatomic and spatial relationships, which decreases the complexity and increases the safety of this procedure. However, inappropriate and unnecessary use of fluoroscopy during ureteroscopy has the potential to expose the patient, surgeon, and staff to significant unnecessary radiation exposure. Unlike preoperative imaging, where the radiologists and technicians control radiation protocols, intraoperative use of fluoroscopy is under urologic control. There are several fluoroscopy reduction strategies including behavioral changes such as increased situational awareness, shorter pedal activations, and maintaining appropriate distance from the radiation source for both the surgeon and patient. There are also technical adjustments that can be made including use of last image hold, lowering of the kVp and mAs, use of fixed versus automatic brightness control settings, use of a laser-guided C-arm, use of pulsed instead of continuous fluoroscopy, and the use of shielding and collimation.

In a study of situational awareness, Ngo and colleagues provided surgeons with feedback regarding their fluoroscopy utilization (as well as comparison amongst their peers) and found a 24% reduction in fluoroscopy times ($p=0.002$) despite unchanged operative times [83]. Other ways to enhance situational awareness include providing fluoroscopy time in the operative report, ensuring an audible signal is generated during pedal depression, setting an alarm every 1 min to allow the surgeon to gauge fluoroscopy use, and employing only surgeon activation of the fluoroscopy pedal.

Another well-documented method to decrease fluoroscopy time is the use of the "last image hold" function which may reduce exposure by up to 60% [68]. Early C-arm machines provided only real-time images and if the foot pedal was not depressed there was no screen image. All modern C-arms have a last image hold function that allows the surgeon to carefully scrutinize the image without incurring any additional radiation exposure. Although some steps during ureteroscopy like passing a wire beyond an impacted stone may require dynamic fluoroscopy, most tasks can be effectively performed by viewing a static image.

Another principal to reduce radiation exposure during fluoroscopy is the inverse square law between exposure and distance. If the distance from the source is doubled, the radiation exposure decreases by a factor of four. This applies to the patient, urologist, and the staff members. The fluoroscopy machine should always be used with the spacer present at the radiation source to prevent the operator from moving the source too close to the patient. All operating room members should work at the greatest distance from the source that allows the safe performance of their clinical duties.

Collimation is another strategy for reducing the amount of radiation that escapes from the source by restricting the radiation solely to the area of interest. Similar to collimation, shielding limits the radiation exposure to the area of interest and may reduce exposure by 80% [68, 84]. Shielding is significantly underutilized in urology but has been employed with pregnant patients [85]. Shields are made out of lead or other dense materials with thicker shields providing greater protection. The most common apron worn by staff members covers the front of the surgeon in an attempt to reduce the weight but may allow exposure when the surgeon is not facing the source. Alternatively, a wrap-around skirt and vest provide circumferential coverage while distributing the weight over the hips and shoulders. This distribution of weight is important as 64.2% of endourologists have orthopedic problems including 38.1, 27.6, and 14.2% with back, neck, and knee or hip problems, respectively. These problems correlated with surgeon age and case volume [86].

Although most urologists wear a lead apron (97%) the use of thyroid shields (68%) and lead glasses (17.2%) is more variable [86]. Reasons listed by endourologists for noncompliance included unavailability (81.6%), carelessness and disbelief of the harmful effects of radiation (36.7%), lack of knowledge about radiation hazards and lack of proper measures of protection (10.2%) [86]. It has been documented that the scatter to the lens is relatively low at 1.9 mGy ± 0.5 during endourological procedures [87]. When combined with environmental background exposures this can become substantial over the career of a busy endourologist's practice. This ocular radiation can be substantially reduced using lead glasses. In a study performed by Chodick and colleagues, in 35,000 radiation technologists followed for almost 20 years the authors concluded that the amount of radiation required to cause cataracts is as low as centi-sieverts and not the 2 Sv previously assumed to be necessary [88].

Thyroid shields can also be utilized to decrease the amount of radiation to the neck area of the urologic surgeon. Since the amount of radiation needed to cause cancer of the thyroid is currently unknown it is wise to use shielding. A 0.5 mm lead equivalent thyroid shield reduced radiation of the thyroid from 0.46 to 0.02 mSv [89].

Another technique to reduce radiation exposure in ureteroscopy patients is through alteration of the machine settings utilized during fluoroscopy. Fluoroscopy machines can be operated using automatic brightness control settings

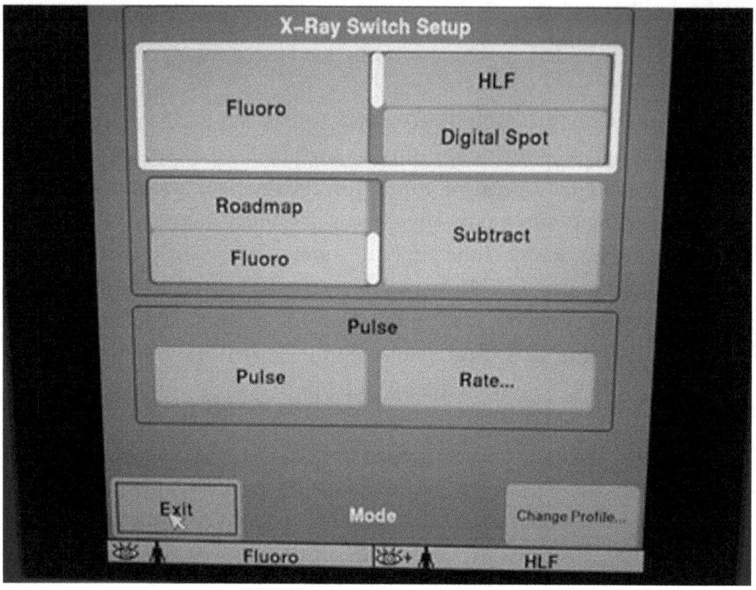

Fig. 20.1 Sample screen employed to shift from continuous to pulsed mode

where the machine automatically adjusts the mA and kVp to provide optimal image quality based upon the density of objects within the field of interest [90]. One highly effective method for reducing radiation exposure is to intentionally decrease the kVp slightly while modestly decreasing the mA using fixed manual settings. During ureteroscopy the visualization of guidewires, ureteroscope position and dense stones can all be performed easily even with a low quality image. Use of intentionally lowered fixed settings also prevents the "whited out" image which can occur using automated settings if the C-arm sensor encounters dense structures such as the bar on the fluoroscopy table, equipment resting on the patient or a dense region of contrast [91]. These settings can be intentionally reduced to the lowest level that still provides adequate image quality to perform the task at hand.

Another alteration that can be applied to the fluoroscopic machine is the use of a pulsed rate rather than continuous fluoroscopy. In continuous fluoroscopy X-rays are continuously created and captured on a video camera display at a rate of 30 frames per second [92]. In contrast, the operator can manually adjust the number of frames per second in pulsed rate fluoroscopy. Pulsed rate fluoroscopy has been employed in cardiology, radiology, and gastroenterology and shown to provide adequate images while significantly reducing radiation exposure [93–95]. The pulsed mode works particularly well when using single spot films to confirm guidewire, ureteroscope, and stent position. In order to employ pulsed fluoroscopy one must only alter the settings on the fluoroscopy machine (Figs. 20.1 and 20.2).

The optimal strategy for fluoroscopy reduction may combine many of the previously mentioned measures into an integrated protocol. In a study performed by Greene and colleagues several of the previously discussed measures were combined in an attempt to reduce fluoroscopy time [96]. In addition, use of a laser-guided C-arm, use of a designated fluoroscopy technician, timing the fluoroscopy activation with end expiration, and substitution of visual and tactile cues instead of reliance upon fluoroscopy during the steps of ureteroscopy were employed. The laser-guided C-arm allowed activation of the C-arm after the machine was correctly positioned to eliminate the fluoroscopy required to position the X-ray beam (Fig. 20.3). Use of a designated fluoroscopy technician allowed the development

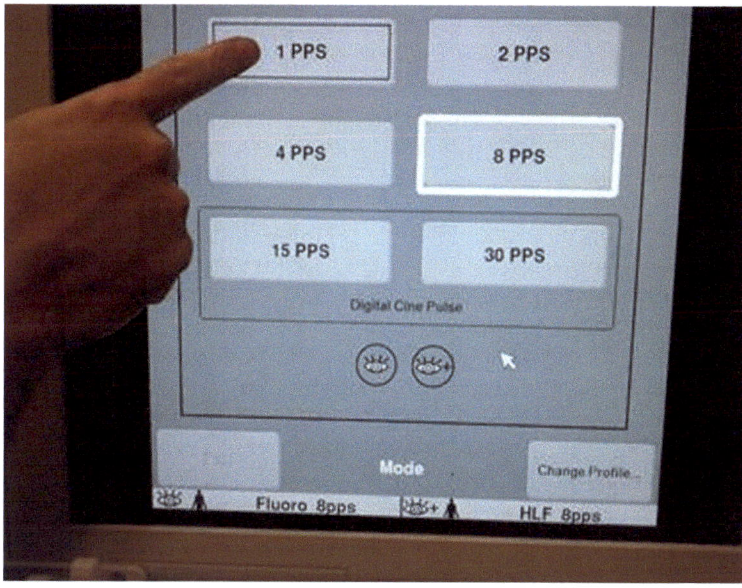

Fig. 20.2 Rate selections available in the pulsed mode

of expertise in beam localization and adjustment of low-dose settings to optimize the image quality at intentionally lowered fixed kVp and mA levels. Tactile and visual cues were substituted for fluoroscopic cues during the passage of guidewires, ureteroscopes, and stents. For example if the second wire was noted to be the same length as the first wire, it was assumed that the tips were in the same location without fluoroscopic confirmation (Fig. 20.4). Implementation of this simple protocol reduced fluoroscopy time during ureteroscopy from 86.1 to 15.5 s (an 82% reduction) with no difference in operative time, stone-free rates or complications [96].

Radiation in Children

The first study to evaluate low-dose radiation in humans was performed by Alice Stewart [97]. She determined that in utero exposure to 10–20 mSv in a pregnant woman increased the incidence of cancer and leukemia by 50% in the child at 10 years. Similarly, Monson and colleagues determined that children exposed to prenatal diagnostic X-rays had a 1.5 times higher risk of dying from leukemia than unexposed children [98]. In a case–control twin study by Harvey and colleagues it was found that twins with leukemia or other childhood cancers were twice as likely to be exposed to X-rays in utero as twins who were free from disease [99]. Children represent a unique and highly radiation sensitive population. The tissues in children and adolescents have higher water content and subsequently require proportionally greater radiation to penetrate a similar thickness compared to an adult [100].

The risk of radiation induced malignancy is five times greater after obtaining a CT in children compared to adults due to DNA damage in rapidly replicating cells [101]. Knowledge of the potential harm that radiation can cause in children gave rise to the ALARA principle (As Low As Reasonably Achievable) [102] which holds as its premise that radiation should always be kept to the lowest possible level that will provide adequate diagnostic information for the ordering physician. Additionally, the urologic surgeon should keep in mind that the pediatric patient may experience a CT body dose between 29 and 68 mSv when scanned at 100–300 mAs [103]. It has been estimated that ionizing radiation may be linked to 58,000 excess lifetime fatal cancers

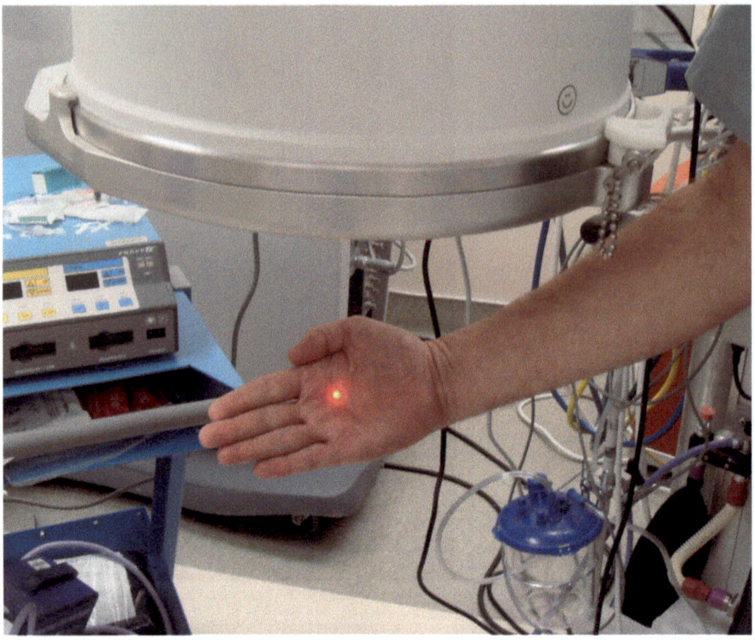

Fig. 20.3 Laser-guided C-arm used to position fluoroscopy without machine activation

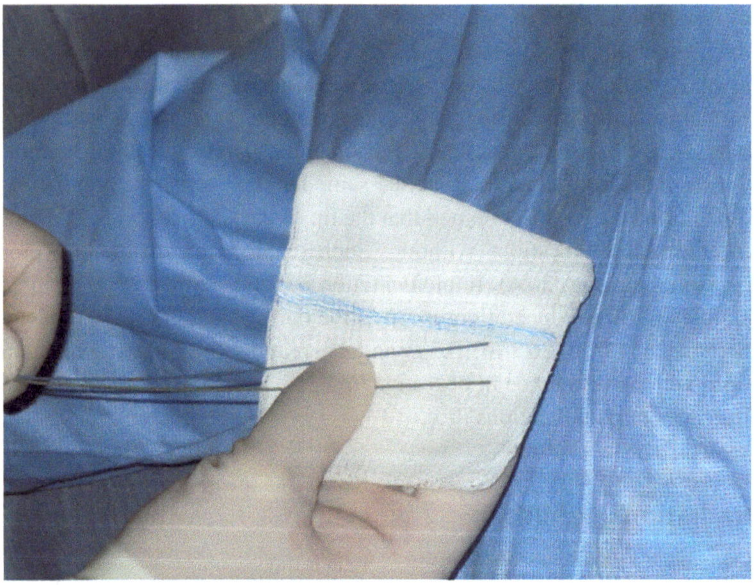

Fig. 20.4 Using tactile and visual cues, the second wire is placed without using additional fluoroscopy

among the 6.5 million pediatric patients in the USA who underwent 18.1 million abdominal CT scans in 2006 [102].

Also concerning is the fact that the incidence of pediatric urolithiasis has been steadily increasing. Routh and colleagues found that the annual incidence of pediatric urolithiasis increased by 10.6% between 1999 and 2008 [104]. Similarly, VanDervoot compared the incidence of pediatric urolithiasis between 1994 and

1996 with 2003–2005 demonstrating a 4.6-fold increase in incidence [105]. In pediatric ureteral calculi patients, two-thirds have spontaneous passage of stones <5 mm [106].

In addition to the previously described methods of improving radiation safety a different paradigm should be considered when evaluating children for urolithiasis. In a retrospective review of 42 patients by Johnson and colleagues, nearly 90% of the patients treated in their study for symptomatic urolithiasis could have completed their evaluation and treatment without computed tomography [107].

Radiation Safety in Pregnant Patients

The incidence of urolithiasis in pregnant patients is unknown however it is estimated between 1 in 244 and 1 in 2000 pregnancies [108]. In no other population is the issue of radiation safety more important. If an embryo is exposed to 50–100 mGy prior to implantation (0–2 weeks after conception) the result is typically the death of the embryo. Exposure to 200 mGy of radiation during the organogenesis phase (2–8 weeks after conception) may result in congenital abnormalities of the skeleton, eyes, and genitals. If the fetus is exposed to >60 mGy during the fetal period (8–15 weeks) the result can be severe mental retardation and microcephaly. Finally, if the fetus is exposed to 250–280 mGy of radiation after 16–25 weeks, mental retardation may result [85].

In a pregnant patient presenting with flank pain the optimal initial imaging modality should be a renal and bladder ultrasound. If neither a stone nor hydronephrosis is identified, no further urologic imaging is routinely required. Despite having the benefit of no radiation exposure to the patient, the sensitivity of 34% and specificity of 86% are poor in pregnant patients [109]. In patients presenting with hydronephrosis the difficult diagnostic dilemma is whether this hydronephrosis is physiologic or due to obstruction. Physiologic hydronephrosis is present in 90% of pregnant women by 6–10 weeks and does not resolve until 4–6 weeks postpartum [110]. Other factors which may help identify ureteral obstruction from physiologic hydronephrosis include a change in resistive indices and absence of the ipsilateral ureteral jet [111, 112]. Lastly, transvaginal ultrasound can be utilized if the presence of obstruction is equivocal with abdominal ultrasound. Laing and colleagues identified distal ureteral stones in 100% of pregnant patients that presented with symptoms consistent with urolithiasis [113]. With pregnancy, the use of conservative management results in stone passage in 70–80% of the patients [114, 115].

If it is determined that ionizing radiation will assist in the diagnosis of ureteral obstruction then a limited IVP is an excellent second line imaging modality. Stothers and Lee were able to detect ureteral stones in 16/17 pregnant patients utilizing a scout film, a 30 s film and 20 min film [109]. In a study performed by White and colleagues, 20 pregnant patients underwent a low-dose CT scan (mean 7.1 mGy) for evaluation for suspected urolithiasis. Stones were identified in 13 of 20 patients [116]. It is possible that as experience mounts with the use of low-dose CT in pregnant patients, the mAs and kVp could be substantially reduced without compromising stone detection. Patients with obstructing stones accompanied by refractory pain or infection should progress to timely surgical decompression.

Traditionally, before 22 weeks of gestation, percutaneous nephrostomy tube placement was considered ideal management because nephrostomy tubes could be changed at regular intervals without general anesthesia. The placement of ureteral stents was thought to be appropriate for the later stages of pregnancy [108]. However, due to relatively rapid encrustation (4–8 weeks) and the need for frequent exchanges, both of these options may be suboptimal for long-term management.

Evidence is mounting that ureteroscopy with laser lithotripsy may be a viable first-line treatment for urolithiasis in pregnant patients and may be performed throughout pregnancy [85, 117, 118]. Akpinar and colleagues successfully performed ureteroscopic laser lithotripsy in seven pregnant patients between 1997 and 2003 [119]. Typically in pregnant patients there is minimal use of fluoroscopy and the entire procedure can be performed using ultrasound [120, 121].

Since these patients typically have physiologic hydronephrosis, ureteral dilation is commonly not necessary and small flexible ureterscopes can easily traverse the ureteral orifice [122]. These pregnant patients should have a multidisciplinary management receiving input from a high-risk obstetrician, urologist, and radiologist. Prior to any ionizing radiation or surgical treatment a thorough counseling and informed consent should be documented.

Conclusion

Medical imaging is essential for state-of-the-art diagnosis, surgical treatment, and follow-up in individuals undergoing ureteroscopy. It is important that the urologic surgeon considers the potential risks and benefits of all imaging modalities prior to employing them. It is vitally important that urologists work together with radiologists to maximize diagnostic accuracy while minimizing radiation exposure through the use of alternative nonionizing imaging studies, by spacing out ionizing studies and through the development and implementation of low-dose CT protocols. By adhering to the ALARA principle and the principles outlined for the safe utilization of fluoroscopy, the endoscopic surgeon can achieve optimal outcomes with a significant reduction in risk for both the patient and staff. In this manner the surgeon can fulfill the Hippocratic Oath "To first do no harm."

References

1. Young HH, Frontz WA, Baldwin JC. Congenital obstruction of the posterior urethra. J Urol. 1919;3:289–365. J Urol. 2002;167(1):265–67; discussion 268.
2. Kavoussi L, Clayman RV, Basler J. Flexible, actively deflectable fiberoptic ureteronephroscopy. J Urol. 1989;142(4):949–54.
3. Higashihara E, et al. Laser ureterolithotripsy with combined rigid and flexible ureterorenoscopy. J Urol. 1990;143(2):273–4.
4. Grasso M, Bagley D. A 7.5/8.2 F actively deflectable, flexible ureteroscope: a new device for both diagnostic and therapeutic upper urinary tract endoscopy. Urology. 1994;43(4):435–41.
5. Lee CI, Haims AH, Monico EP, Brink JA, Forman HP. Diagnostic CT scans: assessment of patient, physician, and radiologist awareness of radiation dose and possible risks. Radiology. 2004;231:393–8.
6. Doctors "shocked" by radiation overexposure at Cedars-Sinai. http://abcnews.go.com/Health/CancerPreventionAndTreatment/doctors-shocked-radiation-exposure/story?id=8818377. Accessed 8 Dec 2011.
7. Radiation overdoses from CT scans lead to maladies in patients. http://www.cleveland.com/nation/index.ssf/2010/08/radiation_overdoses_from_ct_sc.html. Accessed 23 Oct 2011.
8. Illinois medical malpractice blog. http://medicalmalpractice.levinperconti.com/radiation_injury/. Accessed 23 Oct 2011.
9. Brenner DJ, Hall EJ. Computed tomography–an increasing source of radiation exposure. N Engl J Med. 2007;357(22):2277–84.
10. de Berrington Gonzalez A, et al. Projected cancer risks from computed tomographic scans performed in the United States in 2007. Arch Intern Med. 2009; 169(22):2071–7.
11. White Paper: Initiative to Reduce Unnecessary Radiation Exposure from Medical Imaging. http://www.fda.gov/Radiation-EmittingProducts/RadiationSafety/RadiationDoseReduction/ucm199994.htm. Accessed 8 Dec 2011.
12. Greene R. Fleischner Lecture. Imaging the respiratory system in the first few years after discovery of the X-ray: contributions of Francis H. Williams, M.D. AJR Am J Roentgenol. 1992;159(1):1–7.
13. Leucutia T. Heuristic gems from the American Radium Society. Am J Roentgenol Radium Ther Nucl Med. 1974;121(3):653–60.
14. Coppes-Zantinga AR, Coppes MJ. Madame Marie Curie (1867–1934): a giant connecting two centuries. AJR Am J Roentgenol. 1998;171(6):1453–7.
15. Langland OE, Langlais RP. Early pioneers of oral and maxillofacial radiology. Oral Surg Oral Med Oral Pathol Oral Radiol Endod. 1995;80(5): 496–511.
16. Feinendegen LE. Evidence for beneficial low level radiation effects and radiation hormesis. Br J Radiol. 2005;78(925):3–7.
17. Wolff S. The adaptive response in radiobiology: evolving insights and implications. Environ Health Perspect. 1998;106 Suppl 1:277–83.
18. Calabrese EJ, Baldwin LA. Toxicology rethinks its central belief. Nature. 2003;421(6924):691–2.
19. Puskin JS. Perspective on the use of LNT for radiation protection and risk assessment by the US Environmental Protection Agency. Dose Response. 2009;7(4):284–91.
20. Hoel DG, Li P. Threshold models in radiation carcinogenesis. Health Phys. 1998;75(3):241–50.
21. Questions and answers about biological effects and potential hazards of radiofrequency electromagnetic fields. http://transition.fcc.gov/Bureaus/Engineering_Technology/Documents/bulletins/oet56/oet56e4.pdf. Accessed 24 Dec 2011.

22. Ng KH. Non-ionizing radiations- sources, biological effects, emissions, and exposures. Proceedings of the International Conference on Non-ionizing Radiation at UNITEN. Oct. 20th-22nd, Kajang, Selangor, Malaysia. 2003. p. 1–16.
23. Groves AM, et al. 16-detector multislice CT: dosimetry estimation by TLD measurement compared with Monte Carlo simulation. Br J Radiol. 2004;77(920): 662–5.
24. Jacobi W. The concept of the effective dose–a proposal for the combination of organ doses. Radiat Environ Biophys. 1975;12(2):101–9.
25. Frequently asked questions. http://www.radprocalculator.com/FAQ.aspx. Accessed 23 Dec 2011.
26. Hendrick RE. Radiation doses and cancer risks from breast imaging studies. Radiology. 2010;257(1): 246–53.
27. Jaworowski Z. Radiation risk and ethics. Phys Today. 1999;52(9):24–9.
28. Standards for protection against radiation: Nuclear Regulatory Commission. Final rule. Fed Regist. 1991;56(98):23360–474.
29. Wrixon AD. New ICRP recommendations. J Radiol Prot. 2008;28(2):161–8.
30. Koenig TR, Mettler FA, Wagner LK. Skin injuries from fluoroscopically guided procedures: part 2, review of 73 cases and recommendations for minimizing dose delivered to patient. Am J Roentgenol. 2001;177(1):13–20.
31. Koenig TR, et al. Skin injuries from fluoroscopically guided procedures: part 1, characteristics of radiation injury. AJR Am J Roentgenol. 2001;177(1): 3–11.
32. Miller DL, et al. Minimizing radiation-induced skin injury in interventional radiology procedures. Radiology. 2002;225(2):329–36.
33. Smith JC, et al. Ultra-low-dose protocol for CT-guided lung biopsies. J Vasc Interv Radiol. 2011;22(4):431–6.
34. Paulino AC, et al. Normal tissue development, homeostasis, senescence, and the sensitivity to radiation injury across the age spectrum. Semin Radiat Oncol. 2010;20(1):12–20.
35. Sodickson A, et al. Recurrent CT, cumulative radiation exposure, and associated radiation-induced cancer risks from CT of adults. Radiology. 2009;251(1): 175–84.
36. Sampaio FJB, BA, Bohle A, Billis A, et al. Urological survey: editorial comment re: computed tomography—an increasing source of radiation exposure. Int Braz J Urol. 2007;33(6):854–77.
37. Delongchamp RR, et al. Cancer mortality among atomic bomb survivors exposed in utero or as young children. Radiat Res. 1997;147(3):385–95.
38. Jellison FC, et al. Effect of low dose radiation computerized tomography protocols on distal ureteral calculus detection. J Urol. 2009;182(6):2762–7.
39. Pierce DA, Preston DL. Radiation-related cancer risks at low doses among atomic bomb survivors. Radiat Res. 2000;154(2):178–86.
40. Preston DL, et al. Solid cancer incidence in atomic bomb survivors: 1958–1998. Radiat Res. 2007;168(1):1–64.
41. Brenner DJ, et al. Cancer risks attributable to low doses of ionizing radiation: assessing what we really know. Proc Natl Acad Sci U S A. 2003;100(24): 13761–6.
42. Abdominal X-ray procedure & cost information. http://newchoicehealth.com/Directory/Procedure/81/Abdominal%20X-Ray. Accessed 8 Dec 2011.
43. Heidenreich A, Desgrandschamps F, Terrier F. Modern approach of diagnosis and management of acute flank pain: review of all imaging modalities. Eur Urol. 2002;41(4):351–62.
44. Mettler FA, et al. Effective doses in radiology and diagnostic nuclear medicine: a catalog. Radiology. 2008;248(1):254–63.
45. Levine JA, et al. Ureteral calculi in patients with flank pain: correlation of plain radiography with unenhanced helical CT. Radiology. 1997;204(1): 27–31.
46. Tamm EP, Silverman PM, Shuman WP. Evaluation of the patient with flank pain and possible ureteral calculus. Radiology. 2003;228(2):319–29.
47. Passerotti C, et al. Ultrasound versus computerized tomography for evaluating urolithiasis. J Urol. 2009;182(4):1829–34.
48. Pfister SA, et al. Unenhanced helical computed tomography vs intravenous urography in patients with acute flank pain: accuracy and economic impact in a randomized prospective trial. Eur Radiol. 2003; 13(11):2513–20.
49. Chen MYM, Zagoria RJ. Can noncontrast helical computed tomography replace intravenous urography for evaluation of patients with acute urinary tract colic? J Emerg Med. 1999;17(2):299–303.
50. Grisi G, et al. Cost analysis of different protocols for imaging a patient with acute flank pain. Eur Radiol. 2000;10(10):1620–7.
51. Katayama H, et al. Adverse reactions to ionic and nonionic contrast media. A report from the Japanese Committee on the Safety of Contrast Media. Radiology. 1990;175(3):621–8.
52. Goldenberg I, Matetzky S. Nephropathy induced by contrast media: pathogenesis, risk factors and preventive strategies. CMAJ. 2005;172(11):1461–71 (vol 173(10), p. 1210, 2005).
53. Dalrymple NC, et al. The value of unenhanced helical computerized tomography in the management of acute flank pain. J Urol. 1998;159(3):735–40.
54. Ng WH, Lee PSF, Chan HCA, et al. Cost effectiveness analysis of protocol driven intravenous urogram performed by radiographers. J HK Coll Radiol. 2003;6:86–9.
55. Shokeir AA, et al. Diagnosis of ureteral obstruction in patients with compromised renal function: the role of noninvasive imaging modalities. J Urol. 2004;171(6):2303–6.
56. MRI cost & MRI procedure introduction. http://newchoicehealth.com/MRI-Cost. Accessed 8 Dec 2011.

57. Vrtiska TJ. Quantitation of stone burden: imaging advances. Urol Res. 2005;33(5):398–402.
58. Sandhu C, Anson KM, Patel U. Urinary tract stones—part 1: role of radiological Imaging in diagnosis and treatment planning. Clin Radiol. 2003; 58(6):415–21.
59. Hoppe H, et al. Alternate or additional findings to stone disease on unenhanced computerized tomography for acute flank pain can impact management. J Urol. 2006;175(5):1725–30.
60. Jaffe TA, et al. Radiation dose for body CT protocols: variability of scanners at one institution. Am J Roentgenol. 2009;193(4):1141–7.
61. McNicholas MMJ, et al. Excretory phase CT urography for opacification of the urinary collecting system. Am J Roentgenol. 1998;170(5):1261–7.
62. Silverman SG, Leyendecker JR, Amis ES. What is the current role of CT urography and MR urography in the evaluation of the urinary tract? Radiology. 2009;250(2):309–23.
63. Caoili EM, et al. Urinary tract abnormalities: initial experience with multi-detector row CT urography. Radiology. 2002;222(2):353–60.
64. Stabin M, et al. Radiation-dosimetry for technetium-99 m-MAG3, technetium-99 m-DTPA, and iodine-131-OIH based on human biodistribution studies. J Nucl Med. 1992;33(1):33–40.
65. Taylor A, Schuster DM, Alazraki A, editors. Clinician's guide to nuclear medicine. 1st ed. Reston: Society of Nuclear Medicine, Inc.; 2000. p. 45–56.
66. Chen MYM, Pope Thomas L. Jr, Ott DJ. Basic radiology. 1st ed. McGraw-Hill Companies, Inc. New York, 2004. p. 15–8.
67. Jamal JE, et al. Perioperative patient radiation exposure in the endoscopic removal of upper urinary tract calculi. J Endourol. 2011;25(11):1747–51.
68. Bagley DH, Cublergoodman A. Radiation exposure during ureteroscopy. J Urol. 1990;144(6):1356–8.
69. Krupp N, et al. Fluoroscopic organ and tissue-specific radiation exposure by sex and body mass index during ureteroscopy. J Endourol. 2010;24(7): 1067–72.
70. Giblin JG, et al. Radiation risk to the urologist during endourologic procedures, and a new shield that reduces exposure. Urology. 1996;48(4):624–7.
71. Ferrandino MN, et al. Radiation exposure in the acute and short-term management of urolithiasis at 2 academic centers. J Urol. 2009;181(2):668–72. discussion 673.
72. Kocher KE, et al. National trends in use of computed tomography in the emergency department. Ann Emerg Med. 2011;58(5):452–62.e3.
73. Miller OF, Kane CJ. Time to stone passage for observed ureteral calculi: a guide for patient education. J Urol. 1999;162(3 Pt 1):688–90. discussion 690–1.
74. Hamm M, et al. Low dose unenhanced helical computerized tomography for the evaluation of acute flank pain. J Urol. 2002;167(4):1687–91.
75. Zilberman DE, et al. Low dose computerized tomography for detection of urolithiasis-its effectiveness in the setting of the urology clinic. J Urol. 2011;185(3): 910–4.
76. Poletti PA, et al. Low-dose versus standard-dose CT protocol in patients with clinically suspected renal colic. Am J Roentgenol. 2007;188(4):927–33.
77. Jin DH, et al. Effect of reduced radiation CT protocols on the detection of renal calculi. Radiology. 2010;255(1):100–7.
78. Heldt JP, et al. Ureteral calculi detection accuracy using low-dose computed tomography protocols is compromised in overweight and underweight patients. J Endourol. 2011;25:A93–A4.
79. Kalra MK, et al. Detection of urinary tract stones at low-radiation-dose CT with Z-axis automatic tube current modulation: phantom and clinical studies. Radiology. 2005;235(2):523–9.
80. O'Malley ME, et al. Comparison of low dose with standard dose abdominal/pelvic multidetector CT in patients with stage 1 testicular cancer under surveillance. Eur Radiol. 2010;20(7):1624–30.
81. Chow LC, et al. Split-bolus MDCT urography with synchronous nephrographic and excretory phase enhancement. Am J Roentgenol. 2007;189(2):314–22.
82. Dahlman P, et al. Optimization of computed tomography urography protocol, 1997 to 2008: effects on radiation dose. Acta Radiol. 2009;50(4):446–54.
83. Ngo TC, et al. Tracking intraoperative fluoroscopy utilization reduces radiation exposure during ureteroscopy. J Endourol. 2011;25(5):763–7.
84. Ionising radiation safety. http://www.e-radiography.net/radsafety/radsafety.htm. Accessed 8 Dec 2011.
85. Cocuzza M, et al. Use of inverted fluoroscope's C-arm during endoscopic treatment of urinary tract obstruction in pregnancy: a practicable solution to cut radiation. Urology. 2010;75(6):1505–8.
86. Elkoushy MA, Andonian S. Prevalence of orthopedic complaints among endourologists and their compliance with radiation safety measures. J Endourol. 2011;25(10):1609–13.
87. Hellawell GO, et al. Radiation exposure and the urologist: what are the risks? J Urol. 2005;74(3):948–52. discussion 952.
88. Chodick G, et al. Risk of cataract after exposure to low doses of ionizing radiation: a 20-year prospective cohort study among US radiologic technologists. Am J Epidemiol. 2008;168(6):620–31.
89. Tse V, et al. Radiation exposure during fluoroscopy: should we be protecting our thyroids? Aust N Z J Surg. 1999;69(12):847–8.
90. Reilly AJ, Sutton DG. A computer model of an image intensifier system working under automatic brightness control. Br J Radiol. 2001;74(886):938–48.
91. Nakamura A, et al. Increased radiation dose by automatic exposure control system during fluoroscopy and angiography of pelvis due to contrast material in the bladder: experimental study. Radiat Med. 2004;22(4):225–32.
92. Bushberg J, Seiberd JA, Leidholdt EM, et al. The essential physics of medical imaging. 2nd ed. Philadelphia: Lippencott Williams & Wilkins; 2002.

93. Herrmann K, et al. Initial experiences with pulsed fluoroscopy on a multifunctional fluoroscopic unit. Rofo. 1996;165(5):475–9.
94. Holmes DR, et al. Effect of pulsed progressive fluoroscopy on reduction of radiation-dose in the Cardiac-Catheterization Laboratory. J Am Coll Cardiol. 1990;15(1):159–62.
95. Hernandez RJ, Goodsitt MM. Reduction of radiation dose in pediatric patients using pulsed fluoroscopy. Am J Roentgenol. 1996;167(5):1247–53.
96. Greene DJ, et al. Comparison of a reduced radiation fluoroscopy protocol to conventional fluoroscopy during uncomplicated ureteroscopy. Urology. 2011;78(2):286–90.
97. Stewart A, Webb J, Hewitt D. A survey of childhood malignancies. Br Med J. 1958;1(5086):1495–508.
98. Monson RR, MacMahon B. Radiation carcinogenesis: epidemiology and biological significance prenatal X-ray exposure and cancer in children. New York: Raven; 1984.
99. Harvey EB, et al. Prenatal X-ray exposure and childhood cancer in twins. N Engl J Med. 1985;312(9): 541–5.
100. Alzen G, Benz-Bohm G. Radiation protection in pediatric radiology. Dtsch Arztebl Int. 2011;108(24): 407–14.
101. Brenner D, et al. Estimated risks of radiation-induced fatal cancer from pediatric CT. AJR Am J Roentgenol. 2001;176(2):289–96.
102. Bertell R, Ehrle LH, Schmitz-Feuerhake I. Pediatric CT research elevates public health concerns: low-dose radiation issues are highly politicized. Int J Health Serv. 2007;37(3):419–39.
103. Nickoloff E. Current adult and pediatric CT doses. Pediatr Radiol. 2002;32(4):250–60.
104. Routh JC, Graham DA, Nelson CP. Epidemiological trends in pediatric urolithiasis at United States freestanding pediatric hospitals. J Urol. 2010;184(3): 1100–4.
105. VanDervoort K, et al. Urolithiasis in pediatric patients: a single center study of incidence, clinical presentation and outcome. J Urol. 2007;177(6): 2300–5.
106. Pietrow PK, et al. Clinical outcome of pediatric stone disease. J Urol. 2002;167(2):670–3.
107. Johnson EK, et al. Are stone protocol computed tomography scans mandatory for children with suspected urinary calculi? Urology. 2011;78(3):662–6.
108. Srirangam SJ, Hickerton B, Van Cleynenbreugel B. Management of urinary calculi in pregnancy: a review. J Endourol. 2008;22(5):867–75.
109. Stothers L, Lee LM. Renal colic in pregnancy. J Urol. 1992;148(5):1383–7.
110. McAleer SJ, Loughlin KR. Nephrolithiasis and pregnancy. Curr Opin Urol. 2004;14(2):123–7.
111. Shokeir AA, Mahran MR, Abdulmaaboud M. Renal colic in pregnant women: role of renal resistive index. Urology. 2000;55(3):344–7.
112. Di Salvo DN. Sonographic imaging of maternal complications of pregnancy. J Ultrasound Med. 2003;22(1):69–89.
113. Laing FC, et al. Distal ureteral calculi: detection with vaginal US. Radiology. 1994;192(2):545–8.
114. Lewis DF, et al. Urolithiasis in pregnancy. Diagnosis, management and pregnancy outcome. J Reprod Med. 2003;48(1):28–32.
115. Loughlin KR, Ker LA. The current management of urolithiasis during pregnancy. Urol Clin North Am. 2002;29(3):701–4.
116. White WM, et al. Low-dose computed tomography for the evaluation of flank pain in the pregnant population. J Endourol. 2007;21(11):1255–60.
117. Travassos M, et al. Ureteroscopy in pregnant women for ureteral stone. J Endourol. 2009;23(3):405–7.
118. Lifshitz DA, Lingeman JE. Ureteroscopy as a first-line intervention for ureteral calculi in pregnancy. J Endourol. 2002;16(1):19–22.
119. Akpinar H, et al. Ureteroscopy and holmium laser lithotripsy in pregnancy: stents must be used postoperatively. J Endourol. 2006;20(2):107–10.
120. Loughlin KR. Management of acute ureteral obstruction in pregnancy utilizing ultrasound-guided placement of ureteral stents. Urology. 1994;43(3):412.
121. Jarrard DJ, Gerber GS, Lyon ES. Management of acute ureteral obstruction in pregnancy utilizing ultrasound-guided placement of ureteral stents. Urology. 1993;42(3):263–7. discussion 267–8.
122. Semins MJ, Trock BJ, Matlaga BR. The safety of ureteroscopy during pregnancy: a systematic review and meta-analysis. J Urol. 2009;181(1):139–43.
123. Radiation basics. http://hps.org/publicinformation/ate/faqs/radiation.html. Accessed 22 Dec 2011.
124. SI radiation measurement units: conversion factors. http://www.stevequayle.com/ARAN/rad.conversion.html. Accessed 23 Dec 2011.
125. Radiation safety guide. http://web.princeton.edu/sites/ehs/radsafeguide/rsg_app_e.htm#10. Accessed 23 Dec 2011.
126. The millisievert and milligray as measures of radiation dose and exposure. http://www.mun.ca/biology/scarr/Radiation_definitions.html. Accessed 23 Dec 2011.
127. How are different amounts of radiation expressed? http://www.radiation-scott.org/radsource/2-0.htm. Accessed 23 Dec 2011.
128. Brenner DJ. Are X-ray backscatter scanners safe for airport passenger screening? For most individuals, probably yes, but a billion scans per year raises long-term public health concerns. Radiology. 2011;259(1): 6–10.
129. Medvedev G. Chernoybl notebook. Novy Mir. 1989;(6):3–108.
130. Weinberg HSH, Korol AB, Kirzhner VM, Avivi A, et al. Very high mutation rate in offspring of Chernobyl accident liquidators. Proc Biol Sci. 2001; 268(1471):1001–5.

21 The Role of Pre-stenting for Ureteroscopy

Samih Al-Hayek and Timothy D. Averch

Introduction

Many authors have investigated the role of ureteric stents after ureteroscopy. However, only few studies have evaluated the use of pre-stenting. This is defined as the insertion of a ureteral stent, by a separate procedure, prior to undertaking a planned ureteroscopy. This chapter discusses the advantages, disadvantages, and technical aspects of placing a stent before ureteroscopy.

Indications and Principles of the Ureteral Stent Effect

Early studies have shown that an indwelling stent causes reversible ureteral dilatation but the mechanism is not well understood [1–3]. It was reported that ureteric contractions are reduced in a stented porcine model. After 6 weeks of stenting, there were incomplete contractions and the ureter had lost its ability to respond to diuresis, which would normally increase the frequency and strength of contractions [4].

This principle led some urologists to stent tight ureters after unsuccessful ureteroscopy to facilitate subsequent ureteric manipulation for stone treatment [5]. Theoretically, a wider ureter can accommodate a larger ureteric access sheath, which in turn could provide better irrigation, better view and removal of larger stone fragments allowing for better success and shorter operative time. This can potentially minimize ureteric injury. Ureteropelvic junction (UPJ) would also become wider allowing easier stone retrieval with baskets.

In many cases, stents are placed in emergency circumstances as a temporary measure to relieve acute obstruction, infection, or uncontrolled pain due to stones. Ureteroscopy or extracorporeal shock wave lithotripsy (ESWL) could then be applied to treat the stone(s) electively at a later date making use of the advantages that are mentioned above.

Advantages of Pre-stenting

Effect on Ureteroscopy Success, Stone-Free Rate, and Reoperation Rate

The first reported benefit of pre-stenting was in 1990 by Jones et al. [5], where they placed a stent in failed rigid ureteroscopy (9.5–11 Fr) for ureteric stones. Out of 42 failed cases, 30 had stent placed for 2–4 weeks and 12 did not. Stone size was comparable between the two groups. Subsequent ureteroscopy was successful in 21 of the 30 stented cases (70%) compared to only 5 of the 12 (42%) non-stented group ($p=0.015$). Two

S. Al-Hayek, M.D., F.R.C.S.(Urol.) (✉)
T.D. Averch, M.D.
Department of Urology, University of Pittsburgh Medical Center, 3471 Fifth Avenue, Kaufmann Building, Suite 700, Pittsburgh, PA 15213, USA
e-mail: salhayek@hotmail.com

M. Monga (ed.), *Ureteroscopy: Indications, Instrumentation & Technique*, Current Clinical Urology, DOI 10.1007/978-1-62703-206-3_21, © Springer Science+Business Media New York 2013

of the pre-stented (6.6%) and 3 (25%) of the non-stented group needed ureterolithotomy.

The same advantage was reported by Rubenstein et al. [6]. The authors compared 36 patients who had been pre-stented to 79 with no stent. Using 6.9 or 7.5 Fr semirigid or flexible ureteroscope, stone clearance was achieved in 67% in the pre-stented and 47% in the non-stented group ($p = 0.048$). Clearance was defined as no residual stones visualized on computed tomography (CT) (79%) or intravenous urography (IVU) with tomography (20%) at a mean follow up of 10 weeks. There was no difference in stone size (31 in total had stones of >9 mm), stone location or number between the two groups. The pre-stenting allowed the use of larger access sheath (14–16 Fr) in 38% of the cases compared to 16% if not stented ($p = 0.003$).

In children, Hubert and Palmer [7] used stents to passively dilate the ureter before ureteroscopy to avoid the need for active dilatation. The authors found that the stent did not only dilate the ureteric orifice but also dilated the whole of the ureter including the known physiological sites of ureteral narrowing (the iliac vessels and UPJ) allowing for complete evaluation of the entire ureter successfully. Active dilatation of the ureter using balloon or rigid dilators in children has been reported to cause vesico-ureteral reflux and stricture formation of the ureteric orifice [8–10].

Chu et al. compared 45 pre-stented cases with 59 matched non-stented cohort. Inserting a stent before ureteroscopy improved the stone-free rate [11]. However, the difference did not reach statistical significance ($p = 0.83$). Stone-free rate (SFR) was defined as no residual fragment >2 mm on ultrasound scan (USS) or plain kidney ureters and bladder (KUB) X-ray. Those who were pre-stented for stone burden of ≥1 cm had significantly lower reoperation rate ($p = 0.001$). The difference was more apparent for proximal ureteric ($p = 0.02$) or renal stones ($p = 0.03$).

In another recent study by Lumma et al. [12], 474 patients underwent 550 ureteroscopies using semirigid and flexible ureterorenoscopes. 486 were pre-stented and 64 were not. Stone-free rate (SFR) defined as no stones on KUB or IVU was dependent on stone size. The pre-stented patients had higher clearance rate but only for mid, proximal or renal stones at 67.1% compared to 34.5% for non-stented group. They concluded that pre-stenting is not indicated for distal ureteric stones.

Shields et al. [13] reviewed 150 pre-stented and 71 non-stented patients who underwent rigid and or flexible ureteroscopy for urolithiasis. Stones were comparable at 1.3 and 1.2 cm in pre-stented and non-stented patients, respectively. Although there was a tendency to have a higher SFR in the pre-stented cohort compared to the non-stented (88.7% vs. 83.1%), this was not statistically significant ($p = 0.25$). SFR was defined as no stones on CT and KUB during the 12 weeks postoperative follow-up period except for punctate (1 mm) in renal papillae. The pre-stenting had allowed more use of ureteric access sheaths (57% compared to 35% in the pre-stented and non-stented cohort, respectively, $p = 0.002$).

Some other authors mentioned briefly the effect of having a stent prior to ureteroscopy but did not look into it in detail. Fabrisio et al. [14] reported that pre-stented ureters were more dilated but did not state if that had any effect on success rate and they had not reported the stone size. Hollenbeck et al. [15] compared the success rate of ureteroscopy for stones above and below the pelvic brim. The authors reported that pre-stented patients were less likely to need ureteral dilatation but no statistical analysis had been performed. Perlmutter et al. [16] found that pre-stenting had dilated the ureter allowing for better success rate when treating renal stones ureteroscopically but no further details were given.

Effect on Operative Time

Two studies reported on the effect of having a stent prior to ureteroscopy on the operative time. In the previously mentioned studies, Chu et al. [11] measured the operative time of first ureteroscopy (OTFU) by dividing the operative duration by the stone size. Pre-stented group had significantly shorter OTFU at 93.3 min compared to 123.6 min in the non-stented patients ($p = 0.008$). Total operative time was also compared. This included the time for ureteral stent placement as a separate procedure. The total operative time was significantly shorter in pre-stented patients when stone burden was >1 cm (148.5 vs. 256.7 in presented and non-stented patients, respectively, $p=0.01$). The duration was not significantly different if the stone was 1 cm or less. Median time for stent placement was 10.2 min.

Lumma et al. [12] found that being pre-stented extended the operative time by 4.9 min (43.3 for pre-stented compared to 38.4 min in non-stented). They attributed the difference to the time needed to remove the stent before performing the ureteroscopy. However, only 31 out of the 550 (5.6%) had stones of >1 cm.

Effect of Pre-stenting on Complication Rate

Pre-stenting did not seem to affect the complication rate [6, 17]. Hubert and Palmer [7] reported no side effects in pre-stented children and no significant stent side effects that required the need for anti-cholinergics.

However, Lumma et al. [12] reported that pre-stenting has reduced the complications when treating mid, proximal ureteric, and renal stones. The complication rate was 17.2% in non-stented compared to 7.2% in pre-stented group. Pre-stenting did not affect the complication rates when dealing with distal ureteric stones and if anything, complications tended to be slightly higher (3.5% and 3.1% in pre-stented and non-stented cases, respectively). Ureteric perforation was observed in 13 of 486 (2.7%) pre-stented patients and in 6 of 64 (9.4%) non-stented cohort.

Effect of Pre-stenting on Cost

To our knowledge, there is only one study that reported on the implication of pre-stenting on cost-effectiveness. Chu et al. [17] reviewed 45 pre-stented ureteroscopy cases and compared them to 59 matched non-stented cohort. The stent procedure was done either in the operating room or in the office under local anesthesia. The surgeon fees, the anesthesia base cost, the staff cost, and the operating room reimbursements were calculated. The patient costs associated with lost work-days were also estimated. The total healthcare cost of pre-stented patients included the cost of the pre-ureteroscopy stenting procedure.

The median cost in patients with <1 cm was $12,344 and $10,872 ($p=0.006$) in the pre-stented and non-stented groups, respectively. However, for stone burden of >1 cm, the cost was $17,706 and $27,806 ($p=0.03$) in the pre-stented and non-stented patients, respectively. This indicated that placement of stent before undertaking ureteroscopy is cost effective when treating stones of >1 cm. Pre-stenting, however, increased the cost when used in the treatment for stones of <1 cm.

Disadvantages of Pre-stenting

It seems that pre-stenting has several advantages. However, it is not commonly practiced. This might be due to the inconvenience of having to undertake two procedures, one for the stent and one to deal with the stone(s). However, the stent procedure is usually done with sedation and as a day case, therefore having a minimum impact on the patients' activities.

The main reason for avoiding pre-stenting is due to the stents' side effects. Side effects have been reported to range widely and differ from one patient to another. In a study by Joshi et al. [18], 62 of 85 patients (73%) completed a validated [19] ureteral stent symptoms questionnaire (USSQ). Of those, 78% reported bothersome urinary symptoms including frequency, urgency, dysuria, incontinence, and hematuria. More than 80% of the patients reported pain affecting their daily activities. Nearly a third of the patients (32%) reported sexual dysfunction and 58% reported reduced work capacity. In the same study, comparative health status and cost utility analysis was undertaken using the EuroQol questionnaire [20]. This showed significantly reduced patient satisfaction with the treatment following stent insertion.

Technical Aspects: What Stent, What Size, and How Long for?

With the limited data about use of stents before ureteroscopy, little is reported about the ideal duration to keep the stent in before undertaking the actual ureteroscopy procedure, the type of stent to use, the size and whether to perform the procedure under general (GA), or local anesthetic (LA).

Jones et al. [5], who first reported on using a stent before ureteroscopy, used 5–7 Fr polytetrafluorethylene stents. They kept the stent for 2–4 weeks. Hubert and Palmer [7] used 4.8 Fr double J stent for their pediatric population. They left the stent in for a period of 2–8 weeks (median of 3 weeks). Lumma et al. [12] used size 6 Fr but no comments made about the type or the duration. The procedure was done under sedation. Rubenstein [6] mentioned that the stent procedure was done under GA but no mention to the size, type, or the duration of the stent. Shields [13] used size 6–8.5 Fr stents. The stent was left for a minimum of 2 weeks but the maximum duration was not stated. Chu et al. [11] reported a wide range of how long the stent was kept in (7–67 weeks with median of 19.5 weeks). This was attributed to the fact that outside urologists placed some of these stents. Few weeks lapsed for the patients to be referred and scheduled for definitive ureteroscopy. The stents pre-placed by the authors were done under Monitored Anesthesia Care (MAC), approximately 2 weeks before the planned ureteroscopy.

How Common Is Pre-stenting in Clinical Practice?

The small number of reports regarding pre-stenting makes it difficult to determine how common this has been used in practice. A survey was conducted by Auge et al. [21] to investigate the practice pattern for stent placement after routine ureteroscopy for stone surgery. The survey showed that stent placement before ureteroscopic stone surgery was uncommon. 76.2% reported pre-stenting in 10% of the time or less. This practice is less common among young urologists who have recently completed their residency. None of the urologists with fewer than 2 years of experience performed pre-stenting. 2% of the urologists with 2–10 years of experience used pre-stenting, while 10% of those with more than 10 years of experience pre-stented more than 50% of the time.

Summary and Conclusions

Taking into account the small number of published studies, most authors reported benefit from pre-stenting in allowing access to ureteral and renal stones after failed ureteroscopy. This applies to both adults and children. Some centers showed general improvement in stone-free rates. Others showed improvement in specific groups such as mid, proximal, and renal but not distal ureteric stones. Two studies showed tendency to improve the stone clearance but did not reach statistical significance. A contributing problem may be that authors used different criteria to define stone free and relied on different investigations to confirm this including KUB, USS, IVU, or CT.

Other benefits of pre-stenting were reduced operative time and the reduction in the need for reoperation in patients with a stone burden of >1 cm. This was associated with lower cost compared to non-stented patients. In children, passive dilatation with pre-stenting seems to help avoid the risk of developing ureteral stricture or reflux that could result from active dilatation.

Pre-stenting did not seem to be associated with increased complications. Authors tended not to report on the side effect from the stents except in the pediatric population where the authors commented that children tolerated the stent well with no need for medications.

Unfortunately, there was not enough data to determine the ideal duration of keeping the stent in before undertaking the therapeutic procedure for the stone but all authors kept the stent for minimum of 2 weeks. Also, there was no agreement on stent size or type.

In conclusion, placing a stent is indicated when ureteroscopy fails due to a narrow ureteric orifice or difficult access. This passively dilates the ureter and seems to improve the stone-free rate, especially in more proximal stones. The benefit extends to a shorter operative time and less cost in the presence of large stone burden.

References

1. Wiseman JL. Observations of the stimulating influence of temporary rubber splinting on regeneration following ureteral resection. Br J Urol. 1934;6:11–6.
2. Drake WM, Carroll J, Bartone L, et al. Evaluation of materials used as ureteral splints. Surg Gynecol Obstet. 1962;114:47–57.
3. Weinberg SL. Ureteral, function 11. The ureteral catheter and the ureterometrogram. Invest Urol. 1985;12:255.
4. Kinn AC, Lykkeskov-Andersen H. Impact on ureteral peristalsis in a stented ureter: an experimental study in the pig. Urol Res. 2002;30:213–8.
5. Jones BJ, Ryan PC, Lyons O, et al. Use of the double pigtail stent in stone retrieval following unsuccessful ureteroscopy. Br J Urol. 1990;66:254–6.
6. Rubenstein RA, Zhao LC, Loeb S, et al. Prestenting improves ureteroscopic stone-free rates. J Endourol. 2007;21:1277.
7. Hubert KC, Palmer JS. Passive dilation by ureteral stenting before ureteroscopy: eliminating the need for active dilation. J Urol. 2005;174:1079–80. discussion 1080.
8. Bassiri A, Ahmadnia H, Darabi MR, Yonessi M. Transureteral lithotripsy in pediatric practice. J Endourol. 2002;16:257.
9. Jayanthi VR, Arnold PM, Koff SA. Strategies for managing upper tract calculi in young children. J Urol. 1999;162:1234.
10. Busaidy SS, Prem AR, Medhat M. Paediatric ureteroscopy for ureteric calculi: a 4-year experience. Br J Urol. 1997;80:797.
11. Chu L, Sternberg KM, Averch TD. Preoperative stenting decreases operative time and reoperative rates of ureteroscopy. J Endourol. 2011;25(5):751–4.
12. Lumma PP, Schneider P, Strauss A, Plothe KD, Thelen P, Ringert RH, Loertzer H. Impact of ureteral stenting prior to ureterorenoscopy on stone-free rates and complications. World J Urol. 2011; Oct 29.
13. Shields JM, Bird VG, Reid G, et al. Impact of preoperative ureteral stenting on outcome of ureteroscopic treatment for urinary lithiasis. J Urol. 2009;182: 2768–74.
14. Fabrizio MD, Behari A, Bagley DH. Ureteroscopic management of intrarenal calculi. J Urol. 1998;159: 1139.
15. Hollenbeck BK, Schuster TG, Faerber GJ, et al. Comparison of outcomes of ureteroscopy for ureteral calculi located above and below the pelvic brim. Urology. 2001;68:351.
16. Perlmutter AE, Talug C, Tarry WF, et al. Impact of stone location on success rates of endoscopic lithotripsy for nephrolithiasis. J Urol. 2007;71:214.
17. Chu L, Farris CA, Corcoran AT, Averch TD. Preoperative stent placement decreases cost of ureteroscopy. Urology. 2011;78(2):309–13.
18. Joshi HB, Stainthorpe A, MacDonagh RP, et al. Indwelling ureteral stents: evaluation of symptoms, quality of life and utility. J Urol. 2003;169:1065.
19. Joshi HB, Newns N, Stainthorpe A, et al. Ureteral stent symptom questionnaire: development and validation of a multidimensional quality of life measure. J Urol. 2003;169:1060.
20. EuroQol—a new facility for the measurement of health-related quality of life. The EuroQol Group. Health Policy. 1990;16(3):199–208.
21. Auge BK, Sarvis JA, L'Esperance JO, et al. Practice patterns of ureteral stenting after routine ureteroscopic stone surgery: a survey of practice urologists. J Endourol. 2007;21:1287.

Semirigid Ureteroscopy: The Cleveland Clinic Approach

22

Mark J. Noble and Wahib E. Isac

This chapter contains video segments that can be found on the accompanying DVD

Introduction

The original, rigid ureteroscope pioneered the ability to endoscopically remove ureteral stones in a minimally invasive fashion. These first instruments were modeled after the design of rigid cysto-panendoscopes but were longer and narrower, in the 10–12 F range. Thus, they utilized a rod lens system to transfer the image from the tip of the scope to the eyepiece, and significant bending or deflection of the instrument usually resulted in a "half-moon" eclipsing of the endoscopic image and at times cracking of the optics with subsequent need to rebuild and repair the telescope [1–3].

Hence, the semirigid ureteroscope utilizing fiber optic bundles, which are fairly flexible, provided the ability to manufacture a rigid scope that could be bent to some degree without damage, in order to traverse bends in the course of the urethra, the lower ureter, and even the upper ureter in favorable circumstances [4]. This proved a major advance in rigid ureteroscopic design and is commonly used today. Another advance was the incorporation of a digital chip into the tip of the instrument, thus dispensing with the fiber optic bundles entirely, and lightening the lens (or surgeon's) end of the instrument since no camera would be connected any longer, as it can now be built into the leading end or tip of the scope [5]. Finally, we are seeing thinner diameter ureteroscopes that often fit through a ureteral orifice without the need to first dilate the orifice. This enables a quicker, less traumatic procedure.

Indications

Ureteroscopy is indicated in the diagnosis and treatment of ureteral and renal calculi [6], neoplasms [7–9], stricture or other ureteric obstructions, unexplained hematuria, removal of migrated ureteral stents or other foreign bodies, and ureteral fistula [4, 10–17]. While commonly used in adults, ureteroscopy is also applicable to patients in the pediatric population as a primary intervention for ureteral and at least some renal calculi [18–24].

While early reports show reasonably successful outcomes using ureteroscopy with ultrasound guidance (no fluoroscopy was used) for treatment of acute ureteral calculi during pregnancy (≅70% success, with some stones simply pushed back into the kidney followed by stenting and delayed treatment after delivery), more recent papers reveal improved success for ureteroscopy during pregnancy (≅90% success), probably due to

M.J. Noble, M.D. (✉)
Surgery Division, Urology Department, Glickman Urologic Institute, Cleveland Clinic, 9500 Euclid Avenue, Cleveland, OH 44195, USA
e-mail: noblem@ccf.org

W.E. Isac, M.D.
Urology Department, Minimally Invasive Surgery, Cleveland Clinic Foundation, Cleveland, OH, USA

M. Monga (ed.), *Ureteroscopy: Indications, Instrumentation & Technique*, Current Clinical Urology, DOI 10.1007/978-1-62703-206-3_22, © Springer Science+Business Media New York 2013

refinements in ureteroscopic instruments [25–27]. Some therefore consider ureteroscopic stone intervention a plausible first-line therapy during pregnancy, based on these results.

If a patient is morbidly obese, such that technical factors and/or medical risk factors preclude shock-wave lithotripsy or percutaneous access to the urinary tract (i.e., the need for continuous anticoagulants), then ureteroscopy becomes the preferred intervention for treatment of stones and certain other lesions in the urinary tract, within the practical limitations of the ureteroscopic instrumentation that is currently available. As technology enables further refinement of ureteroscopic instrumentation, it is conceivable the "envelope" will be pushed further in terms of what is possible with ureteroscopy.

Semirigid vs. Flexible Ureteroscopy

Why would a urologic surgeon sometimes prefer a semirigid instrument to a flexible one? In what instances might a semirigid ureteroscope be more advantageous? For what diseases are these ureteroscopes best suited? To answer these questions, it is necessary to directly compare the flexible and rigid instruments in a functional way. For the next several paragraphs, please refer to data in Table 22.1 describing currently available semirigid ureteroscopes and their specifications [28, 29].

Consider: A semirigid ureteroscope is self-supporting due to a strong, thin-walled, metal outer tube that encloses the components of the telescope. It only needs to include a working channel and fiber bundles (to transmit light and an image). However, a flexible ureteroscope must in addition contain a deflection mechanism (whose cable occupies space within the instrument). Also, the flexible jacket of the device requires bendable, reinforcing layers that tend to be thicker than the metal comprising a semirigid telescope; without reinforcing layers, the flexible ureteroscope might wear out (fatigue) too quickly from repeated flexing and extending. In this vein, a semirigid instrument might be expected to have a narrower outer diameter than a flexible one. In reality, most are at least as thick, and they utilize their additional space within to contain a larger working channel, a greater number of optical fibers, or both.

While smaller sizes and newer designs are continually being developed and might be in production at the time of publication of this treatise, flexible ureteroscopes today are between 5.3 and 7.5 F (outer diameter of the tip), while adult semirigid ureteroscopes are between 4.5 and 8.4 F tip diameter [5].

But the above sizes are somewhat misleading; the tip of the smallest currently available semirigid ureteroscope (the Richard Wolf Model 8701 "Needle Ureteroscope") actually describes the size of the absolute tip of the scope, including the lens, but excluding the bevel (beak) which contains the working/irrigation 3 F channel; just a few millimeters from the tip, the slope of the beak augments the total diameter to 6.5 F [30]. In contrast, the Olympus flexible ureteroscope (URF-P5) is truly 5.3 F diameter for a significant portion of the instrument's length [31]. Both designs become thicker, as one progresses from the tip to the ocular, in order to provide more support and durability for the instrument. In addition, the semirigid scopes usually have a 5–12° look-down angle at the usually beveled tip of the scope, while the flexible scope tends to view straight ahead (0° angle).

Most manufacturers of semirigid ureteroscopes provide a choice of two lengths, 33 and 43 cm, enabling the urologist to pick the scope most appropriate to the task at hand. A short, semirigid scope might be better in a female; when one combines the length of the urethra with the distance from the vesical neck to the ureteral orifice, and then the ureteral length itself (up to the uretero-pelvic junction), it would be rare for the total distance to exceed 33 cm. However, for the male patient, the length of the urethra, plus the distance from the vesical neck to the ureteral orifice, and of course adding the length of the ureter, one might need a 43 cm long ureteroscope

Table 22.1 Specifications and comparison of some currently available semirigid ureteroscopes[a]

Company	Stryker	Storz	Olympus	Olympus	Wolf	Wolf	Gyrus/ACMI	Gyrus/ACMI
Scope name/series	SRU-6/SRU6X	27001K/L	OES 4000 dual	OES pro single	E-Line offset/ultrathin	Needle	Bagley	Slimline
Working length	33/43 cm	34/43 cm	33/43 cm	33/43 cm	31/43 cm	31/43 cm	33/43 cm	33/43 cm
Tapered shaft	Yes	Yes	Yes	Yes	Yes	Yes	Yes	Yes
Tip size	6.9Fr	7/8Fr	7.5Fr	6.4Fr	6/8Fr	4.5Fr	6.9Fr	7/7.7Fr
Pixel quantity	30,000	N/A	N/A	50,000	20,000/50,000	N/A	N/A	N/A
Eyepiece	Straight	Offers both	Offers both	Offers both	Angled	Angled	Straight	Angled
Single/dual channel	Dual	Single	Dual	Single	Single	Single	Dual	Single
Working channel size(s)	3.4/2.5Fr	5Fr	N/A	6.4Fr	4/5Fr	3.4Fr	3.4/2.3Fr	5.4Fr
Direction of view	12°	6°	7°	7°	5°/12°	5°	5°	5°

N/A = Specification not available

[a]Data obtained via personal communications and on-line listed specifications of various semirigid ureteroscopes

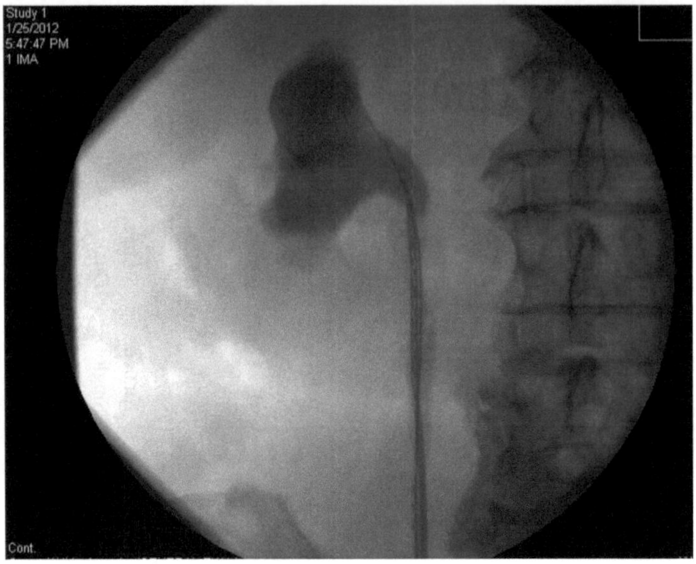

Fig. 22.1 A semirigid ureteroscope was easily passed alongside a safety guide wire in order to treat an acquired uretero-pelvic junction stricture in this patient. The instrument can be seen in the lower renal pelvis after the stricture was opened with a laser; contrast was instilled through the scope and there was only slight extravasation as contrast passed down the ureter alongside the ureteroscope

unless one is only working in the distal portion of the ureter. Figure 22.1 depicts a semirigid ureteroscope that was easily advanced to the patient's right uretero-pelvic junction (UPJ); such is usually possible in patients with normal anatomy and whose psoas muscles are not unduly bulky.

Flexible ureteroscopes are approximately 54–70 cm long, and this enables the surgeon to reach fully into all branches of the renal collecting system, even in a male patient with morbid obesity. But the surgeon usually sees better with a semirigid ureteroscope than with a flexible scope under most conditions. The optical resolution is nearly always better (30–50,000 pixels vs. 3–6,000 pixels, although the "chip on the tip" flexible scopes may correct this discrepancy in the next 3–5 years) [28, 32, 33], and the saline irrigant tends to flow more quickly, due to larger working channels (3.6 F for most flexible ureteroscopes vs. 4.5 F for most semirigid ureteroscopes); both factors can help with difficult situations such as active bleeding, compared to a flexible scope.

Introduction of a flexible ureteroscope is possible, even without a wire, but it tends to be difficult for those surgeons not practiced with such techniques. If a stone is fairly distal in the ureter, manipulation of a flexible ureteroscope can be difficult due to lack of purchase; i.e., the very nature of the flexible scope can allow buckling to occur, with subsequent loss of access into the ureter (Fig. 22.2). A semirigid ureteroscope provides its own inherent stability, and one thus has greater control over the tip, and consequent treatment of a stone or other lesion, while working in the lower ureter (Fig. 22.3).

This author has had several instances performing laser lithotripsy where the unexpected happened: A Holmium:YAG laser failed in the midst of ureteral stone fragmentation during semirigid ureteroscopy, and no substitute laser device was immediately available. One option would have been to place a stent and complete the procedure another day, or keep the patient under anesthesia until another laser could be secured (>1 h delay). However, a Lithoclast was available and the procedure was safely completed using that device. Though laser is sometimes more effective and has a lower complication rate, pneumatic lithotripsy is still a reasonably safe alternative [12–17]. Due to limited flexibility of the pneumatic wire, the Lithoclast cannot currently be used with flexible ureteroscopes or with semirigid ureteroscopes lacking a straight-entry working channel.

A semirigid ureteroscope becomes difficult to use in a patient whose pelvic floor lacks elasticity. A patient with advanced cancer in the pelvis, one who has scar tissue from previous pelvic

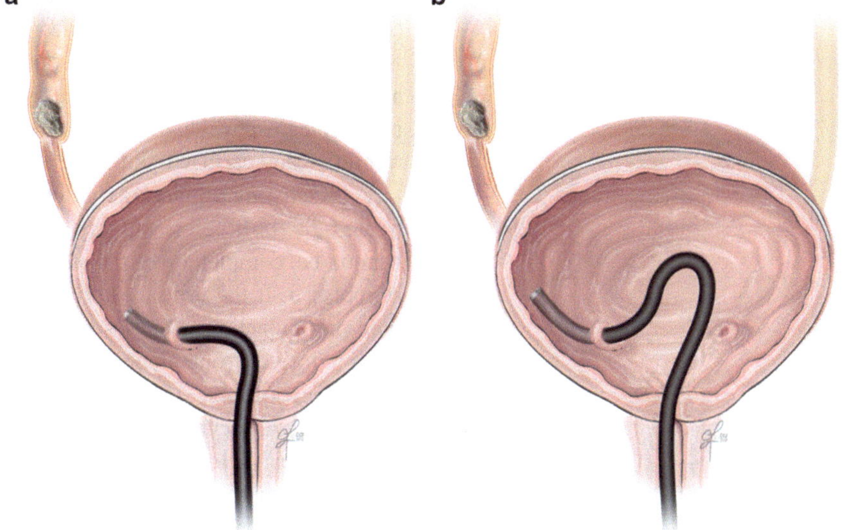

Fig. 22.2 This illustrates the sometimes encountered difficulty stabilizing a flexible ureteroscope when treating a distal ureteral calculus; pushing on the instrument may result in curling within the bladder rather than advancement of the device up the ureter, so control is thus limited in these instances

surgery, or one who has received previous pelvic radiation with subsequent fixation of organs and tissues, can prove more challenging for insertion of a semirigid ureteroscope. If one cannot pass the instrument initially, but the surgeon still wishes to utilize a semirigid rather than flexible ureteroscope, there are two "tricks" this author has found helpful at times. The first is to insert the semirigid instrument over a stiff glide wire, or even over an Amplatz Super-Stiff Guidewire. The wire helps direct the tip of the instrument and the stiffer wires tend to "straighten out" the angles and thus facilitate passage. One can also adjust the angle and/or position of one or both legs of the patient; sometimes this "straightens" the ureter as it relaxes the psoas and other muscles [34].

Interestingly, a semirigid ureteroscope can be utilized successfully in situations where angulation and/or tortuosity might be thought to totally preclude ureteral access. For example, a patient with prior surgery to correct vesico-ureteral reflux, as with the Cohen cross-trigonal technique, can usually undergo successful semirigid ureteroscopy despite the altered anatomy, if one uses a ureteral balloon dilating catheter (Uromax®, Boston Scientific, Inc.), the controlled expansion, stiff (when inflated under pressure) balloon usually eliminates curves and angles, thus permitting a straighter path even after deflation, and thus enabling passage of a semirigid ureteroscope [4, 35]. This technique can be applied to renal allograft transplant ureters (i.e., ones implanted in the dome or lateral bladder wall) as well [36, 37].

Semirigid ureteroscopy would be difficult (but not always impossible) when accessing the lower ureter through a bladder substitute (ileal conduit, Studor or Indiana Pouch, etc.). Such access is easier with a flexible ureteroscope and in many instances, requires antegrade insertion of a guidewire through a nephrostomy puncture, in order to instrument the ureter in a retrograde manner in patients with these types of anatomic alterations [38].

Patient Preparation, Set-Up, and Equipment

Patients should be prepared for ureteroscopy as for any surgical procedure that requires anesthesia. A complete history and physical examination

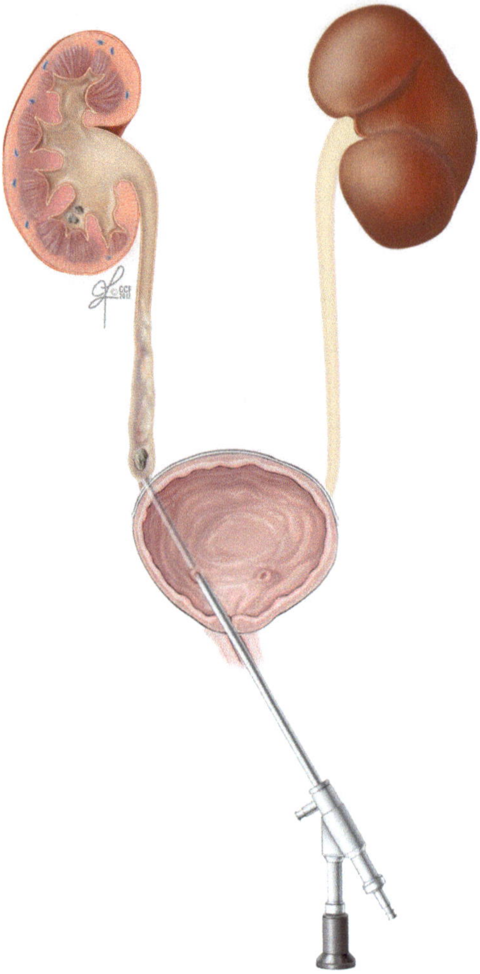

Fig. 22.3 A semirigid ureteroscope is self-stabilizing when used to access a lower third ureteral stone, and thus the tip can be readily controlled, in contrast to a flexible ureteroscope (previous illustration)

should be obtained, and pertinent laboratory studies are usually ordered (a complete blood count and at least a basic chemistry, plus urinalysis). If the urinalysis shows pyuria, bacteriuria, positive nitrite, or otherwise is suggestive of a urinary tract infection, then a urine culture should be requested reporting *any* growth of uropathogens. Standard informed consent is obtained as per any surgical procedure, commensurate with the rules for the institution where the ureteroscopy is to be performed.

In select cases (patients with symptoms and/or comorbid medical conditions that increase the likelihood of heart disease), an electrocardiogram (EKG) should be ordered if one was not done within the preceding 6 months, and any major abnormalities should be addressed by the patient's primary care physician, or by a cardiologist, to minimize any cardiac risk for surgery.

A preexisting urinary tract infection should be treated 24–48 h before surgery, or if bacteriuria cannot be completely eliminated, it should be suppressed. If the urine is sterile preoperatively, then prophylactic antibiotics should be administered before instrumentation of the upper urinary tract, according to the current American Urological Association (AUA) Guidelines [39]. In most cases, such will consist of a fluoroquinolone (FQL) or trimethoprim-sulfa (TMP-SMX), given with a sip of water an hour before surgery, or intravenously, so-as to enable adequate blood and urine levels before instrumentation. For patients allergic to these antibiotics, an aminoglycoside with a cell-wall inhibitor (i.e., a penicillin-type drug, a cephalosporin, or vancomycin) will provide good coverage of most uropathogens.

When a patient has had a joint replacement within the previous 2 years, when a patient is immunosuppressed (i.e., on chemotherapy, HIV positive, etc.), or when a patient has a prosthetic heart valve, he/she may be more susceptible to infection either of their implanted prosthetic device, or to urosepsis, so attention to the AUA Guidelines for Antimicrobial Prophylaxis is strongly recommended [39]. Anticoagulants are not routinely stopped prior to diagnostic ureteroscopy or laser lithotripsy of ureteral stones at our institution, but they might require temporary cessation if tissue is to be incised [40, 41].

Except in cases of pregnancy, fluoroscopy is routinely used for guidance of guidewires, ureteroscopic instruments, and stents during the procedure. Personnel should wear adequate protective coverage, including lead aprons, and the operating room should contain lead shielding in its walls and door(s). The operating surgeon(s) should additionally use protective eyewear (leaded glasses) if performing a high-volume of fluoroscopic procedures, as cataracts are a long-term risk after recurrent radiation exposure to one's eyes [42, 43].

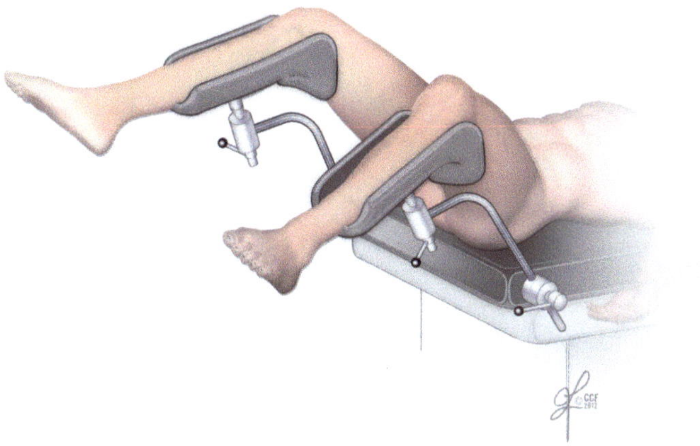

Fig. 22.4 The dorsal lithotomy position allows good access to the genitalia and facilitates semirigid ureteroscopy. This author finds nearly all patients can have suitable access with the semirigid instrument, without extending, lowering, or modifying leg position. Frozen hip and/or knee joints interfere with this patient position and would necessitate either a flexible ureteroscopic or percutaneous approach to the ureter

The patient should normally be in the dorsal lithotomy position (Fig. 22.4) or a modified dorsal lithotomy position where the ipsilateral leg (to the side being operated upon) is lowered and extended [44]. This latter position has been found by some to make the semirigid ureteroscopy easier and faster; it is thought that the ureter is better aligned for insertion of the instrument. The patient should not be able to move during insertion of a semirigid ureteroscope, as sudden patient movement could result in perforation or other complications. Thus, a good degree of muscle relaxation with general anesthesia or an adequate level of spinal or epidural anesthesia (with motor block) is preferred, although it has been reported that one can perform semirigid ureteroscopy under local anesthesia in very select patients [45].

A routine cystoscopy/panendoscopy set-up (flexible or rigid) is arranged on a sterile field with standard drapes and the following additional items: The surgeon's preferred guide wires, 50 ml or more of radiographic contrast, an open-ended ureteral catheter (usually 5 or 6 F size), a 12 or 14 F foley catheter, 10 and 20 ml syringes, and a pressure irrigation system with room temperature or body temperature saline. A single-action pump system or a pressure bag surrounding the saline for irrigation is the most commonly used methods for pressure irrigation through the ureteroscope. At our institution, we have not found any observable difference in outcome with room temperature saline vs. warmed (body temperature) saline for irrigation.

The length and size/type of ureteroscope should be appropriate to the location of the stone (or lesion) and the patient's anatomy. A video camera imaging system is almost mandatory; otherwise, the surgeon must be a "contortionist" to keep his or her eye at the ocular end of the semirigid ureteroscope while advancing it into the lower ureter. Further, a camera system facilitates teaching, permits an assistant to better coordinate manipulation of a basket or other instrument, and keeps the operator's face away from the ureteroscope's working port, thus reducing the possibility of being sprayed in the face with a mixture of saline and the patient's bodily fluids. It is more helpful if the video monitor and fluoroscopy monitor can be in close proximity, but as long as they are both easily visible for the urologic surgeon while performing the procedure, they will be adequate to the task at hand.

Technique

With the patient prepped and draped in the dorsal lithotomy position, standard cystourethroscopy is performed and the anatomic landmarks delineated. Assuming no preexisting ureteral stent is

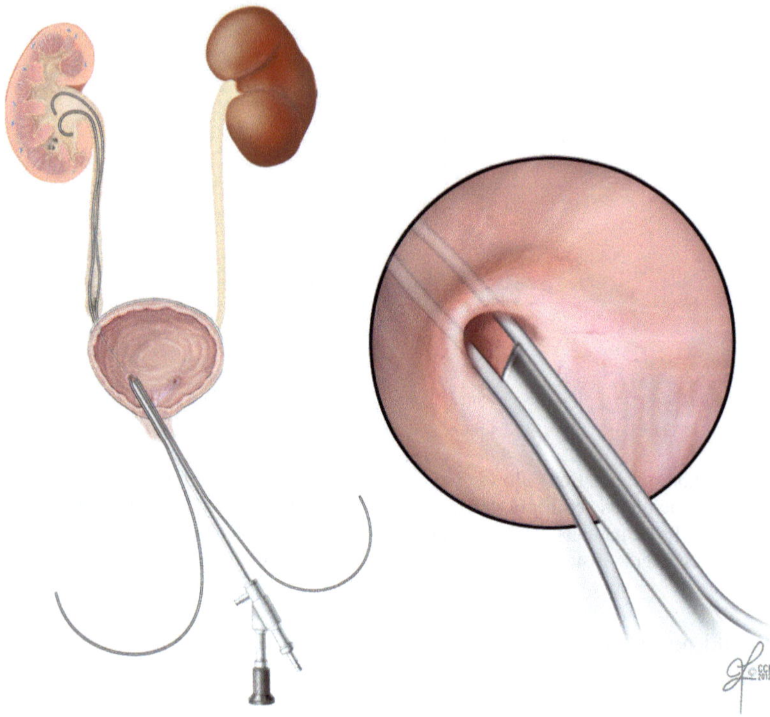

Fig. 22.5 The semirigid ureteroscope is advanced between two wires into the ureteral orifice ("Ladder Technique")

in place, the ureteral orifice of interest is cannulated with a 5 Fr open-ended ureteral catheter and retrograde pyelography is performed using radiographic contrast (Renografin-60®, Conray-60®, Ultravist-300®, Isovue-300®, or equivalent) diluted 50:50 with sterile water or normal saline. This will verify the location of the stone(s) and demonstrate the presence of stricture or other lesions that might affect the surgeon's ability to safely insert the semirigid ureteroscope. If the patient is morbidly obese, sometimes it is necessary to dilute the contrast less, or even to use undiluted contrast, just to properly see the ureter on the fluoroscope (not usually an issue with newer, more powerful fluoroscopes that have improved resolution but sometimes necessary with older units).

A 0.035″ stiff-shaft glide wire is then advanced through the ureteral catheter into the renal collecting system using fluoroscopic guidance. The cysto-panendoscope and ureteral catheter are both removed over the wire, leaving the wire in place. Usually with semirigid ureteroscopy, only one wire is needed as a safety, so this wire is clipped to the drapes as a safety wire. Should a second wire be needed for the "ladder technique" or some other purpose, a dual lumen catheter may be placed over the wire and a second, identical wire advanced through the second lumen using fluoroscopic guidance, the dual lumen catheter is removed over the two wires, and one wire is clipped to the drapes as a safety wire. The second wire can be used as a "working wire" to pass a balloon dilating catheter or even to pass the ureteroscope. Or, it can also be clipped to the drapes as a second safety or stabilizing wire, permitting the ureteroscope to be passed between the two glide wires into the distal ureter, as shown in Fig. 22.5 ("ladder technique").

If a preexisting ureteral stent is present, then using graspers through the cystoscope, the stent is brought out to the urethral meatus and cannulated with a 0.035″ stiff-shaft glide wire, or other guide wire per surgeon's preference. The stent is exchanged over the wire for a dual lumen ureteral catheter and a retrograde pyelo-ureterogram is performed via the second lumen. Once stone location is verified, a second identical glide wire, if needed, may be advanced through the dual lumen catheter as described above.

There are some surgeons who prefer to pass a safety wire alongside a preexisting stent before removing the stent, fearing possible loss of access if the stent is clogged with debris thus blocking advancement of a wire through the stent. The "alongside" technique usually works well, but on occasion a wire cannot be inserted alongside the stent and the stent must first be removed. This type of problem is sometimes encountered when the stent fits snugly through a tight ureteral stricture or alongside an impacted stone. Regardless, a safety wire is important in virtually all semirigid ureteroscopy cases, as it provides an exit strategy should one need to terminate the procedure prematurely, for any reason.

After one or two wires have been placed, a 12 or 14 F foley catheter is inserted per urethra, the balloon inflated 5 or 10 ml with sterile water, and the foley allowed to drain into the catch pocket of the drapes. This will help keep the bladder decompressed and it also may make it easier to insert the semirigid ureteroscope, especially through the male urethra, provided there are no urethral strictures. The author has observed that placing the foley catheter on slight tension while inserting the ureteroscope into the urethra often helps with its passage into the bladder.

Regardless of whether the patient be male or female, great care should be exercised to avoid creating a false passage in the urethra. The tip of the semirigid ureteroscope is quite tiny, almost sharp, and if the scope is advanced without viewing the lumen of the urethra at all times, it is very easy to make a mucosal tear, a perforation, or a false channel in the urethra. Such may later lead to urethral stricture or other complications and due care and diligence must be used to avoid this mishap. As previously mentioned, a pressure bag surrounding a bag of sterile, normal saline, single action pump, or other suitable device should be used to provide irrigation fluid for the ureteroscope. Should irrigating fluid be absorbed due to a lengthy procedure via pyelovenous or pyelolymphatic backflow, or even perforation, normal saline is far safer than water, glycine solution, or other irrigants.

Once the ureteroscope is in the bladder, the surgeon follows the safety wire(s) to the ureteral orifice. Sometimes, if visualization is obscured due to bleeding, fluoroscopy can help one to direct the tip of the ureteroscope close to the wire(s) and ureteral orifice of interest, thus enabling direct visualization despite bleeding from the prostate or other source. The ureteroscope is advanced under direct vision into the ureteral orifice, alongside the safety wire (or between both wires if the "ladder technique" is utilized with two wires). If only using one wire, sometimes pressing the end of the scope against the wire helps open up the ureteral orifice in order that the tip of the scope may be advanced into the distal ureter. It is also helpful to dim the light source to approximately ¼ or 1/3 strength (if it is not the automatic dimming type). This cuts down on reflectivity within the ureteral lumen and reduces glare.

With modern, tapered, semirigid ureteroscopes, it is rare for a ureteral orifice to be overly narrow and restrict insertion of the ureteroscope into the distal ureter. But on occasion, it is necessary to utilize a balloon dilating catheter (15 F diameter × 4 cm or 10 cm length Uromax®, Boston Scientific, or equivalent), to enlarge the ureteral orifice sufficiently in order to insert the ureteroscope. It is important when doing this not to advance the balloon past the ureteral stone or lesion of interest. Otherwise, expanding the balloon might compress such into (or even through) the wall of the ureter and this makes it much more difficult to treat. Sometimes a complete perforation might ensue, obviously an undesirable endpoint.

Once the ureteroscope is advanced up the ureter, the stone (or tumor, or other lesion of note) can be visualized and treated. A stone, if impacted, would ordinarily be fragmented using a Holmium® laser (fiber diameter 200 or 365 μm) with power setting at 8–10 W. Once the pieces are small enough, they can be removed using a stone basket or other suitable device to seize one or several fragments, then backing the ureteroscope out of the ureter into the bladder, then releasing them into the bladder lumen. The fragments can be irrigated out of the bladder at the end of the procedure and can be ignored for the time-being. The ureteroscope is reintroduced and additional fragments retrieved to the bladder, and so forth, until all stone pieces have been cleared. "Blow-back" up the ureter all the way into the kidney is rarely a problem for stones being fragmented in the distal one-third of the ureter, though it is not uncommon for more proximal stones, and it would be difficult to retrieve these without switching to a flexible ureteroscope.

Results

Stone clearance rates in the past decade using semirigid ureteroscopes have generally improved, and complication rates have decreased, compared with reports from the initial years when rigid and semirigid ureteroscopy commenced as a minimally invasive procedure. Possibly these improvements are due to better instrumentation, more years of experience, a combination of the two, or perhaps one or more other factors. But as can be seen in Table 22.2, there has been a noticeable improvement in stone clearance rates over time.

In fact, if one reviews these and other published patient outcomes, the success for distal third ureteral stones in both adults and children using semirigid ureteroscopy, Holmium:YAG or Lithoclast devices, is in the 95–99% range, with rates in the 80–90% for stones in the upper third (and intermediate results for stones in the middle third). Laser lithotripsy generally has a lower complication rate, but due to the lower cost of pneumatic methods, Lithoclast lithotripsy through a semirigid ureteroscope is still utilized in many countries with acceptably low complication rates and good success rates.

One should therefore expect a lower ureteral calculus to be cleared with better than 95% success on the first attempt, using semirigid ureteroscopy as described, and pre-supposing an experienced urologic surgeon who regularly performs the procedure. In our institution, this number is between 98 and 99%, and it is very rare indeed that we need to prematurely halt the procedure, place a stent, and try again a week or two later due to edema, bleeding, or other factors that technically interfere with the success of the procedure.

Table 22.2 Results with semirigid ureteroscopy[a]

Author	Year	# of patients	Complications	Success (%)
Ford, TF [3]	1983	10	Unknown	70
Gelet, A [53]	1985	49	15%	72
Daniels, GF [54]	1988	99	27%	77
Ibarluzea, G [55]	1989	120	Unknown	74
Tello Royloa, C [56]	1992	106	19.7%	85[b]
Hernandez, D [57]	1993	399	5.7–9.0%	85–93[c]
Devarajan, R [58]	1998	265	4.1%	90
Pascual Samaniego, M [59]	2002	354	3.05%	93–99[d]
Satar, N [18]	2004	33[e]	0%	94
Tugcu, V [60]	2006	375	Unknown	96
Hong, YK [17]	2009	341	2.6–4.9%	80–97[f]

[a]Not an all-inclusive list; small percentages in some series included disease entities other than stones
[b]Small percentage were secondary treatments of stones post-ESWL
[c]Greater success in Steinstrasse compared to discrete ureteral calculi
[d]Best results in distal third of ureter, worst in proximal third
[e]Pediatric series, mean age 7.4 years
[f]Best results in distal third of ureter, worst in proximal third

Pitfalls and Complications

The most frequent, major complication of semirigid ureteroscopy is perforation, particularly of the ureter, although this can occur in the urethra or in the bladder (or even in the renal collecting system, if the instrument is used in that location). In one series of 979 patients, semirigid ureteroscopy with pneumatic lithotripsy (Lithoclast device) resulted in a perforation rate of 1.7%, and such complications nearly always could be managed with a long-term (i.e., 6 weeks) indwelling ureteral stent, with an ultimately good result [46].

Another major complication in that series was ureteral avulsion, occurring at a rate of 0.4%. This type of injury usually requires a reconstructive procedure, either a uretero-ureterostomy for upper or mid-ureteral injuries or a ureteral reimplantation (with or without Boari Flap) for distal avulsion, although in one reported case of very distal avulsion, ureteral stenting followed by transurethral resection of necrotic tissue avoided an open (or laparoscopic) procedure and gave a good result [47]. In at least one comparative series of laser lithotripsy vs. pneumatic lithotripsy, the perforation rate was significantly lower with laser lithotripsy, but no direct comparison for avulsion vis-à-vis the two techniques has been reported for any large series [16].

Late stricture formation following semirigid ureteroscopy is estimated to occur in less than 2% of cases, and the rate is most likely even less when the smaller (7.5 F) semirigid instruments are used in contrast to the larger diameter (10 F) instruments [48]. The majority of these strictures can be managed endoscopically, but some might require an open or laparoscopic reconstructive procedure at a later date. In some instances, it is unclear if the stricture resulted from reactive changes and damage due to the ureteral stone, from passage of the ureteroscope, from damage to the ureteral wall, from use of a laser or pneumatic device, or from several of these in combination.

Minor complications for semirigid ureteroscopy include retrograde migration of stone(s), mucosal tears, infection, and/or prolonged bleeding. While more frequent in incidence than the major complications noted above (ranging from 4 to 27%, depending on the series and methodology) [16, 49, 50], nearly all can be managed without an open (or laparoscopic) surgical procedure. An indwelling stent for one or several weeks, a secondary procedure (to treat proximally migrated stones), and/or postoperative use of antibiotics almost always successfully solves such problems.

There are no rigorously performed, objective studies relating to chronic pain syndromes following upper urinary tract instrumentation, but it is the author's experience that such problems are exceedingly rare. Before consigning such patients to the pain management specialists, it is best to be certain no residual stone fragments or other, surgically solvable etiologies exist, even if a repeat endoscopy and/or CT scan is required.

Conclusions

Semirigid ureteroscopy has advanced to the point where this author considers it the procedure of choice for stones and other lesions in the ureter below the pelvic brim (the distal one-third of the ureter). While there is at least one prospective study where shock wave lithotripsy (ESWL) proved as successful [51], one often cannot determine at the time of ESWL if the procedure was completely effective in fragmenting and clearing a stone (whereas one can virtually always know the stone was broken and cleared when it is performed under direct vision), so a patient can avoid such uncertainty by means of a practiced surgeon using a ureteroscope to clear the stone problem.

Semirigid ureteroscopy can be successfully utilized in select instances above the pelvic brim (middle or upper third of the ureter) in many cases as well, provided care is taken with its insertion and manipulation (i.e., one never "forces" the instrument). Its advantages include better optics and better irrigant flow in comparison to most, if not all, flexible ureteroscopes, plus the instrument is more stable, particularly when working in the lowermost ureter. Although not referenced, most agree that semirigid instruments are more durable than flexible ureteroscopes, so the net cost is usually less. Finally, the complication rates are very low, usually below 3%, and the success rates are nearly 100%, for distal ureteral stones treated with the semirigid ureteroscope [52].

One can foresee continued refinement of these instruments, with built-in cameras (obviating the need for lenses or separate cameras), and perhaps the application of robotic technology permitting suturing or other manipulations by means of these instruments. There is little doubt that semirigid ureteroscopy will remain an important part of the urologist's armamentarium for the foreseeable future.

References

1. Lyon ES, Huffman JL, Bagley DH. Ureteroscopy and ureteropyeloscopy. Urology. 1984;23:29–36.
2. Chailley J, Besancenez A. Ureteral lithiasis: excision by ureteroscopy. J Urol (Paris). 1983;89:639–41.
3. Ford TF, Watson GM, Wickham JE. Transurethral ureteroscopic retrieval of ureteric stones. Br J Urol. 1983;55:626–8.
4. Ferraro RF, Abraham VE, Cohen TD, Preminger GM. A new generation of semirigid fiberoptic ureteroscopes. J Endourol. 1999;13:35–40.
5. Delvecchio FC. Chapter 36: Access to the ureter: rigid ureteroscopy. In: Smith AA, Badlani G, Preminger GM, Kavoussi LR, editors. Smith's textbook of endourology. Chichester: Wiley-Blackwell; 2012.
6. Aboumarzouk OM, Kata SG, Keeley FX, Nabi G: Extracorporeal shock wave lithotripsy (ESWL) versus ureteroscopic management for ureteric calculi. Cochrane Database Syst Rev: CD006029.
7. Chen GL, Bagley DH. Ureteroscopic surgery for upper tract transitional-cell carcinoma: complications and management. J Endourol. 2001;15:399–404. discussion 409.
8. Chen GL, El-Gabry EA, Bagley DH. Surveillance of upper urinary tract transitional cell carcinoma: the role of ureteroscopy, retrograde pyelography, cytology and urinalysis. J Urol. 2000;164:1901–4.
9. Chen GL, Bagley DH. Ureteroscopic management of upper tract transitional cell carcinoma in patients with normal contralateral kidneys. J Urol. 2000;164:1173–6.
10. el Khader K, Koutani A, el Yazidi A, Ibn Attya A, Hachimi M, Lakrissa A. Rigid ureteroscopy. Apropos of 88 cases. Ann Urol (Paris). 1998;32:33–7.
11. Narang V, Sinha T, Karan SC, Sandhu AS, Sethi GS, Srivastava A, Talwar R, Adlakha N. Ureteroscopy: savior to the gynecologist? Ureteroscopic management of post laparoscopic-assisted vaginal hysterectomy ureterovaginal fistulas. J Minim Invasive Gynecol. 2007;14:345–7.
12. Aghamir SK, Mohseni MG, Ardestani A. Treatment of ureteral calculi with ballistic lithotripsy. J Endourol. 2003;17:887–90.
13. Moyano Calvo JL, Huesa Martinez I, Ramirez Mendoza A, Davalos Casanova G, Aparcero Rodriguez E, Morales Lopez A, Maestro Duran JL. Ambulatory ureteroscopy and pneumatic lithotripsy. Our experience after 1803 ureteral stones. Arch Esp Urol. 2004;57:539–44.
14. Jeon SS, Hyun JH, Lee KS. A comparison of holmium:YAG laser with Lithoclast lithotripsy in ureteral calculi fragmentation. Int J Urol. 2005;12:544–7.
15. Zeng SM, Chang JP, Wang F, Wu F. Treatment of ureteral calculi with ballistic lithoclast. Zhongguo Yi Xue Ke Xue Yuan Xue Bao. 2005;27:374–6.
16. Tipu SA, Malik HA, Mohhayuddin N, Sultan G, Hussain M, Hashmi A, Naqvi SA, Rizvi SA. Treatment of ureteric calculi—use of Holmium:YAG laser lithotripsy versus pneumatic lithoclast. J Pak Med Assoc. 2007;57:440–3.
17. Hong YK, Park DS. Ureteroscopic lithotripsy using Swiss Lithoclast for treatment of ureteral calculi: 12-years experience. J Korean Med Sci. 2009;24:690–4.
18. Satar N, Zeren S, Bayazit Y, Aridogan IA, Soyupak B, Tansug Z. Rigid ureteroscopy for the treatment of ureteral calculi in children. J Urol. 2004;172:298–300.
19. El-Assmy A, Hafez AT, Eraky I, El-Nahas AR, El-Kappany HA. Safety and outcome of rigid ureteroscopy for management of ureteral calculi in children. J Endourol. 2006;20:252–5.
20. Herndon CD, Viamonte L, Joseph DB. Ureteroscopy in children: is there a need for ureteral dilation and postoperative stenting? J Pediatr Urol. 2006;2:290–3.
21. Lesani OA, Palmer JS. Retrograde proximal rigid ureteroscopy and pyeloscopy in prepubertal children: safe and effective. J Urol. 2006;176:1570–3.
22. Minevich E, Sheldon CA. The role of ureteroscopy in pediatric urology. Curr Opin Urol. 2006;16:295–8.
23. Erturhan S, Yagci F, Sarica K. Ureteroscopic management of ureteral calculi in children. J Endourol. 2007;21:397–400.
24. Gedik A, Orgen S, Akay AF, Sahin H, Bircan MK. Semi-rigid ureterorenoscopy in children without ureteral dilatation. Int Urol Nephrol. 2008;40:11–4.
25. Lemos GC, El Hayek OR, Apezzato M. Rigid ureteroscopy for diagnosis and treatment of ureteral calculi during pregnancy. Int Braz J Urol. 2002;28:311–5. discussion 316.
26. Lifshitz DA, Lingeman JE. Ureteroscopy as a first-line intervention for ureteral calculi in pregnancy. J Endourol. 2002;16:19–22.
27. Akpinar H, Tufek I, Alici B, Kural AR. Ureteroscopy and holmium laser lithotripsy in pregnancy: stents must be used postoperatively. J Endourol. 2006;20:107–10.

28. Payne DA, Keeley Jr FX. Chapter 34: Rigid and flexible ureteroscopes: technical features. In: Smith AA, Badlani G, Preminger GM, Kavoussi LR, editors. Smith's textbook of endourology. Chichester: Wiley-Blackwell; 2012.
29. Noble M Personal communication and on-line listed specifications of semi-rigid ureteroscopes; 2012.
30. Wolf R pp Richard Wolf USA product information for the Needle Semi-rigid Ureteroscope Model 8701; 2012.
31. Olympus, pp URF-P5 Flexible Ureteroscope; 2012
32. Grasso M, Bagley D. Small diameter, actively deflectable flexible ureteropyeloscopy. J Urol. 1998; 160:1648–54.
33. Abdelshehid C, Ahlering MT, Chou D. Comparison of flexible ureteroscopes: deflection, irrigant flow and optical characteristics. J Urol. 2005;173:2017–21.
34. Lezrek M, Ammani A, Bazine K, Assebane M, Kasmaoui el H, Qarro A, Beddouch A, Alami M. The split-leg modified lateral position for percutaneous renal surgery and optimal retrograde access to the upper urinary tract. Urology. 2011;78:217–20.
35. Wallis MC, Brown DH, Jayanthi VR, Koff SA. A novel technique for ureteral catheterization and/or retrograde ureteroscopy after cross-trigonal ureteral reimplantation. J Urol. 2003;170:1664–6. discussion 1666.
36. Basiri A, Simforoosh N, Nikoobakht M, Hosseini Moghaddam MM. The role of ureteroscopy in the treatment of renal transplantation complications. Urol J. 2004;1:27–31.
37. Basiri A, Nikoobakht MR, Simforoosh N, Hosseini Moghaddam SM. Ureteroscopic management of urological complications after renal transplantation. Scand J Urol Nephrol. 2006;40:53–6.
38. Delvecchio FC, Kuo RL, Iselin CE, Webster GD, Preminger GM. Combined antegrade and retrograde endoscopic approach for the management of urinary diversion-associated pathology. J Endourol. 2000;14: 251–6.
39. Antibiotic prophylaxis for urologic procedures, Best Practice Guidelines, American Urological Association, February; 2012.
40. Watterson JD, Girvan AR, Cook AJ, Beiko DT, Nott L, Auge BK, Preminger GM, Denstedt JD. Safety and efficacy of holmium:YAG laser lithotripsy in patients with bleeding diatheses. J Urol. 2002;168: 442–5.
41. Kuo RL, Aslan P, Fitzgerald KB, Preminger GM. Use of ureteroscopy and holmium:YAG laser in patients with bleeding diatheses. Urology. 1998;52:609–13.
42. Prins R, Dauer LT, Colosi DC, Quinn B, Kleiman NJ, Bohle GC, Holohan B, Al-Najjar A, Fernandez T, Bonvento M, et al. Significant reduction in dental cone beam computed tomography (CBCT) eye dose through the use of leaded glasses. Oral Surg Oral Med Oral Pathol Oral Radiol Endod. 2011;112:502–7.
43. Cousin AJ, Lawdahl RB, Chakraborty DP, Koehler RE. The case for radioprotective eyewear/facewear. Practical implications and suggestions. Invest Radiol. 1987;22:688–92.
44. Korkes F, Lopes-Neto AC, Mattos MH, Pompeo AC, Wroclawski ER. Patient position and semi-rigid ureteroscopy outcomes. Int Braz J Urol. 2009;35:542–7. discussion 548–50.
45. Rittenberg MH, Ellis DJ, Bagley DH. Ureteroscopy under local anesthesia. Urology. 1987;30:475–8.
46. Aridogan IA, Zeren S, Bayazit Y, Soyupak B, Doran S. Complications of pneumatic ureterolithotripsy in the early postoperative period. J Endourol. 2005;19: 50–3.
47. Sawazaki H, Yoshikawa T, Takahashi T, Taki Y, Takeuchi H. Ureteral avulsion: a rare complication of ureteroscopy. Hinyokika Kiyo. 2007;53:641–4.
48. Yaycioglu O, Guvel S, Kilinc F, Egilmez T, Ozkardes H. Results with 7.5F versus 10F rigid ureteroscopes in treatment of ureteral calculi. Urology. 2004;64:643–6. discussion 646–7.
49. Wang Y, Hou J, Wen D, OuYang J, Meng J, Zhuang H. Comparative analysis of upper ureteral stones (>15mm) treated with retroperitoneoscopic ureterolithotomy and ureteroscopic pneumatic lithotripsy. Int Urol Nephrol. 2010;42:897–901.
50. Marchant F, Storme O, Osorio F, Benavides J, Palma C, Ossandon E. Prospective trial comparing shock wave lithotripsy and ureteroscopy for management of distal ureteral calculi. Actas Urol Esp. 2009;33: 869–72.
51. Pearle MS, Nadler R, Bercowsky E, Chen C, Dunn M, Figenshau RS, Hoenig DM, McDougall EM, Mutz J, Nakada SY, et al. Prospective randomized trial comparing shock wave lithotripsy and ureteroscopy for management of distal ureteral calculi. J Urol. 2001; 166:1255–60.
52. Krambeck AE, Murat FJ, Gettman MT, Chow GK, Patterson DE, Segura JW. The evolution of ureteroscopy: a modern single-institution series. Mayo Clin Proc. 2006;81:468–73.
53. Gelet A, Martin X, Henriet M, Devonec M, Canton F, Codas H, Dubernard JM. Technic and results of ureteroscopy for ureteral lithiasis. Apropos of 54 ureteroscopies. J Urol (Paris). 1985;91:251–5.
54. Daniels Jr GF, Garnett JE, Carter MF. Ureteroscopic results and complications: experience with 130 cases. J Urol. 1988;139:710–3.
55. Ibarluzea G, Jorge A, Garcia Tabar P, Astobieta A, Gurtubai I, Aurtenetxe JJ. Our experience in the endoscopic treatment of ureteral lithiasis. 120 cases of transurethral ureterorenoscopy. Actas Urol Esp. 1989; 13:190–2.
56. Tello Royloa C, Rodriguez Vela L, Rioja Sanz C, Gil Sanz JM, Urruchi Fernandez P, Gonzalvo Ibarra A, Rioja Sanz LA. Rigid ureteroscopy. Results and complications. Actas Urol Esp. 1992;16:398–401.
57. Hernandez D, Larrea Masvidal E, Castillo M, Garcia C, Valdes C, Baez D, Ramirez L. Ureteroscopy. Our results and complications. Arch Esp Urol. 1993;46: 405–9.

58. Devarajan R, Ashraf M, Beck RO, Lemberger RJ, Taylor MC. Holmium:YAG lasertripsy for ureteric calculi: an experience of 300 procedures. Br J Urol. 1998;82:342–7.
59. Pascual Samaniego M, Calleja Escudero J, Rivero Martinez MD, Rivera Ferro J, Trueba Arguinarena FJ, Fernandez del Busto E. Endoscopic treatment of ureteral lithiasis. Our experience with 360 retrograde uretero-renal endoscopies in the last ten years. Actas Urol Esp. 2002;26:339–44.
60. Tugcu V, Gurbuz G, Aras B, Gurkan L, Otunctemur A, Tasci AI. Primary ureteroscopy for distal-ureteral stones compared with ureteroscopy after failed extra-corporeal lithotripsy. J Endourol. 2006;20:1025–9.

Semirigid Ureteroscopy Step-by-Step: The Tulane Approach

23

Christopher E. Keel and Raju Thomas

This chapter contains video segments that can be found on the accompanying DVD

Introduction

Ureteroscopy has become an integral part of urologic care and practice. Currently, ureteroscopy is a procedure, which is performed worldwide for the management of indications ranging from ureteral stones by fragmentation and extraction, ureteral lesion evaluation and biopsy, and for the treatment of ureteral strictures. Thus, the ureteroscope is both a diagnostic and therapeutic armamentarium for the practicing urologist.

Technological innovations have led to the introduction of the semirigid ureteroscope. Harold Hopkins, MD developed the rod-lens system for rigid endoscopes in 1960 [1] and Richard Wolf (Richard Wolf Medical Instruments, Vernon Hills, IL) designed the first ureteroscope, which was rigid, and 13 Fr in diameter [2]. The rigid ureteroscope was also introduced with an offset eyepiece to facilitate usage of fragmentation devices such as the ultrasonic lithotripter. A major advancement in ureteroscopy was incorporating the fiber optic bundles with the rod-lens system to develop the semirigid ureteroscope, which is now available in various sizes and from several manufacturers. Candela Laser Corporation developed the first available semirigid ureteroscope in 1989. Miniaturization of the semirigid ureteroscope often negates the need to dilate the ureteral orifice, saving time, and decreasing morbidity. Such semirigid scopes represented a significant advance in the endourologic management of ureteral pathology [3].

C.E. Keel, D.O. • R. Thomas, M.D., F.A.C.S., M.H.A. (✉)
Department of Urology, Tulane University School of Medicine, 1430 Tulane Avenue, SL-42, New Orleans, LA 70112, USA
e-mail: rthomas@tulane.edu

Indications

While initially utilized in the treatment of ureteral calculi, the benefits of ureteroscopy have now been observed in areas of urologic oncology and obstructive uropathy as well. Ureteroscopic indications, thus, now include the diagnosis and treatment of stones, tumors, and strictures. With excellent stone-free rates, decreased morbidity and complications, with relatively few contraindications; ureteral endoscopic treatments have become favorable primary treatment options by both the patient and the surgeon [4].

Required Equipment

When performing semirigid ureteroscopy, there are a few items required that one should consider essential. Customarily, one must have all the equipment needed to perform standard rigid cystoscopy (Fig. 23.1). In addition, when choosing a semirigid ureterscopic approach we recommend having access to a variety of guide-wires (GW)

M. Monga (ed.), *Ureteroscopy: Indications, Instrumentation & Technique*, Current Clinical Urology,
DOI 10.1007/978-1-62703-206-3_23, © Springer Science+Business Media New York 2013

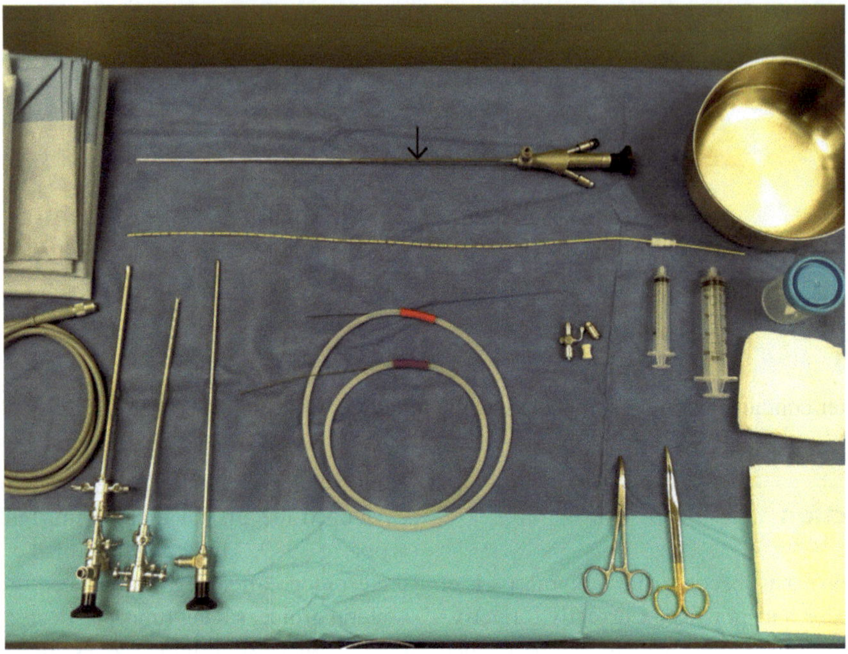

Fig. 23.1 Basic semirigid ureteroscopy (*arrow*) setup

and baskets, ureteral catheters, a ureteral balloon dilator, or fascial dilators, and should stone management or endoureterotomy be planned, a Holmium laser with 200–400 μm fibers should be available.

The essential paraphernalia, such as stone baskets and ureteral stents, needed for rigid and semirigid ureteroscopy is listed elsewhere in this book.

Techniques for Passage of Semirigid Ureteroscope: A Step-by-Step Approach

As mentioned in the previous chapter on rigid ureteroscopy, one must be cognizant of the anatomy of the ureter as it hugs the lateral aspect of the pelvis, crosses over the iliac vessels, and traverses on top of the psoas muscle, finally descending into the renal fossa lateral to the great vessels. Thus, the natural course of the ureter makes several tortuous turns creating several pressure points. This anatomic awareness is crucial in not only navigating up the ureter but also in preventing complications. An informed consent elaborating the benefits, risks, and other treatment options should be discussed and obtained prior to initiating the procedure. Sterile urine is essential prior to ureteroscopy and should also be included in the preoperative evaluation.

The technique required for passing the semirigid ureteroscope is one that, with care, can be easily mastered. It is an extension of an urologist's cystoscopic skills, though with a different set of indications and potential adverse events. It should be introduced into the ureter with caution, as a semirigid ureteroscope should be treated as a "weapon." The room set up should be the same as for cystoscopy with the video and fluoroscopic monitors ergonomically placed for the operating surgeon. Normal saline is the preferred irrigation solution and the option of using a pressure bag should be available. Other pressure irrigation devices are commercially available and their use is discussed below.

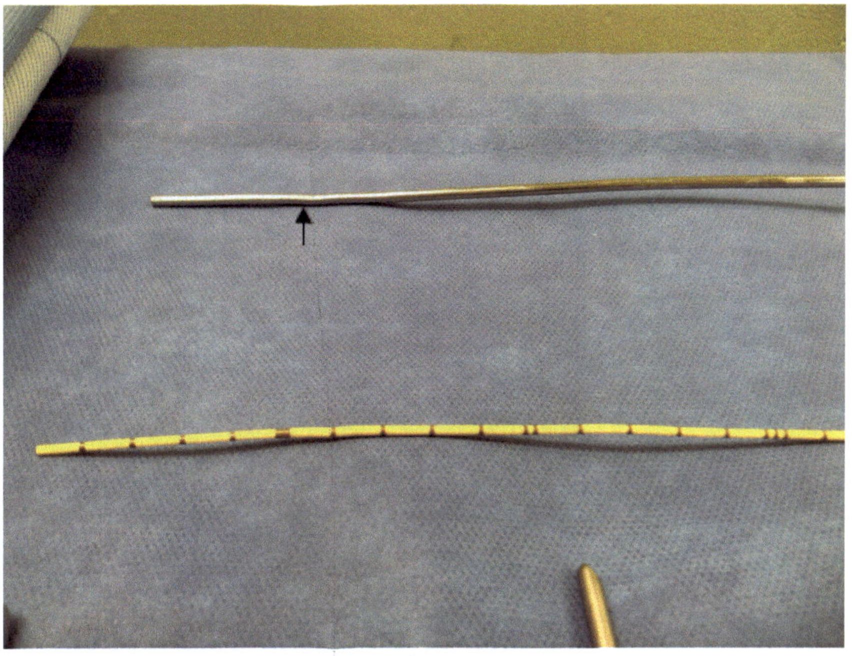

Fig. 23.2 Image shows the diameter comparison of the semirigid ureteroscope (*arrow*) and a 5 Fr ureteral catheter

After confirming the correct side and performing a cystoscopic examination of the bladder, a GW is placed into the ureteral orifice and its position confirmed by fluoroscopy. We recommend that semirigid ureteroscopy be performed along side the stiffest wire possible, such as an Amplatz Super Stiff™ (Boston Scientific, Natick, MA). However, it is best to place a floppy tipped GW, such as a Bentson™ GW (Cook Medical, Bloomington, IN) initially and exchange this, if needed, using a ureteral catheter, to prevent ureteral trauma or perforation. There are a variety of GWs from different manufactures that one can utilize.

At this point one has established access to the ureter and kidney, it is imperative that it not be compromised and thus securing this GW, coiled, to the contralateral side by a hemostat to the drape prevents migration of the wire and inadvertent dislodgement. This GW is considered the lifeline of the procedure, especially if there are any adverse events.

The technique for passing the semirigid ureteroscope is similar to that of a rigid ureteroscope, however it should be performed with extreme caution. Depending on the manufacturer and the size, the tip of the ureteroscope is much more pointed than that of the rigid ureteroscope and thus can easily create a false passage in the ureter (Fig. 23.2). It is also incumbent on the operator to maintain the sterility of the scope as its length can easily inadvertently contaminate the surgical field, beyond the sterile area.

The passage of the semirigid ureteroscope starts by placing the tip within the urethra. The scope is then advanced into the bladder maintaining the urethral lumen in the center of the visual field. When passing the scope on a male, the sphincter and prostate may act as a fulcrum and the movements to facilitate passage may seem exaggerated when compared to cystoscopy or in females. As long as the urethral lumen is maintained within the center of the field, access to the bladder can be accomplished even with large prostates.

Once inside the bladder, access to the ureter is achieved by locating the GW and placing the scope tip underneath it. This serves to elevate the ureter and open the ureteral orifice. The scope is then advanced carefully, again maintaining the lumen within the field of vision on the video monitor.

Fig. 23.3 Fluoroscopic image showing the semirigid ureteroscopy proximal to the iliac vessels

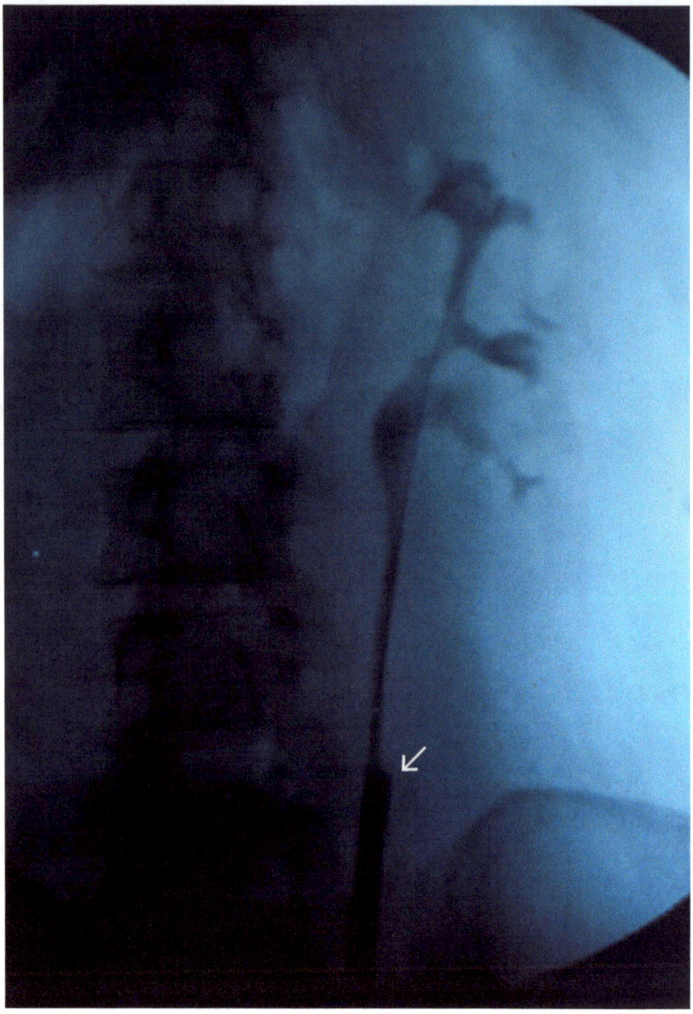

Any resistance met during passage, or lack of progress, should be evaluated and consideration given as to the safety to proceed. If one begins to create a false passage, as determined by raising of a flap of mucosa, an alternative method of treatment such as flexible ureteroscopy or introducing a ureteral stent and returning at a later date to obtain passive dilation of the ureter should be considered.

Many authors recommend limiting rigid and semirigid ureteroscopy to diagnose or treat ureteral pathology distal to the iliac vessels. However, with caution one can advance the semirigid ureteroscope into the proximal ureter (Fig. 23.3). Factors such as muscular (large psoas muscles) body habitus, obesity, and prior lower ureteral surgery will make passage of the semirigid ureteroscope challenging, if not impossible. This is when the flexible ureteroscope, as described elsewhere in this book, may become a better treatment option. If either of these issues is encountered, passive dilation by ureteral stent placement may be required. Thus, it is important to preoperatively counsel the patient that future staged treatments may be required. It is also important to caution users, particularly those accustomed to the rigid ureteroscope, that bending the semirigid ureteroscope can be significant without losing visual acuity. Thus, periodic evaluation with fluoroscopy should confirm safe passage.

If no problems are encountered, the semirigid ureteroscope can be safely passed from the distal ureter into the proximal ureter, and in many patients one can access the renal pelvis and even the upper calyx. When the anticipated area of interest is reached, the pathology is visualized before treatment is initiated or a biopsy taken. This is when ureteral calculi can be basketed or fragmented and basketed. Also, if a ureteral tumor is encountered this can't only be biopsied but also treated. Unfortunately, all semirigid ureteroscopic procedures do not always proceed as planned. Individual patient variability will introduce challenging scenarios, which will need caution, skill, and experience to overcome. As with any endoscopic procedure, problems will be encountered. Below we have listed common challenges that one will face when performing semirigid ureteroscopy.

Overcoming Problems

Accessing the Ureter

Often one is met with the inability to gain access into the ureteral orifice. If this occurs there are several options left to the surgeon.

In females or children after placing a GW, we have found that passage of a 10 Fr fascial dilator normally used for percutaneous tract dilation, can easily dilate the ureteral orifice allowing for an adequate diameter to accommodate passage of the ureteroscope (Fig. 23.4). This fascial dilator has a tip with adequate flexibility to be safely passed over a GW, under fluoroscopy, but enough rigidity to prevent kinking of the GW.

If one encounters resistance passing the fascial dilator or when operating on a male patient, we prefer the use of a ureteral balloon dilator [5]. This is performed by placing the balloon with radiographic markers over the wire and using dilute contrast to inflate the balloon up to 4 mm (12 Fr) in size.

If both of these techniques fail and there is no progress in advancing the ureteroscope, one is left with the option of placing a ureteral stent to allow passive dilation for subsequent ureteroscopy. Rarely one may cautiously perform an ureterotomy utilizing the Holmium laser for severely stenotic intramural ureter.

Intra-ureteral Problems

Difficult Scope Passage

Once within the ureter, one may still encounter situations, which make passage of the semirigid ureteroscope challenging. As mentioned earlier, several authors advocate limiting semirigid

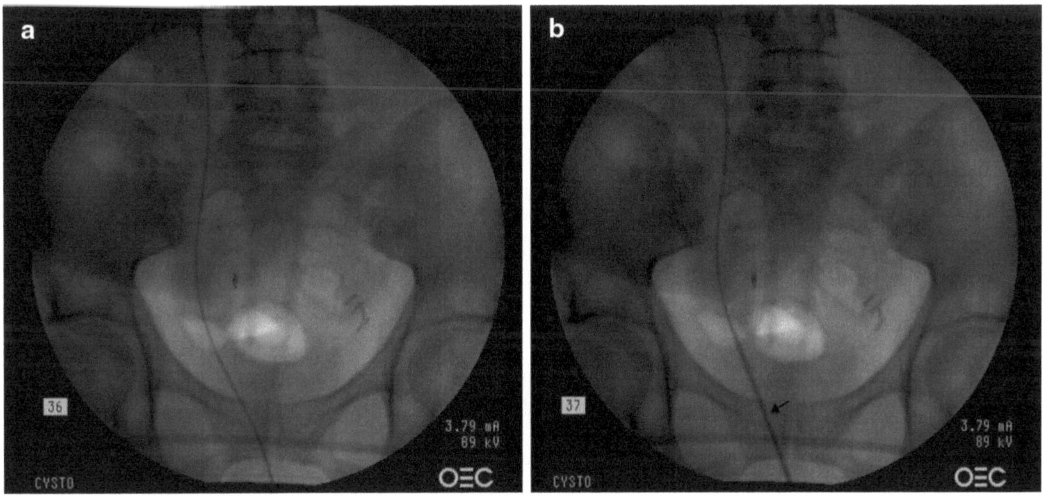

Fig. 23.4 (**a**) Guide-wire seen in the right ureter. (**b**) 10 Fr Fascial dilator seen over guide-wire (*arrow*)

ureteroscopy to the distal ureter. We, however, believe that the entire ureter can be safely accessed with the above-mentioned precautions.

When passing the ureteroscope into the proximal ureter, the iliac vessels and/or the psoas muscle can present a challenge. The "Railroad" technique that can be used, generally allows safe passage over these structures with minimal difficulty. This technique involves placing a second GW through the working channel of the ureteroscope. Once in place, the scope is carefully advanced, rotating the scope as needed, to adjust the position of the scope's beak to pass between the two wires. When using this technique, most ureteral narrowing's can be navigated safely.

Poor Visualization

Problems with visualization can often occur within the ureteral lumen. This happens for several reasons. One limitation is that of the working space to allow for adequate flow of irrigation fluid, because this space becomes smaller as one approaches a stone, tumor, or other obstruction. Additionally, the irrigation channel of the ureteroscope is small, and in some ureteroscopes this is shared with the working channel, meaning that wires or fibers placed within the working channel limit the volume of irrigation fluid available. Fortunately, ureteroscopes with two working channels, one for irrigation and one for instrumentation are now available.

When the surgeon encounters poor visibility the first thing to ensure is that there is adequate pressure, for visualization, within the irrigation bag. If this is not the source, ensure that all instruments are removed from the working channel and that there is no kinking of the irrigation tubing. Additionally, one must ensure that the semirigid ureteroscope is not bent or kinked, which can be confirmed by fluoroscopy. In rare cases poor visualization persists. If this happens, the use of a Single Action Pumping System™ (Boston Scientific, Natick, MA) may be beneficial. This pump connects to the irrigation bag and the surgical assistant can use this device to increase the pressure and volume of the irrigation. In some cases, even this technique may be inadequate and then one should consider ureteral stent placement and a subsequent procedure. Caution is advised with this technique so as not to dislodge any ureteral calculi or fragments because of the irrigation pressure.

The surgeon should remain cognitive of the potential for pyelo-venous and pyelo-lymphatic backflow when using high-pressure irrigation. We recommend the lowest possible pressure be used to ensure adequate visualization.

Stone Treatment

Once access has been established and the stone has been visualized (Fig. 23.5), the surgeon has to make a decision regarding basketing or fragmentation and subsequent basketing. The surgeon must use the minimal amount of irrigation necessary to facilitate passage of the ureteroscope when approaching a stone with proximal hydroureter. Failure to do so may result in the stone being pushed proximally into the kidney making the semirigid ureteroscope impractical.

After encountering the stone there are several choices for treatment. Holmium laser lithotripsy is the most common form of lithotripsy currently employed, though there still remain other forms. If the Holmium laser is not available then other options such as, EHL (electrohydraulic lithotripter) or pneumatic lithotripter can be utilized instead. The laser fiber is extended clearing the beak of the scope. The fiber is then used to contact the stone. The Holmium laser is a contact laser and failure to contact the stone will not result in adequate stone fragmentation.

There are two techniques that can be used when performing intracorporeal lithotripsy within the ureter. For smaller stones it may be advantageous to "paint" the stone, carefully removing the outer parameter of the stone to allow extraction. If the stone is large and/or impacted it is more common to fragment the stone into pieces, at which point the "painting" technique can be used. Fragmentation is usually performed by dividing the stone or stone fragments into sections, using the laser to split the stones into halves. The GW can be used as a metric to gauge the size of the fragments and determine the ability to extract them. Great care must be taken to prevent damage to the GW or ureteral mucosa

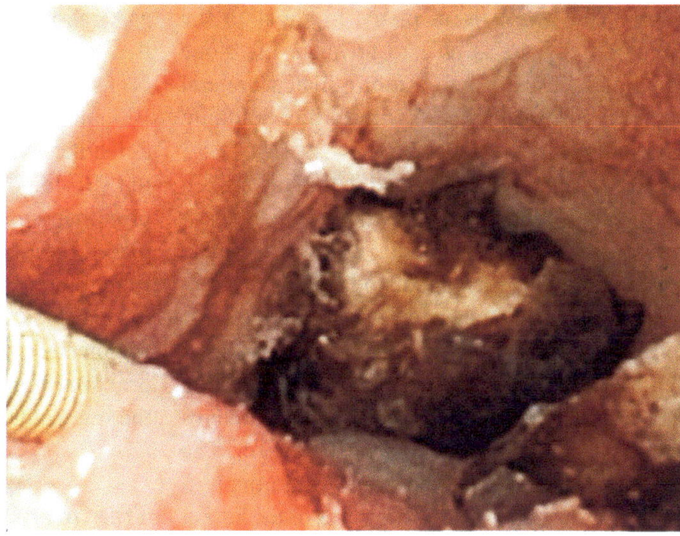

Fig. 23.5 Fragmental ureteral stone within the ureteral lumen

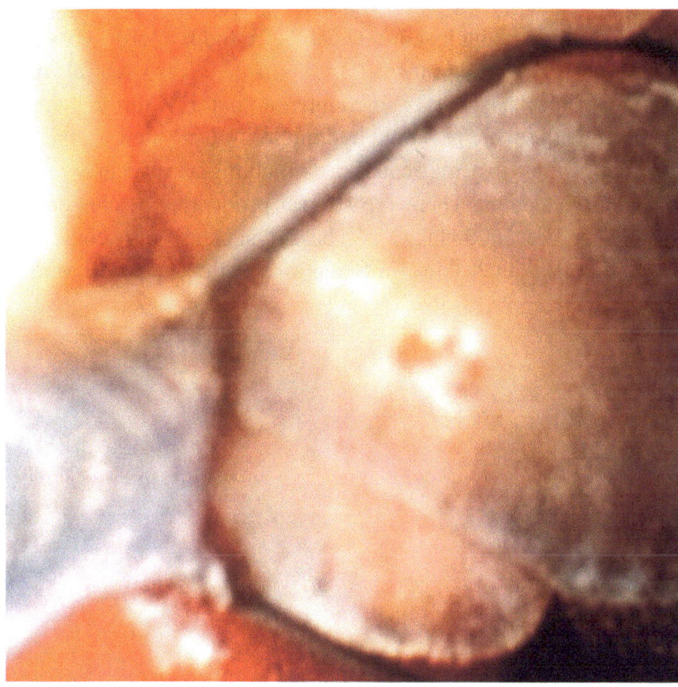

Fig. 23.6 Stone being extracted

from the laser fiber, as this can lead to postoperative ureteral stricture [6].

If the stone is small enough to be extracted it can simply be placed in a basket and removed (Fig. 23.6). We prefer the use of the tipless nitinol basket such as NCircle Basket™ (Cook Medical, Blomington, IN) to prevent ureteral trauma. When removing the stone or stone fragments, one must be careful not to cause further damage to the ureter. For example, if any resistance is met, one should discontinue extraction. Failure to do so can lead to perforation, stricture or possible avulsion of the ureter distal to the stone with unwanted sequelae.

If the surgeon encounters impaction of the stone several options should be considered. First of all, ensure that a GW is in place proximal to the stone. Often, one is able to advance the stone proximally, usually into a more dilated ureteral segment, and then proceed with further holmium laser lithotripsy.

If a basketed stone is lodged within the basket, and cannot be extracted, extracorporeal disassembly of the basket will usually facilitate removal of the basket and dislodge the stone.

However, if the impacted stone cannot be dislodged, then the basket is extracorporeally disassembled and the ureteroscope is removed leaving the disassembled basket in place. The ureteroscope is reintroduced alongside the basket. The calculus is reached and the stone within the basket is fragmented or one of the wires of the basket may be severed. Care must be taken to cut the basket wire only in one place to prevent pieces of the basket from being lost and becoming a nidus for future stone formation.

Often times a stone is encountered that is impacted with severe proximal hydoureter. When this occurs lithotripsy may cause proximal migration of the calculus. There are several products available to prevent this. Use of a basket, such as the Escape Basket™ (Boston Scientific, Natick, MA) allows the stone to be fragmented within the basket. Other options include the use of a backstop device such as NTrap™ (Cook Medical, Bloomington, IN), Stone Cone™ (Boston Scientific, Natick, MA), or the BackStop™ liquid (Boston Scientific, Natick, MA) can prevent proximal stone migration. These devices are placed through the working channel of the semirigid ureteroscope and the scope is then offloaded. It is then reintroduced and the stone is fragmented. These backstop devices prevent proximal migration and can assist in extracting the fragments.

Treatments of Tumor or Stricture

The techniques for treatment of ureteral strictures or tumors are similar to the treatment of stones. Ureteral tumors (Fig. 23.7) can be biopsied through the semirigid ureteroscope either by ureteroscopic biopsy forceps or brushing, though the accuracy of such small pathologic specimens can be challenging. We have found that flexible ureteroscopic biopsy forceps using the BIGOpsy™ (Cook Medical, Bloomington, IN) is sometimes

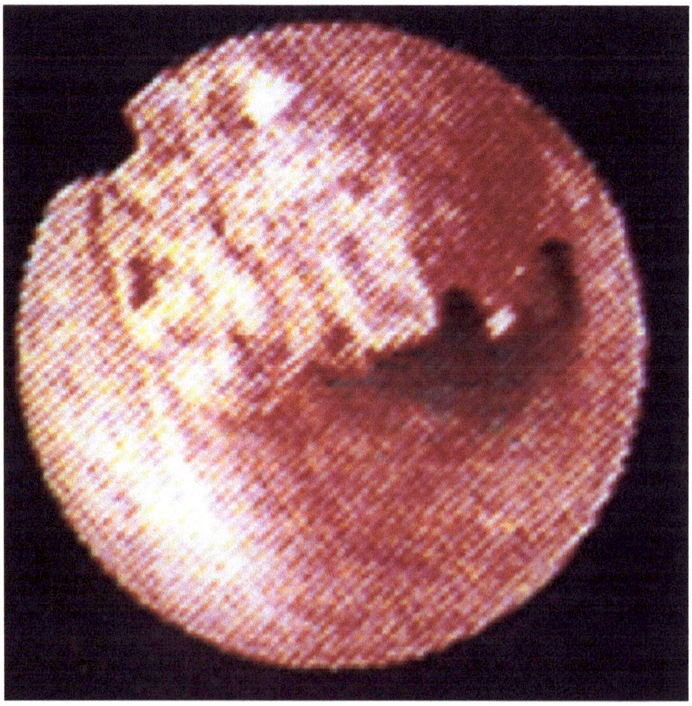

Fig. 23.7 Image shows a papillary tumor within the lumen of the ureter

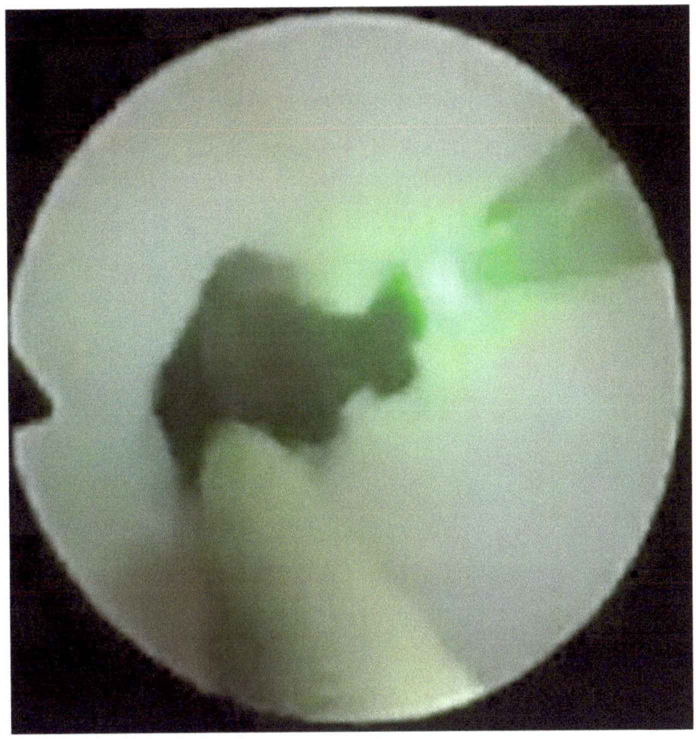

Fig. 23.8 Image demonstrating the use of a holmium laser to perform an endoureterotomy for a left ureteral stricture

superior to other ureteroscopic biopsy forceps. The holmium laser can be used to ablate tumors much in the same way a stone is treated. Alternatively, papillary lesions can be snared at their base and removed in a basket followed by holmium laser ablation of their base [7, 8].

Both primary and secondary ureteral strictures can be treated using a semirigid ureteroscope (Fig. 23.8) [9]. Caution is advised, if the lumen is obliterated, an endoureterotomy is not feasible and the procedure should be abandoned. Further discussion of the technique is listed elsewhere in this book.

What If?

Occasionally, even with the greatest care, ureteral trauma does occur. This is evident by the raising of a mucosal flap, the presence of extravasation on retrograde urography, or visualization of periureteral fat. When this is encountered, immediate cessation of the procedure is recommended [10]. Placement of a ureteral stent is performed and the patient is returned to the operating theater on another date for completion of the planned procedure, and reimaging the patient is recommended. Continuation of the procedure in the face of ureteral trauma increases the risk for ureteral stricture, avulsion, and postoperative complications.

Conclusion

Semirigid ureteroscopy is a key component of urologic practice today. Having adequate instrumentation, paraphernalia, and experience will increase success and minimize adverse events for the patient.

References

1. Bagley DH, Huffman JL, Lion ES. Combined rigid and flexible ureteropyeloscopy. J Urol. 1983;130:243–4.
2. Bagley DH. Ureteroscopy. AUA Update Series. 1994;13:206–11.
3. Ferraro RF, Abraham VE, Cohen TD, Preminger GM. A new generation of semi rigid fiberoptic ureteroscopes. J Endourol. 1999;13:35–40d.

4. Preminger GM, Tiselius HG, Assimos DG, et al. 2007 guideline for the management of ureteral calculi. J Urol. 2007;178:2418–34.
5. Thomas R. Rigid ureteroscopy: pitfalls and remedies. Urology. 1988;32:328–34.
6. Lane BR, Singh D, Meraney A, Streem SB. Novel endourologic applications for holmium laser. Urology. 2005;65:991–3.
7. Soderdahl D, Fabrizio M, Rahman N, et al. Endoscopic treatment of upper tract transitional cell carcinoma. Urol Oncol. 2005;23:114–22.
8. Park S, Hong B, Kim C, Ahn H. Impact of tumor location on prognosis of transitional cell carcinoma of the upper urinary tract. J Urol. 2004;171:621–5.
9. Thomas R. Choosing the ideal candidate for ureteroscopic endoureterotomy. J Urol. 1993;149:314.
10. Schuster TG, Hollenbeck BK, Faerger GJ, Wolf Jr JS. Ureteroscopic treatment of lower pole calculi: comparison of lithotripsy in situ and after displacement. J Urol. 2002;168:43–5.

Flexible Ureteroscopy: Access Sheath

24

Bodo E. Knudsen

This chapter contains video segments that can be found on the accompanying DVD

Introduction

An expanding role of flexible ureterorenoscopy for the management of upper urinary tract renal stones and tumors has developed over the past decade [1, 2]. This has been driven by improvements in flexible endoscope design, miniaturization of instruments, and the development of the holmium:YAG laser as the gold standard for intracorporeal lithotripsy [3, 4].

The development of the ureteral access sheath (UAS) has served to further advance flexible ureteroscopy. Takayasu and Aso first described the use of a UAS in 1974 [5]. Since then it has been demonstrated to be a cost-effective tool allowing safe and efficient reentry into the ureter and upper collecting system while improving vision, reducing intrarenal pressures, and providing better patient outcomes [6].

Advantages

The use of a UAS during flexible ureteroscopy provides several advantages in comparison to when a UAS is not used (Table 24.1). With the UAS in proper position, the flow of irrigation in the kidney is improved due to irrigation fluid to continuous flow in through the ureteroscope channel and flow out through the UAS. Having adequate flow during the procedure is important during laser lithotripsy or tumor ablation, as it will help keep the field of view clear allowing the surgeon to visualize the target. For example, laser lithotripsy will create many small stone fragment, the so-called holmium storm, and without an access sheath this cloud of stone fragments can severely impair visibility. By allowing continuous, low pressure irrigation, the stone fragments and dust-like debris can be washed from the kidney and out through the access sheath. Similarly, some bleeding may occur either during laser lithotripsy or during tumor ablation. Improved irrigation through the access sheath will flush out any blood in the collecting system thereby keeping a clear visual field. Similarly, patients who have a history of stones or urothelial cell tumors may present with hematuria. Flexible ureteroscopy in these patients may be challenging if a UAS is not used due to the blood in the urine impairing visualization. In these patients, the initial returns through the access sheath after it is placed are often very dark. However, with irrigation through the ureteroscope the blood in the field usually clears quickly, facilitating visualization.

The correct placement of the UAS allows maintaining low intrarenal pressures during

B.E. Knudsen, M.D., F.R.C.S.C. (✉)
Department of Urology, Wexner Medical Center, The Ohio State University, Columbus, OH, USA
e-mail: bodo.knudsen@osumc.edu

M. Monga (ed.), *Ureteroscopy: Indications, Instrumentation & Technique*, Current Clinical Urology,
DOI 10.1007/978-1-62703-206-3_24, © Springer Science+Business Media New York 2013

Table 24.1 Advantages of the ureteral access sheath

	Indwelling preoperative stent	No preoperative stent
Male	13/15 F or 14/16 F, 45 cm	11/13 F or 12/14 F, 45 cm
Female	13/15 F or 14/16 F, 35 cm	11/13 F or 12/14 F, 35 cm

flexible ureterorenoscopy. Maintaining intrarenal pressure below 40 ccH_2O during flexible ureteroscopy prevents pyelovenous and/or pyelolymphatic backflow during the procedure. Rehman et al., studied intrarenal pressures in cadaveric kidneys using 10/12, 12/14, and 14/16 F UAS, and compared this to controls without a UAS. With the ureteroscope in place, irrigation was run at pressures of 50, 100, and 200 cmH_2O. Without a UAS, intrarenal pressures rose to 52–59 cmH_2O, high enough to cause pyelovenous and pyelolymphatic backflow. With the use of a UAS lower pressures were observed. The 10/12 F access resulted in pressures of 22–29 cmH_2O, while the larger 12/14 and 14/16 F sheaths had lower pressures with measurements of 17.5–19.5 and 14.5–19.5 mmH_2O, respectively [7]. This suggests, at least in terms of intrarenal pressure management, that a 12/14 F UAS strikes the best balance between size of the sheath and effectiveness.

During treatment of upper tract urothelial cell carcinoma, a properly selected and deployed UAS may aid in preventing extravasation of tumor cells by maintaining low intrarenal pressures. The sheath may also reduce the exposure of the lower portions of the ureter to tumor cells as it effectively covers the urothelium and promotes the flow of irrigation out through the sheath directly rather than around it.

With a UAS in position, the surgeon is able to introduce and remove the ureteroscope at will during the procedure. When a tumor is being investigated, multiple biopsies with larger instruments such as a back-loading biopsy forceps can be performed. However, the greatest advantage may be in the treatment of renal calculi. After laser lithotripsy of an upper ureteral or renal stone, the surgeon is able to basket extract the fragments through the UAS in an attempt to render the patient stone-free. The size of the fragments removed is limited by the diameter of the access sheath. The access sheath protects the ureter from the inadvertent removal of fragments that are too large and that could get trapped in the ureter, or worse, avulse the ureter if a sheath were not used. If fragments are attempted to be removed that are too large for the sheath, they are then further reduced in size with laser lithotripsy before further removal is attempted.

Removal of the fragments has several potential benefits for the patient. When the patient passes the fragments they may experience episodes of renal colic. Worse, if the fragments became obstructed, further intervention may be required including possible stent placement or further lithotripsy. If the fragments fail to pass and they remain in the kidney, then they could become the nidus for future stone formation [8, 9]. In a nonrandomized study, L'Esperance et al. demonstrated that the use of a UAS resulted in an 12% higher stone-free rate as compared to procedure where an access sheath was not used (79% vs. 67% SFR, respectively) [10].

Kourambas et al. performed a study that randomized 59 patients who were scheduled to undergo ureteroscopy into two groups—one with a UAS and one without. The majority (85%) of the procedures were performed for stone disease. They determined that there was a statistically significant reduction in the mean operating time by 10.5 min when an access sheath was employed during the procedure. Furthermore, despite the cost of the access sheath, the overall cost per patient was reduced by $350 in the cases where the sheath was used. Contrary to L'Esperance's data, this study showed no difference in the stone-free rate between the two groups. This may be due to the lack of stone basketing in the access sheath arm. Short-term follow-up did not reveal an increased rate of ureteral strictures in the access sheath arm of the study [6].

Ischemia

A concern with the placement of a UAS has been whether ischemia to the ureter can occur. In an animal study, Lallas et al. studied the potential for ischemia in porcine ureters after the placement of an access sheath using laser Doppler flowmeter. Access sheaths of 10/12, 12/14, and 14/16 F were placed and measurements were taken at 5 min intervals from the proximal ureters. Blood flow was reduced in all ureters at the first 5 min interval, but the greatest reduction in blood flow occurred with the larger 12/14 and 14/16 F sheaths, where flow decreased greater than 50% by 15 min. However, blood flow subsequently increased to 70% of baseline levels by the 70 min mark. Histologic exam of the ureters taken at 72 h after the procedure showed no evidence of ischemia or necrosis [11]. This suggests that despite the initial decrease in blood flow, the impact is transient and the reduction is not enough to induce ischemic necrosis.

Stricture Risks

The transitory reduction in ureteral blood flow raises the question as to whether there could be an increased risk of stricture formation in patients who undergo ureteroscopy with a UAS. To date, no randomized data has shown this to be a risk. In a nonrandomized study, Delvecchio et al. reviewed the records of 150 patients who underwent ureteroscopy with the use of a UAS. Sixty-two of these patients had follow-up in excess of 3 months. In this subgroup, only one patient developed a stricture suggesting that the overall stricture rate is similar to previously published stricture rates after ureteroscopy without a sheath [12, 13].

Stent or No Stent

The debate whether to place a stent after ureteroscopy has continued over the last decade. Several studies have shown that in uncomplicated ureteroscopy that routine stenting is not indicated and that unstented patients had decreased pain, narcotic use, and morbidity [14, 15]. However, this work was done prior to the widespread use of UASs and these studies do not discuss the use of a UAS. The placement of a UAS can result in some minor trauma to the ureter during insertion as well as transient ischemia [11]. Rapaport et al. reported in a nonrandomized series of patients that 37% of patient who underwent a ureteroscopy with a UAS returned for an unscheduled emergency visit in the postoperative period vs. 14% of patients who underwent ureteroscopy without an access sheath. They recommended that a stent be placed after all ureteroscopy cases involving a UAS [16]. It is not entirely clear what led to the increased rate of ER visits in the group that had a UAS placed during surgery, but transient colic for spasm or edema of the ureter is a possible explanation.

Reducing Scope Damage

The limited durability and high cost of repair of modern flexible ureteroscopes is a financial hurdle that can be difficult to overcome for some centers wishing to adopt the technology [17]. In a nonrandomized study using historical controls, Pietrow et al. reported that when UAS were used, they were able to double the number of procedures before repairs to their endoscopes were needed as compared to when no access sheath was used (27.5 uses) [18]. Several factors could be contributing to this. When a UAS is not used, the flexible ureteroscope is usually passed up over a guide wire (railroad technique). This can result in damage to the endoscope channel from the wire, especially with wires that have a rigid back end. Small perforations to the channel of the ureteroscope will lead to leaks that will further damage the endoscope. Small flaps in the channel can also be created that may make the passage of instruments difficult. Furthermore, when the resistance is encountered during the advancement of the ureteroscope, the scope can buckle from the force. Given the delicate design of these scopes, this may also lead to further damage. Buckling of the scope is prevented when it is advanced through a UAS.

Properties of Different Access Sheaths

There are a wide variety of commercially available UASs that differ in their physical properties. The properties of the sheath may impact how clinically effective they are. Monga et al. evaluated in a bench study eight UAS to determine their resistance to buckling and kinking as well as lubriciousness (coefficient of friction). They determined that the Applied Forte XE (Applied Medical, Rancho Santa Margarita, CA) and Cook Flexor sheaths (Cook Medical, Bloomington, IN) were the most resistant to kinking as well as most lubricious (Fig. 24.1). The Cook Flexor also had the greatest resistance to buckling [19]. By resisting kinking, the lumen of the access sheath may be less likely to collapse during a procedure. Having a lower coefficient of friction, may allow the access sheath to slide up the ureter more easily but could also make it more susceptible to slipping backwards during a procedure. Resistance to buckling may allow the sheath to pass easier when some resistance is encountered, such as at the ureteral orifice or pelvic brim.

Using this data, a prospective randomized trial was performed comparing these two sheaths in a clinical study. Fifty-four patients were

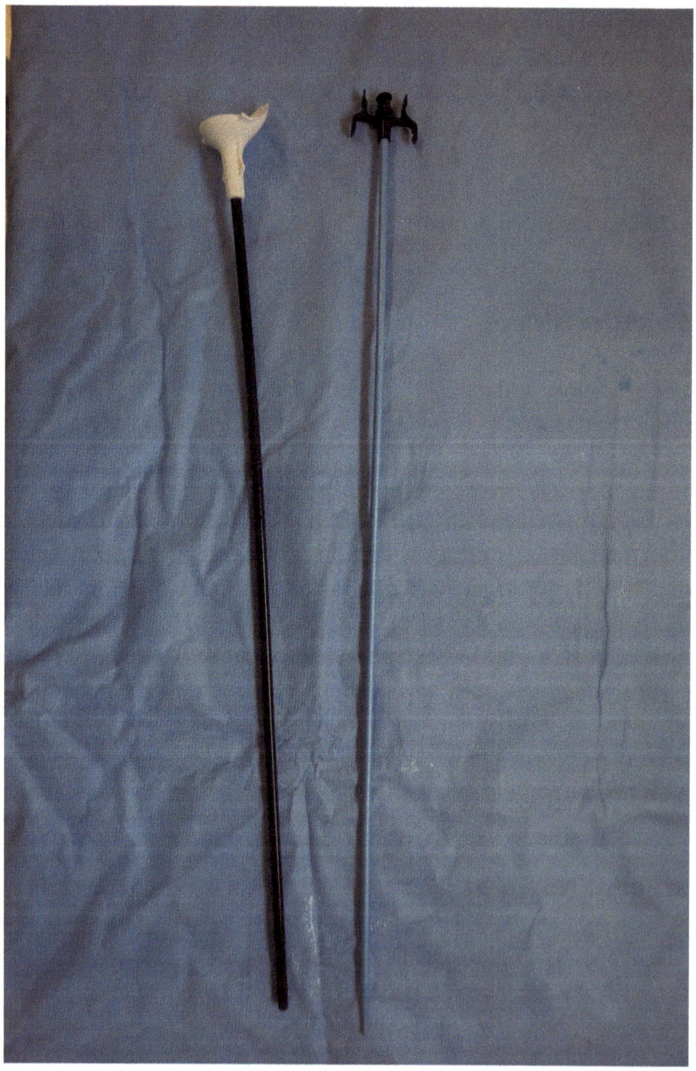

Fig. 24.1 UAS showing inner obturator and outer sheath

randomized to flexible ureteroscopy procedures with either a 12/15 F Applied Access Forte XE or 12/14 F Cook Flexor. Both of these sheaths are reinforced with an embedded coil system and feature a hydrophilic coating. The overall device failure rate for the Applied Access Forte XE was 44% vs. no failures for the Cook Flexor. Buckling (25%), kinking (25%), and difficulty passing instruments (13%) were the causes of failure for the Applied sheath. Of note, in procedures where the Applied sheath failed, the Cook Flexor sheath was then attempted to be placed. In all cases the Cook Flexor was successfully placed. The Cook Flexor was also scored higher subjectively by the surgeon in terms of ease of placement, instrument passage, and ease of stone extraction. The authors speculated that the larger outer diameter of the Applied sheath (15 F vs. 14 F) and the length and configuration of the tip of the sheath may have been a factor in the outcome of the study [20].

A follow-up study evaluated "next-generation" UASs in terms of buckling and kinking. Sheaths evaluated including the Cook Flexor (12/14 F, 35 cm), ACMI UroPass (12/14 F, 38 cm) (Gyrus ACMI, Southborough, MA), Bard Aquaguide (11/13 F, 35 cm) (Bard Medical, Covington, GA), and Boston Scientific Navigator (11/13 and 13/15 F, 36 cm) (Boston Scientific, Natick, MA). The Cook Flexor was again the most resistant to buckling requiring 5.1 N to buckle, followed by the ACMI at 3.2 N, the Bsci-13/15 at 2.9 N, the Bard at 2.8 N, and the Bsci-11/13 at 2.0 N. The smaller diameter of the Bard and BSci 11/13 appear to make them more prone to buckling. The Bard sheath was the most prone to kinking, requiring only 9 N/mm to do so. The BSci 13/15 kinked at 30 N/mm, the BSci 11/13 at 41 N/mm, the Cook at 42 N/mm, and the least likely to kink was the ACMI at 83 N/mm. All sheaths tested had hydrophilic coatings and showed similar coefficient of frictions [21].

Our own clinical experience has been that kinking of the sheath during a procedure is rarely seen with a modern coil reinforced access sheath UAS but buckling can be encountered with advancement of the sheath. Passing the UAS over an Amplatz superstiff guide wire may reduce the incidence of buckling, but care must be taken to not exert too high of a force in order to avoid trauma to the ureter. Study has shown that experienced urologists use up to 6.6 N when placing an access sheath [22]. While the exact force needed to perforate a ureter while advancing an access sheath over a guide wire is variable depending on both the type of UAS used as well as individual patient factors, a CT-1 needle requires 4.7 N of force to perforate a human ureter [23].

UAS and Flexible Ureteroscopes Facilitating Other Procedures

The use of a flexible ureteroscope combined with a UAS can be advantageous during percutaneous stone procedures. By placing a UAS in a retrograde fashion at the start of a percutaneous nephrolithotomy (PCNL), the access sheath allows for small stone fragments to pass out through the sheath and not become lodged in the ureter. This also assists in maintaining low pressures within the renal collecting system during the procedure. A flexible ureteroscope can be advanced up into the kidney during the procedure to visualize the best calyx prior to percutaneous puncture. Contrast or air can be injected through the scope to facilitate puncture, but the tip of the scope can also serve as the fluoroscopic target. With the scope in position, the puncture of the needle is directly visualized as it enters into the collecting system. The guide wire can also be captured with a stone basket passed through the endoscope and withdrawn out through the UAS [24]. The flexible ureteroscope with laser lithotripsy and basket extraction can also be used to clear residual stone burden that could not be reached in an antegrade fashion during the PCNL procedure. This may reduce the need for multiple nephrostomy tracts in patients with large or complex stone burdens [25].

Radially Dilating Balloon

A novel UAS that incorporates a radially dilating balloon has been reported. The proposed advantages of a radially dilating balloon incorporated into the UAS are that it eliminates the shearing forces associated with axial dilation. This is a reported advantage to using balloon dilation vs. radial dilation during PCNL and may translate to similar findings with UAS placement [26]. Harper et al. reported their experience placing a balloon expandable ureteral access (BEUS) and compared it to placement of a conventional sheath (Cook Flexor, 12/14 F) in ten farm pigs. The BEUS is 9.5 F in nonexpanded form and after placement it expands to have an inner diameter of 12 F and an outer diameter of 14 F. The study demonstrated that the BEUS required less maximum (0.36 lb vs. 1.48 lb) and less mean force (0.11 lb vs. 0.49 lb) to place vs. the conventional UAS. The flow rate through the BEUS was also slightly improved over the conventional UAS (90.0 cc/min vs. 80.6 cc/min). Blinded reviewers also scored the BEUS superior for less total urothelial tear length (1.2 cm vs. 2.6 cm) and less damage to the ureter overall [27]. This type of access sheath design holds promise as an advancement over current designs. However, some changes to the technique of access sheath placement may be required. It would be important to ensure that there are no unrecognized strictures in the ureter prior to placement. If a tight stricture were to be encountered that the sheath could not dilate, it would require pulling the expanded sheath through the stricture. It is unclear as to how much force this would place on the ureter but the concern would be that enough force could be generated to risk of avulsion of the ureter. This force would be variable depending on both the location of the stricture and other patient factors. By performing a retrograde ureterogram prior to the placement of the sheath, one would be able to identify a previously unrecognized stricture and treat it appropriately prior to placement of the BEUS.

UAS Facilitating the Treatment of Large Intrarenal Calculi

Kidney stones larger than 2.0 cm have traditionally been treated with PCNL, which has been shown to be both safe and effective [28]. However, PCNL may be difficult or impossible in some select patient populations such as those that are morbidly obese, have anatomic deformations making percutaneous access to the kidney difficult, are on chronic anticoagulation, or simply refuse PCNL. In addition, PCNL has associated morbidity and typically requires at least an overnight hospital stay [29]. The development and expanding use of the UAS, along with advancements in flexible ureteroscopes and holmium:YAG laser fibers, has allowed surgeons to become increasingly more aggressive in treating larger stone burdens ureteroscopically [17, 30–32]. Hyams et al. conducted a retrospective multicenter review of patients undergoing flexible ureterorenoscopy with holmium:YAG laser lithotripsy for stone 2–3 cm in size. A UAS was used in 67% of cases and 84% of patients had a single-staged procedure. Overall complication rates were low for this select group of patients but stone-free rates were low with only 47% being stone-free and 66% having fragments ≤2.0 cm [2]. Riley et al. reported their experience treating 22 patients with stones greater than 2.5 cm utilizing flexible ureterorenoscopy with holmium:YAG laser lithotripsy using a UAS in all patients (13/15 F). Patients underwent an average of 1.82 procedures with only five patients requiring one procedure. Complications were low and the overall stone-free rate, defined as fragments <2.0 mm, was 90.9% [33]. The higher stone-free rate in the latter study is likely multifactorial, however with the higher percentage of patients treated using an UAS, it lends support to the use of a sheath in patients with larger stone burdens.

It appears that flexible ureteroscopy with holmium:YAG laser lithotripsy using a UAS is a viable treatment alternate for select patients with large stone burdens. Future randomized trails comparing PCNL with URS with laser lithotripsy and UAS are needed to better define the relative pros and cons of these two procedures.

Technique: Renal Stones

At our institution we routinely use UAS for the treatment of renal stones. For patients who do not have a preoperative stent, a 12/14 F UAS is

Table 24.2 Advantages of a ureteral access sheath

Decreased intrarenal pressure
Improved visualization
Ability to perform multiple passes with the ureteroscope
Protection of the ureter when stone fragments extracted
Reduce tumor cell exposure in the lower urinary tract during biopsy or ablation
Reduced wear and tear on endoscopes

selected and for patients with a preoperative stent, especially with a larger stone burden, a 14/16 F UAS is used. For women, a 35 cm length is selected unless they are less than 152 cm in height, in which case a 28 cm sheath is used. For men, a 45 cm length UAS is selected (Table 24.2). The procedure is initiated by first passing a hydrophilic tipped wire up the ureter with a flexible cystoscope. A scout image of the kidney should be taken and saved for reference. The bladder is emptied with a straight catheter. If a concomitant ureteral stone is suspected, the distal ureter is dilated with an 8–10 coaxial dilator and the ureter inspected with a sub-7.0 F semirigid ureteroscope. If no ureteral stone is suspected, then a retrograde pyelogram is performed through a 5 F open-ended catheter. A retrograde pyelogram may demonstrate the stone as a filling defect, identify other pathology, and importantly it will delineate the anatomy of the upper ureter and UPJ which will guide placement of the UAS. The 8–10 coaxial dilator is used to place a second wire, this time an Amplatz Superstiff. The hydrophilic-tipped wire is clipped to the drape as a safety wire and the Superstiff wire is used to advance the access sheath. Using a Superstiff wire reduces the risk of the wire kinking and buckling during advancement of the UAS. The UAS should be wet thoroughly with water prior to passing it to activate the hydrophilic coating. The UAS is advanced up to level of the UPJ if possible, but if there is significant angling of the ureter at the UPJ care must be taken to not over advance the sheath, as the rigid tip of the sheath can injure the ureter or kidney. Advancement of the sheath should always be down under fluoroscopic guidance (Fig. 24.2). Once in place, the inner obturator and Superstiff wire are removed. The sheath is then secured with a 2.0 silk suture to the patient's inner thigh. This prevents the UAS from sliding out during the procedure, reducing potential ureteral trauma from the access sheath being repositioned without the inner obturator in place. Using a pressurized irrigation system, the kidney is then carefully inspected with the flexible ureteroscope. Fluoroscopy can aid in this process and all calyces should be visualized. Once the targets are visualized, the holmium:YAG optical laser fiber can be loaded into the scope. Care should be taken to ensure that the scope is straight when the fiber is passed through it, so as not to damage the fragile inner channel. A sub-300 μm core sized fiber is used to maximize flow through the endoscope, not limit deflection, and decrease the wear and tear on the deflection mechanism. Laser energy settings of 0.6 J at a frequency of 6 Hz is the typical starting setting. If the stone appears to be very dense, higher energy and pulse rates are selected as needed. After fragmentation of the stone, the pieces are removed systematically with a 1.5 F tipless nitinol stone basket. Care must be taken to not attempt to extract stone pieces that are too large, as injury to the ureter could ensue. After the fragments are removed, the UAS is slowly withdrawn while the ureter is simultaneously inspected with the ureteroscope. This is done to ensure that no stones were missed in the ureter and that no other pathology of the ureter is seen. With the sheath removed, another retrograde pyelogram is performed, a 6 F ureteral stent is placed, and the bladder is emptied.

Our practice is to leave the stent in place for approximately 7 days. Patients with radiopaque calculi undergo a KUB prior to stent removal to ensure that there are not any significant residual fragments. After the stent is removed, patient return for follow-up 8 weeks later with a renal ultrasound, to ensure stability of the upper tracts.

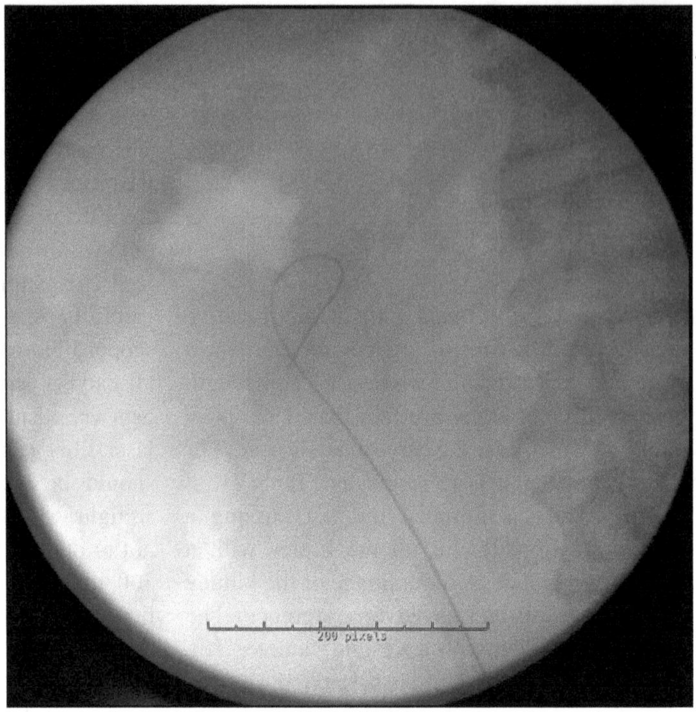

Fig. 24.2 Access sheath and safety wire in place

Conclusion

The development of the UAS has facilitated the use of flexible ureteroscopy to treat upper tract pathology such as renal calculi and tumors. Properly employed, UAS promote safe, low pressure procedures with excellent visualization, reduced scope wear, and the ability to easily pass the scope multiple times as needed. Future refinement of the UAS may see the adoptions of radially dilating sheaths.

References

1. Best SL, Nakada SY. Flexible ureteroscopy is effective for proximal ureteral stones in both obese and nonobese patients: a two-year, single-surgeon experience. Urology. 2011;77(1):36–9.
2. Hyams ES, et al. Flexible ureterorenoscopy and holmium laser lithotripsy for the management of renal stone burdens that measure 2 to 3 cm: a multi-institutional experience. J Endourol. 2010;24(10):1583–8.
3. Khanna R, Monga M. Instrumentation in endourology. Ther Adv Urol. 2011;3(3):119–26.
4. Sofer M, et al. Holmium:YAG laser lithotripsy for upper urinary tract calculi in 598 patients. J Urol. 2002;167(1):31–4.
5. Takayasu H, Aso Y. Recent development for pyeloureteroscopy: guide tube method for its introduction into the ureter. J Urol. 1974;112(2):176–8.
6. Kourambas J, Byrne RR, Preminger GM. Does a ureteral access sheath facilitate ureteroscopy? J Urol. 2001;165(3):789–93.
7. Rehman J, et al. Characterization of intrapelvic pressure during ureteropyeloscopy with ureteral access sheaths. Urology. 2003;61(4):713–8.
8. Candau C, et al. Natural history of residual renal stone fragments after ESWL. Eur Urol. 2000;37(1):18–22.
9. Rebuck DA, et al. The natural history of renal stone fragments following ureteroscopy. Urology. 2011; 77(3):564–8.
10. L'Esperance JO, et al. Effect of ureteral access sheath on stone-free rates in patients undergoing ureteroscopic management of renal calculi. Urology. 2005; 66(2):252–5.
11. Lallas CD, et al. Laser Doppler flowmetric determination of ureteral blood flow after ureteral access sheath placement. J Endourol. 2002;16(8):583–90.
12. Abdel-Razzak OM, Bagley DH. Clinical experience with flexible ureteropyeloscopy. J Urol. 1992;148(6): 1788–92.
13. Delvecchio FC, et al. Assessment of stricture formation with the ureteral access sheath. Urology. 2003; 61(3):518–22. discussion 522.

14. Denstedt JD, et al. A prospective randomized controlled trial comparing nonstented versus stented ureteroscopic lithotripsy. J Urol. 2001;165(5):1419–22.
15. Hosking DH, McColm SE, Smith WE. Is stenting following ureteroscopy for removal of distal ureteral calculi necessary? J Urol. 1999;161(1):48–50.
16. Rapoport D, Perks AE, Teichman JM. Ureteral access sheath use and stenting in ureteroscopy: effect on unplanned emergency room visits and cost. J Endourol. 2007;21(9):993–7.
17. Knudsen B, et al. Durability of the next-generation flexible fiberoptic ureteroscopes: a randomized prospective multi-institutional clinical trial. Urology. 2010;75(3):534–8.
18. Pietrow PK, et al. Techniques to maximize flexible ureteroscope longevity. Urology. 2002;60(5):784–8.
19. Monga M, Gawlik A, Durfee W. Systematic evaluation of ureteral access sheaths. Urology. 2004;63(5):834–6.
20. Monga M, et al. Prospective randomized comparison of 2 ureteral access sheaths during flexible retrograde ureteroscopy. J Urol. 2004;172(2):572–3.
21. Pedro RN, et al. Physical characteristics of next-generation ureteral access sheaths: buckling and kinking. Urology. 2007;70(3):440–2.
22. Pedro RN, et al. Ureteral access sheath insertion forces: implications for design and training. Urol Res. 2007;35(2):107–9.
23. Pedro RN, et al. In vitro evaluation of ureteral perforation forces. Urology. 2007;70(3):592–4. discussion 594–5.
24. Patel MB, Mason BM, Hoenig DM. Retrograde endoscopic-assisted percutaneous renal access: a novel "lasso" technique to achieve rapid secure access to the collecting system. J Endourol. 2008;22(4):591–6. discussion 596.
25. Landman J, et al. Combined percutaneous and retrograde approach to staghorn calculi with application of the ureteral access sheath to facilitate percutaneous nephrolithotomy. J Urol. 2003;169(1):64–7.
26. Benway BM, Nakada SY. Balloon dilation of nephrostomy tracts. J Endourol. 2008;22(9):1875–6. discussion 1887, 1889.
27. Harper JD, et al. Comparison of a novel radially dilating balloon ureteral access sheath to a conventional sheath in the porcine model. J Urol. 2008;179(5):2042–5.
28. Duvdevani M, et al. Third prize: contemporary percutaneous nephrolithotripsy: 1585 procedures in 1338 consecutive patients. J Endourol. 2007;21(8):824–9.
29. Michel MS, Trojan L, Rassweiler JJ. Complications in percutaneous nephrolithotomy. Eur Urol. 2007;51(4):899–906. discussion 906.
30. Breda A, et al. Flexible ureteroscopy and laser lithotripsy for single intrarenal stones 2 cm or greater—is this the new frontier? J Urol. 2008;179(3):981–4.
31. Mues AC, Teichman JM, Knudsen BE. Evaluation of 24 holmium:YAG laser optical fibers for flexible ureteroscopy. J Urol. 2009;182(1):348–54.
32. Takazawa R, Kitayama S, Tsujii T. Successful outcome of flexible ureteroscopy with holmium laser lithotripsy for renal stones 2 cm or greater. Int J Urol. 2011;19(3):264–7.
33. Riley JM, Stearman L, Troxel S. Retrograde ureteroscopy for renal stones larger than 2.5 cm. J Endourol. 2009;23(9):1395–8.

25 Flexible Ureteroscopy: Wireless and Sheathless

Jacob H. Cohen, Seth D. Cohen, and Michael Grasso III

This chapter contains video segments that can be found on the accompanying DVD

Introduction

No-touch ureteroscopy, also termed "wireless and sheathless" ureteroscopy, was first introduced as means of mapping the upper urinary tract urothelium in those who had undergone prior endoscopic therapy of an urothelial malignancy. Minimizing incidental trauma from a guide wire or dilator was found to be particularly helpful in performing a meticulous endoscopic evaluation in this select patient population. Bagley was the first to describe a no touch or atraumatic diagnostic technique [1, 2]. A small diameter semirigid ureteroscope was first employed under direct vision inspecting the distal ureter, and then over a guide wire passed only into the distal ureter, the flexible ureteroscope was placed to complete the more proximal ureteral and intrarenal inspection. Improvements in the mechanics of flexible ureteroscopes, including smaller tip diameter, exaggerated tip deflection, and a larger deflecting radius allow for the intubation of the ureteral orifice and the complete upper urinary tract inspection to be performed solely with a flexible endoscope, commonly without the assistance of a potentially traumatic guide wire.

Direct flexible ureteroscope access to the upper urinary tract involves identifying, intubating, and traversing the intramural ureter under direct vision without the use of a guide wire or an access sheath which might obscure a distal ureteral lesion. Achieving upper tract urinary access with this technique was described in 2004 by Johnson et al. [3]. Atraumatic evaluation of the upper urinary tract is particularly useful in those undergoing diagnostic ureteroscopy with a history of upper tract urothelial malignancies. In this setting, use of a ureteral access sheath may obscure small ureteral tumors, and a guide wire may cause mucosal trauma and erythema, rendering a diagnostic evaluation difficult. With the safety and efficacy of this technique in diagnostic applications, the indications for no-touch ureteroscopy have expanded to include a variety of therapeutic indications including tumor therapy and endoscopic lithotripsy. Herein, a review of the current techniques and results associated with wireless and sheathless flexible ureteroscopy will be presented.

J.H. Cohen, M.D., M.P.H. • S.D. Cohen, M.D.
Department of Urology, Lenox Hill Hospital, 4 East, 100 E. 77th Street, New York, NY 10075, USA

M. Grasso III, M.D. (✉)
Department of Urology, Lenox Hill Hospital, 4 East, 100 E. 77th Street, New York, NY 10075, USA

Department of Urology, Medical College of New York, Valhalla, NY 10595, USA
e-mail: mgrasso3@earthlink.net

M. Monga (ed.), *Ureteroscopy: Indications, Instrumentation & Technique*, Current Clinical Urology, DOI 10.1007/978-1-62703-206-3_25,

Instrumentation

The early 1990s saw the advent of the two-way, actively deflectable, flexible ureteroscope, ushering in the era of modern, flexible ureteroscopy. New generation flexible ureteroscopes possess many design advantages that facilitate no-touch ureteroscopy, such as smaller tip diameter, increased primary active deflection, and greater shaft durometer (stiffness).

No-touch ureteroscopy requires the smallest tip diameter fiberoptic flexible ureteroscopes, typically having a 7.5 Fr tip diameter and a shaft diameter of 8.1–8.5 Fr (Fig. 25.1). Digital ureteroscopes tend to be of a larger diameter and less deflectable making intramural intubation more challenging. The smallest diameter endoscopes also help facilitate irrigant drainage around the instrument, minimizing over-distension of the renal collecting system. The standard 3.6 Fr working channel allows placement of accessory instruments with adequate simultaneous irrigation. Increased ureteroscope shaft stiffness prevents buckling in the bladder and distal ureter, thus facilitating greater control of the ureteroscope tip.

One-to-one torquability (rotating the flexible ureteroscope at the handle facilitates the same degree of tip rotation) and logical active deflection (lever down leads to tip down) of up to 270° facilitate accurate placement of the flexible ureteroscope throughout the upper urinary tract (Fig. 25.2). Active tip deflection by depressing the endoscope lever is enhanced by passive distal shaft deflection, often required to access the lower pole. With the instrument hand lever maximally depressed, the instrument is advanced causing buckling at a predetermined shaft segment. This maneuver, termed passive deflection, is useful in placing endoscope accessories into a particularly dependant lower pole calyx. Accessory equipment, such as a 365-μm laser fiber and a 2.4 Fr Nitinol basket decrease tip deflectability, but their application is enhanced with this maneuver.

Technique

Ureteroscopy begins with cystoscopic evaluation of the bladder to both evaluate the lower urinary tract urothelium and define the location and caliber of the ureteral orifices. A 5-Fr open-ended ureteral catheter and real-time fluoroscopy are employed for a contrast-based retrograde pyelogram, defining ureteral and calyceal anatomy. The bladder is then drained completely, and the flexible ureteroscope passed into the bladder. Sufficient irrigant (typically 50–60 cc) is instilled

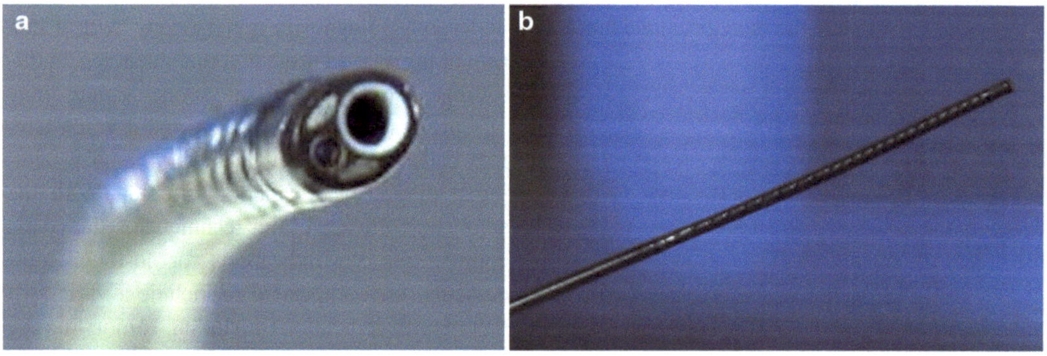

Fig. 25.1 Cross-section view of a flexible ureteroscope showing the optical system and 3.6 Fr working channel (**a**). Figure 23.1a from Cohen JH, Grasso III, M. Ureteroscopy for Upper Ureteric and Renal Stones: Overcoming Difficulties with the Flexible Approach. In: Difficult Cases in Endourology Al-Kandari A, Desai M, Shokeir AA, Shoma AM, Smith AD, editors. New York. Springer Science+Business Media; 2013. Reprinted with permission. Modern fiberoptic flexible ureteroscopes typically have a 7.5 Fr tip diameter, a shaft diameter of 8.1–8.5 Fr (**b**)

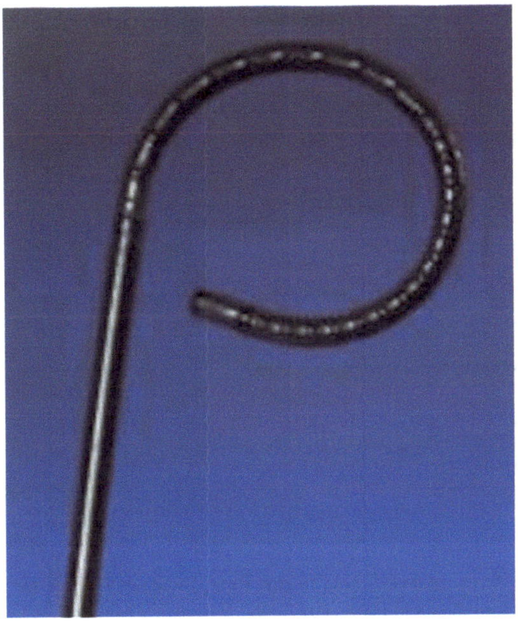

Fig. 25.2 270° tip deflection is demonstrated. Figure 23.1b from Cohen JH, Grasso III, M. Ureteroscopy for Upper Ureteric and Renal Stones: Overcoming Difficulties with the Flexible Approach. In: Difficult Cases in Endourology Al-Kandari A, Desai M, Shokeir AA, Shoma AM, Smith AD, editors. New York. Springer Science + Business Media; 2013. Reprinted with permission

to lift the back wall of the bladder off of the trigone, which aids in identifying the ureteral orifice. If the bladder is over distended, the intramural tunnel is compressed, making ureteral cannulation with the endoscope challenging.

The ureteral orifice is gently cannulated with the flexible ureteroscope under direct vision and then directed proximally (Fig. 25.3). If a ureteral peristaltic wave is encountered, retrograde passage is transiently paused until the wave has passed. Once in the kidney, a complete mapping of the collecting system is routinely performed. Instillation of dilute radio-opaque contrast thru the working channel of the ureteroscope can be employed as a map for subsequent endoscopic inspection. Lower pole calyces can be challenging to visualize, particularly if associated with a narrow or angled infundibulum. The combination of maximal active tip deflection with passive proximal shaft buckling (i.e., secondary deflection) will often help facilitate endoscope placement in this setting (Fig. 25.4).

Irrigant is employed thru the working channel of the endoscope to clear the optical lens of debris and to distend the collecting sufficiently for inspection. A simple irrigation system commonly

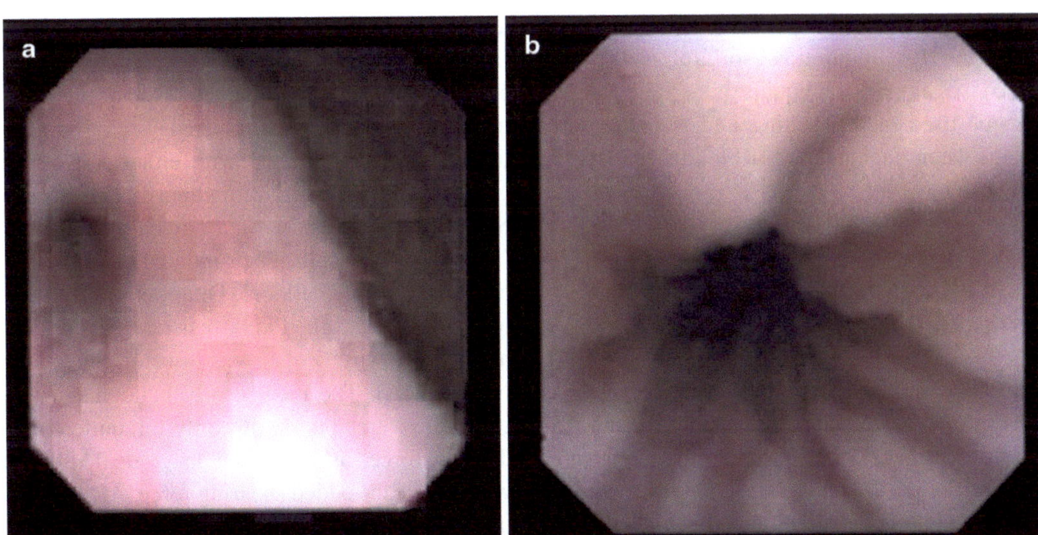

Fig. 25.3 View of the right ureteral orifice through the ureteroscope (**a**). A peristaltic wave is encountered in the mid-ureter (**b**)

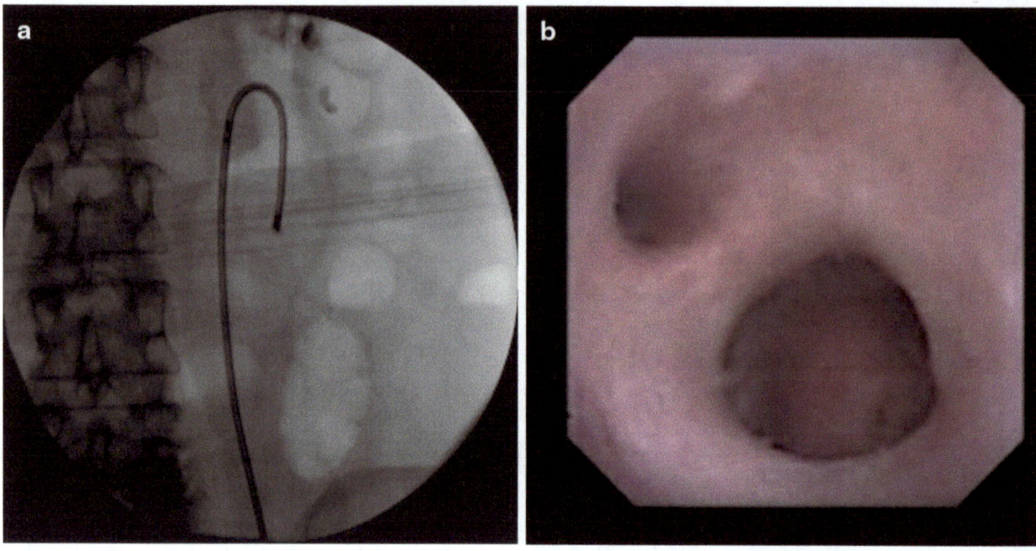

Fig. 25.4 Secondary active and passive deflection is required to achieve access to this right, lower-pole calyx (**a**). Endoscopic view of anterior and posterior mid-pole calyxes from the renal pelvis (**b**)

employed is based on two refillable 60 cc syringes joined to a 3-way stopcock attached to the endoscope with standard Luer-lock ended tubing (Fig. 25.5). The assistant instills sufficient irrigant to clear the optical field, varying the pressure and flow as needed based on the clinical presentation. Normal saline is the most common irrigant employed for diagnostic ureteroscopy and endoscopic lithotripsy. If electrocautery is to be employed for fulguration, sorbitol is the preferred irrigant. Small aliquots of sterile water can also be used in this setting and is particularly useful when encountering a bloody endoscopic field of view.

Difficult Endoscope Access: Broadening the Algorithm

No-touch flexible ureteroscopic access is employed when technically feasible for the reasons previously defined. Commonly, a tight ureteral orifice or a tortuous intramural ureter will prohibit endoscope placement. In this setting a flexible tipped guide wire is passed thru the working channel of the endoscope and the distal ureter is intubated under direct vision. This maneuver frequently facilitates endoscope passage thru a tortuous or kinked segment of the ureter, straightening the ureter while providing increased shaft rigidity. Once the narrowed or tortuous segment is traversed, the guide wire is removed and the remainder of the ureter and collecting system inspected without a wire in place.

If the intramural ureter is narrowed, a common finding in young males, and a guide wire alone will not facilitate access, intramural dilation is required (Fig. 25.6). Dilators with the smallest caliber outer diameter cause the least ureteral trauma and are preferred. The intramural ureter is actively dilated with either a 6–12 Fr graduated dilator (i.e., Nottingham dilator, Boston Scientific, Natick Mass.), or a balloon dilator (5 Fr delivery sheath, 12 Fr inflated outer diameter, 4–10 cm long balloon). Dilation is performed over a teflon sheathed kink-resistant, nickel-titanium guide wire (Zebra wire, Boston Scientific, Natick, MA). The more costly balloon dilation can be less traumatic with only circumferential dilating force, as compared to gradual dilators which have the added shearing force. After active intramural dilation, the flexible ureteroscope is then passed over the guide wire to begin the endoscopy.

If the flexible ureteroscope cannot traverse the ureteral orifice after active dilation, a mucosal lip

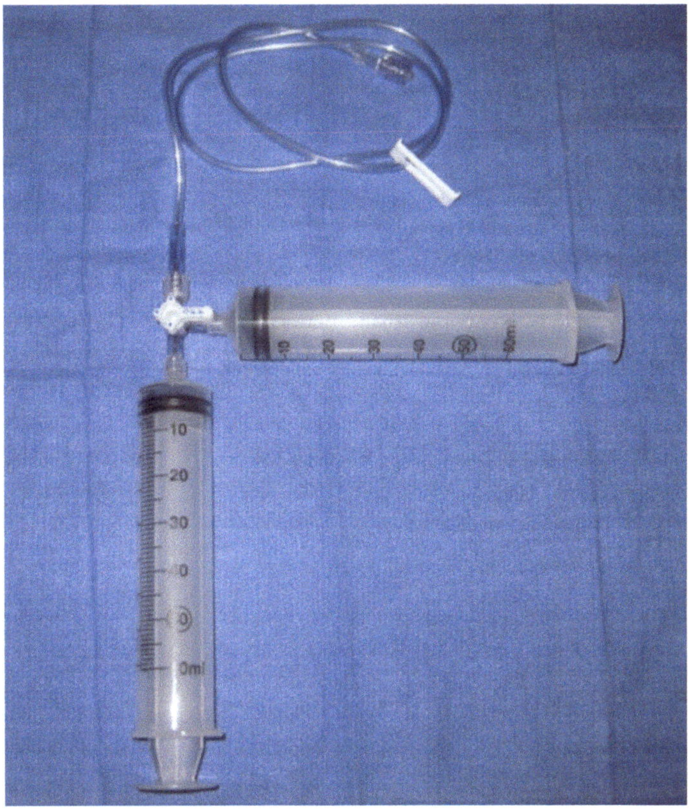

Fig. 25.5 Two 60 cc syringes connected through a 3-way stopcock to Luer-lock extension tubing allows variation in pressure and flow while irrigating

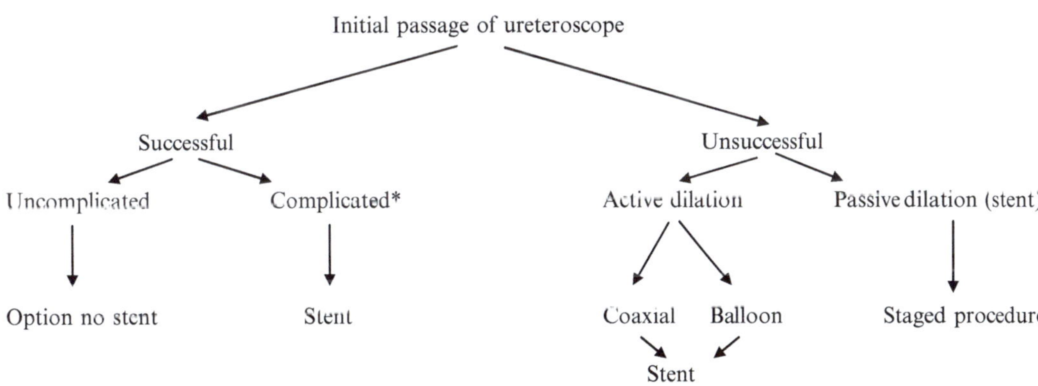

Fig. 25.6 Procedural algorithm. *Asterisk*: Complicated defined by prolonged procedure, infection, ureteral edema/trauma, congenital obstructive anomaly, or significant residual stone burden. Figure 23.2 from Cohen JH, Grasso III, M. Ureteroscopy for Upper Ureteric and Renal Stones: Overcoming Difficulties with the Flexible Approach. In: Difficult Cases in Endourology Al-Kandari A, Desai M, Shokeir AA, Shoma AM, Smith AD, editors. New York. Springer Science+Business Media; 2013. Reprinted with permission

or fold may be inhibiting progress. In that setting a small caliber semirigid ureteroscope is employed to inspect this segment. The passage of the graduated semirigid endoscope will also facilitate ureteral dilation in this setting. There are certain clinical presentations where after the aforementioned maneuvers, the endoscope will not pass proximally. Patients with prior retroperitoneal surgery or radiotherapy causing marked ureteral fibrosis may prohibit diagnostic ureteroscopy.

In this setting, performing a staged procedure by first placing an ureteral stent to facilitate passive dilatation of the ureter over time is a useful technique.

Management of Upper Urinary Tract Urothelial Tumors

Atraumatic ureteroscopic examination of the upper urinary tract is crucial in the setting of diagnosing and treating upper urinary tract tumors. No-touch flexible ureteroscopy, if technically feasible, facilitates a pristine inspection of the urothelium, minimizing bleeding and inadvertent urothelial trauma. In addition, the application of an access sheath in this setting may disrupt a papillary lesion or obscure distal ureteral tumors and thus are infrequently employed, particularly during diagnostic endoscopic mapping (Fig. 25.7).

Cystoscopic mapping of the lower urinary tract urothelium, bladder barbotage for cytological evaluation, and retrograde pyelograms are

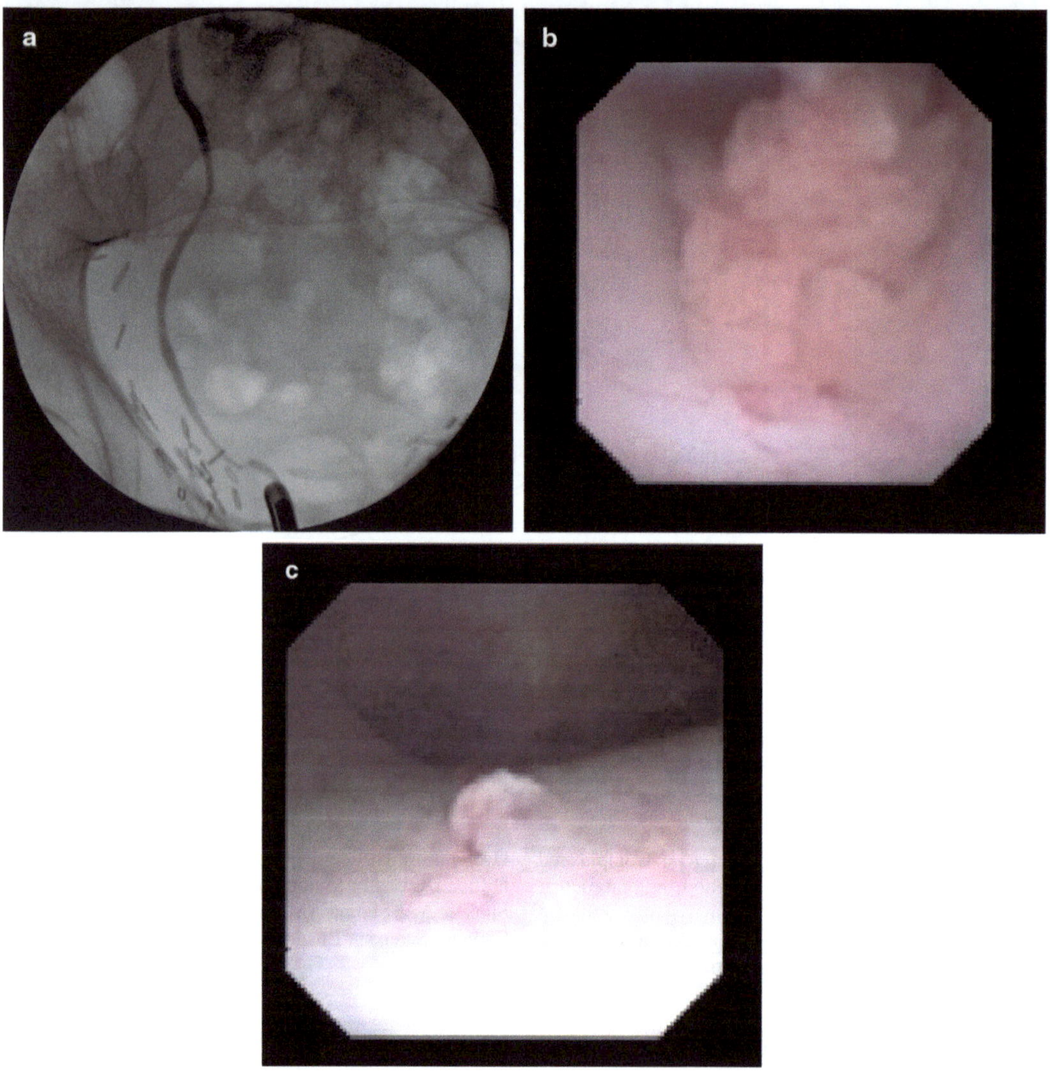

Fig. 25.7 Normal retrograde pyelogram in a patient with a history of prior pelvic surgery and upper tract urothelial cancer (**a**). No-touch ureteroscopy was performed, revealing a 5 mm right distal ureteral tumor that did not manifest as a filling defect on the retrograde pyelogram (**b**). A 1 mm tumor in the renal pelvis easily appreciated with atruamatic inspection of the upper urinary tract without prior sheath or wire placement (**c**)

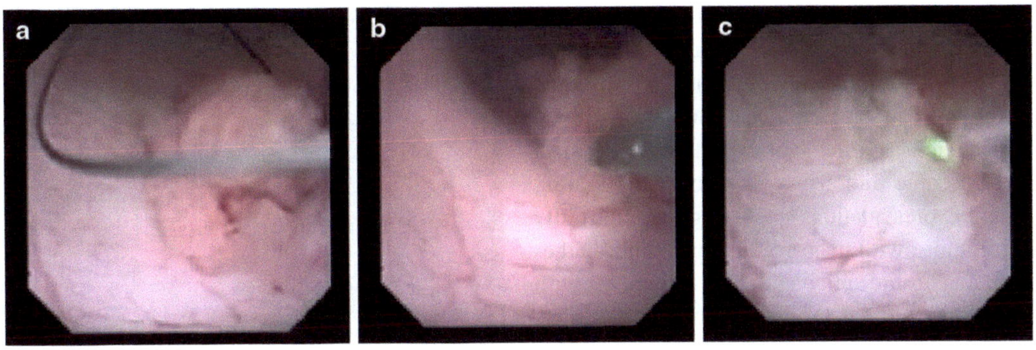

Fig. 25.8 A 2.4 Fr basket is placed around the tumor (**a**). The tumor is pulled free and the tumor, basket, and ureteroscope are withdrawn down the ureter as a unit (**b**). The tumor base is then coagulated using holmium laser energy (**c**)

performed prior to diagnostic ureteroscopy. A small aliquot of dilute contrast is instilled thru a 5 Fr angiographic ureteral catheter under real-time fluoroscopic guidance to opacify the collecting system. Over distension of the collecting system may cause extravasation and mucosal changes, potentially obscuring small or flat lesions.

Obtaining an adequate biopsy specimen is paramount to accurately diagnosing upper urinary tract tumors and crafting a treatment plan. Papillary tumors are best biopsied with a flat-wire 2.4 Fr stainless steel Segura basket (Boston Scientific, Natick, MA). The flexible ureteroscope is withdrawn with the engaged specimen under vision, as extracting the basket through the working channel of the ureteroscope will shear off specimen (Fig. 25.8). For large and vascular lesions, it is often helpful to first coagulate the tumor base with laser energy or electrocautery to minimize hematuria associated with the biopsy. Flat lesions are biopsied with a cup biopsy forceps (Piranha biopsy forceps, Boston Scientific, Natick, MA) with the small specimens prepared and evaluated using cytologic cell block technique [4]. Obtaining a barbotage specimen of saline obtained thru the working channel of the endoscope after biopsy will increase the sensitivity of the cytologic evaluation [5].

Once an ureteroscopic biopsy has been performed, tumor therapy can proceed in the appropriate setting. The indications for ureteroscopic therapy have broadened with the best results in those with modest sized, lower grade lesions [6, 7]. Ureteroscopic resection of an upper urinary tract urothelial lesion is performed with either electrocautery or laser energy, with the intent to remove all visible tumor. Small caliber 2 Fr electrocautery electrodes are employed to both resect and coagulate lesions. Holmium laser energy is an efficient means of clearing papillary tumor fronds, employing low power setting of 0.6 J and frequency of pulsation of 5 Hz to coagulate small bleeding sites as tumor is ablated. ND:YAG (neodymium) laser energy can be employed simultaneously with holmium to obtain deeper tissue coagulation. Twenty watts of Nd:YAG power for 15–20 s will both coagulate and also cause deeper tissue necrosis as compared to holmium, and as such should be used with caution in the ureter in light of a relatively high risk of subsequent structure [8]. Staged ureteroscopic resection is employed commonly for large tumors, and to help facilitate topical therapies.

Postoperative ureteral stenting is employed after ureteroscopic tumor therapy based in part on the complexity of the procedure and the volume of tumor treated. In cases where active dilation was employed for access, or when an intrarenal chemotherapy is planned, a ureteral catheter is placed at the termination of ureteroscopic therapy.

Ureteroscopic Lithotripsy

Flexible ureteroscopic lithotripsy is a common therapy for upper urinary tract calculi, and is particularly useful for extracorporeal shock wave

(ESWL) failures and in those patients who are not candidates for the more invasive percutaneous nephrostolithotomy (PCNL). Ureteroscopic lithotripsy can be employed for various stone compositions, often irrespective of size. Ureteroscopic lithotripsy is useful in treating complex presentations including the morbidly obese, those with uncorrectable bleeding diathesis or on chronic anticoagulation, or patients with other comorbidities limiting their ability to tolerate more invasive procedures. A relative contraindication to flexible ureteroscopic lithotripsy is active pyelonephritis, potentially with pyonephrosis, where primary drainage and staged endoscopic lithotripsy are the best course.

The holmium laser is the most common lithotrite employed thru the flexible ureteroscope, delivering laser energy in a pulsatile fashion through flexible, low water density quartz fibers. Holmium laser energy fragments all stones irrespective of composition, with higher power required for the more dense calcium oxalate monohydrate and brushite calculi. Laser fibers of 365 or 200-μm diameter are commonly used. Larger fibers have an exponentially larger spot size and efficiency in fragmentation, while smaller diameter fibers maximize irrigant flow and endoscope deflectability, which is particularly useful when treating dependant lower pole calculi. Laser settings for lithotripsy often begin at 1 J and 5 Hz frequency of pulsation. For particularly dense calcium oxalate monohydrate stones, higher settings may be used, with the caveat that increased kinetic energy will be transmitted to the stone, making it more difficult to pin and fragment smaller pieces. Once primary fragmentation is complete, lowering the laser settings will help efficiently pulverize residual. Laser fiber strippers should be available to optimize the fiber tip as it is degraded during active lithotripsy.

Small caliber (1.3–2.4 Fr) nitinol baskets are employed to extract representative fragments for stone analysis after ureteroscopic lithotripsy. The nitinol basket's soft and moldable spherical shape is useful in both extracting and disengaging stone fragments (Fig. 25.9). Nitinol graspers (1.9 Fr Graspit, Boston Scientific, Natick, MA or 1.7 Fr Engage, Cook Urology, Spencer, IN) can disengage calculi more easily and are particularly useful in relocating calculi from a lower pole location to a more easily accessible cephalad calyx where a larger laser fiber can be employed to maximize efficient lithotripsy.

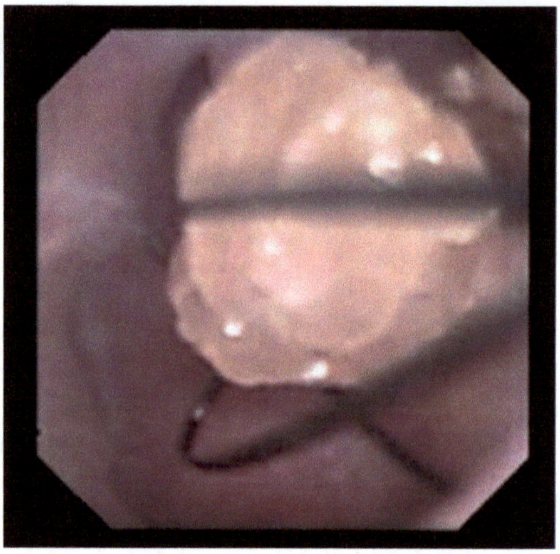

Fig. 25.9 A zero-tipped nitinol basket is used to grap a cystine stone fragment. The basket's helical shape conforms to the shape of the ureter. The operating surgeon must ensure that stone fragments are small enough to be withdrawn atraumatically

Continuous bladder drainage during ureteroscopic lithotripsy is commonly performed by placing a small diameter 14 Fr foley catheter to gravity drainage beside the ureteroscope. Decompressing the bladder will help clear the optic field and minimize intramural ureteral pressure which can limit ureteroscopic maneuverability.

At the conclusion of endoscopic lithotripsy, an ureteral stent is placed if intramural ureteral dilation was required for endoscope access, significant edema from impacted stones was encountered, infectious debris was noted endoscopically, or if significant stone debris remains requiring passive ureteral dilation to help facilitate subsequent clearance. Routine ureteral stenting is not otherwise performed, especially if no-touch ureteroscopic access is employed.

Special Stone Situations: Impacted Ureteral Stones, Lower Pole Stones, and Large Calculi

The application of the actively deflectable, flexible ureteroscope for an impacted, proximal ureteral stone is a common but clinically challenging presentation. Significant mucosal edema may surround the calculus, limiting visualization (Fig. 25.10). In this setting, it is paramount to place the laser fiber centrally on the stone to limit ureteral wall trauma. Rather than completely fragmenting the stone in situ, the preferred technique is to centrally fragment and disimpact the calculus, moving it to a more cephalad intrarenal location to complete the lithotripsy. This will help minimize fragments remaining in the inflamed ureteral segment, which can become submucosal and can be associated with ureteral fibrosis [9]. Placing the patient in a head-down position with the ipsilateral side raised will help direct disimpacted stone fragments cephalad, away from a dependant lower pole calyx.

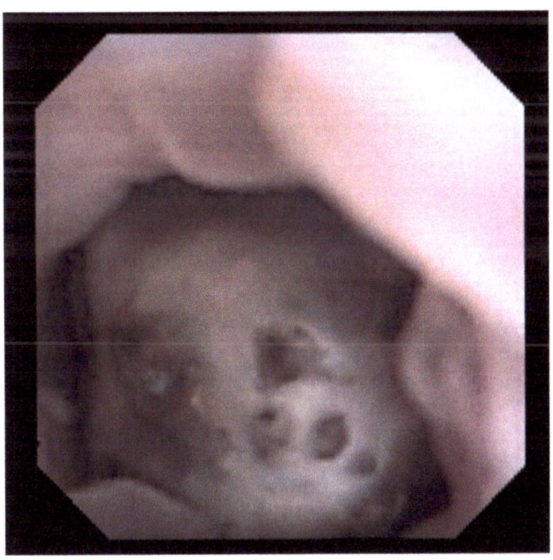

Fig. 25.10 A 1.8 cm, impacted proximal ureteral stone with a characteristic appearance of calcium oxalate monohydrate. There is significant ureteral edema. Figure 23.4a from Cohen JH, Grasso III, M. Ureteroscopy for Upper Ureteric and Renal Stones: Overcoming Difficulties with the Flexible Approach. In: Difficult Cases in Endourology Al-Kandari A, Desai M, Shokeir AA, Shoma AM, Smith AD, editors. New York. Springer Science+Business Media; 2013. Reprinted with permission

For lower pole stones, the endoscopist must chose to either fragment in situ in the lower pole and remove fragments, or to move the stone (if it is small enough) to the upper pole where fragmentation can proceed more efficiently. It can be challenging to place a relatively stiff laser fiber into a dependant, medial lower pole calyx associated with a long, narrow infundibulum. Small nitinol baskets and graspers inhibit endoscope deflection less and are easier to manipulate thru a maximally deflected ureteroscope. They are particularly useful in moving lower pole stones to a more cephalad location where they can be fragmented more easily with larger diameter caliber laser fibers. If the lower pole stone is too large to extract, in situ lithotripsy is employed to create moveable fragments which are promptly relocated and then treated to completion.

Flexible ureteroscopy lithotripsy can be employed for large, noninfectious branching stone burdens (>2 cm). Ureteroscopic lithotripsy in this setting creates stone dust that coats the urothelium, eventually limiting visualization and often necessitating staged therapy. Keys to success when treating large calculi ureteroscopically include moving fragments cephalad to maximize laser parameters, while maintaining continuous bladder drainage during ureteroscopic lithotripsy. Between staged ureteroscopic lithotripsy sessions, and in particular for stone compositions like cystine or uric acid that are in part dissolvable, retrograde catheters are employed for topical therapy to clear stone dust (Fig. 25.11). Inflow is performed thru a 6 Fr Cobra catheter positioned with it tip in a dependant lower pole location where debris tends to collect. Outflow is obtained with a 6 or 8 Fr single pigtail catheter positioned in a superior calyx. Both catheters are secured to a urethral foley, and are irrigated by hand if blocked by debris.

Irrigant choice depends on stone composition (Table 25.1), and the rate is adjusted from 50 to 100 cc/h based on patient tolerance. Irrigation is promptly stopped and the patient reassessed if symptoms of obstruction are noted or if the patient has a significant rise in temperature. After

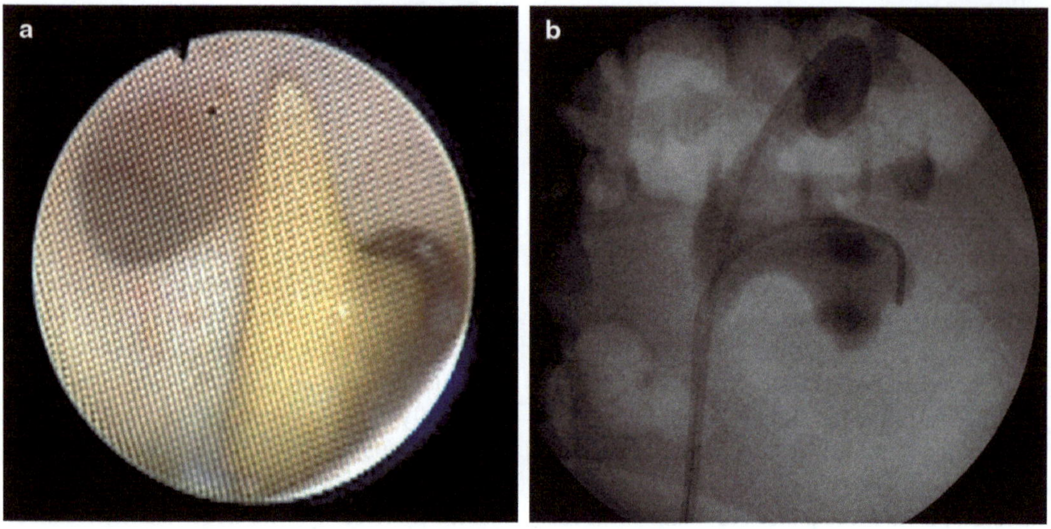

Fig. 25.11 A 2.5 cm lower pole partial staghorn calculus in a patient with cystinuria (**a**). Between stated ureteroscopic lithotripsy sessions, retrograde catheters are employed for topical therapy to clear stone dust. Inflow is performed thru a 6 Fr Cobra catheter with its tip in a dependant lower pole location, where debris tends to collect. Outflow is obtained thru a 6 or 8 Fr single pigtail catheter positioned in a superior calyx (**b**). Figure 23.5 from Cohen JH, Grasso III, M. Ureteroscopy for Upper Ureteric and Renal Stones: Overcoming Difficulties with the Flexible Approach. In: Difficult Cases in Endourology Al-Kandari A, Desai M, Shokeir AA, Shoma AM, Smith AD, editors. New York. Springer Science+Business Media; 2013. Reprinted with permission

Table 25.1 Irrigant choice for intrarenal irrigation

Stone type	Irrigant choice	Effect
Cystine	THAM-E and Mucomyst[a]	Clear dust and debris
Uric acid	THAM-E	Dissolve fragments, clear dust and debris
Calcium-based	Saline and gentamicin	Clear dust and debris

[a]THAM-E is pH-10 trometamol *tris*-hydroxymethyl aminomethane, Mucomyst is *N*-acetylcysteine

an interval of irrigation, most frequently 36–48 h, a second stage of endoscopic lithotripsy is employed to treat residua. Interval irrigation improves visualization during the second session. In addition, the passive ureteral dilation from the irrigation catheters helps facilitate passage of remaining debris, with many patients being rendered stent-free thereafter.

Results and Complications

In 2006, Johnson et al. reviewed 460 consecutive upper urinary-tract procedures performed by a single surgeon using a 7.5 Fr actively deflectable, flexible ureteroscope [3]. Procedures were performed for a variety of therapeutic indications, including evaluation and treatment of essential gross hematuria, upper-tract urothelial tumors, ureteral strictures, endoscopic lithotripsy, and ureteropelvic junction (UPJ obstruction). A stent was in place or had been previously placed in 108 of the procedures (24 %). Only 52 of the remaining 352 procedures (11 %) required any form of ureteral dilation to facilitate ureteral access. Two hundred and twenty-seven (48 %) wireless and sheathless procedures were performed, identifying and intubating the ureteral orifice under direct vision in atraumatic fashion. Inability to access the lower pole was rare, observed in only 1.5 % of procedures.

Grasso et al. published a multi-institutional study of retrograde ureteropyeloscopic lithotripsy of large upper tract stones, including many partial

Table 25.2 Comparison of ureteroscopic complications

	Blute et al. [14]	Abdel-Razzak and Bagley [15]	Harmon et al. [16]	Grasso et al. [17]
Year	1988	1992	1997	2000
Procedures	346	290	209	1,000
Minor complications	(%)	(%)	(%)	(%)
Colic/pain	–	9	3.5	4.2
Fever	6.2	6.9	2	1.3
False passage	0.9	–	–	0.4
Hematuria minor	0.5	2.1	0	0.8
Prolonged	0.3	1.0	0	0.8
Extravasation	0.6	1.0	–	–
UTI	–	1.0	–	1.7
Pyelonephritis	–	–	–	1.0
Major complications	(%)	(%)	(%)	(%)
Major perforation	4.6	1.7	1.0	0
Stricture	1.4	0.7	0.5	0.4
Avulsion	0.6	0	0	0
Urinoma	0.6	–	0	0
Urosepsis	0.3	0	0	0
CVA	–	–	0.5	0.1
DVT	–	–	–	0.1
MI	–	–	–	0.1

UTI urinary tract infection, *CVA* cerebrovascular accident, *DVT* deep venous thrombosis, *MI* myocardial infarction
From [17], reprinted with permission from Elsevier Limited

staghorn calculi, treating these stones with direct ureteral access without an access sheath. Stone clearance was 95 % with a 5 % complication rate [10]. Other series of flexible ureteroscopic lithotripsy for large upper urinary tract stone burdens (>2 cm) describe stone clearance rates of 90 % or greater, yet all utilized ureteral access sheaths to facilitate repeated access up and down the ureter [11–13]. The complication rates in these series ranged from 0 to 20 %. Therefore, even with the most complex stone burdens, Grasso et al. showed a ureteral access sheath was not necessary to achieve an excellent stone clearance rate with minimal complications.

Improvements in instrumentation and refinement in technique have decreased complications from flexible ureteroscopy. Reported complication rates are low, ranging from 1 to 5 %. Infectious events, such as pyelonephritis, are the most commonly reported complication, and are minimized by ensuring a sterile, preoperative urine and appropriate antibiotic prophylaxis. Gross hematuria is infrequent, and may be treated with mild supportive measures.

If small diameter endoscopes are employed and contemporary described technique is used, major complications such as ureteral perforation, avulsion, and stricture are infrequent (Table 25.2). In a published series of 1,000 consecutive ureteroscopies by a single urologist, of which 491 were endoscopic lithotripsies, there were no perforations or avulsions, and the ureteral stricture rate was 0.4 % [14].

Conclusion

Newer generation flexible ureteroscopes, with their greater deflectability, miniaturization, and improved tip control are key to the atraumatic inspection of the entire urothelium. Flexible ureteroscopy without use of an access sheath or guide wire is a feasible and safe technique for diagnostic and also therapeutic procedures. When practiced with the described technique, no-touch flexible ureteroscopy allows the least traumatic intervention for upper tract urinary pathology possible.

References

1. Keeley Jr FX, Bibbo M, Bagley DH. Ureteroscopic treatment and surveillance of upper urinary tract transitional cell carcinoma. J Urol. 1997;157(5):1560–5.
2. Bagley DH. Ureteroscopic laser treatment of upper urinary tract tumors. J Clin Laser Med Surg. 1998;16(1):55–9.
3. Johnson GB, Grasso M. Exaggerated primary endoscope deflection: initial clinical experience with prototype flexible ureteroscopes. BJU Int. 2004;93(1):109–14.
4. Bian Y, Ehya H, Bagley DH. Cytologic diagnosis of upper urinary tract neoplasms by ureteroscopic sampling. Acta Cytol. 1995;39(4):733–40.
5. Keeley FX, Kulp DA, Bibbo M, McCue PA, Bagley DH. Diagnostic accuracy of ureteroscopic biopsy in upper tract transitional cell carcinoma. J Urol. 1997;157(1):33–7.
6. Grasso M, Fraiman M, Levine M. Ureteropyeloscopic diagnosis and treatment of upper urinary tract urothelial malignancies. Urology. 1999;54(2):240–6.
7. Johnson GB, Fraiman M, Grasso M. Broadening experience with the retrograde endoscopic management of upper urinary tract urothelial malignancies. BJU Int. 2005;92(2):110–3.
8. Schmeller NT, Hofstetter AG. Laser treatment of ureteral tumors. J Urol. 1989;141(4):840–3.
9. Grasso M, Liu JB, Goldberg B, Bagley DH. Submucosal calculi: endoscopic and intraluminal sonographic diagnosis and treatment options. J Urol. 1995;153(5):1384–9.
10. Grasso M, Conlin M, Bagley D. Retrograde ureteropyeloscopic treatment of 2 cm or greater upper urinary tract and minor staghorn calculi. J Urol. 1998;160(2):346–51.
11. Breda A, Ogunyemi O, Leppert JT, Lam JS, Schulam PG. Flexible ureteroscopy and laser lithotripsy for single intrarenal stones 2 cm or greater—is this the new frontier? J Urol. 2008;179(3):981–4.
12. Ricchiuti DJ, Smaldone MC, Jacobs BL, Smaldone AM, Jackman SV, Averch TD. Staged retrograde endoscopic lithotripsy as alternative to PCNL in select patients with large renal calculi. J Endourol. 2007;21(12):1421–4.
13. Hyams ES, Munver R, Bird VG, Uberoi J, Shah O. Flexible ureterorenoscopy and holmium laser lithotripsy for the management of renal stone burdens that measure 2 to 3 cm: a multi-institutional experience. J Endourol. 2010;24(10):1583–8.
14. Blute ML, Segura JW, Patterson DE. Ureteroscopy. J Urol. 1988;139(3):510–2.
15. Abdel-Razzak OM, Bagley DH. Clinical experience with flexible ureteropyeloscopy. J Urol. 1992;148(6):1788–92.
16. Harmon WJ, Serson PD, Blue ML, Patterson DE, Segura JW. Ureteroscopy: current practice and long-term complications. J Urol. 1997;157(1):28–32.
17. Grasso M. Ureteropyeloscopic treatment of ureteral and intrarenal calculi. Urol Clin North Am. 2000;27(4):623–31.

Upper Tract Urothelial Carcinoma: Ureteroscopic Biopsy and Specimen Preparation

26

Kelly A. Healy, Nir Kleinmann, Marluce Bibbo, and Demetrius H. Bagley

This chapter contains video segments that can be found on the accompanying DVD

Abbreviations

UTUC	Upper tract urothelial carcinoma
CSS	Cancer specific survival
RNU	Radical nephroureterectomy
CKD	Chronic kidney disease
MDCTU	Multidetector computed tomographic urography
OS	Overall survival
BTA	Bladder tumor antigen
FDP	Fibrin/fibrinogen degradation product
FISH	Fluorescence in situ hybridization
RPG	Retrograde ureteropyelogram
FU	Flexible ureteroscope
F	French
Ho	Holmium
Nd	Neodymium
YAG	Yttrium aluminum garnet
WL	White light
CROES	Clinical research office of the endourological society
NBI	Narrow band imaging
TUR	Transurethral resection
PHH3	Phospho-histone
H&E	Hematoxylin and eosin

K.A. Healy, M.D. • N. Kleinmann, M.D.
D.H. Bagley, M.D., FACS (✉)
Department of Urology and Radiology, Thomas Jefferson University, 1025 Walnut Street, Suite 1112 College Building, Philadelphia, PA 19107, USA
e-mail: demetrius.bagley@jefferson.edu

M. Bibbo, M.D., Sc.D.
Cytopathology Division, Pathology Department, Thomas Jefferson University, Philadelphia, PA, USA

Introduction

Upper tract urothelial carcinoma (UTUC) is a relatively uncommon malignancy, which accounts for only 5% of urothelial tumors and 8% of renal tumors [1]. The estimated annual incidence of UTUC in Western countries is approximately one to two new cases per 100,000 inhabitants. Compared to 15% of bladder tumors, 60% of UTUC are invasive at the time of diagnosis [2–4]. Overall 5-year cancer specific survival (CSS) is approximately 75% but is highly stage dependent. While the 5-year CSS exceeds 90% for pTa and T1 disease, this declines to 74.7%, 54%, and 12.2% for pT2, pT3, and pT4 disease, respectively [5]. Radical nephroureterectomy (RNU) with bladder cuff excision is the gold standard treatment for UTUC and may be performed using an open, laparoscopic, or robotic-assisted approach. However, with advancements in ureteroscopes as well as ablative devices, ureteroscopic resection has emerged as an attractive alternative nephron-sparing option in carefully selected patients with acceptable long-term outcomes [6–8]. Though initially reserved for patients with absolute indications for nephron preservation [9–12], ureteroscopic management

M. Monga (ed.), *Ureteroscopy: Indications, Instrumentation & Technique*, Current Clinical Urology,
DOI 10.1007/978-1-62703-206-3_26,

is now electively done in those with a normal contralateral kidney [13, 14] with renal maintenance in approximately 70–80% of cases [11, 15]. Recently, the risks of chronic kidney disease (CKD) have become increasingly recognized and CKD is associated with a wide range of causes of increased mortality, particularly cardiovascular [16–18]. As such, emphasis has been placed on nephron preservation, specifically partial nephrectomy for renal cell carcinoma [19–21]. These same arguments can be extrapolated to UTUC. The concept of renal preservation is also appealing due to the risk of panurothelial recurrences. The appropriate selection of patients for conservative management is imperative. Currently, accurate staging remains a challenge and grade serves as a surrogate for stage. Thus, obtaining an accurate tissue diagnosis is a critical step in the decision making process for UTUC patients.

Historically, intravenous excretory urography was used to evaluate patients with suspected UTUC. However, multidetector computed tomographic urography (MDCTU) has emerged as the gold standard imaging study for evaluation of the upper urinary tract [22–26]. Overall, MDCTU is highly accurate in identifying UTUC. For polypoid lesions between 5 and 10 mm, MDCTU has demonstrated 96% sensitivity and 99% specificity. Sensitivity decreases to 89% for polypoid lesions <5 mm and 40% for polypoid lesions <3 mm. Nonetheless, the identification of flat lesions remains a challenge until they have massively infiltrated the renal parenchyma. In addition to detecting the tumor, CTU has the potential advantage of providing information regarding the stage. Several studies have also found that hydronephrosis on preoperative imaging was associated with invasive tumor and worse oncologic outcomes [27]. Alternatively, magnetic resonance urography (MRU) may be utilized in patients who cannot undergo MDCTU due to either intravenous contrast allergies or azotemia [28]. Compared to MDCTU, MRU is less sensitive with a detection rate of 75% for tumors <2 cm [29]. Importantly, MRU is contraindicated in patients with severe renal impairment (creatinine clearance <30 mL/min) due to the rare but serious risk of nephrogenic systemic fibrosis [30]. In such cases, noncontrast CT scan in combination with retrograde pyelography can be used instead of MRU to diagnose UTUC.

Despite technologic advancements, imaging studies alone are insufficient to definitively diagnose UTUC and proceed with RNU. While imaging may be highly suggestive of UTUC, a filling defect may represent a wide range of benign entities including a polyp, blood clot, fungus ball, inflammatory lesion, or poorly calcified radiolucent stone such as a matrix calculus. Endoscopic visualization alone is also inadequate to direct treatment decisions. In one series, ureteroscopic appearance was only 70% accurate in determining the malignancy or grade of an upper tract tumor [31]. Another group found that among patients managed endoscopically with a visual diagnosis only, 21% developed grade 3 UTUC during follow-up [32]. However, not all cases of UTUC warrant radical extirpative surgery. The treatment decision is carefully guided by tumor grade which serves as a surrogate for tumor stage. Low grade, low volume tumors have responded well to nephron-sparing endoscopic approaches. In fact, endoscopic resection confers equivalent overall survival (OS) and CSS to RNU in patients with low grade disease; on the other hand, patients with high grade disease fair poorly regardless of the approach [6]. Ureteroscopy with biopsy and possibly resection has been the most accurate technique to date for grading and potentially staging upper tract lesions [33–35].

Herein, we describe our techniques for the ureteroscopic biopsy and specimen handling of upper urinary tract tumors. In doing so, patients may be appropriately selected for a nephron-sparing ureteroscopic laser ablation vs. extirpative surgery with RNU and bladder cuff excision for the management of UTUC.

The Role of Urine Studies in Diagnosis of UTUC

The ideal urine study for the diagnosis of UTUC is obtained using noninvasive techniques and demonstrates both high sensitivity and specificity. Cytologic examination of voided urine was shown to have an overall sensitivity of approximately 30% for the detection of bladder urothelial carcinoma. Importantly, this is highly grade dependent with a sensitivity for grade 1, grade 2, and grade 3 tumors of 12%, 26%, and 64%, respectively [36]. Voided urine cytology is even less sensitive in detecting UTUC [37]. Given the low sensitivity of voided urine for urothelial carcinoma, particularly UTUC, investigators have evaluated alternative methods of urine collection to improve the diagnostic yield. Early studies by Bibbo et al. found an improvement of the sensitivity for UTUC by examining urine obtained by ureteral catheterization with barbotage or brushing [38]. A positive cytology may be valuable in staging because it has been associated with advanced pathologic disease [39]. In addition to urine cytology, multiple alternative urine-based markers have been evaluated for the diagnosis and follow-up of urothelial carcinoma, predominantly among bladder cancer patients. Several urinary markers have demonstrated superior sensitivities but higher false-positive rates compared to cytology [36, 40]. Among UTUC patients, select studies have assessed the utility of alternative markers including Immunocyt™, bladder tumor antigen (BTA), fibrin/fibrinogen degradation product (FDP), and fluorescence in situ hybridization (FISH).

Immunocyt™ is an immunocytochemical diagnostic tool which traces three monoclonal antibodies (19A211, M344, and LDQ10) directed against three antigens (two mucins and a carcinoembryonic antigen) that are expressed by urothelial carcinoma [41]. Initial studies in urothelial carcinoma of the bladder found an overall sensitivity and specificity for voided urine Immunocyt™ of 86.1% and 80%, respectively. Immunocyt™ also maintained a higher sensitivity (84–96%) than cytologic analysis (4–56%) for detecting grade 1 and 2 tumors [41, 42]. Given these promising results, investigators then evaluated Immunocyt™ for the detection of UTUC. Lodde et al. prospectively assessed the clinical performance of Immunocyt™ in 37 patients with suspected UTUC [43]. These authors reported a higher overall sensitivity of Immunocyt™ for detecting UTUC compared to cytologic analysis in voided and ureteral urine. Compared to voided urine cytology, Immunocyt™ from voided urine was more sensitive in detecting both grade 1 (33% vs. 0%) and 2 (100% vs. 17%) tumors. However, Immunocyt™ was less sensitive than cytology in detecting grade 3 tumors (71% vs. 100%). Similarly, upper tract Immunocyt™ was more sensitive for grade 1 and 2 tumors, while cytology was more sensitive for grade 3. The combination of cytologic analysis and Immunocyt™ yielded outstanding results with 100% sensitivity and specificity. Based on these findings, the authors concluded that Immunocyt™ complements cytologic analysis in detecting UTUC, primarily due to its high sensitivity for low grade tumors.

The clinical performance of the BTA test for the detection of UTUC has also been studied. This is a qualitative latex agglutination assay which detects the presence of basement membrane complexes exfoliated in the urine in patients with urothelial carcinoma [44–46]. Several studies have demonstrated the BTA test to have superior sensitivity to urinary cytology in the diagnosis of primary and recurrent bladder cancer, ranging from 50 to 82% [47, 48]. However, the BTA test was poor at identifying upper tract tumors. Zimmerman et al. found 60% sensitivity and 40% specificity of the BTA test using ureteroscopically sampled urine specimens [44]. Due to these poor test characteristics, the authors concluded that the BTA test had no clinical value for diagnosing UTUC.

Another alternative urine-based marker is FDP, which is a lateral flow immunoassay using monoclonal antibodies to detect elevated urinary FDPs previously described in patients with bladder cancer [49–51]. In prospective studies among bladder cancer patients, FDP had a higher overall sensitivity (81%) compared to either BTA (28%) or urinary cytology (35%) [51]. In a preliminary, prospective study, Siemens et al. reported that FDP demonstrated excellent test characteristics, for both voided urine and ureteral washing, with an overall high sensitivity of 100% (BTA 50%, cytology 29%) and accuracy of 83% (BTA 62%, cytology 59%) at the expense of decreased specificity of 67% (BTA 73%, cytology 86%) [48].

FISH analysis of voided bladder urine has emerged as a common diagnostic study for bladder cancer. This assay uses fluorescent probes that detect four chromosomal anomalies typical of bladder cancer, specifically chromosomes 3, 7, 17, and the 9p21 band [52, 53]. Although FISH has demonstrated a higher sensitivity [54–56] than urine cytology, it has not obviated the need for direct cytoscopic evaluation in diagnosing bladder cancer. Several studies have examined voided FISH as an adjunct for detecting UTUC, but the sensitivity has varied widely from 35 to 87.5% [43, 57–60]. Three smaller studies showed encouraging results [43, 57, 58]. In an early study, Lodde et al. analyzed 37 patients with symptomatic or radiographic evidence of UTUC and noted 75% sensitivity [43]. Importantly, of the 16 patients confirmed to have UTUC, 13 underwent radical extirpative surgery while only 3 were managed endoscopically. Among 16 patients with suspected UTUC, Akkad et al. found 87.5% sensitivity [57]. Marin-Aguilera et al. reported 76.7% sensitivity vs. 36% for cytology [58]. Nevertheless, the majority of patients in their series (21/30) subsequently underwent open RNU. While these UTUC series document a high sensitivity of voided FISH, the results must be interpreted with caution since a significant portion of their patients ultimately underwent radical extirpative surgery and are likely distinct from those who underwent endoscopic treatment. That is, their study cohorts may be predominantly comprised of patients with higher volume and higher grade disease, in which voided cytology and FISH may demonstrate improved test characteristics for higher grade or bulkier tumors.

To date, the two largest cohorts bring the utility of voided FISH for the diagnosis of UTUC into question [59, 60]. Chen and Grasso evaluated 94 consecutive FISH specimens from voided urine or selective samples obtained in the operating room endoscopically [59]. Voided specimens demonstrated a poor sensitivity (35%). This improved for bladder washings and selective upper tract washings to 67% and 65%, respectively. Although invasive sampling may increase the diagnostic yield, FISH alone does not appear to be a reliable noninvasive test for the detection of UTUC. Most recently, Johannes et al. evaluated a total of 67 voided urine FISH specimens from 35 patients with a known history of UTUC who previously qualified for a strict endoscopic surveillance and resection protocol [60]. Overall FISH yielded 56% sensitivity and 80% specificity, while cytology had 33% sensitivity for detecting UTUC lesions. After excluding patients with concurrent bladder tumor, the sensitivity and specificity of FISH were 54% and 78%, respectively compared to 18% sensitivity and 100% specificity for bladder cytology. Of note, in this series the majority of patients had low grade (79%) and low volume tumor since they qualified for the strict endoscopic protocol. Based on these disappointing test characteristics, the authors concluded that voided FISH did not provide acceptable sensitivity to eliminate direct ureteroscopic evaluation. Therefore, voided FISH has limited value in the diagnosis and surveillance of UTUC.

At this point, currently available urine-based markers alone are inadequate to definitively diagnose or perform surveillance of UTUC. Direct endoscopic evaluation remains the gold standard diagnostic technique and, simultaneously, provides the opportunity to selectively treat low volume, low grade tumors.

Endoscopic Evaluation and Biopsy Technique

Endoscopic evaluation of the urinary tract begins with cystoscopy to assess for any concomitant lower urinary tract pathology. First, cystoscopy is performed to evaluate the entire urethra, prostate, and bladder. This is typically done using both a 30° and 70° lens. Cystoscopy is a basic but critical step since new or recurrent bladder tumors occur in 20–44% of patients after ureteroscopic treatment [61]. A urine sample is also obtained for cytology. Next, retrograde ureteropyelogram (RPG) is performed on the affected side as well as the contralateral side with dilute (30%) iodinated contrast (Fig. 26.1). Recurrences in the contralateral upper tract are observed in 5–10% of patients [61] and, thus, bilateral RPGs are typically

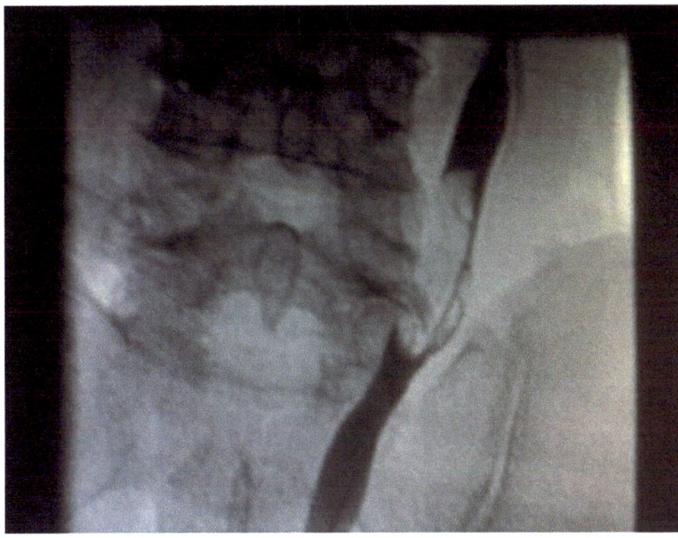

Fig. 26.1 A retrograde ureteropyelogram demonstrates a 3 cm ureteral tumor

done. We strongly prefer to use an appropriately sized cone tip catheter, most commonly 8 F. This provides an excellent seal of the ureteral orifice and thereby prevents leakage of contrast into the bladder. In contrast, an open-ended catheter may not satisfactorily distend the upper tract to identify filling defects. Moreover, an open-ended catheter is usually inserted over a guidewire, which may traumatize the unexamined urothelium. Care must be taken not to over distend the collecting system or use excessively dense contrast material, which may obscure subtle filling defects.

After examining the lower urinary tract, the entire upper urinary tract is thoroughly surveyed using one of two "no touch techniques." This refers to visual inspection of the entire urothelium prior to any instrumentation; even guidewire introduction may incur trauma and cause bleeding, which impairs visualization and confounds inspection. Using the first "no touch technique," a small caliber semirigid ureteroscope is inserted into the bladder and used to cannulate the ureteral orifice under direct vision [62, 63]. The scope is advanced as far proximally as possible without significant torque or angulation. While in a female the semirigid ureteroscope may often be passed to the renal pelvis without difficulty, the scope typically cannot be passed beyond the level of the mid-ureter at the iliac vessels in most patients. The initial use of a radially dilating semirigid ureteroscope to inspect the distal and mid ureter facilitates subsequent insertion of the flexible ureteroscope (FU). The semirigid ureteroscope is then removed and a guidewire is left in place at the level last inspected. Over this wire, a FU is inserted under fluoroscopic guidance. At this step, care must be taken to prevent inadvertent proximal migration of the wire, which again may cause urothelial injury. Dilation of the ureter should also be avoided to minimize the risk of trauma from both the guidewire and the dilation itself. Due to the miniaturization of ureteroscopes, it is rarely necessary to formally dilate the ureter. In fact, Hudson et al. found that the ideal FU outer diameter is 7.5 F to minimize the need for ureteric dilation, as <1% of cases failed to pass without formal dilation using this size scope [64]. However, digital ureteroscopes have a distal digital chip-based camera (CCD or CMOS), or "chip on the tip" technology which necessitates a larger endoscope outer diameter of nearly 10 F and therefore may require dilation before scope insertion.

Utilizing the second "no touch technique," the semirigid ureteroscope is not used at all. Instead, the FU is exclusively employed for the entire inspection using a wireless, sheathless approach [65]. Under direct vision, the FU is inserted into the bladder, throughout the ureter,

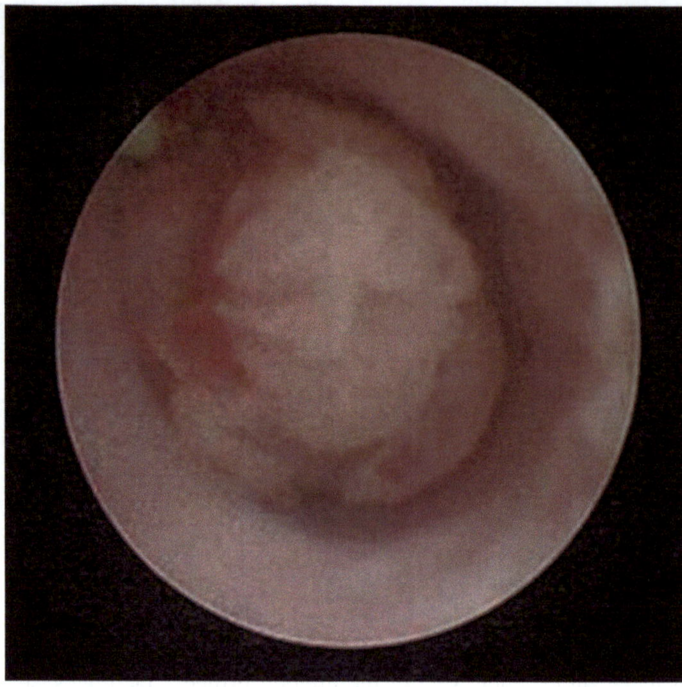

Fig. 26.2 Endoscopic view of ureteral neoplasm

and the intra-renal collecting system. Importantly, this is only possible with the appropriately sized endoscopes and a patent ureteral lumen.

The FU is then advanced under direct vision throughout the ureter and any small ureteral tumors are biopsied and treated as they are encountered using the techniques described below (Fig. 26.2). Commonly, such small lesions may be avulsed with scope advancement, which may induce bleeding and/or make it difficult to identify the lesions later during the procedure. If a large ureteral tumor is encountered, it may be helpful to advance the ureteroscope beyond the lesion to survey the more proximal ureteral segment to identify other tumors. In some instances, it may be difficult to identify the ureteral lumen itself to pass the tumor. It can be useful to follow the contour of the ureteral wall and, in select cases, to pass a hydromer-coated guidewire beyond the tumor to gain proximal access. While a no touch technique is preferred, a guidewire is utilized anytime there is concern in being able to reaccess the ureter.

Next, the collecting system is entered and a renal pelvis aspirate is obtained and sent fresh in normal saline for cytology. This is done by connecting a large Luer lock syringe (50–60 mL) directly to the irrigation port (Fig. 26.3). Then, systematic pyeloscopy is performed and the entire intra-renal collecting system is inspected. Severe deflection may be required to reach lower pole calices and thereby induce premature bleeding. For this reason, inspection should proceed in a cranial to caudal fashion in order to minimize bleeding and optimize visualization. In order to inspect the lower pole calices in most kidneys, the ureteroscope must deflect at least 170° [61]. However, in most currently available fiberoptic ureteroscopes, the deflection has been increased to approximately 300° to compensate for the loss of deflection with working instruments in place.

Following a survey of the entire intra-renal collecting system, any tumors are then sampled for microscopic analysis. Over the years, various devices have been introduced to biopsy upper tract tumors including baskets, forceps, brushes, snares, and graspers. The two most commonly utilized devices include the 3 F cup biopsy forceps and the stainless steel flat wire basket (Fig. 26.4) [62]. The small cup forceps are available in several designs of 1-mm diameter. These are ideally suited for sampling smaller, sessile, or

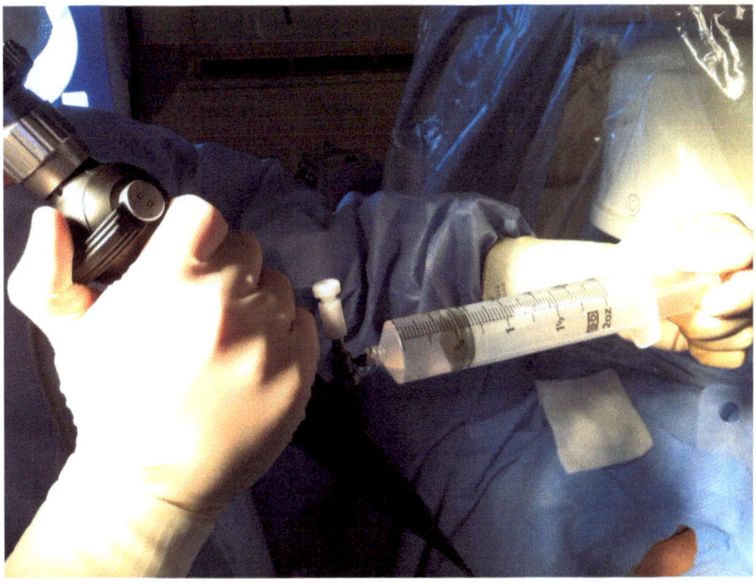

Fig. 26.3 Obtaining a renal pelvis aspirate by connecting a large Luer lock syringe (50–60 mL) directly to the irrigation port of the flexible ureteroscope

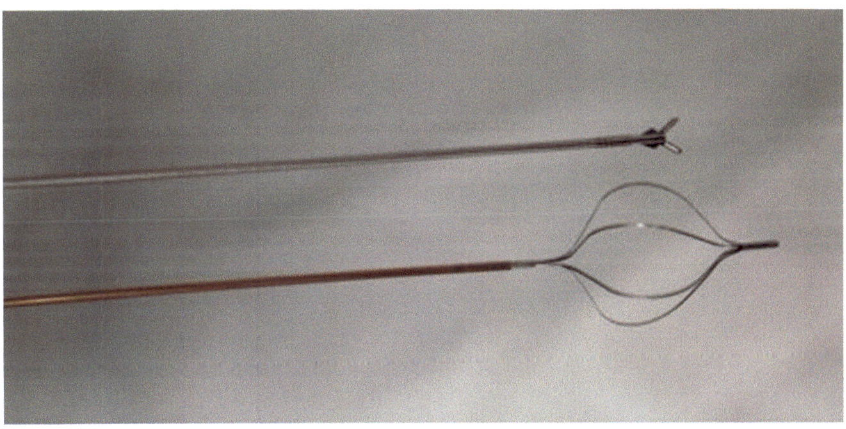

Fig. 26.4 The two most commonly used ureteroscopic biopsy devices are the cup biopsy forceps and flat wire basket

nonpapillary lesions. If the sample is entirely contained within the cup, the device may be withdrawn through the working channel. Then, the device is replaced and multiple samples are taken in a similar fashion to ensure sufficient specimen for cytologic evaluation. However, if the tissue fragment extends beyond the extent of the cup, the entire unit consisting of FU, forceps, and biopsy should be removed to preserve the largest specimen possible. The endoscope is then replaced and additional biopsies are obtained. Depending on the FU utilized, the shaft stiffness of the cup forceps often limits the deflection to approximately 90–100° [61]. This can pose obvious challenges when attempting to biopsy lower pole lesions.

Alternatively, the stainless steel flat wire basket is effective for more sizable, papillary, and friable tumors [62]. The tumor is trapped between the angles of the wire. Next, the basket is closed snugly but not completely. It is then used to avulse a piece of tissue. In this way, a large

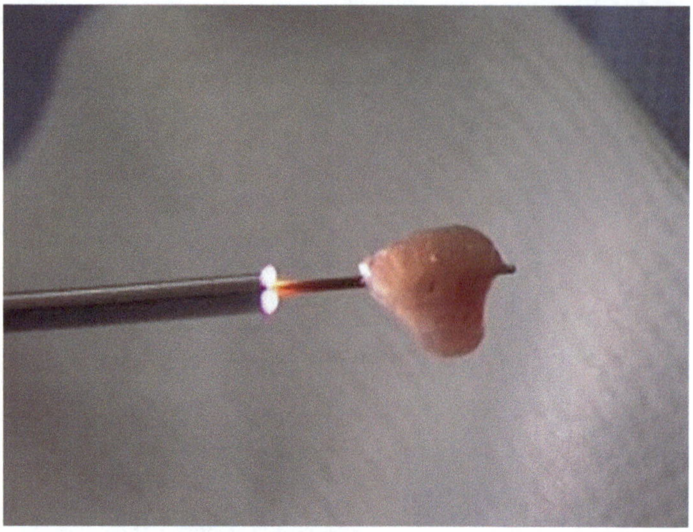

Fig. 26.5 A large piece of tumor is shown hanging from the flat wire basket. The entire unit consisting of tumor, basket, and ureteroscope is withdrawn to preserve the largest specimen possible

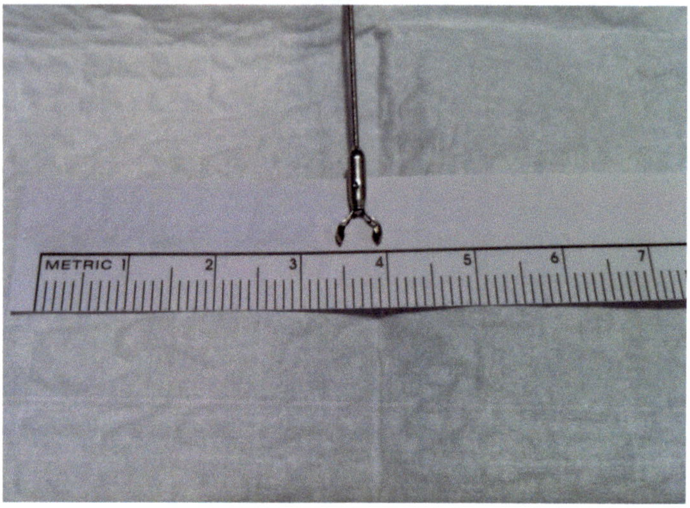

Fig. 26.6 Back-loading biopsy forceps with 2 mm cup

sample measuring up to several millimeters may be retrieved. In contrast to the cup forceps, samples obtained with the flat wire basket should not be withdrawn through the working channel since most of the tissue would be sheared off and lost. Instead, the entire unit consisting of FU, basket, and biopsy should always be withdrawn to maintain the largest tissue specimen possible (Fig. 26.5). Again, the FU is reinserted and multiple biopsies are taken. Using the flat wire basket, large tumors can be mechanically debulked quite effectively. In fact, the flat wire basket may be utilized to biopsy tumors measuring several centimeters in diameter.

Other devices are largely ineffective and thus seldom used. Unlike the flat wire basket, the nitinol round wire baskets do not have enough grasping edge to capture tumor well. The brush is also very poor in retrieving tissue. When viewed directly endoscopically, the brush can be seen moving the tissue but not actually sampling it. Wire pronged graspers may be useful for papillary tumors if other devices are not available or cannot reach the tumor. Recently, a larger cup forceps with a 2 mm cup has been introduced (Fig. 26.6). However, two key points warrant discussion. First, it must be back-loaded through the working channel of the FU. In turn, the

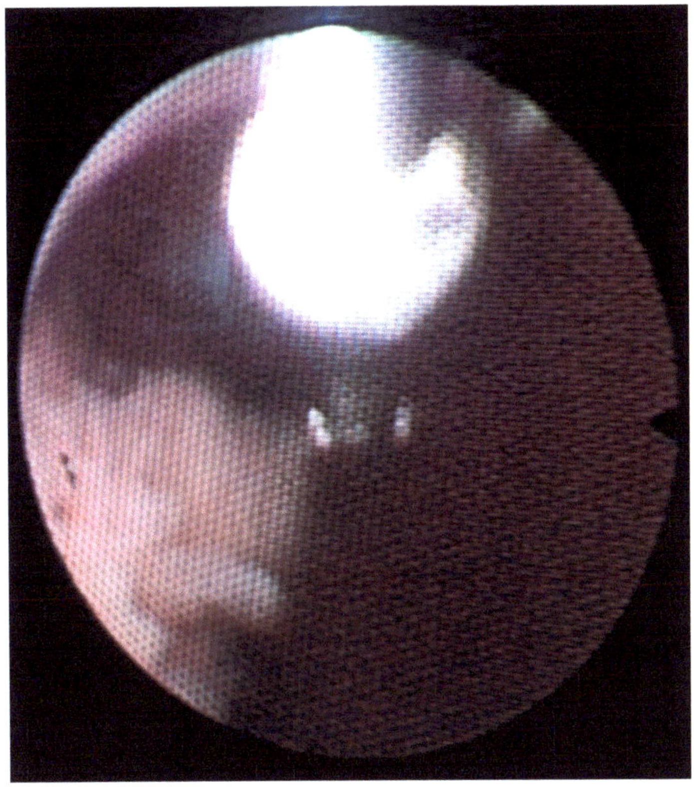

Fig. 26.7 The visual field is obscured by the back-loading biopsy forceps

back-loading biopsy forceps and the FU must be placed through a ureteral access sheath. If this device is employed, we recommend first carefully inspecting the ureter with a no touch technique to evaluate for ureteral lesions prior to access sheath insertion. Second, the larger cup forceps obscure the visual field when opened (Fig. 26.7). Despite these obvious disadvantages, the larger cup forceps appear to offer better deflection characteristics compared to the small cup forceps and flat wire basket (Fig. 26.8). However, the amount of tissue retrieved using the flat wire basket is significantly larger (Fig. 26.9).

After ureteroscopic biopsy, the tissue sample is transferred directly from the cup forceps or flat wire basket into a specimen container with normal saline (Fig. 26.10). By minimizing the number of specimen transfers, the chance of specimen loss is reduced. Cytologic preservative known as Saccomanno fixative is added if specimen delivery to the Cytopathology laboratory may be delayed. Fresh specimens are hand delivered to the laboratory, where they are evaluated using the cytospin smear technique. Importantly, all samples are processed as cytology specimens to avoid tissue loss during preparation [66]. Cytopathologic techniques for handling and interpreting the ureteroscopic biopsy specimens will be discussed in detail later in this chapter. Multiple samples are taken with either device to obtain sufficient tissue for pathologic analysis. This includes not only multiple samples of the tumor itself, but also post-biopsy and post-laser aspirates.

Once adequate tissue sample has been obtained, the tumor is then treated. Advances in laser technologies have transformed the endoscopic management of upper tract tumors. In particular, the holmium (Ho) and neodymium (Nd):yttrium aluminum garnet (YAG) lasers allow for the safe and efficacious treatment of UTUC [61]. Laser ablation and resection will be described in detail in subsequent chapters. Briefly, the Ho:YAG laser is a pulsed device with a wavelength of 2,100 nm. Because the

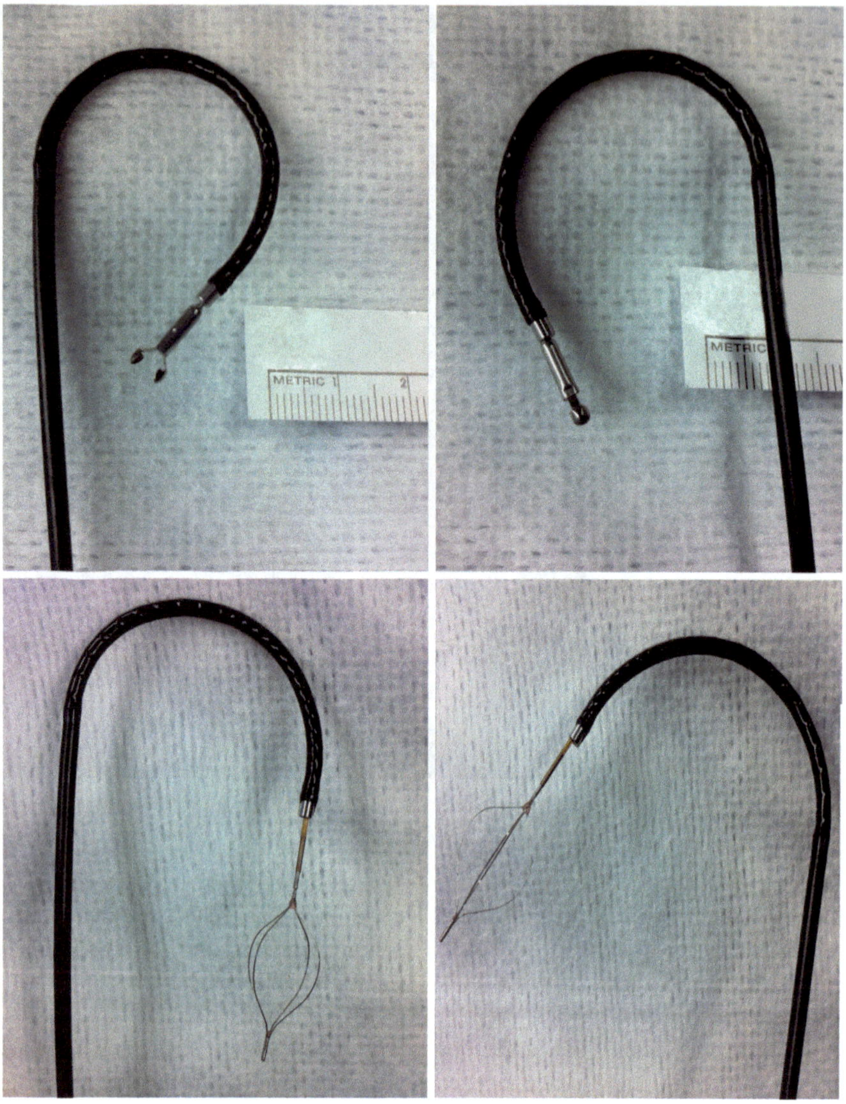

Fig. 26.8 Superior deflection characteristics of the back-loading biopsy forceps compared to the flat wire basket

holmium energy penetrates tissue only 0.5 mm, its tissue effect is relatively superficial and visible endoscopically. The Ho:YAG laser has a dominant ablative effect, but may also be used to coagulate tumors by defocusing the laser beam on the tissue. On the other hand, the Nd:YAG laser is a continuous wave device with a wavelength of 1,064 nm. This penetrates ten times deeper than Ho:YAG, with a depth of penetration up to approximately 5–10 mm. Unlike Ho:YAG, it is more difficult to determine the depth of penetration during treatment. Due to the increased risk of ureteral stricture formation, use of Nd:YAG should be avoided within the ureter. Even within the kidney, Nd:YAG should be applied cautiously as indiscriminate use may lead to infundibular stenosis. While the Ho:YAG both ablates and coagulates tissue, the Nd:YAG only coagulates. However, it is particularly effective at coagulating bleeding sites and large tumors up to several centimeters in diameter. In contrast to the Ho:YAG which is a contact laser, the Nd:YAG does not require direct contact of the laser fiber with the neoplasm. This property may be advantageous for tumors which are difficult to reach. These two lasers are best used in combination. In fact,

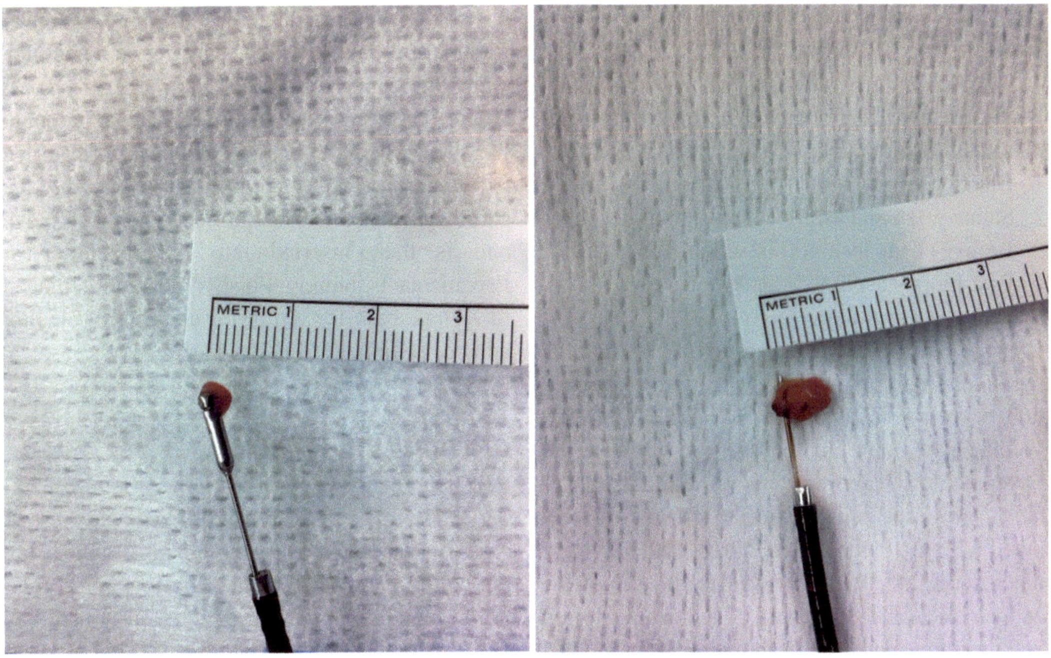

Fig. 26.9 Larger sample obtained by using flat wire basket compared to back-loading biopsy forceps

Fig. 26.10 The specimen is transferred directly into a small specimen cup containing normal saline without fixative solution and then delivered to the Cytopathology laboratory

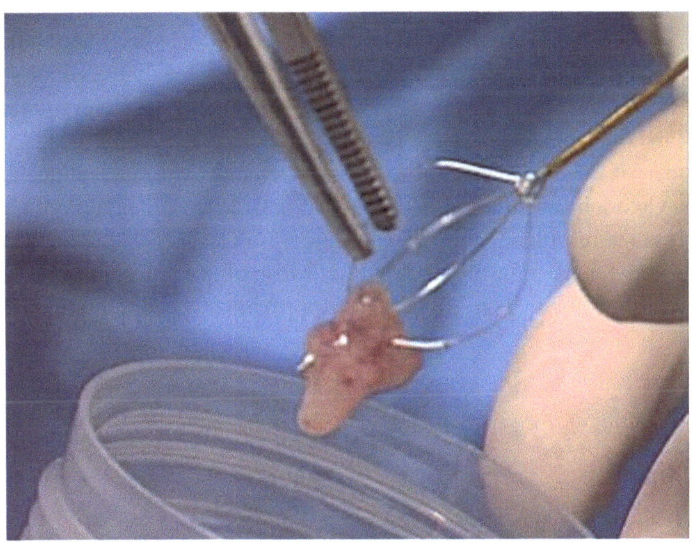

the Ho and Nd:YAG lasers are available in a combined unit with a dual foot switch. This allows for rapid interchange and selective application of each laser to exploit their unique properties. Most commonly, a 200 or 365 μm laser fiber is employed.

Notably, special Ho:YAG lasers have been developed with variable pulse duration [61]. While the typical pulse duration for holmium laser lithotripsy of urinary calculi is 350 μs, the variable pulse duration laser allows for the pulse length to be increased to 700 μs. The longer pulse delivers the same energy over a longer time, which in turn improves coagulation. Hence, this type of holmium laser is ideal for treating ureteral tumors.

Specimen Handling

By the end of the procedure the following samples should be obtained:

1. Bladder urine.
2. Saline wash and aspirate from site of lesion(s).
3. Biopsy of the lesion(s) in saline.
4. Post-biopsy aspirate.
5. Post-laser aspirate.

One of the most crucial principles in handling the tissue for pathologic diagnosis is close collaboration with the cytopathologist. Delivering the specimens without fixation, fresh in saline, to the Cytopathology laboratory is of utmost importance for tissue preservation. Samples are prepared with the cytospin technique. If there is any macroscopically visible tissue in the sample, a cell block is also prepared. This sample often demonstrates both the architecture of the neoplasm and the individual cells, to allow grading of urothelial carcinoma.

Cytospin Technique

First, Saccomanno fixative is added to the specimen. If the specimen appears grossly hematuric, a Cytorich red solution is first added in order to lyse the red blood cells. The specimen is centrifuged for 10 min at 1,200 RPM. Most of the supernatant is then discarded. Approximately 3–5 mL of the supernatant is placed into a special funnel apparatus, which contains a specimen slide, and centrifuged for 10 min at 1,300 RPM. At the end of this process, the cells are adherent to the slide. The slide is disassembled and air dried for 10 min, placed in alcohol 95% to remove the carbowax contained in the Saccomanno fixative and is then inserted into the machine for Papanicolaou staining. Finally, the slide is placed in Xylene bath for 2 min for clearing of alcohol and coverslipped (Fig. 26.11a).

Cell Block Preparation

A cell block can be prepared whenever there is any visible tissue in the sample. This is done using the pellet obtained following the first centrifugation. The pellet is transferred to a fenestrated bag and wet with formalin. The bag is wrapped and placed in a cassette, which is immersed in Formalin solution. The specimen is processed in several solutions, including two fixations in Formalin, dehydration from 70% alcohol through three absolute alcohol solutions, and clearing of alcohol in Xylene solution. It is then extracted from the bag and embedded in wax, sliced, and adhered to a glass slide. Lastly, the slides are stained with hematoxylin and eosin (H&E) and prepared as a histologic specimen. Architectural details of the lesion can often be demonstrated using cell block preparation (Fig. 26.11b).

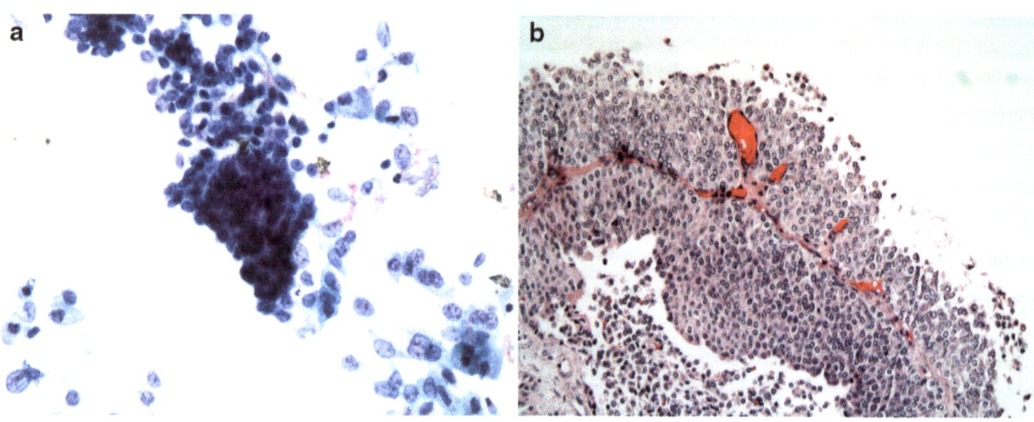

Fig. 26.11 (**a**) Grade 2 tumor in cytology specimen. (**b**) The cell block shows the histology of the same tumor

Table 26.1 Samples collected for cytology during ureteroscopic biopsy

1. Bladder urine
2. Aspirate of ureter or renal pelvis urine
3. Biopsy of tumor(s)
4. Post-biopsy renal pelvis aspirate
5. Post-laser renal pelvis aspirate

Table 26.2 Handling of biopsy specimens

1. Large specimen if possible (and multiple specimens)
2. Place in normal saline
3. Deliver fresh to cytology laboratory
4. Cytospin preparation
5. Cell block if possible
6. Communicate with cytopathologist

Using this systematic approach to ureteroscopic biopsy and specimen preparation, we have significantly improved our diagnostic yield. By handling all specimens in the Cytopathology laboratory, we increased our yield for diagnostic yield from 40% to approximately 90% [66].

There has been concern that the ureteroscopic biopsies may not reflect the actual pathology, particularly the tumor grade. However, considering tumor grade, several series have demonstrated a biopsy concordance of approximately 80–90% between the endoscopic and final pathologic specimens [34, 35]. Moreover, the accuracy may be enhanced by providing the pathologist with multiple samples and, ideally, macroscopically visible samples to be used for cell block preparation. Importantly, all samples should be delivered to the Cytopathology laboratory in normal saline as rapidly as possible to keep them fresh without cellular degradation (Tables 26.1 and 26.2).

Adjunctive Measures in Ureteroscopic Biopsy and Tissue Preparation

Visual Aids During Ureteroscopy

Despite advances in FU, challenges remain in the diagnosis of UTUC. White light (WL) imaging is imperfect in detecting the presence and limits of urothelial lesions in both the lower and upper urinary tract. New developments in optical diagnostics have been introduced to overcome these limitations [67]. One such optical imaging technique is narrow band imaging (NBI). NBI filters WL into two narrow bandwidths of 415 nm (blue) and 540 nm (green), which are strongly absorbed by hemoglobin. As a result, the contrast between normal urothelium and vascular structures is enhanced. Due to the vascular nature of urothelial carcinoma, NBI enhances the contrast between superficial tumors and normal mucosa. Notably, NBI does not require the instillation of fluorescent agents and therefore no special patient preparation. Rather, it simply requires the flip of a filter switch.

Initially, NBI was evaluated for the diagnosis of urothelial carcinoma of the bladder and showed proven benefit. Earlier studies showed that NBI cystoscopy significantly improved the detection of primary and recurrent nonmuscle invasive bladder cancer compared to standard WL cystoscopy [68–71]. More recently, NBI-assisted transurethral resection (TUR) was found to decrease the residual tumor rate significantly compared to a matched cohort of standard WL-TUR (15.0% vs. 30.5%, respectively) [72]. At the present time, the clinical research office of the endourological society (CROES) is conducting a multicenter, international randomized trial on the impact of NBI-assisted TUR on recurrence rates. For urothelial carcinoma of the bladder, it appears that NBI improves the detection rate as well as the completeness of treatment.

By extrapolating these findings to the upper tract, it seems plausible that NBI may similarly aid in the diagnosis of UTUC. Bagley et al. evaluated whether NBI-aided fiberoptic FU enhanced detection of recurrent UTUC over WL [73]. A total of ten patients with prior history of low grade UTUC underwent surveillance using WL and then NBI (Fig. 26.12). Direct biopsies were performed of any suspicious lesions, which were then laser resected. Pathology interpretations were then correlated with the corresponding WL and NBI findings. Of a total of ten biopsies obtained from seven upper urinary tracts, nine were warranted based on WL alone. NBI failed to

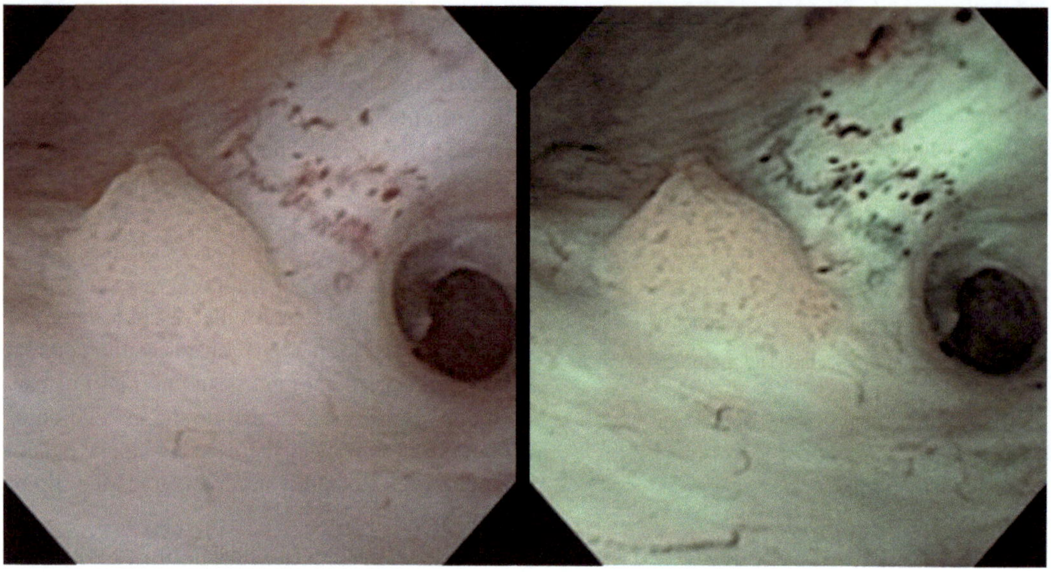

Fig. 26.12 Renal upper pole papillary tumor on white left (*left*) vs. narrow band imaging (*right*). Cytopathology showed low grade urothelial carcinoma

detect any occult UTUC not seen on WL. The overall sensitivity for the detection of upper tract abnormalities was equivalent for NBI (90%) vs. WL (89%) fiberoptic FU. Hence, the authors concluded that NBI-assisted fiberoptic FU offered no significant advantage in surveillance for UTUC.

On the other hand, Traxer et al. subsequently found NBI to be a valuable diagnostic tool for UTUC [74]. These authors performed NBI and WL digital FU in 27 patients, including 14 patients with known history of UTUC as follow-up and 13 patients with suspected UTUC. Subjectively, NBI significantly improved the endoscopic visualization of the tumors by providing a detailed description of their vascular architecture as well as tumor limits. Objectively, NBI detected the extended limits of three tumors (8.5%) in three patients. NBI also detected five additional tumors (14.2%) in four patients. In this study, NBI considerably improved the tumor detection rate by 22.7% compared to WL.

Although the results are mixed, future larger studies of NBI-aided ureteroscopy are needed to elucidate the role of this optical technology in the management of UTUC.

Alternative Staining Techniques

Ureteroscopic biopsies are typically small and delicate. Careful biopsy technique and tissue handling are paramount for obtaining a tissue diagnosis. Alternative fixative and preservative solutions as well as stains are being evaluated in an attempt to further improve the diagnostic yield of ureteroscopic biopsies. Bultitude et al. assessed whether Bouin's fixative could improve the interpretation of ureteroscopic biopsies [75]. This is a noncoagulant picrate solution which is routinely utilized to fix testicular biopsies because the nuclear detail is better preserved by this method. In total, 28 pathological areas were studied in 18 patients. This included two groups of patients: Bouin's group (7 patients, 10 pathological areas) vs. 10% Formalin group (11 patients, 18 pathological areas). All specimens were reviewed by two pathologists in a blinded fashion using an objective scoring system to evaluate five domains: specimen quality/size, specimen processing, architecture, cytoplasmic detail, and nuclear detail. No equivocal results were obtained within the Bouin's group. In contrast, there were two equivocal biopsies within the Formalin group. Furthermore, nuclear detail was better preserved in the specimens fixed in Bouin's solution ($p < 0.001$).

Importantly, the authors highlight that Bouin's solution is useful as either a fixative or staining solution, but it is not suitable as a preservative [75]. Due to tissue shrinkage induced by the picric acid, tissues cannot be stored in Bouin's solution for extended periods of time (>48 h). By staining everything yellow, this solution makes specimen identification easier at the time of sampling and while embedding during processing. Subsequently, the yellow stain is removed with multiple ethanol washes. The specimen is then handled in the same way as a biopsy fixed in formaldehyde. While there are reports in other tissue sites of some limitation in subsequent immunohistochemistry, the authors did not encounter this problem. Based on these findings, the authors concluded that Bouin's fixative improved the assessment of ureteroscopic biopsies. Bouin's fixative not only facilitates specimen identification but also better preserves nuclear details allowing a more accurate pathological assessment.

In addition to alternative fixative solutions, special stains are being studied to aid in pathologic analysis of ureteroscopic biopsies. Grading UTUC in cell blocks may be challenging and interobserver agreement among pathologists is poor. Both mitotic figure counting and nuclear features are important in tumor grading. However, several factors such as apoptosis and artifact may hinder this task. Solomides et al. investigated the use of a mitotic specific marker phospho-histone H3 (PHH3) as an adjunct to H&E stain for grading UTUC in cell blocks [76]. Formalin-fixed paraffin-embedded cell blocks from 61 UTUCs were stained with H&E followed by PHH3-antibody. A total of three pathologists graded tumors in a blinded fashion, first on H&E and then on H&E plus PHH3 stained slides. Gradings were then compared between pathologists and for H&E staining vs. H&E plus PHH3 staining. By adding the PHH3 stain to the H&E stain, the interobserver agreement in grading among the three pathologists improved dramatically and was statistically significant (average pairwise agreement = 80%, overall kappa = 0.69). Therefore, PHH3 immunostain may serve an important role in grading UTUC in small cell block samples.

These preliminary studies are promising and suggest that alternative solutions and stains may improve the diagnostic yield and accuracy of pathologic analysis. Further studies are warranted to explore these techniques in larger patient cohorts.

Conclusion

UTUC is a rare malignancy. Nevertheless, it is a potentially lethal disease, especially when diagnosed in advanced stages. Ureteroscopy with biopsy is an important part of the evaluation whenever a filling defect is encountered or UTUC is suspected. RNU with bladder cuff excision has been considered the gold standard treatment for UTUC. However, ureteroscopic laser treatment has become a promising alternative, especially in patients in whom nephron-sparing procedures are crucial. While ureteroscopic management enables preservation of renal function and avoidance of major surgery, it requires a vigilant surveillance protocol and a compliant patient. Ureteroscopic biopsy and careful specimen preparation are necessary to reach an accurate diagnosis and thereby guide treatment decisions. Close collaboration between the urologist and cytopathologist is essential. Further studies are needed to determine whether new optical imaging technologies and alternative stains may optimize the diagnostic yield of ureteroscopic biopsy for UTUC.

References

1. Flanigan R (2007). Urothelial tumors of the upper urinary tract. In: Wein AJ, Novick AC, Partin AW et al., editors. Campbell-Walsh urology. 9th ed. Philadelphia: Saunders Elsevier. p. 1638–52.
2. Rouprêt M, Zigeuner R, Palou J, et al. European guidelines for the diagnosis and management of upper urinary tract urothelial cell carcinomas: 2011 update. Eur Urol. 2011;59:584–94.

3. Hall M, Womack S, Sagalowsky A, et al. Prognostic factors, recurrence, and survival in transitional cell carcinoma of the upper urinary tract: a 30-year experience in 252 patients. Urology. 1998;52:594–601.
4. Olgac S, Mazumdar M, Dalbagni G, et al. Urothelial carcinoma of the renal pelvis: a clinicopathologic study of 130 cases. Am J Surg Pathol. 2004;28: 1545–52.
5. Margulis V, Shariat S, Matin S, et al. Outcomes of radical nephroureterectomy: a series from the upper tract urothelial carcinoma collaboration. Cancer. 2009;115:1224–33.
6. Gadzinski A, Roberts W, Faerber G, et al. Long-term outcomes of nephroureterectomy versus endoscopic management for upper tract urothelial carcinoma. J Urol. 2010;183:2148–53. http://www.ncbi.nlm.nih.gov/pubmed/20399468. Accessed 16 Feb 2012.
7. Rouprêt M, Hupertan V, Traxer O, et al. Comparison of open nephroureterectomy and ureteroscopic and percutaneous management of upper urinary tract transitional cell carcinoma. Urology. 2006;67:1181–7.
8. Lucas S, Svatek R, Olgin G, et al. Conservative management in selected patients with upper tract urothelial carcinoma compares favourably with early radical surgery. BJU Int. 2008;102:172–6. http://www.ncbi.nlm.nih.gov/pubmed/18341624. Accessed 16 Feb 2012.
9. Deligne E, Colombel M, Badet L, et al. Conservative management of upper urinary tract tumors. Eur Urol. 2002;42:43–8.
10. Sowter S, Ilie C, Efthimiou I, et al. Endourologic management of patients with upper-tract transitional-cell carcinoma: long-term follow-up in a single center. J Endourol. 2007;21:1005–9.
11. Krambeck A, Thompson R, Lohse C, et al. Imperative indications for conservative management of upper tract transitional cell carcinoma. J Urol. 2007;178: 792–7.
12. Rouprêt M, Traxer O, Tligui M, et al. Upper urinary tract transitional cell carcinoma: recurrence rate after percutaneous endoscopic resection. Eur Urol. 2007;51: 709–13.
13. Elliott D, Segura J, Lightner D, et al. Is nephroureterectomy necessary in all cases of upper tract transitional cell carcinoma? Long-term results of conservative endourologic management of upper tract transitional cell carcinoma in individuals with a normal contralateral kidney. Urology. 2001;58:174–8.
14. Chen G, Bagley D. Ureteroscopic management of upper tract transitional cell carcinoma in patients with normal contralateral kidneys. J Urol. 2000;164: 1173–6.
15. Pak R, Moskowitz E, Bagley D. What is the cost of maintaining a kidney in upper-tract transitional-cell carcinoma? An objective analysis of cost and survival. J Endourol. 2009;23:341–6.
16. Wen C, Cheng T, Tsai M, et al. All-cause mortality attributable to chronic kidney disease: a prospective cohort study based on 462 293 adults in Taiwan. Lancet. 2008;371:2173–82.
17. Weiner D, Tighiouart H, Amin M, et al. Chronic kidney disease as a risk factor for cardiovascular disease and all-cause mortality: a pooled analysis of community-based studies. J Am Soc Nephrol. 2004;15:1307–15.
18. Go A, Chertow G, Fan D, et al. Chronic kidney disease and the risks of death, cardiovascular events, and hospitalization. N Engl J Med. 2004;351:1296–305.
19. Campbell S, Novick A, Belldegrun A, et al. Guideline for management of the clinical T1 renal mass. J Urol. 2009;182:1271–9.
20. McKiernan J, Simmons R, Katz J, et al. Natural history of chronic renal insufficiency after partial and radical nephrectomy. Urology. 2002;59:816–20.
21. Thompson R, Boorjian S, Lohse C, et al. Radical nephrectomy for pT1a renal masses may be associated with decreased overall survival compared with partial nephrectomy. J Urol. 2008;179:468–71.
22. Van Der Molen A, Cowan N, Mueller-Lisse U, et al. CT urography: definition, indications and techniques. A guideline for clinical practice. Eur Radiol. 2008;18: 4–17.
23. Dillman J, Caoili E, Cohan R, et al. Detection of upper tract urothelial neoplasms: sensitivity of axial, coronal reformatted, and curved-planar reformatted image-types utilizing 16-row multi-detector CT urography. Abdom Imaging. 2008;33:707–16.
24. Wang L, Wong Y, Chuang C, et al. Diagnostic accuracy of transitional cell carcinoma on multidetector computerized tomography urography in patients with gross hematuria. J Urol. 2009;181:524–31.
25. Wang L, Wong Y, Huang C, et al. Multidetector computerized tomography urography is more accurate than excretory urography for diagnosing transitional cell carcinoma of the upper urinary tract in adults with hematuria. J Urol. 2010;183:48–55.
26. Wang L, Wong Y, Ng K, et al. Tumor characteristics of urothelial carcinoma on multidetector computerized tomography urography. J Urol. 2010;183: 2154–60.
27. Ito Y, Kikuchi E, Tanaka N, et al. Preoperative hydronephrosis grade independently predicts worse pathological outcomes in patients undergoing nephroureterectomy for upper tract urothelial carcinoma. J Urol. 2011;185:1621–6.
28. Takahashi N, Glockner J, Hartman R, et al. Gadolinium enhanced magnetic resonance urography for upper urinary tract malignancy. J Urol. 2010;183:1330–6.
29. Takahashi N, Kawashima A, Glockner JF, et al. Small (<2 cm) upper tract urothelial carcinoma: evaluation with gadolinium-enhanced three-dimensional spoiled gradient-recalled echo MR urography. Radiology. 2008;247:451–7.
30. Natalin R, Prince M, Grossman M, et al. Contemporary applications and limitations of magnetic resonance imaging contrast materials. J Urol. 2010;183:27–33.
31. El-Hakim A, Weiss G, Lee B, et al. Correlation of ureteroscopic appearance with histologic grade of upper tract transitional cell carcinoma. Urology. 2004; 63:647–50.

32. Thompson R, Krambeck A, Lohse C, et al. Endoscopic management of upper tract transitional cell carcinoma in patients with normal contralateral kidneys. Urology. 2008;71:713–7.
33. Keeley F, Bibbo M, Bagley D. Ureteroscopic treatment and surveillance of upper urinary tract transitional cell carcinoma. J Urol. 1997;157:1560–5.
34. Keeley F, Kulp D, Bibbo M, et al. Diagnostic accuracy of ureteroscopic biopsy in upper tract transitional cell carcinoma. J Urol. 1997;157:33–7.
35. Williams S, Denton K, Minervini A, et al. Correlation of upper-tract cytology, retrograde pyelography, ureteroscopic appearance, and ureteroscopic biopsy with histologic examination of upper-tract transitional cell carcinoma. J Endourol. 2008;22:71–6.
36. Lotan Y, Roehrborn C. Sensitivity and specificity of commonly available bladder tumor markers versus cytology: results of a comprehensive literature review and meta-analyses. Urology. 2003;61:109–18.
37. Rife C, Farrow G, Utz D. Urine cytology of transitional cell neoplasms. Urol Clin North Am. 1979;6:519–612.
38. Bibbo M, Gill W, Harris M, et al. Retrograde brushing as a diagnostic procedure of ureteral, renal pelvic and renal calyceal lesions. Acta Cytol. 1974;18:137–41.
39. Brien J, Shariat S, Herman M, et al. Preoperative hydronephrosis, ureteroscopic biopsy grade and urinary cytology can improve prediction of advanced upper tract urothelial carcinoma. J Urol. 2010;184:69–73.
40. Konety B, Getzenberg R. Urine based markers of urological malignancy. J Urol. 2001;165:600–11.
41. Fradet Y, Lockhard C. Performance characteristics of a new monoclonal antibody test for bladder cancer: ImmunoCyt™. Can J Urol. 1997;4:400–5.
42. Mian C, Pycha A, Wiener H, et al. Immunocyt: a new tool for detecting transitional cell cancer of the urinary tract. J Urol. 1999;161:1486–9.
43. Lodde M, Mian C, Wiener H, et al. Detection of upper urinary tract transitional cell carcinoma with ImmunoCyt: a preliminary report. Urology. 2001;58:362–6.
44. Zimmerman R, Bagley D, Hawthorne C, et al. Utility of the Bard BTA test in detecting upper tract transitional cell carcinoma. Urology. 1998;51:956–8.
45. Ianari A, Sternberg C, Rossetti A, et al. Results of Bard BTA test in monitoring patients with a history of transitional cell cancer of the bladder. Urology. 1997;49:786–9.
46. Conn I, Crocker J, Wallace D, et al. Basement membranes in urothelial carcinoma. Br J Urol. 1987;60:536–42.
47. Walsh I, Keane P, Ishak L, et al. The BTA stat test: a tumor marker for the detection of upper tract transitional cell carcinoma. Urology. 2001;58:532–5.
48. Siemens D, Morales A, Johnston B, et al. A comparative analysis of rapid urine tests for the diagnosis of upper urinary tract malignancy. Can J Urol. 2003;10:1754–8.
49. Schmetter B, Habicht K, Lamm D, et al. Results of a multicenter trial evaluation of AuraTek FDP: an aid in the management of bladder cancer patients. J Urol. 1997;158:801–5.
50. McCabe R, Lamm L, Haspel M, et al. A diagnostic-prognostic test for bladder cancer using a monoclonal antibody-based enzyme-linked immunoassay for detection of urinary fibrin(ogen) degradation products. Cancer Res. 1984;44:5886–93.
51. Johnston B, Morales A, Emerson L, et al. Rapid detection of bladder cancer: a comparative study of point of care tests. J Urol. 1997;158:2098–101.
52. Skacel M, Fahmy M, Brainard J, et al. Multitarget fluorescence in situ hybridization assay detects transitional cell carcinoma in the majority of patients with bladder cancer and atypical or negative urine cytology. J Urol. 2003;169:2101–5.
53. Sokolova I, Halling K, Jenkins R, et al. The development of a multitarget, multicolor fluorescence in situ hybridization assay for the detection of urothelial carcinoma in urine. J Mol Diagn. 2000;2:116–23.
54. Halling K, King W, Sokolova I, et al. A comparison of cytology and fluorescence in situ hybridization for the detection of urothelial carcinoma. J Urol. 2000;164:1768–75.
55. Bubendorf L, Grilli B, Sauter G, et al. Multiprobe FISH for enhanced detection of bladder cancer in voided urine specimens and bladder washings. Am J Clin Pathol. 2001;116:79–86.
56. Bollmann M, Heller H, Bánkfalvi A, et al. Quantitative molecular urinary cytology by fluorescence in situ hybridization: a tool for tailoring surveillance of patients with superficial bladder cancer? BJU Int. 2005;95:1219–25.
57. Akkad T, Brunner A, Pallwein L, et al. Fluorescence in situ hybridization for detecting upper urinary tract tumors—A preliminary report. Urology. 2007;70:753–7.
58. Marín-Aguilera M, Mengual L, Ribal M, et al. Utility of fluorescence in situ hybridization as a non-invasive technique in the diagnosis of upper urinary tract urothelial carcinoma. Eur Urol. 2007;51:409–15.
59. Chen A, Grasso M. Is there a role for FISH in the management and surveillance of patients with upper tract transitional-cell carcinoma? J Endourol. 2008;22:1371–4.
60. Johannes J, Nelson E, Bibbo M, et al. Voided urine fluorescence in situ hybridization testing for upper tract urothelial carcinoma surveillance. J Urol. 2010;184:879–82.
61. Bagley D, Grasso M. Ureteroscopic laser treatment of upper urinary tract neoplasms. World J Urol. 2010;28:143–9.
62. Abdel-Razzak O, Ehya H, Cubler-Goodman A, et al. Ureteroscopic biopsy in the upper urinary tract. Urology. 1994;44:451–7.
63. Tawfiek E, Bagley D. Upper-tract transitional cell carcinoma. Urology. 1997;50:321–9.
64. Hudson R, Conlin M, Bagley D. Ureteric access with flexible ureteroscopes: effect of the size of the ureteroscope. BJU Int. 2005;95:1043–4.

65. Johnson G, Portela D, Grasso M. Advanced ureteroscopy: wireless and sheathless. J Endourol. 2006;20: 552–5.
66. Tawfiek E, Bibbo M, Bagley D. Ureteroscopic biopsy: technique and specimen preparation. Urology. 1997;50:117–9.
67. Cauberg E, de Bruin D, Faber D, et al. A new generation of optical diagnostics for bladder cancer: technology, diagnostic accuracy, and future applications. Eur Urol. 2009;56:287–96.
68. Herr H, Donat S. A comparison of white-light cystoscopy and narrow-band imaging cystoscopy to detect bladder tumour recurrences. BJU Int. 2008;102: 1111–4.
69. Bryan R, Billingham L, Wallace D. Narrow-band imaging flexible cystoscopy in the detection of recurrent urothelial cancer of the bladder. BJU Int. 2007; 101:702–6.
70. Naselli A, Introini C, Bertolotto F, et al. Narrow band imaging for detecting residual/recurrent cancerous tissue during second transurethral resection of newly diagnosed non-muscle-invasive high-grade bladder cancer. BJU Int. 2010;105:208–11.
71. Cauberg E, Kloen S, Visser M, et al. Narrow band imaging cystoscopy improves the detection of non-muscle-invasive bladder cancer. Urology. 2010;76: 658–63.
72. Cauberg E, Mamoulakis C, de la Rosette J, et al. Narrow band imaging-assisted transurethral resection for non-muscle invasive bladder cancer significantly reduces residual tumour rate. World J Urol. 2011;29:503–9.
73. Colon-Herdman A, Bagley D. The use of narrow band imaging for the assessment of upper tract urothelial tumors: initial experience. J Endourol. 2010;24 (Abstract) Suppl 1.
74. Traxer O, Geavlete B, de Medina S, et al. Narrow-band imaging digital flexible ureteroscopy in detection of upper urinary tract transitional-cell carcinoma: initial experience. J Endourol. 2011;25:19–23.
75. Bultitude M, Ghani K, Horsfield C, et al. Improving the interpretation of ureteroscopic biopsies: use of Bouin's fixative. BJU Int. 2011;108:1373–5.
76. Solomides C, Birbe R, Bagley D, et al. Does mitosis specific marker PHH3 help grading upper tract urothelial carcinomas in cell blocks? Actol Cytol. 2012; 56(285):8.

Laser Lithotripsy

27

Bingqing Wang, Jinze Qiu, Thomas E. Milner, and Joel M.H. Teichman

Introduction

Since the first introduction of continuous CO_2 laser to fragment human calculi in 1960s [1], intracorporeal laser lithotripsy has become a standard treatment for urinary calculi. During endoscopic laser lithotripsy, an endoscope is inserted into the urinary tract to locate the stone. A laser fiber is passed through the endoscope working channel to deliver laser energy to the stone. The stone is fragmented and the resultant fragments may be removed by basket or may be small enough to pass spontaneously.

The laser is the energy source of lithotripsy. The basic structure of a laser includes three main elements: (a) a gain medium, (b) a resonant optical cavity formed by two reflective mirrors, and (c) an external energy source which excites the gain medium. The gain medium can be gas, liquid, solid, or plasma, which is capable of amplifying the light when it is excited by an external energy source. This external energy source, or pump, can be electric current, chemical energy, or another light source. Upon the excitation of the external energy source, electrons are stimulated to uniformly higher energy states, and release photons with identical energy when they return to their more stable, lower energy states. If the excitation power satisfies the lasing threshold, the number of electrons in the excited state exceeds the number of electrons in lower energy state, resulting in population inversion which amplifies the light. Since the gain medium is usually homogeneous, this amplification process results in the emission of highly coherent light at a single wavelength.

Light amplification is provided by the gain medium in a resonant cavity. The resonant cavity is a box with two reflective mirrors on both ends of the box, as shown in Fig. 27.1. Light is reflected back and forth between the two mirrors and trapped in the resonant cavity. Every time the light travels through the gain media, its power is amplified until the cavity is saturated. The resonant cavity produces highly directional and coherent laser light. In practice, one mirror is a 100% reflector and the other mirror is partially reflective. The partial reflective mirror, sometimes called the output coupler, allows a small portion (usually less than 5%) of light to escape from the resonant cavity, functioning as the output end of the laser cavity.

The basic cavity arrangement mentioned above allows continuous emission of laser energy. For laser lithotripsy, instead of using continuous wave laser, laser light is generally released in a pulsed fashion by various mechanisms, e.g., Q-switching,

B. Wang, B.Sc. • J. Qiu, Ph.D. • T.E. Milner, Ph.D.
Biomedical Engineering Department, The University of Texas at Austin, Austin, TX, USA

J.M.H. Teichman, M.D., F.R.C.S.(C) (✉)
Department of Urologic Sciences, St. Paul's Hospital, University of British Columbia, Burrard Bldg. C307, 1081 Burrard Street, Vancouver, BC, Canada V6Z 1Y6
e-mail: urosec@providencehealth.bc.ca

M. Monga (ed.), *Ureteroscopy: Indications, Instrumentation & Technique*, Current Clinical Urology, DOI 10.1007/978-1-62703-206-3_27, © Springer Science+Business Media New York 2013

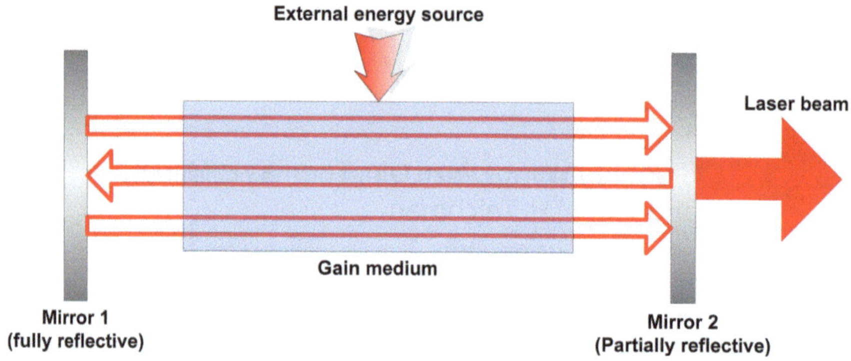

Fig. 27.1 The basic structure of laser includes a gain medium, a resonant optical cavity, and an external energy source which excites the gain medium. The resonant cavity is formed by two reflective mirrors. Mirror 1 is 100% reflective, while Mirror 2 is partly transparent and allows laser light to emit from the cavity

mode-locking, pulsed pumping, etc. The pulse duration plays an important role in deciding the mechanism of lithotripsy. The pulse duration for lithotripsy varies from femtoseconds to milliseconds, and is generally categorized as ultrashort-pulsed (less than 500 ns), short-pulsed (1–10 μs), and long-pulsed (greater than 250 μs) [2].

Physics of Laser Lithotripsy

Depending on the mechanism of laser–target interaction, there are three possible mechanisms: photochemical, photothermal, and photomechanical interactions. Photochemical interactions are characterized by the chemical reactions that are activated, facilitated, or catalyzed by the absorption of light by the target. Photochemical laser mechanism is not currently utilized for lithotripsy. Depending on the duration of laser pulse, photomechanical and/or photothermal interactions occur during laser lithotripsy. In short-pulsed laser lithotripsy (pulse duration ranging from several nanoseconds to several microseconds), the fragmentation of stones is mainly due to photomechanical laser–target interaction, while photothermal interaction is typically seen in long-pulsed laser lithotripsy (pulse duration is several hundred microseconds).

For a photomechanical interaction, the energy of the laser light generates plasma on the surface of the target or in the surrounding media immediately after the onset of laser. The plasma expands to a hemispherical bubble and then collapses or implodes within a few hundred microseconds. During this process, the energy of light is finally converted to mechanical energy in the form of shock waves traveling in all direction. Therefore, a photomechanical interaction is sometimes referred to as a photoacoustic interaction. In the specific application of laser lithotripsy, the pressure of laser-induced shock wave is typically higher than 100 bars. During the photomechanical-type laser lithotripsy, the kidney stones are finally fragmented by mechanical force. As expected, the ablation efficiency is dependent on the mechanical strength of the calculi. It is less efficient in fragmenting relatively hard or "durile" urinary calculi, such as calcium oxalate monohydrate and cystine stones [3]. Q-switched Nd:YAG laser (wavelength: 1,064 nm; pulse duration: tens of nanoseconds), Q-switched alexandrite laser (wavelength: 755 nm; pulse duration: hundreds of nanoseconds), and the flashlamp pumped pulsed dye laser (FPDL, wavelength: around 540 nm; pulse duration: several microseconds) all utilize photomechanical mechanism to fragment kidney stones [4–6]. These lasers produce relatively large fragments (diameter ranging from several hundred microns to several millimeters, fragments larger than 4 mm in diameter were found) during lithotripsy. Plasma is a specific state of matter created by generation of a shared electron cloud and is typically seen with extremely high peak powers created by ultrashort lasers. Not all photomechanical lithotripsy lasers require a plasma to generate photomechanical lithotripsy. In lasers with a pulse duration typically in the range of 1–10 μs, cavitation occurs without plasma formation, and photomechanical lithotripsy occurs.

For long-pulsed laser lithotripsy (pulse duration ranging from 250 to 700 μs), the fragmentation process is dominated by a photothermal mechanism. During a photothermal laser lithotripsy process, a small portion of laser energy is first absorbed by the surrounding media (i.e., water) between fiber tip and stone surface. Water is locally evaporated and forms a local vapor channel. This phenomenon is called the Moses Effect (as in Moses parting the Red Sea). The resulting vapor bubble expands and then collapses, producing weak pressure transients, typically nine bars or less. The magnitude of the pressure transient is significantly weaker than that produced in a photomechanical laser–target interaction and is not capable of fragmenting the stone. The ablation is achieved by the remaining laser energy which is transmitted through the vapor bubble and absorbed directly by the stone. During the 100-μs pulse duration, the laser-induced heat is not able to diffuse away, and is well confined within the irradiation area, causing disruption of the stone lattice and debris ejection. Examples of photothermal interaction include Holmium:YAG (Ho:YAG) and Erbium:YAG (Er:YAG) lithotripsy. Unlike short-pulsed lasers, these long-pulsed lasers are effective for all stone compositions (including durile compositions) and produce relatively small fragments.

Besides photochemical, photomechanical, and photothermal interactions, an emerging approach to efficient stone fragmentation is to harness the multiphoton absorption effects with femtosecond lasers. This technique is currently only available in research laboratories [7]. Although femtosecond laser fires ultrashort laser pulses, femtosecond ablation is characterized by tiny fine debris similar to long-pulsed laser ablation. The ablation process is governed by a plasma-mediated mechanism and is fundamentally distinct from a photomechanical mechanism. During the femtosecond laser lithotripsy process, the calculus is ionized and plasma is generated (i.e., mixture of ions and electrons). After that, incident laser energy is absorbed by free electrons in plasma, exciting electrons and creating additional free electrons [8]. The increased number of high-speed free electrons brings up the local temperature of the stone and disintegrates the stone. Femtosecond laser lithotripsy produces small-sized debris that is mostly less than 1 μm in diameter, significantly smaller than those produced in a photomechanical lithotripsy.

Current Gold Standard: Holmium: YAG Laser Lithotripsy

An ideal laser lithotripsy device should be capable of fragmenting all stone compositions and has a wide safety margin for surrounding tissues. The stone fragments produced from lithotripsy should be reasonably small in size so that they can be passed spontaneously. The fragmentation process should be efficient in order to shorten the duration of surgery. Generally speaking, photothermal lasers provide less efficient fragmentation (slower fragmentation over a longer period of time) than photomechanical lasers [9]. However, photothermal lasers produce smaller fragments and fragment all stone compositions.

One concern during all laser lithotripsy is stone retropulsion. During lithotripsy, stone fragments eject from the surface of a stone. Due to conservation of momentum, the stone moves in the opposite direction of fragment ejection, resulting in stone retropulsion. Strong retropulsion significantly slows down lithotripsy process because the surgeon has to move the endoscope and fiber to the new stone position after laser discharge and stone displacement, potentially making lithotripsy more difficult. Photomechanical lasers generally produce stronger retropulsion than photothermal lasers.

The long-pulse Ho:YAG laser (pulse durations of 250–700 μs, wavelength of 2.1 μm) has been used for intracorporeal laser lithotripsy of urinary calculi since the 1990s, and is considered to be the gold standard modality for laser lithotripsy [10–17]. As mentioned above, the laser–target interaction mechanism for Ho:YAG laser lithotripsy

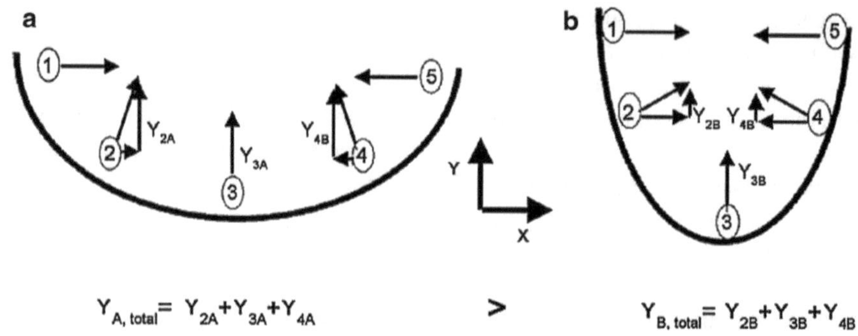

Fig. 27.2 Retropulsion is dependent on the size of optical fiber. (**a**) A wide optical fiber produces a wide and shallow crater with more retropulsion; (**b**) a narrow optical fiber produces a narrow and deep crater with less retropulsion. Reprinted from Lee et al. [22] with permission from Elsevier Limited

is photothermal [18]. The laser produces small-sized fragments [10], fragments all stone compositions, and causes less stone retropulsion compared with short-pulsed lasers [19, 20]. It is clinically safe because Ho:YAG light is highly absorbed by water, reducing collateral damage.

As a trade-off for the production of smaller stone fragments, Ho:YAG lithotripsy is less efficient and requires longer procedure time than photomechanical lasers [15]. The efficiency of Ho:YAG lithotripsy can be improved by increasing laser energy or pulse frequency, but increased pulse energy comes at the cost of larger fragments, increased retropulsion, and fiber tip degradation with energy settings >1.0 J [21]. Thus, the optimal Ho:YAG power setting is largely a balance among fragmentation efficiency, maintaining small stone fragments, and reducing retropulsion.

Previous study shows that retropulsion is greater for larger diameter fibers at a given energy or for larger energies for a given fiber diameter [22, 23]. The relationship of retropulsion on fiber diameter is illustrated in Fig. 27.2. A large-diameter fiber produces a wide and shallow crater, while a thin fiber produces a narrow and deep one. Since stone fragments eject at a normal incident to stone surface, the ejection of fragments from a wide and shallow crater is more uniform in the direction off the stone surface, producing greater momentum to the stone in the opposite direction. Another solution to minimize retropulsion is to use longer pulse duration. A longer pulse duration Ho:YAG laser achieves less retropulsion per pulse, and less retropulsion per unit of stone ablation compared to the "normal" long-pulse Ho:YAG laser [24, 25]. One possible reason is the occurrence of recoil pressure during debris ejection, which is proportional to the radiant power (energy per pulse duration) [26]. As a result, shorter pulse durations with high energy density produce higher retropulsion. To sum up, stone retropulsion during Ho:YAG laser lithotripsy can be reduced by decreasing fiber diameter and increasing the pulse duration.

Clinically, metal-based stabilization or anti-retropulsion devices may be used to reduce retropulsion. The anti-retropulsion device is delivered proximal to the stone before laser energy is applied and prevents retropulsion. Such devices are effective but add operative expense. Metal devices can be damaged potentially by Ho:YAG laser energy. Recently, a reverse thermosensitive material has been proposed as an alternative approach of fixing stones during lithotripsy [27, 28]. The thermosensitive polymer is solid at physiological temperature (37 °C) but becomes liquid when the temperature is lower than 20 °C. Before laser lithotripsy, the polymer is delivered above the stone under low temperature, and thus solidifies as a gel plug at body temperature. During lithotripsy, the solid polymer prevents stone retropulsion. After the laser operation, it can be removed via conventional irrigation. Comparing metal-based anti-retropulsion devices to the reverse thermosensitive polymer, all anti-retropulsion devices here are effective. Some potential advantages of the reverse thermosensitive polymer: it requires no wire to control its position during laser operation, so it does not interfere with the lithotripter and allows a free operative field. In addition, it retains its structure and anti-retropulsion function even if targeted by laser energy.

The ideal power parameters of Ho:YAG lithotripsy are incompletely understood. The efficiency of Ho:YAG lithotripsy can be improved by increasing pulse energy or pulse frequency, both of which increase power. Increased pulse energy produces more lithotripsy per pulse but also produces increased retropulsion and larger stone fragments. Stone retropulsion reduces lithotripsy efficiency because it decouples the fiber tip from the stone surface and increases energy that is absorbed by water between laser tip and stone surface, rather than the stone itself. Prior studies of Ho:YAG laser lithotripsy efficiency favor pulse energy settings less than 1.0 J at high repetition rate [21, 29]. In a recent study, 2.0 J pulse energy setting produces more than four times as much fragmentation as the 0.2 J setting, both at 10 Hz, with only a marginal increase in fragments larger than 1 mm [30]. Total fragmentation (defined as the initial stone mass minus the dominant residual fragment mass) increases as Ho:YAG pulse energy increases. Low pulse energy at a fast repetition rate produces fine, powderized fragmentation debris but overall a slower fragmentation rate compared to using high pulse energy settings at the risk of larger fragmentation chunks. Urologists should select lithotripsy power settings according to desired consequent outcomes. For example, a urologist may want to choose high pulse energy settings to fragment large bladder stones which require lengthy operative time devoted to laser lithotripsy and present less retropulsion due to their large mass, while for smaller stones where retropulsion is the main concern, pulse energy should be turned down to perform a careful ablation with minimal retropulsion and production of tiny debris in the ureter. Anti-retropulsion devices are found to improve the efficiency of lithotripsy, particularly at high pulse energy [30]. With ureteral stone stabilization, high pulse energy settings fragment a stone much more quickly than achieved at low pulse energy settings as retropulsion is negated.

Optical Fibers

Optical fibers are utilized in laser lithotripsy to transmit laser radiation to the calculi with high efficiency. The basic structure of optical fiber consists of a transparent inner core, two to three layers of cladding with lower refractive indices, a buffer layer, and a surrounding jacket. Due to total internal reflection, light will transmit along the fiber core with very low attenuation.

Silica (amorphous silicon dioxide, SiO_2) is the most widely used material for the core. They are clinically used in laser lithotripsy because they are relatively cost-efficient, small, and flexible enough for endoscopic instruments, and they transmit laser light with minimal attenuation. Ho:YAG laser light at 2.1 μm wavelength is highly absorbed by hydroxyl groups; thus it is delivered by low OH silica fiber to reduce light loss and avoid fiber damage [31]. Diameter of the fiber core used for lithotripsy is variable from 150 to 940 μm, normally much smaller than diameter of the collimated laser beam from the laser source. For Ho:YAG wavelengths, fluorine-doped silica which has excellent laser light confinement and small bending radius is the main choice of cladding materials [32].

The laser light irradiated from the laser device is usually collimated, and the diameter of laser beam is often much larger than that of the optical fiber. In order to deliver laser light to the optical fiber, laser light is focused by a convex lens and coupled into the proximal optical fiber tip. To maximize the amount of laser light that is coupled into the fiber, the light has to be focused to the fiber tip with an acceptable divergence angle. In this process, two beam shape parameters are critical to obtain high-efficiency laser–fiber coupling: diameter and numerical aperture (NA) [32, 33]. The diameter of the focused laser beam at fiber surface, or beam waist, should be smaller than the diameter of fiber core to avoid light leakage. However, if the beam diameter is too small, the high energy of the laser light could possibly damage the optical fiber. Thus, a sufficiently large, but smaller than fiber core, beam size is required [34]. The other important parameter, NA, determines the maximal divergence angle that allows a beam to enter the optical fiber [32]. The transmission of light along optical fiber relies on total internal reflection at the core–cladding interface. If the incident angle is larger than the total reflection angle, the light can penetrate the fiber cladding and possibly damage the fiber. The NA of Ho:YAG fibers is 0.2–0.22 [34]. An NA of 0.21 corresponds to a maximum acceptance angle of 12°. The focusing lens should match the NA of optical fiber.

Commercially, an industry standard subminiature version A (SMA) connecter is connected to the proximal end of optical fiber so that fibers with different diameters can easily connect to the same laser source. An SMA connector is designed with an air-filled cavity surrounding the proximal end of the fiber to protect from leakage-related damage [32]. The cavity is made of a polymer material and the shell is usually composed of steel. The SMA connecter protects the optical fiber from mechanical damage and facilitates the alignment of laser–fiber coupling. However, even with the help of SMA connecter, there may still be some axial misalignment of laser and proximal fiber end, especially for small-diameter fibers with core diameter less than 300 μm, which can result in higher order rays, energy attenuation, or fiber damage. For large core fibers, a small misalignment of laser beam from the center of fiber core is sometimes acceptable as long as the beam is focused within the fiber core, but for small-diameter fibers, the partial overlap between laser beam and fiber cladding results in light leakage and fiber damage. Under high power settings, the steel shell of SMA connecter can be vaporized by the energy of stray laser which is not fully coupled into the optical fiber. Over time, the steel vapor will coat the surface of optical fiber and laser source and disrupt their optics structure, leading the failure of laser.

Fiber bending can also affect fiber transmission along optical fiber. Despite total internal reflection, there is still light leakage penetrating fiber cladding. These penetrating light waves, known as evanescent waves, can damage the fiber cladding if they are strong enough. Especially in circumstances of severe fiber deflection, evanescent waves are strengthened due to the reduced incident angle at core–cladding interface. The evanescent light makes more damage on the optical fiber for near-infrared lasers such as Ho:YAG, because their wavelengths are well absorbed by the plastic jacket. Clinically, high-degree fiber bending should be avoided if possible. When treating upper urinary-tract calculi, small-core-diameter fibers (less than 300 μm) are required to pass through the working channel of small caliber ureteroscopes (typically less than 3 mm in diameter). These small-caliber fibers may be bent at high curvatures if the ureteroscope itself is bent, as occurs for example in retrograde ureteronephroscopy of lower pole renal stones. At these extreme bending conditions, more evanescent light leaks into the fiber cladding and can result in fiber damage, or thermal breakdown [32, 35]. Previous studies showed that thermal breakdown occurred at threshold bending diameters from 1 to 3 cm [35]. In general fibers with larger core diameter have lower damage thresholds (easier to fracture even at larger beading diameter). Optical fiber always fractures at the point of maximal bend (smallest bending diameter), suggesting that tight bends increase the risk of thermal breakdown. The optical performance and safety under bending condition greatly vary among fibers from different manufacturers.

At the distal end of the optical fiber, the output light is directly irradiated onto the surface of kidney stones without additional optical elements. During laser lithotripsy, fiber tip degradation can occur especially at high energy settings, typically at pulse energy >1.0 J [29, 36]. The degradation of the fiber tip results in an irregular tip surface, reduced beam transmission through the fiber, less collimated output beam, and finally decreased ablation efficiency. Fiber tip degradation is related to the energy density at the distal end of optical fiber. As a result, the fiber tips degrade faster for small-core-diameter fibers (200–273 μm) and high pulse energies (higher than 1.0 J). Certain stone compositions (uric acid, cystine) are associated with less fiber tip degradation and "burnback" than calcium oxalate and brushite compositions [21, 36].

The positioning of the optical fiber related to the stone also affects the performance of laser lithotripsy. For short-pulsed lasers (pulse duration less than 1 μs) which induce photomechanical laser–target interaction, a separation distance of ~1 mm between the fiber tip and the stone surface is required to yield maximal fragmentation efficiency because the photomechanical mechanism requires space for bubble expansion and collapse which produces pressure transients [4, 37]. Long-pulsed lasers (pulse duration of several hundred microseconds) utilizes photothermal mechanism and is most efficient with direct contact of fiber tip and stone surface in order to minimize the energy loss absorbed by water (Moses Effect) [5, 9, 29, 38, 39].

Future Laser Development

Several lasers are in development and may offer the potential for better laser lithotripsy outcomes. A previous study with free electron lasers shows that lithotripsy is more efficient at wavelengths between 2.9 and 3.1 μm comparing with Ho:YAG wavelength at 2.1 μm [5]. Thus, the Er:YAG laser with a wavelength of 2.9–2.94 μm is potentially a more efficient laser source than Ho:YAG in laser lithotripsy.

Long-pulsed Er:YAG ablation exhibits very similar characteristics as Ho:YAG ablation: little photomechanical effects, similar vapor bubble characteristics, and being capable of fragmenting multiple stone types with symmetric ablation craters [40–42]. In a study, the ablation efficiencies in terms of the crater width, depth, and ablation volume were compared for Er:YAG and Ho:YAG laser lithotripsy at various power settings [42]. The experiment showed that Er:YAG laser produces deeper craters and up to five times larger ablation volumes than Ho:YAG laser for all stone types [42]. The superior drilling makes the Er:YAG laser a more efficient lithotripter than the currently used Ho:YAG laser. Currently, the main factor that limits the clinical application of Er:YAG laser lithotripsy is the lack of clinically useful optical fibers [40]. Unlike Ho:YAG laser, Er:YAG cannot be efficiently transmitted through relatively inexpensive and reusable low OH silica fibers due to their relatively high absorption at Er:YAG wavelength. Fluoride fibers are capable of transmitting Er:YAG light but they are not suitable for clinical application due to their brittleness and hygroscopic structure [40]. Sapphire optical fibers are another option which provide high transmission of Er:YAG light at low power settings, but they do not work well for higher laser power, and they are too expensive for clinical use. It appears that improved fiber delivery is required for Er:YAG lithotripsy to show clinical utility.

Another promising laser candidate for lithotripsy is the thulium fiber laser emitting 1.9 μm [43–46]. Thulium fiber lasers are expected to achieve more fragmentation per unit energy than Ho:YAG laser due to water's much higher absorption coefficient at thulium fiber laser wavelength (1.9 μm). The temporal pulse profile of thulium fiber is rectangular-shaped, so energy is more uniformly delivered to the stone during the ablation process comparing with Ho:YAG laser (Fig. 27.3).

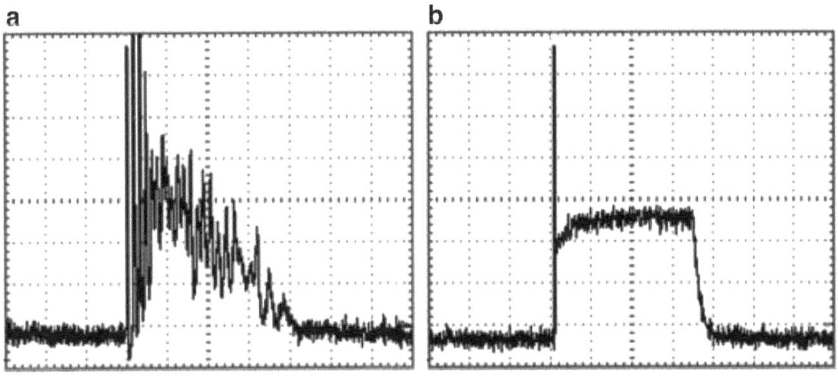

Fig. 27.3 Temporal pulse profiles for (**a**) Ho:YAG laser (220 μs). Large increments = 50 μs; (**b**) modulated thulium fiber laser (1,000 μs). Large increments = 250 μs. Note the more uniform pulse shape for the thulium fiber laser. Reprinted from Blackmon et al. [45] with permission from John Wiley and Sons

In a previous experiment comparing the performance of Ho:YAG and thulium fiber laser lithotripsy, thulium fiber laser fragmented 5–10 times as much stone material as Ho:YAG, both at 70 mJ pulse energies. Currently, power and cost limitations are the main constraints that preclude the clinical utility of thulium fiber laser lithotripsy.

Conclusion

In this chapter, we reviewed the interaction mechanisms of lasers with targets especially urinary calculi during laser lithotripsy. Laser parameters including wavelength, pulse duration, and pulse energy determine the mechanism and characteristics of ablation process. Photomechanical lasers provide higher ablation efficiency while photothermal lasers produce smaller fragments and are effective to all stone compositions. As the current gold standard, photothermal Ho:YAG laser is commonly used in clinical treatment. Stone retropulsion may be minimized by selecting low pulse energy settings or using anti-retropulsion devices. Er:YAG laser and thulium fiber laser are potential future laser candidates to provide more efficient ablation than Ho:YAG lithotripsy.

References

1. Mulvaney W, Beck C. The laser beam in urology. J Urol. 1968;99(1):112.
2. Marks AJ, Qiu J, Milner TE, Chan KF, Teichman JMH. Laser lithotripsy physics. In: Rao NJ, Preminger GM, Kavanagh JP, editors. Urinary tract stone disease. Springer-Verlag, London, 2010. pp. 301–9.
3. Qiu JZ, Teichman JMH, Kuranov RV, Mcelroy AB, Wang T, Paranjape AS, Milner TE. Near infrared femtosecond laser ablation of urinary calculi in water. In: Photonics West 2009. San Jose, CA: SPIE; 2009.
4. Rink K, Delacretaz G, Salathe RP. Fragmentation process of current laser lithotriptors. Lasers Surg Med. 1995;16(2):134–46.
5. Chan KF, Choi B, Vargas G, Hammer DX, Sorg B, Pfefer TJ, Teichman JMH, Welch AJ, Jansen ED. Free electron laser ablation of urinary calculi: an experimental study. IEEE J Quantum Electronics. 2001;7(6):1022–33.
6. Marks AJ, Teichman JMH. Lasers in clinical urology: state of the art and new horizons. World J Urol. 2007;25:227–33.
7. Qiu J, Teichman JMH, Wang T, Neev J, Glickman RD, Chan KF, Milner TE. Femtosecond laser lithotripsy: feasibility and ablation mechanism. J Biomed Opt. 2010;15(2):028001–5.
8. Gamaly EG, Rode AV, Luther-Davies B, Tikhonchuk TV. Ablation of solids by femtosecond lasers: ablation mechanism and ablation thresholds for metals and dielectrics. Phys Plasmas. 2002;9(3):949–57.
9. Chan KF, Pfefer TJ, Teichman JM, Welch AJ. A perspective on laser lithotripsy: the fragmentation processes. J Endourol. 2001;15(3):257–73.
10. Teichman JM, Vassar GJ, Bishoff JT, Bellman GC. Holmium:YAG lithotripsy yields smaller fragments than lithoclast, pulsed dye laser or electrohydraulic lithotripsy. J Urol. 1998;159(1):17–23.
11. Liu MK, Liu PL, Yiu TF, Chan AYT. Clinical experience with holium:YAG laser lithotripsy of ureteral calculi. Lasers Surg Med. 1996;19:103–6.
12. Razvi HA, Denstedt JD, Chun SS, Sales JL. Introcorporeal lithotripsy with the holium:YAG laser. J Urol. 1996;156(3):912–4.
13. Das A, Erhard MJ, Bagley DH. Intrarenal use of the holmium laser. J Urol. 1998;160(2):630–1.
14. Adams DH. Holmium:YAG laser and pulsed dye laser: a cost comparison. Lasers Surg Med. 1997;21(1):29–31.
15. Teichman JMH, Rao RD, Rogenes VJ, Harris MJ. Ureteroscopic management of ureteral calculi: electrohydraulic versus holmium:YAG lithotripsy. J Urol. 1997;158:1357.
16. Teichman JMH, Rao RD, Glickman RD, Harris JM. Holmium:YAG percutaneous nephrolithotomy: the laser incident angle matters. J Urol. 1998;159(3): 690–4.
17. Qiu JZ, Teichman JMH, Milner TE. Ho:YAG laser lithotripsy. Int J Med Biol Front. 2010;17(7):1–10.
18. Chan KF, Vassar GJ, Pfefer TJ, Teichman JMH, Glickman RD, Weintraub ST, Welch AJ. Holmium:YAG laser lithotripsy: a dominant photothermal ablative mechanism with chemical decomposition of urinary calculi. Lasers Surg Med. 1999;25(1):22–37.
19. Marguet CG, Sung JC, Springhart WP, L'Esperance JO, Zhou S, Zhong P, Albala DM, Preminger GM. In vitro comparison of stone retropulsion and fragmentation of the frequency doubled, double pulse Nd:YAG laser and the holmium:YAG laser. J Urol. 2005;173(5):1797–800.
20. Spindel ML, Moslem A, Bhatia KS, Jassemnejad B, Bartels KE, Powell RC, O'Hare CM, Tytle T. Comparison of holmium and flashlamp pumped dye lasers for use in lithotripsy of biliary calculi. Lasers Surg Med. 1992;12:482–9.
21. Spore SS, Teichman JM, Corbin NS, Champion PC, Williamson EA, Glickman RD. Holmium:YAG lithotripsy: optimal power settings. J Endourol. 1999; 13(8):559–66.
22. Lee HO, Ryan RT, Teichman JMH, Kim J, Choi B, Arakeri NV, Welch AJ. Stone retropulsion during holmium:Yag lithotripsy. J Urol. 2003;169(3):881–5.
23. Lee H, Ryan RT, Kim J, Choi B, Arakeri NV, Teichman JMH, Welch AJ. Dependence of calculus retropulsion

dynamics on fiber size and radiant exposure during Ho:YAG lithotripsy. J Biomech Eng. 2004;126(4): 506–15.
24. Kang HW, Lee H, Teichman JMH, Oh JO, Kim J, Welch AJ. Dependence of calculus retropulsion on pulse duration during Ho:YAG laser lithotripsy. Lasers Surg Med. 2006;38(8):762–72.
25. Finley DS, Petersen J, Abdelshehid C, Ahlering M, Chou D, Borin J, Eichel L, McDougall E, Clayman R. Effect of holmium:YAG laser pulse width on lithotripsy retropulsion in vitro. J Endourol. 2005;19(8): 1041–4.
26. Bauerle D. Laser processing and chemistry. Berlin: Springer; 2000.
27. Rane A, Bradoo A, Rao P, Shivde S, Elhilali M, Anidjar M, Pace K, D'A Honey JR. The use of a novel reverse thermosensitive polymer to prevent ureteral stone retropulsion during intracorporeal lithotripsy: a randomized, controlled trial. J Urol. 2010;183(4): 1417–23.
28. Qiu J, Teichman JM, Wang B, Milner TE. Effects of Holmium:YAG energy on BackStop anti-retropulsion polymer; 2012.
29. Vassar GJ, Teichman JMH, Glickman RD. Holmium:YAG lithotripsy efficiency varies with energy density. J Urol. 1998;160(2):471–6.
30. Sea J, Jonat LM, Chew BH, Qiu J, Wang B, Hoopman J, Milner T, Teichman JM. Optimal power settings for holmium:YAG lithotripsy. J Urol. 2012;187(3): 914–9.
31. Teichmann H, Herrmann TR, Bach T. Technical aspects of lasers in urology. World J Urol. 2007;25: 221–5.
32. Nazif OA, Teichman JMH, Glickman RD, Welch AJ. Review of laser fibers: a practical guide for urologists. J Endourol. 2004;18(9):818–29.
33. Harrington JA. Infrared fibers and their applications. Bellingham: SPIE Press; 2004.
34. Marks AJ, Mues AC, Knudsen BE, Teichman JMH. Holmium:yttrium-aluminum-garnet lithotripsy proximal fiber failures from laser and fiber mismatch. Urology. 2008;71(6):1049–51.
35. Knudsen BE, Glickman RD, Stallman KJ, Maswadi S, Chew BH, Beiko DT, Denstedt JD, Teichman JMH. Performance and safety of holmium:YAG laser optical fibers. J Endourol. 2005;19(9):1092–7.
36. Mues AC, Teichman JMH, Knudsen BE. Quantification of holmium:yttrium aluminum garnet optical tip degradation. J Endourol. 2009;23(9):1425–8.
37. Zhong P, Tong HL, Malenbaum J, Cocks FH, Preminger GM. Transient cavitation and acoustic emission produced by different laser lithotripters. J Endourol. 1998;12(4):371–8.
38. Jansen ED, Asshauer T, Frenz M, Motamedi M, Delacretaz G, Welch AJ. Effect of pulse duration on bubble formation and laser-induced pressure waves during holmium laser ablation. Lasers Surg Med. 1996;18(3):278–93.
39. Beghuin D, Delacretaz G, Schmidlin F, Rink K. Fragmentation process during Ho:YAG laser lithotripsy revealed by time-resolved imaging. In: SPIE, San Jose; 1998.
40. Teichman JMH, Chan KF, Cecconi PP, Corbin NS, Kamerer AD, Glickman RD, Welch AJ. Erbium:YAG versus holmium:YAG lithotripsy. J Urol. 2001; 165:876.
41. Chan KF, Lee H, Teichman JMH, Kamerer A, Mcguff HS, Vargas G, Welch AJ. Erbium:YAG laser lithotripsy mechanism. J Urol. 2002;168(2):436–41.
42. Lee H, Kang HW, Teichman JMH, Oh J, Welch AJ. Urinary calculus fragmentation during Ho:YAG and Er:YAG lithotripsy. Lasers Surg Med. 2006;38:39.
43. Fried NM, Murray KE. High-power thulium fiber laser ablation of urinary tissues at 1.94 μm. J Endourol. 2005;19(1):25–31.
44. Fried NM. Thulium fiber laser lithotripsy: an in vitro analysis of stone fragmentation using a modulated 110-watt Thulium fiber laser at 1.94 μm. Lasers Surg Med. 2005;37(1):53–8.
45. Blackmon RL, Irby PB, Fried NM. Holmium:YAG (λ=2,120 nm) versus thulium fiber (λ=1,908 nm) laser lithotripsy. Lasers Surg Med. 2010;42(3): 232–6.
46. Blackmon RL, Irby PB, Fried NM. Thulium fiber laser lithotripsy using tapered fibers. Lasers Surg Med. 2010;42(1):45–50.

Laser Applications, Tumor, and Stricture

28

Adam B. Shrewsberry, Daniel J. Canter, and Kenneth Ogan

Indications

Tumor

Transitional cell carcinoma of the upper urinary tract accounts for approximately 2–5% of all urothelial carcinomas [1, 2]. When urothelial carcinoma is found in the upper tract, the distribution in the kidney and ureter is approximately 3:1 [3]. Traditionally, management of these tumors has consisted of open or laparoscopic nephroureterectomy or, if the lesion is located in the distal ureter, a distal ureterectomy with excision of a bladder cuff and ureteral reimplantation. With the introduction of ureteroscopes and percutaneous techniques in the early 1980s and their continued technological improvements, endoscopic treatment of upper urinary tract urothelial tumors is now possible in selected patients. Nephron-sparing approaches are preferred in patients with bilateral disease, a solitary kidney, preexisting renal insufficiency, or comorbidities that contraindicate major surgery. Furthermore, patients with low-grade, low-stage disease and normal contralateral kidneys may also benefit from endoscopic management. In fact, recent institutional series have shown that endoscopic management of upper tract urothelial carcinoma has equivalent overall, cancer-specific, and metastatic-free survival compared to traditional management (nephroureterectomy) for low-grade and low-stage tumors [4, 5].

A.B. Shrewsberry, M.D. (✉) • D.J. Canter, M.D.
K. Ogan, M.D.
Department of Urology, Emory University, Atlanta, GA, USA
e-mail: adam.shrewsberry@gmail.com

Stricture

In a similar light, ureteroscopic laser treatment of ureteral strictures has become possible with advancements in technique and instrumentation. Often times, intervention is not required when an asymptomatic stricture is associated with stable or absent function in the affected kidney. However, if the stricture results in symptomatic flank pain, recurrent urinary tract infections, and/or deterioration of renal function, treatment of the ureteral stricture is indicated. The three main goals of treating ureteral strictures are ruling out malignancy, preserving renal function, and relieving symptoms.

Preoperative Preparation

Urinary tract infections must be identified and adequately treated with culture-specific antibiotics prior to surgical intervention. There is normally no role for additional laboratory studies prior to treatment. While diagnostic ureteroscopy and stone laser lithotripsy can typically be performed in patients with bleeding diathesis and on

M. Monga (ed.), *Ureteroscopy: Indications, Instrumentation & Technique*, Current Clinical Urology,
DOI 10.1007/978-1-62703-206-3_28,

anticoagulation, we stop warfarin 5 days prior to tumor ablation and stricture incision [6]. Alternatively, patients at high risk are bridged with enoxaparin with the last dose given the night prior to surgery. Patients are usually allowed to continue taking aspirin and clopidogrel prior to the procedure. Finally, preexisting ureteral stents are removed several weeks prior to ureteroscopy to allow for the stent-related inflammation to subside. This provides optimal visualization of the ureter and renal pelvis/calyces to better identify either the boundaries of a stricture or the margins of a tumor and associated satellite lesions. If the patient becomes obstructed following stent removal, a nephrostomy tube is placed for drainage.

Given the level 1b evidence that antibiotic prophylaxis significantly lowers the incidence of perioperative bacteriuria after ureteroscopy, antibiotics are administered within 60 min of upper urinary tract instrumentation [7]. Ampicillin (1–2 g IV) and gentamicin (5 mg/kg IV) are typically the prophylactic antibiotics chosen unless contraindicated. Patients with penicillin allergies are given vancomycin (1 g IV). Those patients with renal insufficiency are given either aztreonam (1 g IV) or a fluoroquinolone instead of gentamicin. Antibiotics are typically not continued postoperatively.

Manipulation of the upper tracts often requires coordination with the anesthesia team. Prior to induction, we always request that the patient be intubated, as opposed to the use of a laryngeal mask airway (LMA). This allows for paralysis and subsequent controlled breath holding, if necessary, during laser tumor ablation and stricture incision. This is particularly important in the kidney where there can be significant movement with respiration, making precise tumor ablation difficult. Once general endotracheal anesthesia is induced, the patient is repositioned in the low dorsal lithotomy position and all pressure points are appropriately padded. Alternatively, the patient can be positioned supine for those with ileal conduits or continent catheterizable pouches. Patients are then prepped and draped in the usual, standard fashion.

Instrumentation

Equipment
Fluoroscopy table
Rigid and flexible cystoscopes
Semirigid ureteroscope
Flexible ureteroscope
Disposable
Hydrophilic guidewires
Holmium laser
5-F ureteral catheter
Biopsy forceps
Ureteroscopic Bugbee electrode
JJ-ureteral stent
Contrast solution

Surgical Technique

Both ureteral stricture and upper tract urothelial carcinoma cases begin with a thorough cystoscopic evaluation of the lower urinary tract using a 22-F rigid cystoscope. Use of both a 30° and a 70° lens provides optimal visualization of the entire bladder urothelium and ureteral orifices. If lesions are identified within the bladder at time of cystoscopy, they are biopsied and treated after treatment of the upper tracts. Alternatively, a flexible cystoscope can be used in patients with a urostomy and urinary diversion. In these patients, due to the unpredictable location of the ureterointestinal anastomoses, intravenous indigo carmine (1 ampule) is given at the beginning of the case to aid in localization of the ureteroenteric anastomoses. Regretfully, in some cases the ureter cannot be accessed in a retrograde fashion and the patient must then undergo a percutaneous antegrade approach.

Regardless of the indications for ureteroscopy, a retrograde pyelogram is performed to assist in defining the patient's anatomy and identifying any anatomical abnormalities (Fig. 28.1). A 5-F cone tip catheter is placed through the cystoscope and flushed prior to cannulation of the ureteral orifice. This removes any potential confusion created by air bubbles appearing as filling defects

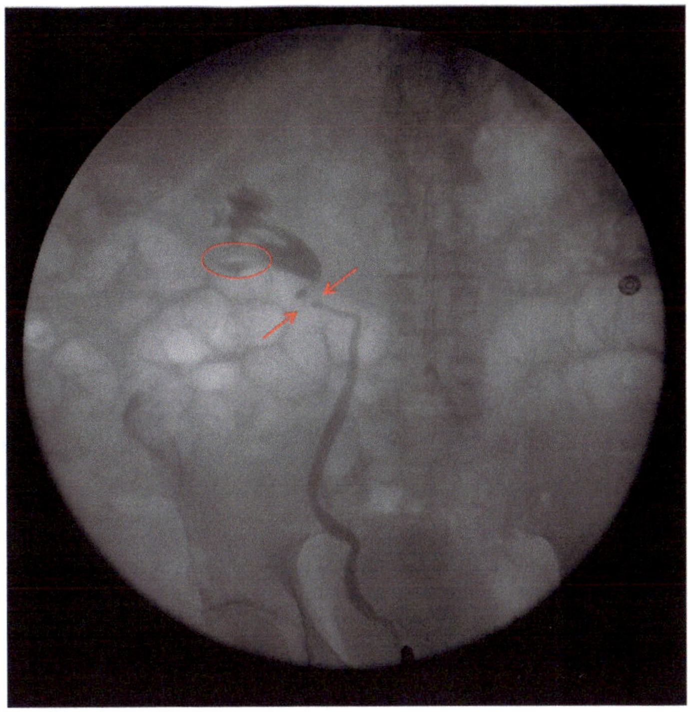

Fig. 28.1 A retrograde is performed at the beginning of the case. A filling defect is clearly identified within the lower pole and proximal ureter. The retrograde pyelogram then serves as a "road map" for the remainder of the procedure

during the retrograde pyelogram. A scout film is taken, the cone tip catheter is inserted into the ureteral orifice, contrast is injected, and fluoroscopic images are obtained. In the case of a ureteral stricture, this helps define location and length. With upper tract transitional cell carcinoma, tumors typically are identified as filling defects. In both situations, the retrograde pyelogram provides a "road map" for the remainder of the case.

Stricture

Following retrograde pyelography, under fluoroscopic guidance, a 0.38 Glidewire (Boston Scientific, Natick, MA) is placed through the cone tip catheter beyond the stricture and coiled within the renal pelvis. For tight strictures, this may need to be accomplished with glidewires in conjunction with angle tipped ureteral catheters. In rare cases when a glidewire cannot bypass a stricture fluoroscopically, attempts can be made under direct endoscopic visualization with a semirigid ureteroscope placed distal to the stricture. If despite all efforts a wire cannot transverse the stricture, the procedure is aborted, and the patient is scheduled for subsequent open repair.

Once the wire is coiled within the renal pelvis, the ureteral catheter and cystoscope are removed, leaving the wire behind. This wire is then exchanged for a stiffer wire, such as a Sensor (Boston Scientific, Natick, MA) or Amplatz (Cook Medical, Bloomington, IN) super stiff wire, which will act as the working wire. In all cases, we prefer to place an additional wire to serve as a safety wire to prevent loss of access. This is achieved with an 8/10-F coaxial dilator, which acts to both dilate the intramural ureter and to introduce the second wire. The 8/10-F coaxial dilator is placed over the original guidewire and the 8-F portion is removed, leaving the 10-F sheath behind. Through this, our safety wire is passed and coiled within the renal pelvis. Fluoroscopy is used throughout this process taking diligent care to minimize exposure to the patient and operative team. Our designated safety wire is then secured to the drapes on the contralateral side to minimize risks of inadvertent removal during the case.

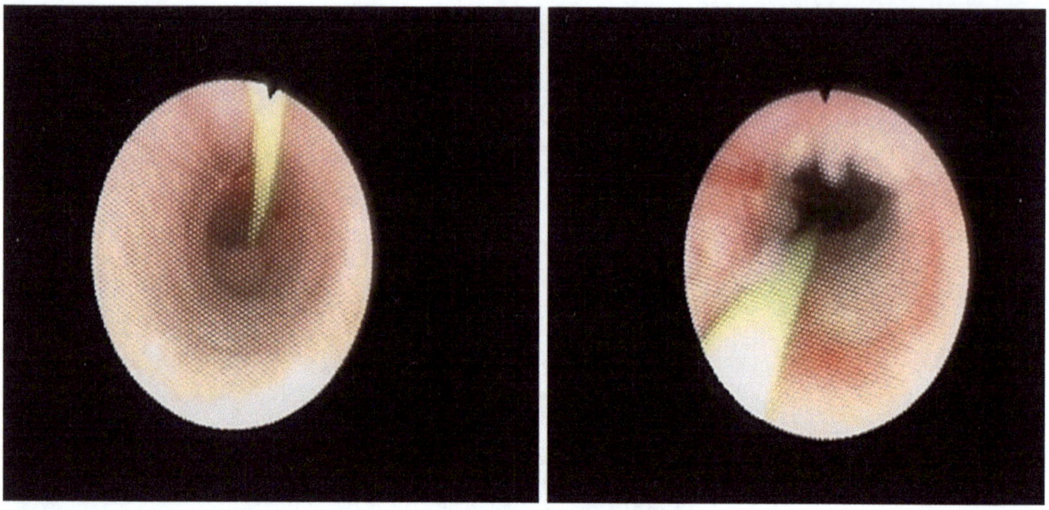

Fig. 28.2 A ureteral stricture is seen in these images, pre- and postendoureterotomy

Once access is obtained, the ureteroscopic equipment is assembled. In order to minimize intrarenal pressure and subsequent pyelovenous backflow during ureteroscopy, we prefer the use of a hand pump irrigator. Additionally, a ureteral access sheath may be used for mid and proximal ureteral strictures to further decrease intrarenal pressures [8]. Irrigation fluid is typically normal saline. However, in our experience, using water for nearly all ureteroscopic cases has been a safe alternative with improved visualization. The ureteroscope is passed over the working wire to the level of the stricture under fluoroscopic guidance. The wire is then removed, leaving the ureteroscope and the safety wire behind. Sometimes traversing the intramural ureter with the ureteroscope is difficult. Using a balloon dilator to dilate the intramural ureter is an option, although this should be done only when necessary.

The length, location, degree of stenosis, and the presence of pulsations are assessed fluoroscopically and endoscopically. Prior to treatment, a biopsy should be performed in patients with a recurrent stricture, a suspicious appearing stricture, a stricture of unclear origin, or a history of urothelial malignancy. Endoureterotomy is then performed under direct vision using an end-firing pulsed holmium laser fiber at a setting of 1 J and 10 Hz (Fig. 28.2). A full thickness incision is made into the periureteral fat. The incision is started proximally and carried distally, taking care to incise the ureter for the entire length of the stricture including normal ureteral margins. When making the incision, it is important to consider the vascular supply to the ureter. Incisions are made laterally for strictures in the proximal and midureter and medially for strictures in the distal ureter to avoid vascular injuries. Following laser incision, the ureteroscope is positioned distal to the stricture and a retrograde ureteropyelogram is performed through the scope. Extravasation of contrast fluoroscopically verifies full thickness incision. The remainder of the ureter is then examined prior to removal of the ureteroscope to confirm there are no additional sites of stricture.

A ureteral stent is then placed over safety wire under fluoroscopic guidance. An endopyelotomy stent can also be used in this situation for temporary internal drainage. Endopyelotomy stents have the advantage of having a larger diameter (10–18 F) at the incised stricture, which in theory may result in higher success rates. However, multiple studies have not demonstrated an advantage when compared to standard stents [9–11]. After full thickness incision of the ureter and stenting, the ureteral wall reforms completely within 2–6 weeks [12]. We therefore typically leave the stent in place for 4–6 weeks.

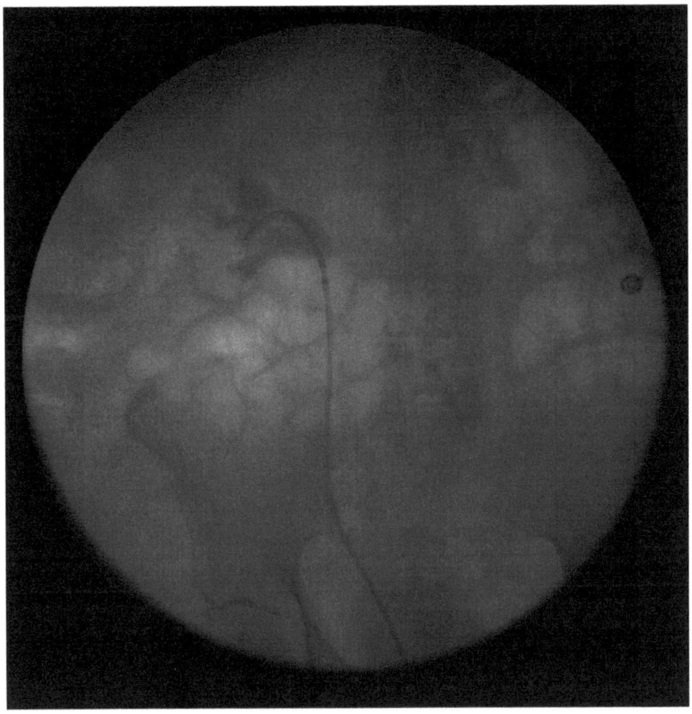

Fig. 28.3 The flexible ureteroscope is employed to perform renoscopy. Here the scope is within the midpole. Using the retrograde pyelogram, the surgeon can ensure complete renoscopy is performed

Tumor

In contrast to the practice of gaining access for ureteral strictures, it is important that no wires are passed prior to complete inspection of the ureter and calyceal system in the evaluation and treatment of upper tract urothelial carcinoma. Any irritation of the urothelium from iatrogenic wire trauma may cause bleeding or mimic a urothelial tumor. Initially, a semirigid ureteroscope is passed into the midureter and complete inspection is performed. Once this has occurred, a guidewire is passed through the semirigid uretperoscope to the midureter but not beyond the previously inspected area. The semirigid ureteroscope is removed and over the wire the flexible ureteroscope is passed. The wire is removed and the flexible ureteroscope is advanced into the renal pelvis under direct visualization. A thorough inspection of the kidney and ureter is performed, using fluoroscopy as an aid in accessing the entire calyceal system (Fig. 28.3).

In general, a distal ureteral pathology can be accessed with a semirigid ureteroscope while a lesion in the mid/proximal ureter or renal collecting system is best approached with a flexible ureteroscope (Fig. 28.4). As with strictures, if tumors are identified in the mid or proximal ureter or kidney, a ureteral access sheath can be used to improve visualization and reduce intrarenal pressure [8]. Once tumors are endoscopically identified, samples are obtained via aspiration adjacent to any visible tumors. Secondly, a barbatoge specimen using normal saline is obtained. For visible tumors, biopsies are taken using the Pirhana (Boston Scientific, Natick, MA) or BIGopsy (Cook Medical, Bloomington, IN) biopsy forceps. Since the BIGopsy forceps need to be back loaded onto the scope, a ureteral access sheath must be used when using this instrument. Alternatively, in an effort to garner more tissue, large papillary tumors can be snared with a wire basket. For flat lesions and those in the ureter, a brush biopsy can be performed. Following

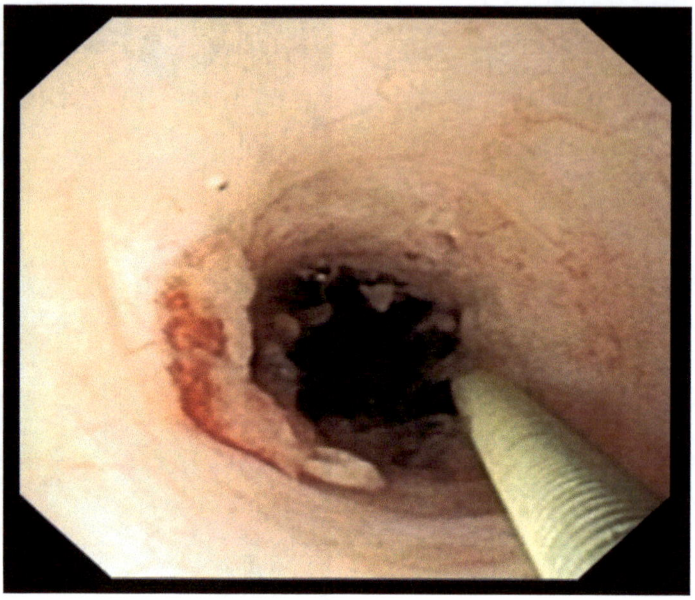

Fig. 28.4 A ureteral tumor is identified in the proximal ureter, which corresponds to the ureteral filling defect in Fig. 28.1

biopsies, fluid should again be aspirated and a barbatoge specimen should be acquired. In all cases, multiple samples should be obtained, and all should be sent to the cytopathology laboratory for analysis. Obtaining specimens as stated above, will improve diagnostic yield. In studies by Kelley and Tawfiek, when these techniques are employed, the ability to grade tumors increases from 42.9 to 97.2% [13, 14].

Once adequate cytology and tissue samples have been obtained, treatment of the tumor can be performed with either cauterization or laser ablation. Details regarding the advantages and disadvantages of the various lasers are covered elsewhere in this book. In brief, the Nd:YAG laser has a greater depth of penetration (4–6 mm) and can be used to coagulate the tumor. The Nd:YAG laser does not need to touch the tumor for effect. The Ho:YAG is a contact laser that has a shallower depth of penetration (less than 0.5 mm) and can be used to ablate the tumor with more control and less risk of perforation. For this reason, the Ho:YAG laser is the laser most often employed. A commonly used setting of the Ho:YAG laser is 0.6–1.0 J at 10 Hz. It is important to remember to only treat the intraluminal tumor as attempts to ablate deep into the wall of the upper tract increases the risk of perforation. Use of the laser also provides a degree of hemostasis. Typically, lesions are ablated from distal to proximal. Otherwise, when treating lesions on a stalk, it is helpful to begin ablation at the more proximal portion of the tissue and work distally. A standard indwelling ureteral stent is typically placed for a period of time depending on the extent of the procedure, although the role of post-treatment stenting has not been studied. If intravesical therapy is planned, placement of a ureteral stent may allow reflux into the upper tracts. Previous investigators have demonstrated on cystography the reflux of contrast into the upper tracts with stents in place prior to successful treatment of upper tract CIS with intravesical BCG [15]. While not covered in this chapter, percutaneous resection of upper tract urothelial carcinoma is generally reserved for tumors larger than 1.5 cm or bulky proximal ureteral tumors.

Postoperative Consideration

Endoscopic treatment of ureteral stricture disease is typically performed on an outpatient basis. Placement of a foley catheter is not indicated.

The ureteral stent typically remains in place for 4–6 weeks although several studies lend evidence that 2 rather than 4 weeks of stenting results in the same success with lower infection rates [16, 17]. Depending on the indication for treatment of the ureteral stricture, imaging studies are typically performed after the stent has been removed and most often include renal ultrasound or renal scintigraphy. If the patient remains asymptomatic, imaging is performed at 3 months (MAG-3 lasix renal scan) and then at 6-month (renal sonogram) intervals for 2 years.

Endoscopic treatment of upper tract urothelial carcinoma is also typically performed on an outpatient basis. Short-term foley catheter placement is indicated only in the case of immediate postoperative instillation of chemotherapeutic agents for concomitant bladder tumors. Strict surveillance of the upper urinary tracts is mandatory and involves ureteroscopy, as current imaging tests are not adequate to detect small recurrences.

Complications

The most common technical complications associated with endoscopic management of upper tract urothelial carcinoma are similar to those seen with any upper tract endoscopic intervention. The most common complications of ureteroscopic management of upper tract urothelial carcinoma are perforation and stricture formation. The rate of ureteral or pelvic perforation is between 0 and 10%, and the stricture rate after ureteroscopic treatment of upper tract urothelial carcinoma ranges from 5 to 14% [5, 18, 19]. Not all ureteral strictures are due to technical reasons and biopsy of the stricture must be performed to rule out malignancy. Once malignancy has been ruled out, these strictures can be managed endoscopically.

General risks of endoscopic laser treatment of ureteral strictures include ureteral perforation, gross hematuria, and infection. Ureteral perforation is uncommon, but when it does occur, the procedure should be terminated, and a ureteral stent should be placed. Perforation is more common in the thinner walled proximal ureter compared to the distal ureter.

New Technology

Digital Ureteroscopes

Significant advancements have been made over the last 10–20 years in the field of ureteroscopy, especially with regards to the design of flexible ureteroscopes. In contrast to fiberoptic ureteroscopes, which suffer from grainy analogue images, digital ureteroscopes have been developed that provide superior resolution and safety [20]. Presumably, the increased resolution will translate into greater precision for the diagnosis and treatment of small urothelial tumors.

Narrow-Band Imaging

Narrow-band imaging (NBI, Olympus American, Inc, Center Valley, PA) is an optical enhancement tool that has the potential to improve detection rates and decrease residual tumor rates in bladder urothelial cancers [21]. NBI uses no fluorescent agents and works by filtering standard white light into two bandwidths of illumination centered on 415 nm (blue light) and 540 nm (green light). This light is subsequently absorbed by hemoglobin and enhances contrast between normal and vascular structures. Since most urothelial tumors are hypervascular, these tumors become more prominent when compared to standard white light endoscopy (Fig. 28.5). Our brief experience with this tool has been promising in identifying small upper tract urothelial lesions and detecting margins of tumors. However, no studies examining NBI use in upper tract urothelial carcinoma have been published.

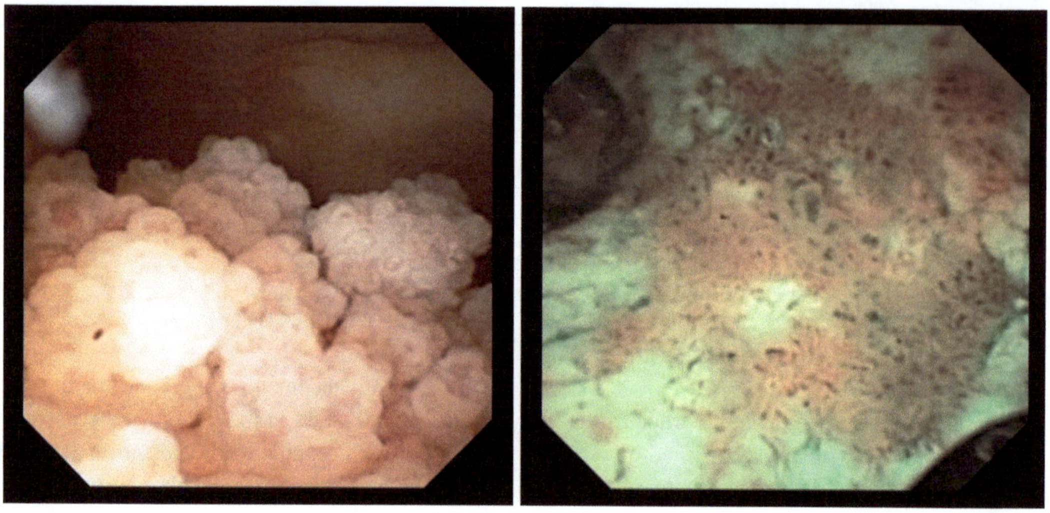

Fig. 28.5 The *left photo* visualizes a tumor with white light endoscopy. The *right photo* visualizes a tumor using Narrow Band Imaging (NBI)

References

1. Charbit L, Gendreau M, Mee S, Cukier J. Tumors of the upper urinary tract: 10 years of experience. J Urol. 1991;146(5):1243–6.
2. Huben R, Mounzer A, Murphy G. Tumor grade and stage as prognostic variables in upper tract urothelial tumors. Cancer. 1988;62(9):2016–20.
3. Williams C, Mitchell J. Carcinoma of the ureter—a review of 54 cases. Br J Urol. 1973;45(4):377–87.
4. Chen G, Bagley D. Ureteroscopic management of upper tract transitional cell carcinoma in patients with normal contralateral kidneys. J Urol. 2000;164(4):1173–6.
5. Elliott D, Segura J, Lightner D, Patterson D, Blute M. Is nephroureterectomy necessary in all cases of upper tract transitional cell carcinoma? Long-term results of conservative endourologic management of upper tract transitional cell carcinoma in individuals with a normal contralateral kidney. J Urol. 2001;58(2):174–8.
6. Kuo RL, Aslan P, Fitzgerald KB, Preminger GM. Use of ureteroscopy and holmium:Yag laser in patients with bleeding diatheses. J Urol. 1998;52(4):609–13.
7. Wolf JS, Bennett CJ, Dmochowski RR, Pearle MS, Schaeffer AJ. Best practice policy statement on urologic surgery antimicrobial prophylaxis. J Urol. 2008;179(4):1379–90.
8. Auge B, Pietrow P, Lallas C, Raj G, Santa-Cruz R, Preminger GM. Ureteral access sheath provides protection against elevated renal pressures during routine flexible ureteroscopic stone manipulation. J Endourol. 2004;18(1):33–6.
9. Siegel J, Smith A. The ideal ureteral stent for antegrade and retrograde endopyelotomy: what would it be like? J Endourol. 1993;7(2):151–4.
10. Meretyk I, Meretyk S, Clayman R. Endopyelotomy: comparison of ureteroscopic retrograde and antegrade percutaneous techniques. J Urol. 1992;148:775–82.
11. Pearle M. Use of ureteral stents after endopyelotomy. J Endourol. 1996;10(2):169–76.
12. Andreoni C, Lin H, Olwenty E, et al. Comprehensive evaluation of ureteral healing after electrosurgical endopyelotomy in a porcine model: original report and review of the literature. J Urol. 2004;171(2):859–69.
13. Keeley FJ, Kulp D, Bibbo M, McCue P, Bagley D. Diagnostic accuracy of ureteroscopic biopsy in upper tract transitional cell carcinoma. J Urol. 1997;157(1):33–7.
14. Tawfiek E, Bibbo M, Bagley D. Ureteroscopic biopsy: technique and specimen preparation. J Urol. 1997;50(1):117–9.
15. Irie A, Iwamura M, Kadowaki K, Ohkawa A, Uchida T, Baba S. Intravesical instillatin of bacille Calmette-Guerin for carcinoma in situ of the urothelium involving the upper urinary tract using vesicoureteral reflux created by a double-pigtail catheter. Urology. 2002;59(1):53–7.
16. Kerbl K, Chandhoke P, Figenshau R, Stone A, Clayman R. Effect of stent duration on ureteral healing following endoureterotomy in an animal model. J Urol. 1993;150(4):1302–5.
17. Mandhani A, Kapoor R, Zaman W, Kumar A, Bhandari M, Gambhir S. Is a 2-week duration sufficient for stenting in endopyelotomy? J Urol. 2003;169(3):886–9.

18. Keeley FJ, Bibbo M, Bagley D. Ureteroscopic treatment and surveillance of upper urinary tract transitional cell carcinoma. J Urol. 1997;157(5):1560–5.
19. Martinez-Pineiro J, Garcia Matres M, Martinez-Pineiro L. Endourological treatment of upper tract urothelial carcinomas: analysis of a series of 59 tumors. J Urol. 1996;156(2):377–85.
20. Andonian S, Okeke Z, Smith A. Digitial ureteroscopy: the next step. J Endourol. 2008;22(4):603–5.
21. Cauberg E, Mamoualakis C, de la Rosette J, de Reijke T. Narrow band imaging-assisted transurethral resection for non-muscle invasive bladder cancer significantly reduces residual tumour rate. World J Urol. 2011;29(4):503–9.

29 Ureteral Stenting or No Stenting

Seth A. Cohen and Roger L. Sur

Introduction

Ureteroscopy has come to the forefront in the surgical management of ureteral calculi. There is significant literature regarding the effectiveness of this modality in clearing stones from the ureter; however, there still remains an active debate regarding the placement of ureteral stents after ureteroscopy. The morbidity of a stent, the resources required for an additional procedure to remove it, as well as the growing body of literature suggesting stentless ureteroscopy is a reasonable option, make it worthwhile to ask when stenting is necessary for optimal surgical outcome and patient care.

S.A. Cohen, M.D.
Urology Division, Surgery Department,
U.C. San Diego Health System, San Diego, CA, USA

R.L. Sur, M.D. (✉)
Division of Urology, Surgery Department,
U.C. San Diego Health System, 200 W Arbor Dr. #8897,
San Diego, CA 92103-8897, USA
e-mail: rlsur@ucsd.edu

What Do Urologists Do?

A survey sent to community and academic urologists to assess the use of ureteral stenting after ureteroscopy for stone surgery was performed demonstrating significant variety in the practice patterns among urologists [1]. Of the 173 respondents, 97% thought patient tolerance of stent discomfort was the most significant issue with indwelling ureteral stents. Approximately 66% of urologists placed a ureteral stent more than 50% of the time after routine ureteroscopy, with 13% of the respondents placing stents 100% of the time. Interestingly 25% of respondents stated that an access sheath would change their use of stents—i.e., 29% would increase their use of stenting and surprisingly 71% would decrease their use of stenting. Half of urologists would place a ureteral stent 100% of the time, if the ureteral orifice was dilated (balloon or coaxial dilator). Despite accumulating evidence suggesting that ureteral stents were likely not necessary after routine ureteroscopy, there appeared to be no consensus in practice patterns. This may have been secondary to a lack of subanalysis regarding stenting for distal ureteral calculi, which the literature has increasingly suggested non-stenting may benefit. Although both community and academic urologists were surveyed, it would have

M. Monga (ed.), *Ureteroscopy: Indications, Instrumentation & Technique*, Current Clinical Urology,
DOI 10.1007/978-1-62703-206-3_29, © Springer Science+Business Media New York 2013

been interesting to note if resident availability influenced academic physicians to embrace non-stenting more frequently. Future research examining an urologist's rationale for stenting would be useful as well—e.g., is it done to prevent readmission, facilitate stone fragment passage, and/or prevent stricture development.

Potential Advantages of Placing a Stent

When considering the reasons for placing a ureteral stent subsequent to ureteroscopy, the literature provides physiologic rationale for placing a stent. Reactive ureteral edema after ureteroscopy and stone manipulation may lead to obstruction, threatening renal function, and causing flank pain. A ureteral stent serves to decompress this system postoperatively. Moreover the rare but recognized risk of ureteral stricture is potentially prevented with ureteral stenting as it promotes ureteral healing [2]. In the setting of ureteral dilation, animal models have shown persistent ureteral edema and upper urinary tract obstruction up to 96 h after dilation; a ureteral stent could potentially decompress this system postoperatively [3, 4]. In addition, it has been postulated that a ureteral stent could aide in passage of residual stone fragments, secondary to passive dilation of the ureter [5–7].

There is also data supporting pre-stenting prior to ureteroscopy to facilitate ease of surgery. A retrospective analysis evaluated the cost-effectiveness of pre-stenting patients prior to ureteroscopy [8]. The retrospective review identified pre-stented and matched control of unstented subjects, with a 19.5 day (range 6–67) median duration of preoperative stent placement. Total healthcare cost for stone clearance in patients with stone burden >1 cm who had been pre-stented was significantly less than the median cost of those not stented, $17,706 and $27,806 $p=0.03$, respectively. Decreased operative time and reoperative rates explained this finding. In those patients with stone burden <1 cm, pre-stenting actually significantly increased the overall cost of stone removal, $12,344 versus $10,872 $p=0.006$.

Potential Disadvantages of Placing a Stent

Indwelling stents have been documented to have significant patient morbidity, with up to 90% of patients with an indwelling ureteral stent complaining of urgency, frequency, flank pain during void, and hematuria [9]. Ureteral stents can fracture, migrate, knot, and encrust, making removal difficult and hazardous for the patient [2]. A large study examining the natural history of 330 ureteral stents in 181 patients demonstrated 47% of the stents were encrusted, with an encrustation rate of 26% at less than 6 weeks, 56% at 6–12 weeks, and 75% at more than 12 weeks, while 14% stents necessitated surgery for removal [10]. The median dwell time for stents that resisted removal was 72 (range 14–124) days and 31 (range 30–60) days for irremovable stents. In rare circumstances retained stents have been found to obstruct the renal unit and to potentially lead to patient death. [11–13]. Thus, the time course of encrustation is associated with increased dwelling time, but appears difficult to predict. Although studies are underway to determine risk factors for encrustation, including proteomic evaluations of stent biofilms, data does indicate that the shorter the interval of placement the lesser the discomfort for the patient [14, 15].

The increased costs associated with ureteral stent placement after ureteroscopy have been documented in previous studies [16, 17]. The costs, however, are not only limited to the ureteroscopy but also to the postoperative period when the stent is cystoscopically removed, given the common practice of performing outpatient cystoscopy to remove ureteral stents [1]. This additional cost of stent removal has been decried as a potential reason to avoid stenting if medically feasible, and some groups have gone as far to devise creative ways to keep this cost down [18].

Quality of Life

In addition to the inconvenience and discomfort of removing an indwelling ureteral stent, one must also consider the impact of an indwelling ureteral stent on patients' health-related quality of life (HRQoL). HRQoL assessment uses measurement instruments, such as surveys, to evaluate aspects of health and well-being as valued by patients, focusing on physical, emotional, and cognitive function, in addition to their abilities to participate in meaningful activities within their workplace, families, and communities [19]. The significance of stent morbidity becomes more compelling when one considers that kidney stone patients have been reported to exhibit higher depression rates than normal population [20].

When determining the appropriate treatment strategy for patients with stone disease, efforts to assess how ureteroscopy and stent placement impact HRQoL could potentially alter practice patterns and patient management. As mentioned, ureteral stents are associated with increased irritative voiding symptoms and hematuria. At this time, there is no stone-specific instrument that has been validated for QoL assessment in nephrolithiasis patients, thus there is no definitive data regarding HRQoL and the use of ureteral stents in lithotripsy. However, informative inquiries have taken place. For instance, a study using the International Prostate Symptom Score (IPSS), International Continence Society (ICS) male and quality of life (QoL), and Bristol Female Lower Urinary Tract Symptoms (BFLUTS) questionnaires to characterize voiding symptoms in 48 patients with indwelling ureteral stents before and after stent removal attempted to validate the morbidity of stents [21]. Not surprisingly mean total IPSS was significantly higher with the stent in situ, compared to after removal, though only the domain "feeling of incomplete emptying" had a statistically significant difference in value. Dysuria and hematuria were additional domains added to the questionnaire and these domains demonstrated significant improvement with stent removal. The ICS and BFLUTS questionnaires found patients to have a higher prevalence of storage symptoms (up to 70%) associated with a high degree of bother and significant dissatisfaction with QoL, with the stent in situ. This data would support the notion that patients suffer decreased QoL with stents in place, yielding another reason to perform stentless ureteroscopy, if safe and feasible.

Objective Data Regarding Stent Placement

Multiple randomized control trials (RCTs) have been performed within the last 10 years examining surgical outcomes in stented versus non-stented patients undergoing ureteroscopy. A multi-center prospective randomized controlled trial was performed in 2001, assessing pain, stone-free rates, and complications in patients undergoing ureteroscopic treatment of distal ureteral calculi (defined as below the iliac vessels on radiographic imaging) in subjects with or without ureteral stents (53 in stented group and 54 in unstented group) [22]. Despite 57% of unstented patients having undergone ureteral balloon or tapered dilation, there was no difference in readmission rate for flank pain (unstented 4 (7.4%) vs. stented 0, $p>0.05$). Furthermore, stented subjects had more postoperative flank pain ($p=0.005$), bladder pain ($p<0.001$), urinary symptoms ($p=0.002$), overall pain ($p<0.001$), and total narcotic use ($p<0.001$) compared to the unstented group. Long-term outcomes did not appear to be affected by lack of stenting as the stone-free rate was similar at 99.1%, and all patients who underwent imaging postoperatively were without evidence of ureteral stricture. The authors concluded uncomplicated ureteroscopy (including lack of significant ureteral trauma or ureteral perforation) for the treatment of distal ureteral calculi, with or without intraoperative distal ureteral dilation, can be safely performed without placement of a ureteral stent.

A 2002 randomized controlled trial evaluated 60 patients, 30 stented, and 30 non-stented, after uncomplicated ureteroscopic lithotripsy with an electrohydraulic lithotripter [23]. Patients without ureteral stents were found to have similar stone-free rates, renal function recovery, pain reduction, and less irritative voiding symptoms as compared to those patients in which stents were placed. After discharge, 1 (3.3%) patient in the non-stented group returned with intolerable flank pain, as opposed to 0 in the stented group. Overall, the authors found it was not necessary to place a ureteral stent routinely after uncomplicated ureteroscopic electrohydraulic lithotripsy, without ureteral dilation, for stones smaller than 1 cm.

In 2004, a randomized controlled trial evaluated 104 patients, 52 stented versus 52 non-stented after uncomplicated ureteroscopic stone removal, without dilation, using pneumatic intracorporeal lithotripsy [24]. No differences were seen in dysuria, hematuria, and frequency/urgency or stricture rates, though the stented group experienced higher pain scores on postoperative day 3. There was no difference in anatomical ureteral narrowing on IVP at 6 months follow-up between the two groups. The authors concluded that when using pneumatic intracorporeal lithotripsy, routine stent placement remained advisable. Of note, this is the only randomized controlled trial to date, in which there was a significantly higher rate of hospital readmission in the non-stented population.

A 2008 study enrolled 43 patients with distal (below the inferior part of the sacroiliac joint) stones larger than 1 cm in a randomized controlled trial comparing stent (21 cases) versus no stent (22 cases) after ureteroscopy with pneumatic lithotripsy [25]. No patients required dilation of the ureteral orifice or intramural ureter. Mean stone size was comparable between the groups (13.28 vs. 12.90 mm). There was no statistically significant difference between the groups for postoperative pain and hematuria, though voiding irritative symptoms were much higher in the stented group. The authors were diligent in removing residual fragments ≥4 mm with additional forceps application. This extra attention given to ensure removal of all residual fragments ≥4 mm may have contributed to the lack of difference in return hospital visits between the stented (1 (4.7%)) and non-stented patients (1 (4.5%)), as opposed to those results found in the previously discussed 2004 study using pneumatic lithotripsy. This highlights the importance of removing large, ≥4 mm fragments, particularly in an unstented patient. Of note, a study in 1998 compared various lithotrites and found fragments ≥4 mm are produced by all types of endoscopic lithotrites, except for the holmium:YAG laser [26]. Thus, when using electrohydraulic or pneumatic lithotrites, it appears to behoove practitioners to diligently remove, when possible, residual fragments ≥4 mm.

A 2008 randomized controlled trial attempted to overcome the limitations of previous trials, which had included small sample size, patient heterogeneity, improper definition of "uncomplicated ureteroscopy," poor documentation of outcomes, and lack of long-term follow-up—all of which compromised the external validity of the results [27]. The definition of "uncomplicated ureteroscopy," was explicitly described as ureteroscopy in adults 18 years or older with stones located in the distal part of the ureter below the iliac vessels, with largest stone diameter of less than 1.5 cm, "no multiple complex stones" no distal ureteral pathology; no intraoperative major complications (e.g., ureteral perforation), and complete stone disintegration or removal. The study was large including 110 stented and 110 unstented subjects. Both patients and surgeons were blinded to group allocation, with the surgeon informed of group allocation when the ureteroscopic portion was completed. All stented patients had ureteral stents in place for 2 weeks. There was no difference in readmission, low-grade fever, flank pain, hematuria, urinary tract infection, time to return to normal physical activity, or postoperative stricture. Dysuria was significantly less in the non-stented group.

Synthesizing the Data: Meta-Analyses

In 2007, Nabi et al. published a meta-analysis of nine randomized controlled trials examining the outcomes with and without stenting after ureteroscopy [28]. The authors found a significantly higher incidence of dysuria (relative risk 2.25, 95% confidence interval (CI) 1.14–4.43) and frequency or urgency (2.00, 95% CI 1.11–3.62).

There was no significant difference in postoperative requirement for analgesia, urinary tract infections, stone-free rate, and postoperative strictures. The authors noted that marked heterogeneity prevented pooling of data for outcomes such as flank pain. Pooled analysis suggested a nonsignificant trend toward a reduced likelihood of unplanned medical visits and hospital admissions in the stented group (RR=0.53, 95% CI 0.17–1.60). They concluded that stenting in uncomplicated ureteroscopy leads to considerable morbidity, but there is still significant uncertainty with the role of stenting due to "lack of standardization of outcome measures, marked clinical heterogeneity, withdrawal after randomization, imprecision in measurement of outcomes (large confidence intervals), and poor reporting of published clinical trials."

In 2008, a systematic review of the same nine randomized controlled trials, reported similar findings to the previous meta-analysis study with respect to stent morbidity and lack of long-term advantages. However, the systematic review concluded stenting in an uncomplicated patient is not mandatory, a slightly different interpretation [29]. The difference in the interpretation of the data may lie in the methodological differences between a systematic review and a meta-analysis, whereas the latter incorporates complex statistical methods of combining evidence.

A combined systematic review and meta-analysis performed in 2011 is one of the most contemporary reports involving 16 randomized controlled trials [30]. No significant differences were found between the groups in fever, urinary tract infection, need for analgesia, unplanned readmission, and late postoperative complications. It is interesting that the authors concluded that routine stenting is not necessary despite the admitted "bias and different quality levels of the included trials" in this meta-analysis. In contradistinction, another recent 2011 meta-analysis of 14 randomized controlled trials demonstrated significant benefit to non-stenting but admitted that the poor quality of available studies resulted in uncertainty in the role of stenting [31]. The authors noted data from the 14 randomized controlled trials were of moderate to poor quality, had clinical heterogeneity (varying sizes of ureteroscopes, different intracorporeal lithotripsy devices, variations in practice), lacked standardized definition of "uncomplicated ureteroscopy," had imprecision in outcomes (large confidence intervals)—all reasons underscoring the need for further investigation.

What Shall We Define as Complex Ureteroscopy?

The results of the aforementioned RCT's and meta-analyses all reserve conclusions for "uncomplicated" ureteroscopy. These conclusions therefore beget the corollary question—what defines "complicated" or "complex" ureteroscopy? The characteristics that define complex ureteroscopy will most likely provide clinical guidelines to elucidate optimal candidates for stentless patients. The current literature unfortunately inconsistently or even fails to define complicated criteria. It is intuitively a multifaceted issue involving patient and stone characteristics, surgical technique as well as surgical equipment variables.

A retrospective evaluation of 219 unstented patients of whom 39 developed postoperative ureteroscopic complications was performed with the goal of determining factors that predict postoperative complications. Of the 39 complications 26 included postoperative obstruction and these were analyzed. The authors concluded that bilateral stentless surgery, history of recent of recurrent urinary tract infections, history of recurrent urolithiasis are the greatest risk factors for postoperative complications. They postulated that a history of urolithiasis and/or urinary tract infections induces abnormal ureteral mechanics, which subsequently predispose these patients to postoperative problems. Prolonged surgical time >45 min with concomitant use of lithotripsy as well as renal pelvic stones were additional risk factors associated with complications [32].

A 2011 retrospective review was performed on patients who had undergone "uncomplicated ureteroscopy" with pneumatic lithotripsy and subsequently required emergent stenting, with the goal of identifying factors to more completely stratify the subset of ureteroscopy patients who require stents [33]. In over 3 years, 276 uncomplicated ureteroscopy procedures were performed; in which 23 (8.3%) patients require emergent ureteral stenting in the initial 24 h secondary to intractable colic pain. All patients had undergone ureteroscopy for what was believed to be a single ureteral calculus through a semirigid ureteroscope. No patient underwent ureteral dilation. Stones were extracted with basket or forceps, with or without pneumatic intracorporeal lithotripsy. Patients were excluded from the review if they had stents placed preoperatively, multiple stones, evidence of active infection, a solitary kidney, or suspected additional ureteral pathologic features (e.g., ureteral stricture). Stones were located in the distal ureter in 11 patients (47.8%), mid-ureter in 6 (26.1%), and proximal ureter in 6 (26.1%). The authors reviewed operative recordings and radiographs and determined that longer operative time, repeated access, large stones, impacted calculi with ureteral wall edema, a mildly narrowed ureteral segment, untreated caliceal small calculi, and a recent history of urinary tract infection were risk factors for postoperative intervention.

Those Situations That Require Further Investigation

In the setting of balloon dilation of the distal ureter, there is no current consensus on whether stenting is necessary. Animal models have found persistent ureteral edema and upper urinary tract obstruction up to 96 h after dilation [3, 4]. However, to our knowledge, limited human data available suggests that stenting after balloon dilation is necessary. The meta-analysis by Nabi et al. demonstrates the inconsistent use of ureteral dilation in the available literature (two studies required dilation, one study excluded subjects who were dilated, three studies did not require dilation) and therefore the unclear need to stent after ureteral dilation [28]. The limited data from the RCT's suggests no untoward effect of dilating, but again the data is too heterogeneous to permit conclusive recommendations. We nevertheless acknowledge the growing body of literature that does support a possible stentless approach to ureteral dilation. A subset analysis by Hollenbeck et al. of their cohorts of stented versus non-stented patients who had undergone ureteral dilation found no difference in the risk of postoperative complications [34]. In 2011, a multi-center prospective randomized control trial enrolled 505 patients undergoing ureteroscopy, with 286 requiring balloon dilation of the ureteral orifice, of which 144 were randomized to be stented and 142 were randomized to receive no stent [35]. In each case of dilation, a 18 Fr-4 cm balloon dilator was applied for approximately 2–3 min. At 1 week postoperatively, patients' pain, dysuria, and urgency were evaluated, in addition to urine culture, plain X-ray, and ultrasounds obtained. At 6 months, follow-up intravenous urogram was obtained to evaluate ureteral narrowing. Although there was no significant difference in pain, infectious complications, unplanned visits, or ureteral narrowing, the irritative symptoms (dysuria and urgency) and hematuria, were more common in the stented group.

Pregnant patients undergoing ureteroscopic management of urolithiasis represent another population for which there is no consensus on postoperative stenting. In 2006, a retrospective review of seven patients found routine insertion of ureteral stents with pullout strings for at least 72 h reduces pain and analgesic use postoperatively [36]. In 2009, Rana et al. reported on a series of 19 pregnant patients who underwent ureteroscopy, 12 (63%) of which were left with postoperative ureteral stents; 2 (11%) developed retained, encrusted stents requiring cystolitholapexy and ureteroscopy for removal [37]. In 2011, Isen et al. published a descriptive analysis of the management of 36 pregnant women with symptomatic ureteric stones [38]. Nine (25%) were managed with ureteroscopic lithotripsy, in which a ureteral catheter was placed at the end of the procedure and withdrawn on the first postoperative day. No significant complications were reported. Thus, the management of stone disease in pregnant patients requires thought and it should be reiterated that indwelling devices, including stents, are associated with increased risks of infection, pain, bacteriuria, dislodgement, and migration—these events during pregnancy may place pregnancy itself at risk [39]. Further studies are needed to elucidate the role of postoperative stent placement in the pregnant population.

Previous literature had reported that patients at highest risk for stricture after ureteroscopy were those with impacted calculi, up to an incidence of 24% in patients with stone impaction greater than 2 months in duration, with the primary risk factor being ureteral perforation at the stone site [40, 41]. Cevik et al. prospectively randomized 60 patients with impacted ureteral stones to undergo ureteroscopic lithotripsy with and without ureteral stent placement [42]. Impacted ureteral stones were defined as stones that did not allow passage of a guidewire at initial attempts before the disintegration of stones at ureteroscopy. Of note, ureteroscopic pneumatic lithotripsy was utilized for distal and middle ureteral impacted calculi, with an 8 French semirigid ureteroscope, without ureteral dilation. Excretory urography was performed 3 months after the procedure. Until postoperative (POD) day 5, narcotic use was more frequently necessary in the non-stent group ($p=0.004$); after POD 5, narcotics were almost unnecessary in the no-stent patients. Stent related irritative symptoms were significantly higher in the stented group (93 vs. 10%, $p<0.001$). Rates of postoperative complications in the stented and no-stent group were otherwise similar: fever (10 vs. 6%, $p=1$), pain delaying discharge (10 vs. 23%, $p=0.299$), emergency department visits (10 vs. 20%, $p=0.472$), and stricture rate (0% in both groups). The authors concluded that routine ureteral stent placement after ureteroscopic lithotripsy for impacted ureteral stones was not necessary in patients without complications.

Conclusions

A multitude of recent evidence in the literature suggest routine stent placement after uncomplicated ureteroscopy may not be necessary, especially for small distal ureteral calculi; however, the current level of evidence leaves some uncertainty to this universal recommendation. Though it is incontrovertible that stents are a source of excess morbidity and that not all patients should be stented, defining those exact patients who are ideal for stentless surgery still requires investigation. Exclusion criteria for the non-stenting recommendation include solitary kidney, renal insufficiency, recent history of urinary tract infection, bilateral ureteroscopy, intraoperative ureteral injury, prolonged surgery, pregnancy, and poor access to postoperative on-call urologic care.

References

1. Auge BK, Sarvis JA, L'Esperance JO, Preminger GM. Practice patterns of ureteral stenting after routine ureteroscopic stone surgery: a survey of practicing urologists. J Endourol. 2007;21(11):1287–91.
2. Knudsen BE, Beiko DT, Denstedt JD. Stenting after ureteroscopy: pros and cons. Urol Clin North Am. 2004;31(1):173–80 [Comparative Study Review].
3. Boddy SA, Nimmon CC, Jones S, Ramsay JW, Britton KE, Levison DA, et al. Acute ureteric dilatation for ureteroscopy. An experimental study. Br J Urol. 1988;61(1):27–31 [Research Support, Non-U.S. Gov't].
4. Moneim AA, Khalaf I. Critical evaluation of acute ureteral dilatation: clinical and experimental study. J Endourol. 1988;2(4):345–53.
5. Drake Jr WM, Carroll J, Bartone F, Cottone RN, Kazal HL, Sumerai S, et al. Evaluation of materials used as ureteral splints. Surg Gynecol Obstet. 1962;114:47–51.
6. Weinberg SL. Ureteral function. II. The ureteral catheter and the urometrogram. Invest Urol. 1975;12(4):255–61 [Research Support, U.S. Gov't, Non-P.H.S.].
7. Jones BJ, Ryan PC, Lyons O, Grainger R, McDermott TE, Butler MR. Use of the double pigtail stent in stone retrieval following unsuccessful ureteroscopy. Br J Urol. 1990;66(3):254–6.
8. Chu L, Farris CA, Corcoran AT, Averch TD. Preoperative stent placement decreases cost of ureteroscopy. Urology. 2011;78(2):309–13.
9. Pollard SG, Macfarlane R. Symptoms arising from Double-J ureteral stents. J Urol. 1988;139(1):37–8.
10. Kawahara T, Ito H, Terao H, Yoshida M, Matsuzaki J. Ureteral stent encrustation, incrustation, and coloring: morbidity related to indwelling times. J Endourol. 2012;26(2):178–82.
11. Ringel A, Richter S, Shalev M, Nissenkorn I. Late complications of ureteral stents. Eur Urol. 2000;38(1):41–4 [Duplicate Publication].
12. Damiano R, Oliva A, Esposito C, De Sio M, Autorino R, D'Armiento M. Early and late complications of

double pigtail ureteral stent. Urol Int. 2002;69(2):136–40.

13. Singh V, Srinivastava A, Kapoor R, Kumar A. Can the complicated forgotten indwelling ureteric stents be lethal? Int Urol Nephrol. 2005;37(3):541–6 [Case Reports].
14. Monga M. The dwell time of indwelling ureteral stents—the clock is ticking but when should We Set the alarm? J Urol. 2011;185(2):387.
15. El-Nahas AR, El-Assmy AM, Shoma AM, Eraky I, El-Kenawy MR, El-Kappany HA. Self-retaining ureteral stents: analysis of factors responsible for patients' discomfort. J Endourol. 2006;20(1):33–7.
16. Netto Jr NR, Ikonomidis J, Zillo C. Routine ureteral stenting after ureteroscopy for ureteral lithiasis: is it really necessary? J Urol. 2001;166(4):1252–4 [Clinical Trial Randomized Controlled Trial].
17. Byrne RR, Auge BK, Kourambas J, Munver R, Delvecchio F, Preminger GM. Routine ureteral stenting is not necessary after ureteroscopy and ureteropyeloscopy: a randomized trial. J Endourol. 2002;16(1):9–13 [Clinical Trial Randomized Controlled Trial].
18. Söylemez H, Sancaktutar AA, Bozkurt Y, Atar M, Penbegül N, Yildirim K. A cheap minimally painful and widely usable alternative for retrieving ureteral stents. Urol Int. 2011;87(2):199–204.
19. Vetter TR. A primer on health-related quality of life in chronic pain medicine. Anesth Analg. 2007;104(3):703–18.
20. Angell J, Bryant M, Tu H, Goodman M, Pattaras J, Ogan K. Association of depression and urolithiasis. Urology. 2012;79(3):518–25.
21. Joshi HB, Okeke A, Newns N, Keeley Jr FX, Timoney AG. Characterization of urinary symptoms in patients with ureteral stents. Urology. 2002;59(4):511–6.
22. Borboroglu PG, Amling CL, Schenkman NS, Monga M, Ward JF, Piper NY, et al. Ureteral stenting after ureteroscopy for distal ureteral calculi: a multi-institutional prospective randomized controlled study assessing pain, outcomes and complications. J Urol. 2001;166(5):1651–7 [Clinical Trial, Multicenter Study, Randomized Controlled Trial, Research Support, Non-U.S. Gov't Research Support, U.S. Gov't, Non-P.H.S.].
23. Chen YT, Chen J, Wong WY, Yang SS, Hsieh CH, Wang CC. Is ureteral stenting necessary after uncomplicated ureteroscopic lithotripsy? A prospective, randomized controlled trial. J Urol. 2002;167(5):1977–80 [Clinical Trial Comparative Study Randomized Controlled Trial].
24. Damiano R, Autorino R, Esposito C, Cantiello F, Sacco R, de Sio M, et al. Stent positioning after ureteroscopy for urinary calculi: the question is still open. Eur Urol. 2004;46(3):381–7. [Clinical Trial Randomized Controlled Trial]. discussion 7–8.
25. Kenan I, Salih B, Suat E, Huseyin E, Vehbi K. Is routine ureteral stenting necessary after uncomplicated ureteroscopic lithotripsy for lower ureteral stones larger than 1 cm? Urol Res. 2008;36(2):115–9.
26. Teichman JM, Vassar GJ, Bishoff JT, Bellman GC. Holmium:YAG lithotripsy yields smaller fragments than lithoclast, pulsed dye laser or electrohydraulic lithotripsy. J Urol. 1998;159(1):17–23.
27. Ibrahim HM, Al-Kandari AM, Shaaban HS, Elshebini YH, Shokeir AA. Role of ureteral stenting after uncomplicated ureteroscopy for distal ureteral stones: a randomized, controlled trial. J Urol. 2008;180(3):961–5 [Randomized Controlled Trial].
28. Nabi G, Cook J, N'Dow J, McClinton S. Outcomes of stenting after uncomplicated ureteroscopy: systematic review and meta-analysis. BMJ. 2007;334(7593):572.
29. Haleblian G, Kijvikai K, de la Rosette J, Preminger G. Ureteral stenting and urinary stone management: a systematic review. J Urol. 2008;179(2):424–30 [Review].
30. Pengfei S, Yutao L, Jie Y, Wuran W, Yi D, Hao Z, et al. The results of ureteral stenting after ureteroscopic lithotripsy for ureteral calculi: a systematic review and meta-analysis. J Urol. 2011;186(5):1904–9.
31. Tang L, Gao X, Xu B, Hou J, Zhang Z, Xu C, et al. Placement of ureteral stent after uncomplicated ureteroscopy: do we really need it? Urology. 2011;78(6):1248–56.
32. Hollenbeck BK, Schuster TG, Seifman BD, Faerber GJ, Wolf Jr JS. Identifying patients who are suitable for stentless ureteroscopy following treatment of urolithiasis. J Urol. 2003;170(1):103–6.
33. Tanriverdi O, Yencilek F, Koyuncu H, Yencilek E, Sarica K. Emergent stenting after uncomplicated ureteroscopy: evaluation of 23 patients. Urology. 2011;77(2):305–8.
34. Hollenbeck BK, Schuster TG, Faerber GJ, Wolf Jr JS. Routine placement of ureteral stents is unnecessary after ureteroscopy for urinary calculi. Urology. 2001;57(4):639–43.
35. Baseskioglu B, Sofikerim M, Demirtas A, Yenilmez A, Kaya C, Can C. Is ureteral stenting really necessary after ureteroscopic lithotripsy with balloon dilatation of ureteral orifice? A multi-institutional randomized controlled study. World J Urol. 2011;29(6):731–6.
36. Akpinar H, Tufek I, Alici B, Kural AR. Ureteroscopy and holmium laser lithotripsy in pregnancy: stents must be used postoperatively. J Endourol. 2006;20(2):107–10 [Comparative Study].
37. Rana AM, Aquil S, Khawaja AM. Semirigid ureteroscopy and pneumatic lithotripsy as definitive management of obstructive ureteral calculi during pregnancy. Urology. 2009;73(5):964–7 [Evaluation Studies].
38. Isen K, Hatipoglu NK, Dedeoglu S, Atilgan I, Caca FN, Hatipoglu N. Experience with the diagnosis and management of symptomatic ureteric stones during pregnancy. Urology. 2012;79(5):1188.
39. Semins MJ, Matlaga BR. Management of stone disease in pregnancy. Curr Opin Urol. 2010;20(2):174–7 [Review].

40. Roberts WW, Cadeddu JA, Micali S, Kavoussi LR, Moore RG. Ureteral stricture formation after removal of impacted calculi. J Urol. 1998;159(3): 723–6.
41. Mugiya S, Nagata M, Un-No T, Takayama T, Suzuki K, Fujita K. Endoscopic management of impacted ureteral stones using a small caliber ureteroscope and a laser lithotriptor. J Urol. 2000;164(2):329–31.
42. Cevik I, Dillioglugil O, Akdas A, Siegel Y. Is stent placement necessary after uncomplicated ureteroscopy for removal of impacted ureteral stones? J Endourol. 2010;24(8):1263–7.

Medical Therapy for Stent Discomfort

30

Zachariah G. Goldsmith, Michael E. Lipkin, and Glenn M. Preminger

Introduction: Scope, Significance, and Physiology of Stent-Related Morbidity

Internal ureteral stents are associated with high rates of morbidity. When surveyed, up to 80% of patients with double-J ureteral stents report bothersome lower urinary tract symptoms and adverse effects on quality of life [1, 2]. Therefore, in addition to adhering to strict indications for stent placement following ureteroscopy, urologists need to be familiar with methods to reduce the morbidity of these devices. This chapter reviews the pathophysiology of stent discomfort and the evidence for medical therapies to reduce stent-related morbidity. Data from multiple clinical trials and recent meta-analyses support the use of alpha blockers in reducing stent discomfort, and these lines of evidence are herein reviewed in detail. In addition, data from preclinical studies and the small number of clinical trials involving other agents are reviewed as well.

Patients with an indwelling internal ureteral stent typically report storage symptoms, including frequency, and urgency with or without incontinence [1]. Dysuria [1, 3] and sexual dysfunction [2] are also reported. Pain is described most commonly in the groin and flank (60%) followed by bladder (38%) and genitalia (32%) [2]. Noninvasive urodynamic studies of patients with indwelling ureteral stents have revealed unobstructed flow rates with minimal post-void residual [1]. Stented patients have reported increased use of pain-medications in addition to spending more time in bed and less time at work [2]. Longitudinal survey administration confirms that these symptoms are reversible following removal of the stent [1, 2].

The prevalence of these symptoms was well characterized in a prospective trial that administered pain assessments to 107 patients randomized to placement of a ureteral stent, or no stent placement, following semirigid ureteroscopy with lithotripsy or basket extraction for distal ureteral stones (mean stone size 6.6 mm) [4]. Patients in the stented group reported significantly higher scores of postoperative flank pain, bladder pain, urinary symptoms, overall pain, and total narcotic use compared to the unstented group. No cases of ureteral stricture were reported in either group, although four patients in the unstented group required hospital readmission for unremitting flank pain and evidence of partial ureteral obstruction. This finding underscores the need for proper patient selection for stent placement following ureteroscopy, and the importance of providing appropriate adjunctive medication to treat stent discomfort.

Although the exact mechanism of stent-related discomfort has not been fully characterized,

Z.G. Goldsmith, M.D., Ph.D. • M.E. Lipkin, M.D.
G.M. Preminger, M.D. (✉)
Division of Urologic Surgery, Surgery Department, Duke University Medical Center, 200 Trent Drive, Room 1572, DUMC 3167, Durham, NC 27710, USA
e-mail: glenn.preminger@duke.edu

M. Monga (ed.), *Ureteroscopy: Indications, Instrumentation & Technique*, Current Clinical Urology,
DOI 10.1007/978-1-62703-206-3_30,

multiple factors have been implicated, including irritation at the level of the trigone, ureteral spasm, and vesicoureteral reflux [1, 5–7]. Fluoroscopic images of a small group of patients with double-J stents in place revealed changes in stent position relative to fixed bony structures when moving from supine to standing, sitting, and bending forward (average 2.3 cm) [8]. This phenomenon may correspond to some patients reporting worsening stent discomfort with movement during the waking hours [1]. In addition, vesicoureteral reflux is present in 56–63% of stented ureters as documented by cystourethrogram studies [9, 10]. During filling, low grade reflux into the ureter was observed, and high grade reflux to the level of the renal pelvis was observed during voiding [9]. In addition, significantly higher rates of reflux were seen with patients in whom stents had been in place for weeks versus those in whom cystourethrograms were obtained immediately following stent placement [10]. These data may provide a mechanism for worsening flank pain experienced with voiding in the presence of a ureteral stent. Infectious or inflammatory processes appear to potentiate the symptoms of ureteral stents as the patients with a positive urine culture obtained during stent placement also report significantly more severe symptoms [11].

Ureteral contraction, like most smooth muscle systems, is mediated primarily by intracellular calcium influx [12]. It has been demonstrated in a porcine model that this process is driven by intrinsic pacemaker cells localized near the palvicalyceal border [13]. In addition, autonomic innervation and a number of hormones and locally active agents, including prostaglandins, serve as regulators of ureteral contractility [14–16]. Alpha-1 adrenergic receptors are located along the entire length of the ureter with the highest concentration in the distal ureter [14, 17]. In a study using dog and rabbit ureters [18], alpha-adrenergic agonists such as phenylephrine were found to have a stimulatory effect on the force and frequency of contraction whereas alpha-antagonists such as phentolamine inhibited this response. In contrast, beta-agonists such as isoproterenol resulted in an inhibitory effect on ureteral contraction. Quantification of alpha-1 receptor expression using semi-quantitative reverse transcriptase polymerase chain reaction (RT-PCR) revealed that the alpha-1d receptor subtype is the most common in all segments of the ureter, with a highest overall density of alpha 1 receptors in the distal ureter [17]. Manipulation of this system with alpha-adrenergic blockers has proven to be an effective therapy for stent discomfort.

Evaluation of Stent-Related Symptoms

A number of instruments have been used to quantify the morbidity and health-related quality of life with ureteral stents. The *u*reteral *s*tent *s*ymptom *q*uestionnaire (USSQ) is an instrument developed specifically to assess ureteral stent discomfort [19]. This instrument assesses six domains, including urinary symptoms, body pain, general health, work performance, sexual matters, and additional problems. Each domain has a sum score, with higher values indicating severity of symptoms. Although completion of this questionnaire requires a significant time investment by patients and investigators, it has been used widely and effectively in a number of clinical trials related to stent discomfort [20–25]. In addition, the bothersome domain of the *I*nternational *P*rostate *S*ymptom *S*core (IPSS), also known as the American Urologic Association Symptom Index [26], has been used as a measure of quality of life in patients with indwelling ureteral stents [27, 28]. Visual analog scales (VAS), often from 0 to 10 or 0 to 5, have also been employed to facilitate self-reported quantification of stent-related symptoms [6, 28–30].

Effects of Stent Design and Stent Placement on Reducing Morbidity

A number of innovations in stent design have been developed in an attempt to minimize patient discomfort. Currently, no ideal stent material or design has been developed to eliminate morbidity [31–33]. At least three randomized trials have been completed comparing stents of different diameter (4.7–6 F). Each of these trials has demonstrated an equivalent degree of patient discomfort with stents of different diameters [29, 34, 35].

Mixed results have been reported from trials assessing the impact of stents manufactured from soft versus firmer materials. A randomized trial involving 130 patients treated with stents made from soft or firm polymers manufactured by the same vendor (Boston Scientific), revealed no significant difference in USSQ scores between the groups [36]. A smaller trial in which 44 patients were randomized to stents from four different manufacturers demonstrated modest improvement in USSQ scores with the Bard Inlay stent compared to the other stents 3 days following stent insertion, although there were no differences in symptoms at postoperative days 1 or 5 [37].

In contrast to stent diameter and material, stent position as well as stent length, have been consistently associated with patient discomfort. Multiple studies have identified an association with the presence of the distal stent coil that crosses the midline, or the presence of an incomplete distal coil, with worsened stent symptoms [6, 11, 25]. These observations have actually been confirmed in a prospective trial in which 120 patients were randomized to placement of a longer stent (26–28 cm) with the distal coil located across the midline of the bony pelvis and proximal coil in the upper calyx versus shorter stents (22–24 cm) with a distal coil that did not cross midline and the proximal coil within the renal pelvis [38]. The same diameter and type of stent (6 F silicone, Cook) was used for all patients. Significantly increased number of patients reported moderate to severe dysuria, urgency, and worsened quality of life in the group with the longer midline-crossing stents. Additional studies have also identified an association between longer stents and higher symptom scores [39], and that stents with less intravesical material (short-loop tail stents) were associated with a trend towards less discomfort [24].

Interestingly, the potential beneficial effects of alpha blockers and anticholinergics on stent discomfort appear to be abrogated in the presence of stents that cross the midline. A randomized 3-arm trial was conducted in which 53 patients following ureteroscopy and stent placement were randomized to standard analgesics, tamsulosin, or tamsulosin plus tolterodine [28]. There was a decrease in IPSS score and storage symptoms in the tamsulosin and tamsulosin plus tolterodine group. However, subgroup analysis revealed that these effects were only significant in patients with properly placed stents. There were no improvements in symptoms with either agent in those patients whose stents were found to cross midline. This finding underscores the need for proper stent length and position in order to optimize the effects of adjunctive medical therapy.

Intravesical Therapies and Drug-Eluting Stents

An additional focus of research has involved administration of local analgesia in the form of intravesical infusion or cystoscopic injection following ureteral stent placement. In one study, 42 patients were randomized to intravesical infusion of ketorolac (10 mg), oxybutynin (10 mg), lidocaine (480 mg), or control immediately after stent placement prior to shock wave lithotripsy [40]. There was a significant improvement in VAS of flank pain at the 1-h timepoint in the ketorolac group versus placebo (0.74 vs. 2.17, $P=0.0085$). The effects of this method appear to be transient, as no significant differences were found in pain scores 24-h after the procedure. In addition, submucosal injection of ropivicaine (50 mg) at five locations around the ureteral orifice and bladder neck prior to stent placement resulted in a trend towards decreased postoperative narcotic use, approaching statistical significance only at the 2-h timepoint following the procedure [30]. A more robust response was observed with submucosal injection of botulin toxin type A (10 U/mL) at three locations around the ureteral orifice following stent placement [41]. A significant decrease in VAS pain score was observed in the Botox group versus control on postoperative day number 7. No complications or adverse effects were noted. In addition, the Botox-treated patients required significantly fewer narcotic pain pills than the control group. However, no significant change in USSQ was noted. These data may suggest a role of detrusor over activity at the level of the trigone in promoting stent discomfort.

An additional focus of research has included the development of drug-eluting ureteral stents to reduce morbidity [31, 33]. These devices have the potential advantages of eliminating the need for separately administered medical adjuvants, and perhaps decreased adverse effects compared to systemically administered medications. A stent loaded with the antibiotic triclosan has been developed and demonstrated resistance to infection with *Proteus mirabilis* in animal models [42, 43]. A paclitaxel-eluting metallic stent has also been developed, and has been shown to reduce ureteral inflammation in porcine studies [44]. In addition, a ketorolac-eluting stent has been developed and studied in a clinical trial [24]. While the safety profile appears favorable, the device was not associated with a significant improvement in symptoms compared to a standard stent in a recent trial. Taken together, these findings suggest that further investigation of drug-eluting ureteral stents is certainly warranted, and may lead to the development of novel devices with less associated morbidity.

Alpha-Adrenergic Blockers

Alpha-stimulatory and beta-inhibitory adrenergic receptors have been well-characterized in the ureter [14, 18, 45]. In porcine models, administration of alpha-1 antagonists resulted in a robust inhibition of ureteral contractility ex vivo [46] and in vivo [47]. In one study, human volunteers were catheterized with a ureteral manometer, and pressure measurements were obtained up to 24 h following the procedure [48]. Treatment with oral tamsulosin (0.4 mg) was shown to reduce the pressure of spontaneous ureteral contractions.

A clinical role of alpha blockers in treating symptoms of ureteral spasm was first reported in a non-placebo controlled trial, in which the non-selective alpha antagonist phentolamine or the beta-antagonist propranolol were administered to patients with acute flank pain and evidence of ureteral obstruction on intravenous pyelogram [49]. A greater proportion of patients in the phentolamine group reported relief of pain (68%) as compared to the propranolol group (3.6%), although neither of the adrenergic agents was as effective as the narcotic pethidine (Demerol).

Since that time, a number of clinical trials have demonstrated beneficial effects of the two alpha blockers tamsulosin (alpha-1 A selective) and alfuzosin (non-subtype specific alpha-1 antagonist) on stent-related morbidity. Two prospective non-placebo controlled trials of tamsulosin (0.4 mg daily) following ureteroscopy with stent placement revealed significantly improved USSQ scores for urinary symptoms and pain [20] as well as improved IPSS score [27] versus the non-tamsulosin group, 1 or 2 weeks postoperatively. These findings have been validated in a larger placebo-controlled trial of 154 patients randomized to 0.4 mg daily tamsulosin versus placebo following ureteroscopic lithotripsy with stent placement for distal ureteral stones [21]. Significantly improved mean urinary symptom USSQ scores were observed in the tamsulosin group versus placebo (20.96 vs. 31.59, $P<0.0001$). In addition, quality of life, as measured using the bother domain of the IPSS, was also significantly improved with tamsulosin versus placebo (1.60 vs. 4.21, $P<0.0001$).

In addition to tamsulosin, a beneficial effect of alfuzosin has been demonstrated in two randomized trials. In a trial of 100 patients with ureteral stones (mean size 7.1–7.6 mm) and hydronephrosis who elected for ureteral stent placement without concomitant ureteroscopy, patients were randomized to alfuzosin (10 mg daily) or placebo following stent placement [22]. Mean urinary symptom USSQ score at 4 weeks postoperatively was significantly improved in the alfuzosin group versus placebo (21.6 vs. 28.1, $P<0.001$). Stent-related pain and number of narcotic tablets consumed were also significantly lower in the alfuzosin group. An additional trial of 66 patients randomized to alfuzosin versus placebo following stent placement revealed significantly decreased proportion of patients reporting painful urination (53% vs. 90%, $P=0.007$) and lower VAS of flank pain (2.55 vs.

4.67, $P=0.017$) in the alfuzosin group at postoperative day 3 [23]. In this trial, no significant difference in narcotic pill consumption was observed. The beneficial effect of alfuzosin was also demonstrated in a 3-arm trial in which patients were randomized to 10 mg alfuzosin, the anticholinergic tolterodine, or placebo following ureteral stent placement [50]. Again, a significant reduction in mean urinary symptom USSQ score was observed in the alfuzosin versus placebo group (22.1 vs. 28.1, $P<0.05$).

The beneficial effects of alpha blockers in reducing stent discomfort have also been confirmed by two well-conducted independent meta-analyses which pooled the results of the above trials. In an analysis by Yakoubi and colleagues [51], four trials (with a total of 341 patients) met the inclusion criteria, which included randomization to alpha blocker or placebo, and the use of the USSQ as an outcome measure. One trial investigating tamsulosin [21] and three trials investigating alfuzosin [22, 23, 50] met these criteria for inclusion. Analysis revealed significant decrease in urinary symptoms and pain, and significant improvement in general health with alpha blocker use. Alpha blockers were not associated with significantly improved scores for the work and sexual function domains of USSQ. In another analysis by Lamb and colleagues [52], an additional trial was included in review, which was not placebo controlled (patients were randomized to tamsulosin versus no therapy) [20], for a total of 416 patients in 5 trials. Again noted was a significant reduction USSQ score for urinary symptoms (mean reduction 8.4 [95% CI, 5.6–11.1]) and body pain (mean reduction 7.2 [95% CI, 2.5–11.8]). The small number of high quality trials with these agents precluded an inverted funnel plot analysis in either meta-analysis, which may assess for publication bias [53]. Notwithstanding these limitations, these data support the use of alpha blockers to reduce stent symptoms in routine clinical practice.

It is important to emphasize that this class of medication, and all other classes reviewed herein, have not received FDA approval for reducing stent-related pain. Of specific note, while tamsulosin and alfuzosin are FDA approved to treat men with symptoms of benign prostatic hyperplasia, neither agent is approved for use in women. Therefore, although there is strong level-one evidence supporting their use from trials, which included men and women, patients should be appropriately counseled on the off-label use of these and all medications offered to reduce stent-related morbidity. Adverse effects of alpha blockers may include orthostatic hypotension, dry mouth, constipation, and dizziness. These adverse effects, when reported in the above studies, appeared to be minor [23, 50]. In addition, no head-to-head trials have compared the efficacy of tamsulosin to alfuzosin in reducing stent morbidity. Both agents appear to reduce USSQ scores relative to placebo by a similar magnitude. It is currently our practice to prescribe tamsulosin 0.4 mg daily for patients with stents placed during treatment of nephrolithiasis.

Anticholinergics

The prevalence of urge symptoms during storage in the presence of a ureteral stent [1, 2] supports a possible role for anticholinergics in alleviating stent discomfort. Two extended release agents have been included in randomized clinical trials with mixed results. In one trial, 60 patients were randomized to receive oxybutynin (extended release, 10 mg daily), phenazopyridine (200 mg three times daily), or placebo, following flexible ureteroscopy with laser lithotripsy and stent placement [54]. A VAS was administered on postoperative days 1, 2 and the day of stent removal. There was no difference in symptom scores or number of narcotic pills consumed among the groups. An additional 3-arm trial randomized patients to tolterodine extended release (4 mg daily), 10 mg alfuzosin, or placebo following ureteral stent placement [51]. In this study, a significant reduction in mean urinary symptom USSQ score was noted in the tolterodine group versus placebo group (22.1 vs. 22.9, $P<0.05$). Of note, the magnitude of this effect was similar to the group which received the alpha blocker alfuzosin. This finding supports further studies to investigate the potential role of anticholinergic medications in reducing the urge component of stent-related symptoms.

Calcium Channel Blockers

The central role of calcium influx in muscle contraction is well established, and calcium channel blockers have long been used in studying ureteral physiology (Weiss [12]). Nifedipine treatment has been shown to reduce contractility of human ureteral explants exposed to a variety of chemical stimulants [55]. More recently, it has been demonstrated that the inhibitory effect of nifedipine is far more potent than that obtained using tamsulosin, in a series of experiments using porcine ureteral explants [56]. In vivo, intraluminal verapamil applied into the ureters of pigs resulted in proximal ureteral dilation [57]. Clinically, a number of trials examining the role of nifedipine with or without concomitant steroids in medical expulsive therapy for ureteral stones have revealed a benefit of these agents in promoting stone passage [58, 59]. However, to our knowledge studies examining the effects of this class of agent on treating stent discomfort have not been published.

Phosphodiesterase Inhibitors

cAMP is known to mediate smooth muscle relaxation, and thus inhibitors of phosphodiesterase (PDE), the enzyme which inactivates cAMP, have been used to induce smooth muscle relaxation in a variety of conditions. A PDE-4 inhibitor (rolipram) has been shown to decrease ureteral peristalsis in vivo in rabbits [60]. In addition, the PDE-5 inhibitors vardenafil, sildenafil, and tadalafil have been shown to induce modest decrease in ureteral contraction of human ureteral segments in vitro [61]. Despite this intriguing data, no clinical studies of PDE inhibitors in alleviating stent discomfort have been identified.

Corticosteroids and Nonsteroidal Anti-inflammatory Drugs

Prostaglandin signaling has been shown to mediate ureteral contraction [15]. In addition, inflammation at the level of the trigone has been suggested as a potential mechanism of stent discomfort [31]. Therefore, a small number of studies have investigated a possible role of anti-inflammatories (corticosteroids and nonsteroidals) in ureteral physiology and stent discomfort. Hydrocortisone has been shown to decrease contractility of porcine ureteral segments in vitro [62]. Clinically, a number of trials focused on medical expulsive therapy for ureteral stones have included corticosteroids as adjuncts to calcium channel blockers or alpha blockers. For example, in a trial of 114 patients with distal ureteral stones 5 mm or greater, patients were randomized to tamsulosin alone, oral glucocorticoid (deflazacort 30 mg daily), both tamsulosin and glucocorticoid, or placebo [59]. A significant increase in stone expulsion rate was demonstrated in the combination group but not in the group that received glucocorticoid monotherapy. The effects of steroids on stent-related morbidity have yet to be specifically investigated. In addition, the possible adverse effect of these agents in potentiating infection following ureteroscopy with stent placement is unclear.

The nonsteroidal cyclooxygenase (COX) inhibitors are widely recognized as inhibitors of prostaglandin synthesis. Both COX-2 and nonselective COX inhibitors have been shown to decrease ureteral contractility in vitro in pig and human ureteral segments [63–66]. Clinically, intravesical infusion of ketorolac (10 mg) immediately after stent placement prior to shock wave lithotripsy resulted in a significant improvement in VAS scores of flank pain versus placebo at 1-h following stent placement [40]. A novel ketorolac-eluting stent was developed in an attempt to reduce stent discomfort. In a multicenter trial, 276 patients were randomized to receive the ketorolac-eluting versus standard stent placed following ureteroscopy [67]. Identical rates of adverse effects were reported in the two groups.

However, in this study there was no significant difference between the two groups in the need for additional interventions for pain, including unscheduled physician contact, change in pain medications, or early stent removal. A trend towards less narcotic pill requirement was observed with the ketorolac-eluting stent, specifically in young men. Further studies with COX inhibitors are certainly warranted, perhaps using alternative formulations of ketorolac for systemic administration.

Summary and Conclusions

A significant number of patients report morbidities associated with indwelling ureteral stents. Multiple studies have reinforced the importance of stent position (proper length that does not cross the midline) in minimizing stent morbidity. Extensive level-one evidence supports the use of alpha blockers (tamsulosin 0.4 mg daily, or alfuzosin 10 mg daily) as medical adjuncts in reducing stent-related morbidity. In addition, a significant benefit was observed with the anticholinergic tolterodine extended release (4 mg daily) in a single randomized trial. When offered to reduce stent-related morbidity, patients should be counseled on the off-label use of these medications. In addition, cystoscopic injection of Botox resulted in a significant improvement in stent-related symptoms in a small pilot study. Future investigation is likely to identify beneficial effects of additional oral medications (including PDE inhibitors) and novel drug-eluting stents to minimize the morbidity of these commonly used devices in urologic procedures. Based on the current evidence base, it is currently our practice to prescribe tamsulosin 0.4 mg daily following stent placement to reduce stent discomfort.

References

1. Joshi HB, et al. Characterization of urinary symptoms in patients with ureteral stents. Urology. 2002;59(4):511–6.
2. Joshi HB, et al. Indwelling ureteral stents: evaluation of symptoms, quality of life and utility. J Urol. 2003;169(3):1065–9. discussion 1069.
3. Hao P, et al. Clinical evaluation of double-pigtail stent in patients with upper urinary tract diseases: report of 2685 cases. J Endourol. 2008;22(1):65–70.
4. Borboroglu PG, et al. Ureteral stenting after ureteroscopy for distal ureteral calculi: a multi-institutional prospective randomized controlled study assessing pain, outcomes and complications. J Urol. 2001;166(5):1651–7.
5. Thomas R. Indwelling ureteral stents: impact of material and shape on patient comfort. J Endourol. 1993;7(2):137–40.
6. Rane A, et al. Have stent-related symptoms anything to do with placement technique? J Endourol. 2001;15(7):741–5.
7. Miyaoka R, Monga M. Ureteral stent discomfort: Etiology and management. Indian J Urol. 2009;25(4):455–60.
8. Chew BH, et al. Pilot study of ureteral movement in stented patients: first step in understanding dynamic ureteral anatomy to improve stent comfort. J Endourol. 2007;21(9):1069–75.
9. Mosli HA, et al. Vesicoureteral reflux in patients with double pigtail stents. J Urol. 1991;146(4):966–9.
10. Yossepowitch O, et al. Assessment of vesicoureteral reflux in patients with self-retaining ureteral stents: implications for upper urinary tract instillation. J Urol. 2005;173(3):890–3.
11. El-Nahas AR, et al. Self-retaining ureteral stents: analysis of factors responsible for patients' discomfort. J Endourol. 2006;20(1):33–7.
12. Weiss RM. Uretral function. Urology. 1978;12(2):114–33.
13. Dixon JS, Gosling JA. The fine structure of pacemaker cells in the pig renal calices. Anat Rec. 1973;175(2):139–53.
14. Malin Jr JM, Deane RF, Boyarsky S. Characterisation of adrenergic receptors in human ureter. Br J Urol. 1970;42(2):171–4.
15. Mastrangelo D, Iselin CE. Urothelium dependent inhibition of rat ureter contractile activity. J Urol. 2007;178(2):702–9.
16. Lipkin M, Shah O. The use of alpha-blockers for the treatment of nephrolithiasis. Rev Urol. 2006;8 Suppl 4:S35–42.
17. Sigala S, et al. Evidence for the presence of alpha1 adrenoceptor subtypes in the human ureter. Neurourol Urodyn. 2005;24(2):142–8.
18. Weiss RM, Bassett AL, Hoffman BF. Adrenergic innervation of the ureter. Invest Urol. 1978;16(2):123–7.
19. Joshi HB, et al. Ureteral stent symptom questionnaire: development and validation of a multidimensional quality of life measure. J Urol. 2003;169(3):1060–4.
20. Damiano R, et al. Effect of tamsulosin in preventing ureteral stent-related morbidity: a prospective study. J Endourol. 2008;22(4):651–6.
21. Wang CJ, Huang SW, Chang CH. Effects of specific alpha-1A/1D blocker on lower urinary tract symptoms due to double-J stent: a prospectively randomized study. Urol Res. 2009;37(3):147–52.

22. Deliveliotis C, et al. Is there a role for alpha1-blockers in treating double-J stent-related symptoms? Urology. 2006;67(1):35–9.
23. Beddingfield R, et al. Alfuzosin to relieve ureteral stent discomfort: a prospective, randomized, placebo controlled study. J Urol. 2009;181(1):170–6.
24. Lingeman JE, et al. Assessing the impact of ureteral stent design on patient comfort. J Urol. 2009;181(6):2581–7.
25. Giannarini G, et al. Predictors of morbidity in patients with indwelling ureteric stents: results of a prospective study using the validated Ureteric Stent Symptoms Questionnaire. BJU Int. 2011;107(4):648–54.
26. Barry MJ, et al. The American Urological Association symptom index for benign prostatic hyperplasia. The Measurement Committee of the American Urological Association. J Urol. 1992;148(5):1549–57. discussion 1564.
27. Navanimitkul N, Lojanapiwat B. Efficacy of tamsulosin 0.4 mg/day in relieving double-J stent-related symptoms: a randomized controlled study. J Int Med Res. 2010;38(4):1436–41.
28. Lee SJ, et al. Stent position is more important than alpha-blockers or anticholinergics for stent-related lower urinary tract symptoms after ureteroscopic ureterolithotomy: a prospective randomized study. Korean J Urol. 2010;51(9):636–41.
29. Erturk E, Sessions A, Joseph JV. Impact of ureteral stent diameter on symptoms and tolerability. J Endourol. 2003;17(2):59–62.
30. Sur RL, et al. Efficacy of intravesical ropivacaine injection on urinary symptoms following ureteral stenting: a randomized, controlled study. J Endourol. 2008;22(3):473–8.
31. Chew BH, Lange D. Ureteral stent symptoms and associated infections: a biomaterials perspective. Nat Rev Urol. 2009;6(8):440–8.
32. Haleblian G, et al. Ureteral stenting and urinary stone management: a systematic review. J Urol. 2008;179(2):424–30.
33. Dellis A, et al. Relief of stent related symptoms: review of engineering and pharmacological solutions. J Urol. 2010;184(4):1267–72.
34. Candela JV, Bellman GC. Ureteral stents: impact of diameter and composition on patient symptoms. J Endourol. 1997;11(1):45–7.
35. Damiano R, et al. Does the size of ureteral stent impact urinary symptoms and quality of life? A prospective randomized study. Eur Urol. 2005;48(4):673–8.
36. Joshi HB, et al. A prospective randomized single-blind comparison of ureteral stents composed of firm and soft polymer. J Urol. 2005;174(6):2303–6.
37. Lee C, et al. Randomized evaluation of Ureteral Stents using validated Symptom Questionnaire. J Endourol. 2005;19(8):990–3.
38. Al-Kandari AM, et al. Effects of proximal and distal ends of double-J ureteral stent position on postprocedural symptoms and quality of life: a randomized clinical trial. J Endourol. 2007;21(7):698–702.
39. Ho CH, et al. Determining the appropriate length of a double-pigtail ureteral stent by both stent configurations and related symptoms. J Endourol. 2008;22(7):1427–31.
40. Beiko DT, et al. Double-blind randomized controlled trial assessing the safety and efficacy of intravesical agents for ureteral stent symptoms after extracorporeal shockwave lithotripsy. J Endourol. 2004;18(8):723–30.
41. Gupta M, et al. Prospective randomized evaluation of periureteral botulinum toxin type A injection for ureteral stent pain reduction. J Urol. 2010;183(2):598–602.
42. Chew BH, Denstedt JD. Technology insight: Novel ureteral stent materials and designs. Nat Clin Pract Urol. 2004;1(1):44–8.
43. Cadieux PA, et al. Triclosan loaded ureteral stents decrease proteus mirabilis 296 infection in a rabbit urinary tract infection model. J Urol. 2006;175(6):2331–5.
44. Liatsikos EN, et al. Application of paclitaxel-eluting metal mesh stents within the pig ureter: an experimental study. Eur Urol. 2007;51(1):217–23.
45. Caine M, Raz S. Some clinical implications of adrenergic receptors in the urinary tract. Arch Surg. 1975;110(3):247–50.
46. Nakada SY, et al. Doxazosin relaxes ureteral smooth muscle and inhibits epinephrine-induced ureteral contractility in vitro. Urology. 2007;70(4):817–21.
47. Danuser H, et al. Systemic and topical drug administration in the pig ureter: effect of phosphodiesterase inhibitors alpha1, beta and beta2-adrenergic receptor agonists and antagonists on the frequency and amplitude of ureteral contractions. J Urol. 2001;166(2):714–20.
48. Davenport K, Timoney AG, Keeley Jr FX. Effect of smooth muscle relaxant drugs on proximal human ureteric activity in vivo: a pilot study. Urol Res. 2007;35(4):207–13.
49. Kubacz GJ, Catchpole BN. The role of adrenergic blockade in the treatment of ureteral colic. J Urol. 1972;107(6):949–51.
50. Park SC, et al. The effects of tolterodine extended release and alfuzosin for the treatment of double-j stent-related symptoms. J Endourol. 2009;23(11):1913–7.
51. Yakoubi R, et al. Is there a role for alpha-blockers in ureteral stent related symptoms? A systematic review and meta-analysis. J Urol. 2011;186(3):928–34.
52. Lamb AD, Vowler SL, Johnston R, Dunn N, Wiseman OJ. Meta-analysis showing the beneficial effect of α-blockers on ureteric stent discomfort. BJUI. 2011;108:1894–902.
53. Tseng TY, et al. How to use a systematic literature review and meta-analysis. J Urol. 2008;180(4):1249–56.
54. Norris RD, et al. A prospective, randomized, double-blinded placebo-controlled comparison of extended release oxybutynin versus phenazopyridine for the management of postoperative ureteral stent discomfort. Urology. 2008;71(5):792–5.

55. Forman A, et al. Effects of nifedipine on the smooth muscle of the human urinary tract in vitro and in vivo. Acta Pharmacol Toxicol (Copenh). 1978;43(2):111–8.
56. Troxel SA, et al. Physiologic effect of nifedipine and tamsulosin on contractility of distal ureter. J Endourol. 2006;20(8):565–8.
57. Ames CD, et al. Pharmacologic manipulation of the porcine ureter: Acute impact of topical drugs on ureteral diameter and peristaltic activity. J Endourol. 2006;20(11):943–8.
58. Borghi L, et al. Nifedipine and methylprednisolone in facilitating ureteral stone passage: a randomized, double-blind, placebo-controlled study. J Urol. 1994; 152(4):1095–8.
59. Porpiglia F, et al. Corticosteroids and tamsulosin in the medical expulsive therapy for symptomatic distal ureter stones: single drug or association? Eur Urol. 2006;50(2):339–44.
60. Becker AJ, et al. The effect of the specific phosphodiesterase-IV-inhibitor rolipram on the ureteral peristalsis of the rabbit in vitro and in vivo. J Urol. 1998;160(3 Pt 1):920–5.
61. Gratzke C, et al. In vitro effects of PDE5 inhibitors sildenafil, vardenafil and tadalafil on isolated human ureteral smooth muscle: a basic research approach. Urol Res. 2007;35(1):49–54.
62. Bandi G, et al. Third prize: Effect of hydrocortisone on porcine ureteral contractility in vitro. J Endourol. 2008;22(6):1169–73.
63. Nakada SY, et al. Selective cyclooxygenase-2 inhibitors reduce ureteral contraction in vitro: a better alternative for renal colic? J Urol. 2000;163(2): 607–12.
64. Wen CC, et al. Ketorolac effectively inhibits ureteral contractility in vitro. J Endourol. 2008;22(4):739–42.
65. Chaignat V, et al. Effects of a non-selective COX inhibitor and selective COX-2 inhibitors on contractility of human and porcine ureters in vitro and in vivo. Br J Pharmacol. 2008;154(6):1297–307.
66. Lee SY, et al. NS-398 (a selective cyclooxygenase-2 inhibitor) decreases agonist-induced contraction of the human ureter via calcium channel inhibition. J Endourol. 2010;24(11):1863–8.
67. Krambeck AE, et al. A novel drug eluting ureteral stent: a prospective, randomized, multicenter clinical trial to evaluate the safety and effectiveness of a ketorolac loaded ureteral stent. J Urol. 2010;183(3): 1037–42.

Postoperative Imaging

31

Gary J. Faerber

Introduction

Ureteroscopy is one of the most common procedures utilized for treatment of upper tract pathology. Advances in fiberoptics, refinements in laser and lithotripsy technology, and miniaturization of the ureteroscopes and the development of specialized ancillary equipment all have resulted in wide-spread use of ureteroscopy. Radiographic imaging is often used as a means of preoperative diagnosis and planning of subsequent ureteroscopic surgery. This chapter will concentrate on the radiologic imaging available for postoperative imaging, and the indications and rationale for imaging following ureteroscopy.

Indications for ureteroscopy include upper tract renal or ureteral calculi, lateralizing hematuria, evaluation of filling defects, treatment of upper tract urothelial tumors. Clearly the most common indication is for treatment of ureteral or renal stones. This chapter will concentrate on postoperative imaging following ureteroscopic treatment of stone disease.

G.J. Faerber, M.D. (✉)
Department of Urology, University of Michigan Hospital and Health Systems, 1500 East Medical Center Drive, Ann Arbor, MI 48109, USA
e-mail: gfaerber@umich.edu

Available Imaging Modalities

There are several imaging modalities available all of which can be used for postoperative imaging. Each has their advantages and disadvantages. Plain abdominal radiograph (KUB) is readily available either in-office or in outpatient or hospital-based radiology units. It is relatively cost-effective, reasonably accurate in identifying residual fragments, very accurate in detecting misplaced or migrated stents, and can be used in patients with nonideal body habitus.

Renal ultrasound is also readily available at the bedside, or in outpatient or hospital-based radiology units, is cost-effective, and very sensitive in detection of hydronephrosis [1, 2]. There is no radiation and is therefore safe to use in instances where radiation exposure is a real or potential concern. Renal ultrasound can detect all types of renal stone, however, its accuracy in detection of residual stone fragments has been questioned [3, 4]. Imaging quality is clearly impacted by body habitus (increased BMI negatively impacts imaging quality and accuracy).

Noncontrast CT (NCCT) is still largely available in free-standing radiology or in-hospital units, but CT availability is becoming more common in large urology group outpatient suites. NCCT is more expensive, but is highly sensitive for detecting residual stones (including stones comprised of uric acid or cysteine, which may

M. Monga (ed.), *Ureteroscopy: Indications, Instrumentation & Technique*, Current Clinical Urology,
DOI 10.1007/978-1-62703-206-3_31, © Springer Science+Business Media New York 2013

not be comprised of visible on plain KUB), hydronephrosis, peri-renal fluid collections, and non-urologic pathology [5–7]. Radiation dose is significantly higher than plain KUB but newer modalities and refinement in technique have significantly decreased radiation exposure [8].

Computed tomographic urography (CTU) is expensive, is time-intensive, requires intravenous contrast (with resultant risk of contrast reaction), and has significantly higher radiation exposure than all the other modalities previously mentioned. In addition to providing imaging seen in NCCT, the CTU can provide useful information on renal function and may provide more detailed structural anatomy. Both NCCT and CTU image quality are less affected by body habitus (except in patients with significant BMI or orthopedic hardware).

Excretory urography (IVP) at one point was the principle radiologic modality for investigating renal function and collecting system anatomy. It is restricted to dedicated radiology units, requires intravenous contrast, and is associated with moderate radiation exposure. Bowel prep prior to the IVP is usually required to further enhance the quality of the imaging and therefore it has less utility in evaluating acute pathology. It has largely been supplanted by NCCT or CTU but probably still has a role in following ureteral stricture disease or complicated ureteral reconstruction.

Nuclear renal imaging is largely available only in hospital-based radiology/nuclear medicine units. Nuclear renal scans provide functional and renal differential function which can be very helpful in determining clinical significance of upper tract dilation. Magnetic resonance imaging (MRI) is very expensive, is available in only specialized outpatient radiologic units or in-hospital radiology suites, and probably has little role for postoperative ureteroscopy.

Routine Postoperative Imaging

Imaging post-ureteroscopy in most instances usually consists of KUB, renal ultrasound, or a combination of the two. Functional studies are usually not indicated for routine follow-up [9]. Some authors have stressed the importance of documenting accurately the presence or absence of residual stone fragments following ureteroscopy based on prognostic implications of having a residual stone. In one study, NCCT was used and stone fragments were followed serially. Approximately 20% of patients experienced a subsequent stone event within 2 years if they had stone fragments ≤4 mm [10]. While this finding is important, using NCCT as a routine follow-up imaging modality is probably not indicated given the healthcare cost and radiation exposure to the patient.

There is controversy whether routine imaging is required at all following routine uncomplicated ureteroscopy. Weizer and associates recommend imaging of the collecting system either with excretory urography, renal ultrasonography, or NCCT at 3 months to determine the presence of silent renal obstruction [11]. Of 241 patients studied retrospectively, 30 (12%) had radiologic detection of obstruction. Of those 30 with postoperative obstruction, 25 (83%) were due to residual stones, 3 (10%) were due to stricture, and 1 (7%) secondary to edema. Pain was the most common presenting symptom of postoperative renal obstruction. Silent obstruction, the most worrisome postoperative sequelae following ureteroscopy, was found in only 2.9% of the entire cohort.

Beiko and associates reported on 89 patients who underwent ureteroscopic holmium:YAG laser lithotripsy who all underwent subsequent postoperative imaging either with ultrasound, intravenous pyelogram or CT [12]. They reported an 8% rate of postoperative obstruction (two from residual stone and four from ureteral stricture). Although their reported rate of silent obstruction was also 2% they recommended against the routine use of postoperative imaging following ureteroscopic laser lithotripsy. They did however, identify risk factors for development of ureteral stricture formation following ureteroscopy and therefore recommended upper tract imaging in patients with chronic stone impaction, significant ureteral trauma during the procedure, preexisting renal function impairment, endoscopic evidence of preexisting stricture, or postoperative pain and/or fever.

Bugg and colleagues recommend that patients require only a KUB for follow-up and functional studies are only necessary in those who present with obstruction and/or pain postoperatively [9]. Adayet and colleagues reported on a post-ureteroscopy stricture rate of 1.4% following 267 procedures on 253 patients. They further subdivided their cohort into uncomplicated ureteroscopy and complicated (stone impaction, balloon dilation, mucosal perforation). None of the uncomplicated ureteroscopies resulted in stricture formation [13]. They recommend selected postoperative imaging in those with symptoms, or who have impaction, perforation or require balloon dilation at the time of ureteroscopy.

The timing of follow-up imaging after ureteroscopy is not standard and has been reported anywhere between 7 days and 3 months [9–13]. Long-term follow-up is suggested for patients with residual stone burden, metabolically active stone disease, ureteral stricture, or hydronephrosis.

Follow-Up Imaging After Uncomplicated Ureteroscopy

The most common radiologic imaging modality following uncomplicated ureteroscopy is a KUB. A KUB immediately prior to or at the time of the patient's postoperative routine visit is usually performed (Fig. 31.1). In these instances a KUB can determine residual stone burden and location of any residual stone, and the proper positioning of the ureteral stent (if present). If patient has significant renal stone burden, then a KUB can assist in determining what subsequent treatment would be necessary (Fig. 31.2).

Ultrasound can be helpful to diagnose the presence of hydronephrosis which may be indicative of ureteral obstruction. While ultrasound is accurate in diagnosing hydronephrosis it is less accurate in determining residual stone burden [4]. The main goal, therefore in using ultrasound, is to determine the presence of hydronephrosis. Using ultrasound in conjunction with a KUB is reasonable; however, the vast majority of patients with obstruction are usually symptomatic. In symptomatic patients an ultrasound would be warranted. A bedside or office ultrasound may be extremely helpful in this clinical scenario (Fig. 31.3). If patients are found to have hydronephrosis, either a CTU, IVP, or cystoscopy with retrograde pyelography may be indicated to further delineate the etiology of the hydronephrosis. The AUA guidelines panel reported an overall incidence of ureteral stricture following ureteroscopy at approximately 1% [14]. The need to search for silent hydronephrosis as a result of ureteral stricture by adding ultrasound to a KUB exam is probably superfluous.

NCCT is probably indicated in patients with non-radiopaque stones (uric acid, cystine). Judicious use of NCCT is warranted given the

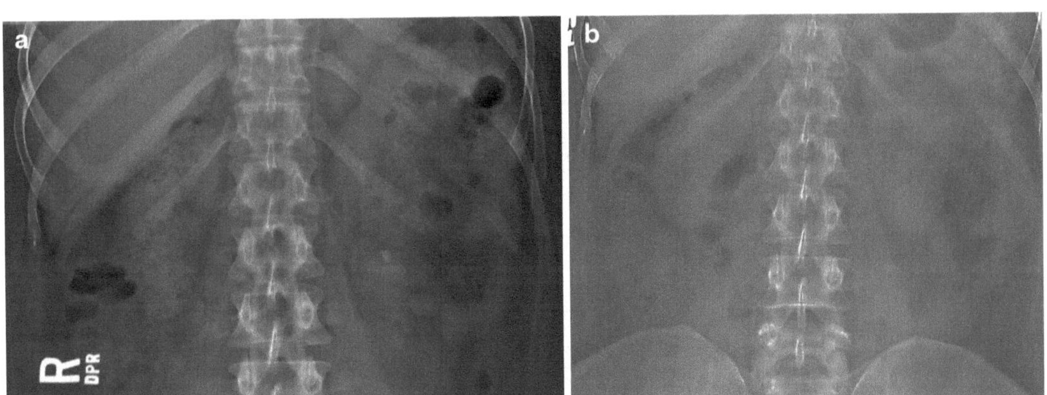

Fig. 31.1 (**a**) Preoperative KUB demonstrated a 6 × 8 mm lower pole renal stone. (**b**) Postoperative KUB demonstrated no residual stone in kidney

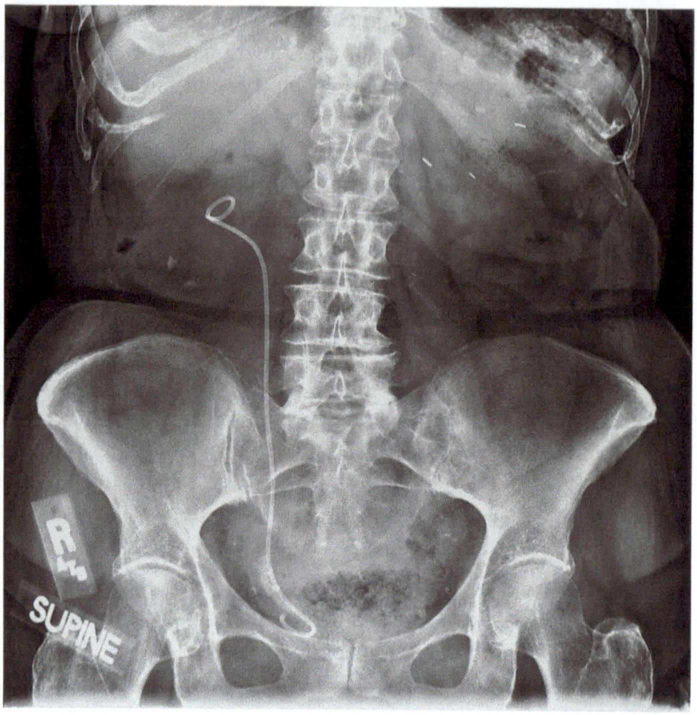

Fig. 31.2 Postoperative KUB demonstrates a ureteral stent in good position with a large steinstrasse. Patient underwent successful ureteroscopic stone removal

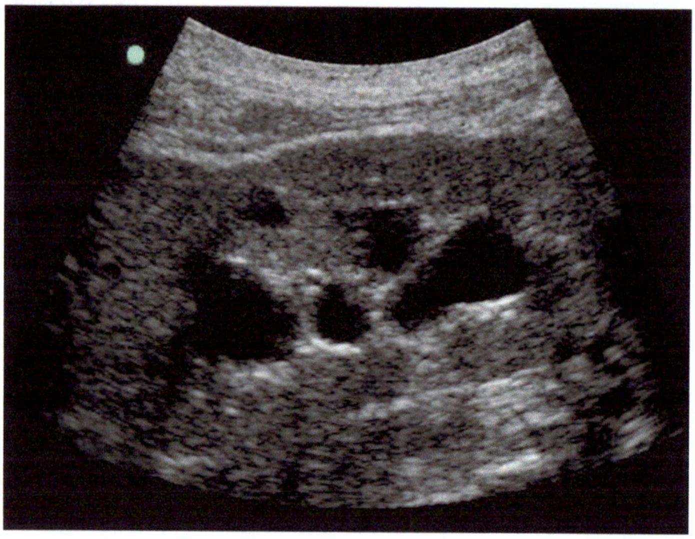

Fig. 31.3 Patient presented with postoperative pain 3 days following teroscopic laser lithotripsy. Bedside ultrasound demonstrated moderate hydronephrosis. KUB demonstrated a 2 mm distal ureteral fragment at the ureterovesical junction. Patient successfully passed the fragment with medical expulsive therapy and follow-up ultrasound revealed resolution of the hydronephrosis

theoretical radiation exposure risk from repeated exams, especially in the pediatric and young adult population [15–17].

Patients who undergo balloon dilation of the ureteral orifice have no greater incidence of postoperative stricture than those who do not undergo balloon dilation [18]. In patients with an atraumatic balloon dilation of the ureteral orifice, no follow-up imaging is required specifically as a result of the balloon dilation.

The use of ureteral sheaths is now a common ancillary procedure used in conjunction with ureteroscopic stone management. Ureteral sheaths facilitate treatment of large stones, provide easy multiple access to the kidney, and decreases intra-operative intrarenal pressure during treatment. In routine cases where a ureteral sheath was used, a follow-up renal ultrasound for detection of hydronephrosis is not indicated. In instances where ureteral splitting of the urothelial lining was noted, a routine follow-up ultrasound 4–6 weeks post-procedure is recommended to rule out silent obstruction in the asymptomatic patient and earlier if patient develops symptoms consistent with ureteral obstruction [19].

Follow-Up Imaging After Complicated Ureteroscopy

Complicated ureteroscopy could be defined as performing a ureteroscopy on a patient with preexisting conditions such as renal insufficiency or a preexisting ureteral stricture, a known impacted stone, intraoperative traumatic balloon dilation, ureteral perforation, or the presence of an impacted stone found at the time of ureteroscopy. In these instances postoperative imaging is definitely warranted. As in uncomplicated ureteroscopy, a KUB at the time of follow-up is helpful to ascertain stent position (usually placed in all of the scenarios listed above for variable time lengths) as well as for residual stone burden. After the stent is removed, an anatomic study such as a renal ultrasound or NCCT is reasonable to obtain at 1–3 months post-stent removal, provided the patient was rendered stone-free initially. These studies can be done earlier if the patient is symptomatic (pain, fever, serum creatinine elevation). Functional studies such as a CTU, IVP, or nuclear renal scan can also be helpful in following patients after a complicated ureteroscopy (Figs. 31.4 and 31.5). In cases of newly diagnosed stricture, worsening hydronephrosis of a preexisting stricture, or symptomatic ureteral stricture, a cystoscopy and retrograde pyelogram is certainly indicated. A cystoscopy and retrograde pyelogram provides a means to ascertain the location, degree, and length of the stricture (Fig. 31.6). It also provides concomitant

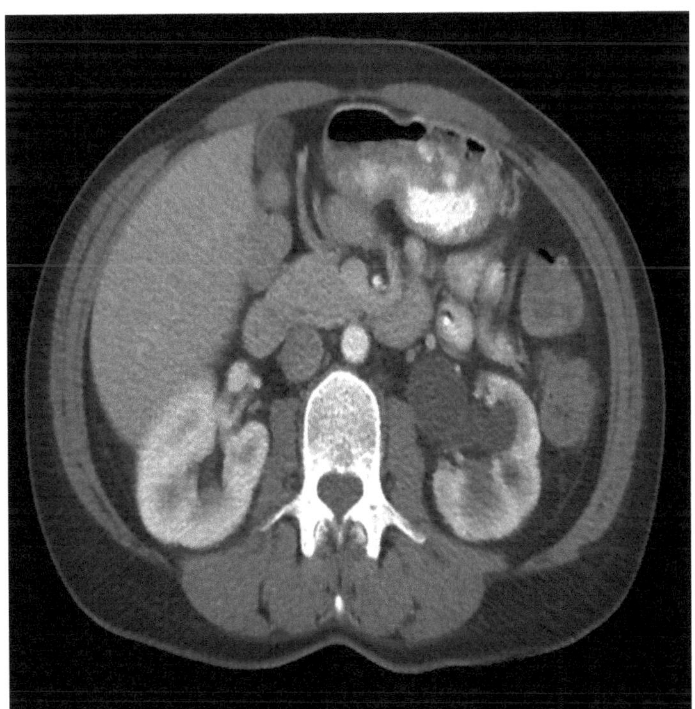

Fig. 31.4 Follow-up NCCT following treatment of a large severely impacted proximal ureteral stone. NCCT demonstrated moderate to severe hydronephrosis despite patient having minimal symptoms

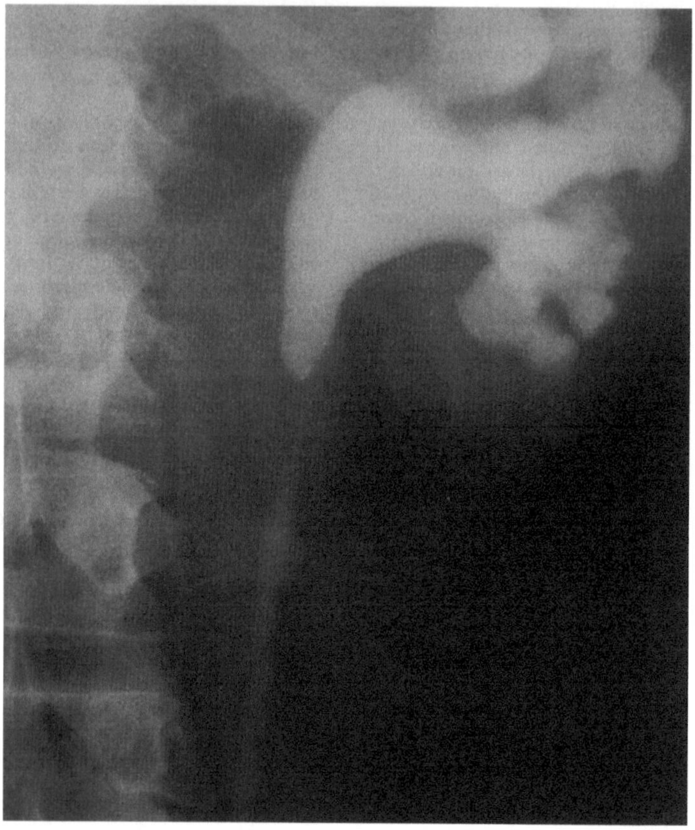

Fig. 31.5 Retrograde pyelography of above patient demonstrated a long proximal ureteral stricture. Patient underwent a difficult but successful open flap pyeloplasty

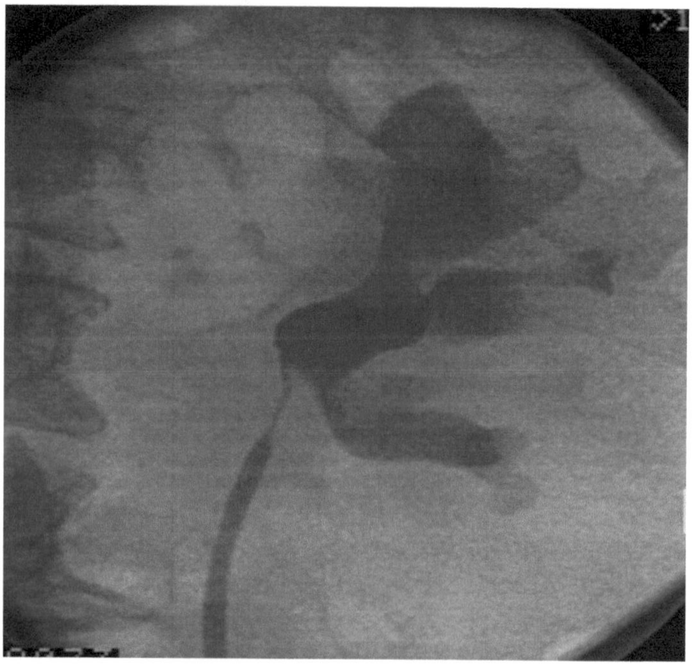

Fig. 31.6 Patient was referred for further management of a complicated proximal ureteral stricture after an ureteroscopic laser lithotripsy which was complicated by a significant perforation at the site of the stone. Patient underwent successful ureterocalycostomy

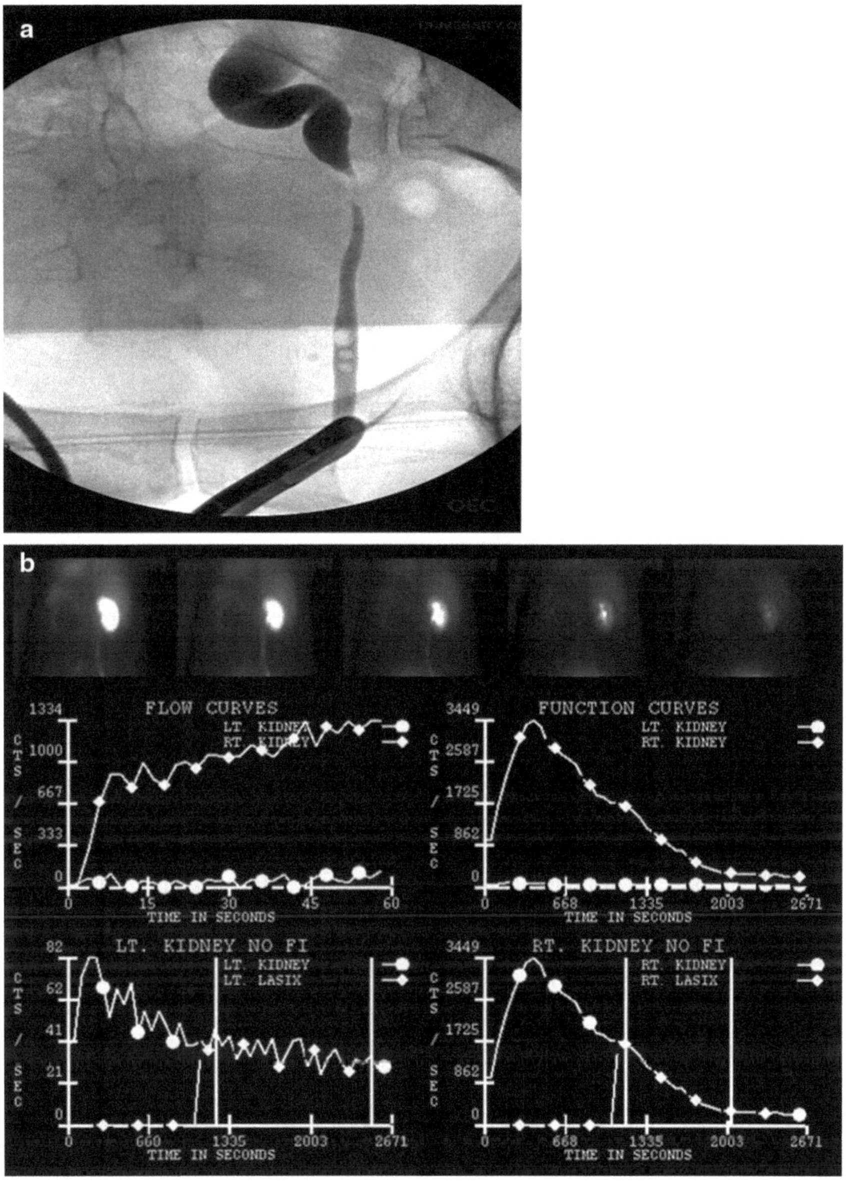

Fig. 31.7 Patient had ureteral perforation at the level of the iliac vessels while performing semirigid ureteroscopy. (**a**) Follow up cystoscopy and retrograde pyelogram demonstrated a severe stricture. (**b**) Renal scan demonstrated differential function of 4% on the affected side. Patient subsequently underwent laparoscopic nephrectomy

treatment options which could be definitive ureteroscopic treatment or temporary relief with placement of a ureteral stent.

Impacted stone or known stricture: In cases of patients with a known ureteral stricture, or with a severely impacted stone who had a perforation at the time of ureteroscopic stone treatment, serial functional exams may be warranted (Fig. 31.7). A 24% stricture rate has been reported in patients who underwent ureteroscopic stone treatment for an impacted stone complicated by ureteral perforation at the site of impaction [20].

Severe Pain Immediately Following Ureteroscopy

Nonroutine imaging may be warranted following ureteroscopy. Significant pain immediately following ureteroscopy is usually not a result of a particular complication but due to the procedure itself. Initially a KUB can be obtained to ensure that a stent, if placed, is in the proper position. If a stent was not used, and known residual stone was left, a steinstrasse or residual ureteral stone causing obstruction may be diagnosed. Postoperative hydronephrosis is a common sequelae following ureteroscopy and therefore a renal ultrasound is often times not helpful in detecting hydronephrosis. In some instances a perinephric fluid collection from extravasation or hematoma can be detected by renal ultrasound. In certain instances a noncontrast CT can be uses to also look for significant perinephric fluid, hematoma, or obstructing ureteral stones. Perinephric stranding following URS is a common and clinically unimportant radiologic finding (Fig. 31.8). While noncontrast CT is the most sensitive radiologic means to diagnose ureteral stones, caution should be used in estimating the size of ureteral stones with noncontrast CT following ureteroscopic lithotripsy. Stone diameter size can be exaggerated with CT due to density averaging (Fig. 31.9). To determine the size of ureteral fragments in a patient with pain following lithotripsy, a KUB is preferred.

Very rarely, severe postoperative bleeding following ureteroscopy can occur. Usually a significant vascular injury is suspected during the procedure itself. If a vascular injury is suspected then angiography may be warranted (Fig. 31.10) [21].

Conclusion

Uncomplicated ureteroscopy requires minimal postoperative imaging. In cases of uncomplicated ureteroscopy in which all stone was removed, no imaging may be necessary. In cases of uncomplicated ureteroscopy with residual stone, a KUB or NCCT may be helpful to ascertain subsequent stone burden. Patients who undergo uncomplicated ureteroscopy who become symptomatic should undergo NCCT or renal ultrasound to rule out newfound hydronephrosis.

Complicated ureteroscopy requires postoperative imaging which usually entails both anatomic and functional radiologic imaging.

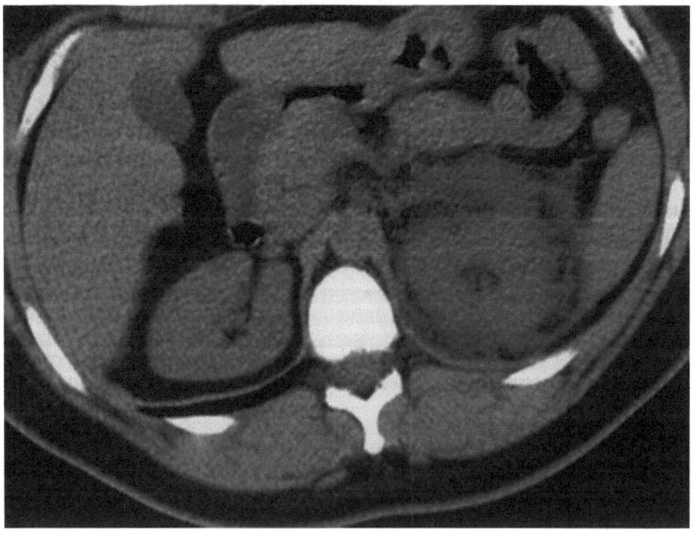

Fig. 31.8 Perinephric stranding seen on NCCT. This is a common radiologic finding after ureteroscopy

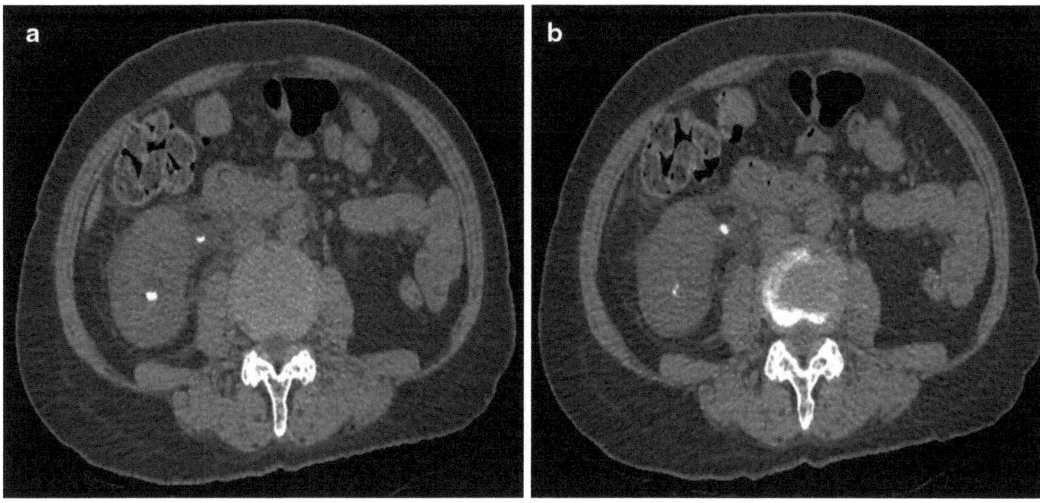

Fig. 31.9 Patient underwent ureteroscopic laser lithotripsy of a 8×6 mm uric acid stone. She presented to an outside emergency room 2 days postoperatively with pain. (**a**) NCCT was performed which was read out as patient having a 2 cm proximal ureteral stone with residual 1 cm stone in lower pole. (**b**) On KUB patient had small stone fragments the largest being approximately 2 mm. She was successfully treated with medical expulsive therapy

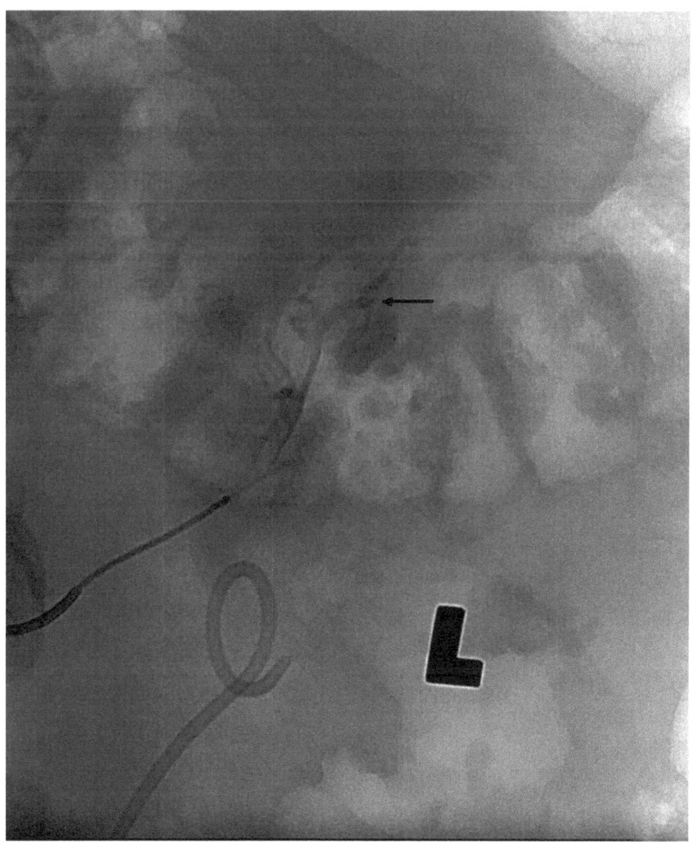

Fig. 31.10 Patient had significant hematuria during ureteroscopic laser lithotripsy which continued post-procedure. Emergent angiogram revealed a minor laceration of a small subsegmental arterial branch of the upper pole adjacent to the calculus (*arrow*). Successful Gelfoam® embolization resulted in immediate resolution of the hematuria

References

1. Moak JH, Lyons MS, Lindsell CJ. Bedside renal ultrasound in the evaluation of suspected ureterolithiasis. Am J Emerg Med. 2012;30:218–21.
2. Edmonds ML, Yan JW, Sedran RJ, McLeod SL, Theakston KD. The utility of renal ultrasonography in the diagnosis of renal colic in emergency department patients. CJEM. 2010;12:201–6.
3. Heidenreich A, Desgrandschamps F, Terrier F. Modern approach of diagnosis and management of acute flankpain: review of all imaging modalities. Eur Urol. 2002;41:351–62.
4. Resorlu B, Kara C, Resorlu EB, Unsal A. Effectiveness of ultrasonography in the postoperative follow-up of pediatric patients undergoing ureteroscopic stone manipulation. Pediatr Surg Int. 2011;27:1337–41.
5. Colistro R, Torreggiani WC, Lyburn ID, Harris AC, Al-Nakshabandi NA, Nicolaou S, Munk PL. Unenhanced helical CT in the investigation of acute flank pain. Clin Radiol. 2002;57:435–41.
6. Hamm M, Knopfle E, Wartenberg S, Wawroschek F, Weckermann D, Harzmann R. Low dose unenhanced helical computerized tomography for the evaluation of acute flank pain. J Urol. 2002;167:1687–91.
7. Miller OF, Kane CJ. Unenhanced helical computed tomography in the evaluation of acute flank pain. Curr Opin Urol. 2000;10(2):123–9.
8. Kluner C, Hein PA, Gralla O, Hein E, Hamm B, Romano V, Rogalla P. Does ultra-low-dose CT with a radiation dose equivalent to that of KUB suffice to detect renal and ureteral calculi? J Comput Assist Tomogr. 2006;30(1):44–50.
9. Bugg Jr CE, El-Galley R, Kenney PJ, Burns JR. Follow-up functional radiographic studies are not mandatory for all patients after ureteroscopy. Urology. 2002;59:662–7.
10. Rebuck DA, Macejko A, Bhalani V, Ramos P, Nadler RB. The natural history of renal stone fragments following ureteroscopy. Urology. 2011;77:564–8.
11. Weizer AZ, Auge BK, Silverstein AD, Delvecchio FC, Brizuela RM, Dahm P, Pietrow PK, Lewis BR, Albala DM, Preminger GM. Routine postoperative imaging is important after ureteroscopic stone manipulation. J Urol. 2002;168(1):46–50.
12. Beiko DR, Beasley KA, Watterson JD, Nott L, Denstedt JD, Razvi H. Upper tract imaging after ureteroscopic holmium:YAG laser lithotripsy: when is it necessary? Can J Urol. 2003;10:2062–7.
13. Adiyat KT, Meuleners R, Monga M. Selective postoperative imaging after ureteroscopy. Urology. 2009; 73:490–3.
14. Preminger GM, Tiselius HG, Assimos DG, Alken P, Buck C, Gallucci M, Knoll T, Lingeman JE, Nakada SY, Pearle MS, Sarica K, Türk C, Wolf Jr JS. EAU/AUA Nephrolithiasis Guideline Panel. 2007 guideline for the management of ureteral calculi. J Urol. 2007;178:2418–34.
15. Slovis TL. The ALARA concept in pediatric CT: myth or reality? Radiology. 2002;223:5–6.
16. Chapple CL, Willis S, Frame J. Effective dose in paediatric computed tomography. Phys Med Biol. 2002; 47:107–15.
17. International Commission on Radiological Protection (ICRP). Publication 87. Managing patient dose in computed tomography. Ann ICRP. 2000;30:1–45.
18. Başeskioğlu B, Sofikerim M, Demirtaş A, Yenilmez A, Kaya C, Can C. Is ureteral stenting really necessary after ureteroscopic lithotripsy with balloon dilatation of ureteral orifice? A multi-institutional randomized controlled study. World J Urol. 2011;29:731–6.
19. Delvecchio FC, Auge BK, Brizuela RM, Weizer AZ, Silverstein AD, Lallas CD, Pietrow PK, Albala DM, Preminger GM. Routine assessment of stricture formation with the ureteral access sheath. Urology. 2003;61:518–22.
20. Roberts WW, Cadeddu JA, Micali S, Kavoussi LR, Moore RG. Ureteral stricture formation after removal of impacted calculi. J Urol. 1998;159:723–6.
21. Miller DC, Faerber GJ. Arterial pseudoaneurysm complicating endoscopic fulguration of upper urinary tract urothelial carcinoma. Urology. 2001;58:799.

Part V

Complex Cases

Ureteroscopic Management of Stones During Pregnancy

32

Vernon M. Pais Jr.

Introduction

The management of stones is typically an orderly endeavor; even the most complex evaluations and subsequent ureteroscopic interventions have a predictable rhythm. The remarkably detailed imaging of computerized tomography grants an unprecedented degree of diagnostic accuracy. Continuously evolving technology combined with the precision of image guidance allows decreasingly invasive surgical access. As such, when treating stones we typically enjoy enviable control of our surgical work environment, putting both patient and physician at greater ease.

In stark contrast, few clinical scenarios generate greater anxiety than renal colic in the pregnant woman. For these patients, all of the advancements in imaging and technology have simply introduced new conflicts, problems, and concerns. Hence, a review of pertinent considerations is warranted. For urologists considering ureteroscopic intervention for stone in the pregnant patient, several important concerns shall be reviewed.

V.M. Pais Jr., M.D. (✉)
Section of Urology, Department of Surgery, Geisel School of Medicine at Dartmouth, 1 Medical Center Drive, Lebanon, NH 03756, USA
e-mail: vmp@hitchcock.org

Epidemiology

A precise definition of the scope of urolithiasis during pregnancy remains elusive, as reports of incidence vary widely. Initially cited to complicate approximately 1 of every 1,500 pregnancies, more recent estimates suggest symptomatic urolithiasis occurs in 1/244 to 1/800 pregnancies [1–4]. These reports arise from geographically disparate regional centers ranging from Michigan to Louisiana to the Pacific Northwest, and employ variable reporting criteria. Therefore, arriving at a "true" incidence may not be feasible although these figures can provide a rough estimate.

Of interest, it has been noted that these do not necessarily arise in an identifiable cohort of recurrent stone formers. Up to 75% presenting with a stone during pregnancy are first time stone formers [2]. Furthermore, among identified stone formers, pregnancy does not appear to increase their rate of stone formation [5].

Symptomatic presentation occurs in the last two trimesters in 87–99%, with the vast majority in the last half of gestation [2, 4]. Symptomatic stones have been confirmed to be equally distributed between left and right sides [4]. In the United States, Caucasians were affected more commonly than either African Americans or Hispanics, consistent with racial distribution of nephrolithiasis in the population at large [2, 3].

M. Monga (ed.), *Ureteroscopy: Indications, Instrumentation & Technique*, Current Clinical Urology, DOI 10.1007/978-1-62703-206-3_32, © Springer Science+Business Media New York 2013

Physiologic Considerations

The extensive physiologic changes of pregnancy are the subject of a large body of work and are well beyond the scope of this chapter. Nonetheless, several physiologic and potentially pathophysiologic changes during pregnancy are pertinent to considerations of stone management during gestation and are highlighted.

Hematologically, leukocytosis (approaching 15,000 mm^3) may be observed and may falsely raise a concern for systemic response to presumed infection. Additionally, a 50% increase in plasma volume with a lesser increase in red blood cells results in a dilutional anemia of pregnancy [6]. Finally, an increase in clotting factors during gestation, diminished fibrinolytic activity, and increased lower extremity venous pressure with reduced venous blood flow due to the gravid uterus result in a hypercoagulable state [7].

Similarly, cardiovascular changes are quite notable. Systemic vascular resistance decreases. With increased demands on blood flow, cardiac output increases 30–50%. There is a subsequent increase in renal plasma flow and glomerular filtration rate, which has been implicated in metabolic urinary changes as noted below. Of particular surgical import, however, is the potential for vena caval compression from the gravid uterus. When the pregnant woman is in the supine position, the potential thus arises for a resultant impairment in venous return and a clinically significant reduction in cardiac output [6].

Important metabolic changes occur in the urine. In general, pregnancy does not connote an increased risk of symptomatic urolithiasis, and as previously noted it does not increase risk of stone events in known stone formers [5]. Nonetheless, increased biochemical risk factors have been identified. In multiple studies, elevated urinary calcium, uric acid, and pH have been observed during pregnancy as compared with postpartum [8, 9]. Elevated supersaturations of calcium phosphate and calcium oxalate were noted as well [8, 9]. These likely underlie the penchant for rapid encrustation of stents during pregnancy. The alkaline urine, while increasing risk of brushite supersaturation is protective against uric acid supersaturation. As such, the predicted increased likelihood of calcium as opposed to uric acid-based stones strongly suggests against a role for empiric alkali dissolution therapies for stones during pregnancy.

Increased production of urinary inhibitors of stone formation has been postulated to explain the absence of increased stone frequency during pregnancy [10]. Included are both citrate and magnesium, which have also been shown by some to be increased during pregnancy [8]. Additionally, thiosulfate is another purported endogenous inhibitor of calcium oxalate nephrolithiasis. Compared with nonpregnant controls, pregnant women have been shown to have progressive increase of urinary thiosulfate throughout gestation [11].

Hormonally, progesterone decreases ureteral peristalsis and may contribute to collecting system dilation [10]. Mechanical obstruction of the ureter at the pelvic brim by the enlarging uterus accentuates this dilatation. Dextrorotation of the gravid uterus along with the suspected protective cushioning of the sigmoid colon over the left ureter predispose to a greater degree of hydronephrosis on the right than the left.

Natural History

Our understanding of the natural history of stones presenting during pregnancy continues to evolve. Initially, Stothers and Lee offered reassurance, reporting in 1992 that in their series of 80 patients, 84% spontaneously passed their stones [4]. A subsequent report noted 64% of a series of 72 pregnancies complicated by urolithiasis passed their stones [12]. Based upon a majority of patients passing their stones, a prejudice against intervention was noted.

More recently, however, this optimistic outlook has been reevaluated. A small series of 18 patients found that only 50% passed their stones, with the remainder requiring ureteroscopic intervention [13]. Applying the most stringent criteria to confirm the presence of stone, Burgess et al. reviewed a series of 90 women with documented urolithiasis during pregnancy and found that only

48% spontaneously passed their stone [14]. Hence, unaided passage of stones presenting during pregnancy can no longer be presumed to be the outcome for the majority of those affected.

Ultimately—and regardless of whether the stone is eventually passed—renal colic poses specific risks during pregnancy. Lewis et al. demonstrated a statistically significant increase in the risk of preterm premature rupture of membranes to 7% of those pregnant women admitted for nephrolithiasis compared with 2.9% of those without stones during pregnancy [2]. Women admitted for stone during pregnancy have also been shown to have nearly twice the risk of preterm delivery [3].

Temporizing Management Strategies

Multiple management options have been employed successfully for women with stones during pregnancy. A brief review of these serves to highlight the role of ureteroscopy.

As for any patient with a ureteral stone, expectant therapy remains a valid treatment option. In 2007 the EAU and AUA jointly released guidelines for the management of ureteral stones. Although specifically delineated for an index, nonpregnant patient, several proposed standards offer important insight into the expectant management of a ureteral stone in the pregnant patient as well. Bacteruria, if present, should be treated. If expectant management is pursued, pain should be appropriately controlled, and there should be no evidence of sepsis or new induction of inadequate renal function [15]. Although these guidelines also discuss the role of medical expulsive therapy with alpha blockers for their index patient, to date the safety and efficacy of medical expulsive therapy in the pregnant patient remain undefined [16].

In those cases in which expectant management is clinically inappropriate or has failed, intervention may then be required. Options include temporizing measures such as stents and nephrostomy, as well as definitive therapies such as ureteroscopy. Both stent and nephrostomy tube have been considered acceptable means of addressing ureteral obstruction during pregnancy, albeit with the goal of delaying, as opposed to delivering, definitive therapy. Either allows immediate decompression of the collecting system, but both have attendant shortcomings.

Cystoscopic ureteral stent placement typically requires transurethral manipulation; nephrostomies are placed percutaneously, often with local anesthesia. Stents are well recognized to cause often poorly tolerated irritative urinary symptoms and flank, suprapubic, and urethral pain. Nephrostomy tubes may have associated flank pain, and—in one series—a 12.5% incidence of sepsis [16, 17]. Furthermore, the hypercalciuria of pregnancy has been implicated in rapid encrustation of both. As such, it has been suggested that stents and nephrostomy tubes should be exchanged as often as every 4 weeks and at least every 8 weeks, subjecting women to potential repeated surgical procedures during pregnancy in order to maintain renal drainage [1, 7]. When this course is taken, arrangements must then still be made during the busy postpartum period to treat the offending stone.

Ureteroscopy

With both the recognition that a majority of patients may not be able to pass their stones during pregnancy and the realization that temporizing measures and their extended courses are poorly tolerated by some, ureteroscopy has been increasingly employed. This now commonly employed endourologic procedure may be applied to the pregnant patient to allow definitive therapy of her stone, with caveats as noted.

Untreated urinary tract infection (UTI) and sepsis are contraindications to ureteroscopy. Proposed relative contraindications include inadequate instrumentation, excessive stone burden, and inexperience of the surgeon [16].

Maternal–Fetal Concerns

When considering surgery in the pregnant patient, concerns necessarily extend beyond the patient herself. Since assessing the issues specific to the safety of the child in utero may be overwhelming for the nonobstetrician, the American College of Obstetrics and Gynecology (ACOG) offers guidance. They recommend that obstetric consultation should be obtained and propose the overarching principle that a pregnant woman should not be denied indicated surgical intervention, regardless of trimester. However, nonurgent surgery is best performed during the second trimester, and truly elective procedures should be postponed until 6 weeks postpartum [18, 19].

If surgical intervention occurs before fetal viability, Doppler confirmation of fetal heart rate before and after the procedure is recommended. After fetal viability has been reached, a greater degree of pre- and postoperative monitoring may be required, including simultaneous monitoring of fetal heart rate and uterine contractions. Of course, if monitoring is performed, a health care provider knowledgeable in its interpretation must be available. The ACOG recommends in this setting that surgery be performed at an institution with neonatal services, and that an obstetrician with cesarean delivery privileges be available. When intraoperative fetal monitoring is considered, five criteria have been set forth: (1) fetal viability, (2) physical ability to position electronic monitoring during the operation, (3) availability of obstetrician to intervene if indications arise, (4) consent for emergency cesarean delivery if required, and (5) surgery would allow safe interruption if needed for emergency delivery [18]. The obstetric consultant would determine the need for such intraoperative monitoring, but the urologist should recognize that in the appropriate setting, ureteroscopy can meet these criteria. Maintenance of a safety wire throughout the procedure allows the immediate placement of a stent and cessation of the procedure if warranted.

Preoperative Considerations

A urine culture should be obtained preoperatively to ensure sterile urine, as untreated UTI or sepsis is a contraindication to ureteroscopy [16]. In the setting of suspected bacterial UTI, consideration should instead be given to upper tract decompression with either stent or nephrostomy tube, with definitive treatment delayed until after adequate treatment of the infection. Based upon urine cultures and in consultation with obstetric service, appropriate antibiotics may be selected. In the absence of suspected UTI, the AUA guidelines committee has recommended that antibiotic prophylaxis be administered prior to ureteroscopy [20].

Cephalosporins and amoxicillin are often used in pregnancy and are considered appropriate alternative agents to otherwise "first line" fluoroquinolones, the role of which in pregnancy remains debated [21]. Given possible fetal exposure and effects, as well as increased maternal GFR and plasma volume of distribution, obstetric and pharmacy input on antibiotic selection may be helpful if available.

From the vantage point of thromboembolism, ureteroscopy has been stratified as a low risk procedure, for which early ambulation is advocated as prophylaxis. However, given that pregnancy is recognized as a hypercoagulable state, intermittent pneumatic compression devices or 5,000 units unfractionated heparin administration may be considered for additional prophylaxis [6, 22, 23].

Anesthetic Considerations

In their issued committee opinion, the ACOG state that there has been no demonstration of teratogenic effects in humans from currently used anesthetic agents administered at standard concentrations [18]. Both regional and general anesthesia may be safely utilized. The choice will depend upon specific patient characteristics, surgical needs, and ultimately the anesthesiologist's recommendation with the goal of maintaining stability of maternal hemodynamics and oxygenation [6]. Progesterone-induced relaxation of the lower esophageal sphincter coupled with mechanical effects of the gravid uterus on the stomach increase the risk of aspiration of gastric contents upon induction of anesthesia, necessitating aspiration precautions [6, 19]. Finally, left lateral tilt of 15–30° reduces direct compression of the inferior vena cava and aorta by the gravid uterus and may help to preserve cardiac output [6, 19].

Procedural Details

Ureteroscopy in the pregnant patient should replicate ureteroscopy in the nonpregnant patient in most facets. Particular points of differentiation include intraoperative image guidance and lithotripsy. A safety wire should be placed if possible. If not—and adequate drainage cannot be obtained—urgent percutaneous nephrostomy may be required, potentially adding to the morbidity of the intervention.

A step-by-step description is presented.

Having attended to preoperative details of management as outlined previously, and with confirmation of safe induction of anesthesia, the patient is placed in a modified dorsal lithotomy position, with a soft radiolucent roll beneath the right side of the pelvis so as to affect the aforementioned left lateral tilt.

Image Guidance

Ureteroscopy is traditionally performed with imaging guidance of wire passage, ureteroscope positioning, and stent placement, with fluoroscopy typically employed. In the setting of pregnancy, however, concerns over fetal exposure to radiation must be considered. Again, the ACOG offers guidance. Citing that exposure to fewer than 5 rad has not been associated with increased observation of fetal anomalies or pregnancy loss, they caution that concerns over radiation exposure should not prevent medically indicated diagnostic radiography studies in the mother [24]. However, they also note that there may be a small risk of carcinogenesis associated with fetal radiation exposure of >1–2 rad, increasing risk of childhood leukemia from a background rate 1/3,000 to 1/2,000. Therefore, they recommend that imaging that does not utilize ionizing radiation (such as ultrasound which has no known adverse fetal effects) should be utilized when appropriate [24].

Fluoroscopy has been estimated to result in an absorbed dose of up to 1.5–2 rad/min [25]. When fluoroscopy is used, several approaches have been described to limit fetal exposure. In all cases, judicious and overall sparing use of fluoroscopic time is recommended. Optimization of the c-arm—taking advantage of the lowest possible dose settings, pulsed fluoroscopy, and a "coned-down" field—will further reduce exposure. In order to shield the pelvis from fluoroscopy, a lead apron may be placed *beneath* the patient's pelvis in order to lie between the c-arm's X-ray tube and the uterus [26]. Another advocated approach is to invert the c-arm with the X-ray tube above the patient. In this case, a lead shield may be placed directly *over* the abdomen to shield the fetus. The shielding therefore remains accessible for manipulation if required [27]. Others have not used imaging at all, simply passing the wire blindly and reserving fluoroscopy for those cases when resistance was encountered [28]. Finally, an imaging-free "follow the wire" technique has been described in which the wire is passed through the ureteroscope and the advancement of the wire is followed step wise under direct ureteroscopic vision until it is beyond the stone [29]. Of note, the report's accompanying editorial raises the concern that the wire may be easily passed submucosally at the site of an impacted stone, and such a complication could be avoided with the judicious use of imaging guidance.

For these reasons, we typically employ intraoperative ultrasound to allow live monitoring of wire positioning, ureteroscope location, and stent placement. A c-arm is available for fluoroscopic monitoring if absolutely required. We discuss that a nephrostomy may have to be placed in the event access to the kidney cannot be obtained.

Placement of Safety Wire

Ultrasound is utilized to identify the kidney and renal pelvis on the affected side. Cystourethroscopy is performed and the affected ureteral orifice is identified. A 0.035 or 0.038 in. wire is then passed into the ureteral orifice and gently advanced until visualized within the renal pelvis on ultrasound.

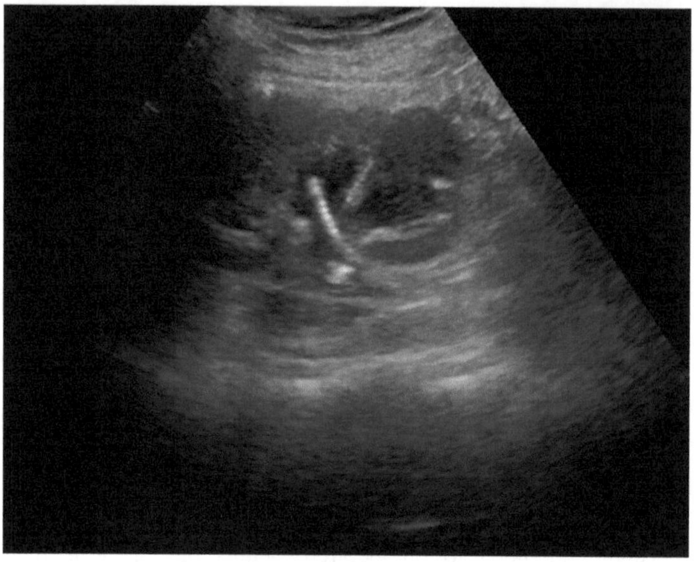

Fig. 32.1 Intraoperative ultrasound monitoring of flexible ureteroscopy

The author typically employs a hydrophilic coated nitinol wire, which allows ease of passage. Furthermore, these have been shown to require greater force to create puncture injury than nonhydrophilic wires, suggesting a less traumatic tip [30]. Although these are routinely secured and utilized as our safety wire, those uncomfortable with the use of a hydrophilic wire in this fashion may exchange it for a nonhydrophilic safety guide wire (with less penchant for dislodgement) thru a five French open-ended ureteral catheter.

Ureteroscopic Inspection

With a safety wire in place and secured, the semirigid ureteroscope may then be used to cannulate the orifice. Typically, a 6.9 F or 6.5 F ureteroscope can be passed readily into the ureteral orifice. With the advent of the 4.5 F "needle" tip ureteroscope (Richard Wolf Medical), ureteral dilation with balloon or tapered dilators and the attendant fluoroscopic monitoring is largely obviated. The ureter can then be inspected alongside the safety wire to the extent allowed by the scope and the patient's anatomy. Although concerns are often raised that the gravid uterus may prevent passage of the ureteroscope, this has not been typically encountered. Thereafter, a flexible ureteroscope is utilized to inspect the more proximal elements of the ureter and renal pelvis (Fig. 32.1). Encountered calculi are extracted if possible; otherwise lithotripsy can be performed.

Lithotripsy

Given the risks entailed and personnel and resources assembled, it is advisable to have appropriate tools for lithotripsy on hand. A stone small enough to allow uncomplicated extraction should be a pleasant surprise as opposed to the expected norm. If a stone is encountered that is too large to safely attempt basket extraction, the ideal lithotripter should have an appropriate tissue safety margin, the flexibility to be delivered via semirigid or flexible ureteroscopes, induce the least peripheral tissue damage, pose the least risk to the fetus, and cause the least reduction in irrigant flow.

Although ultrasonic lithotripters were utilized in one of the earliest reports of ureteroscopy in pregnancy, the authors raised the concern for possible auditory damage to the fetus. No follow-up after birth was available to assess whether fetal hearing had been impaired [31]. Another technology specifically avoided during pregnancy is electrohydraulic lithotripsy, which has been cited

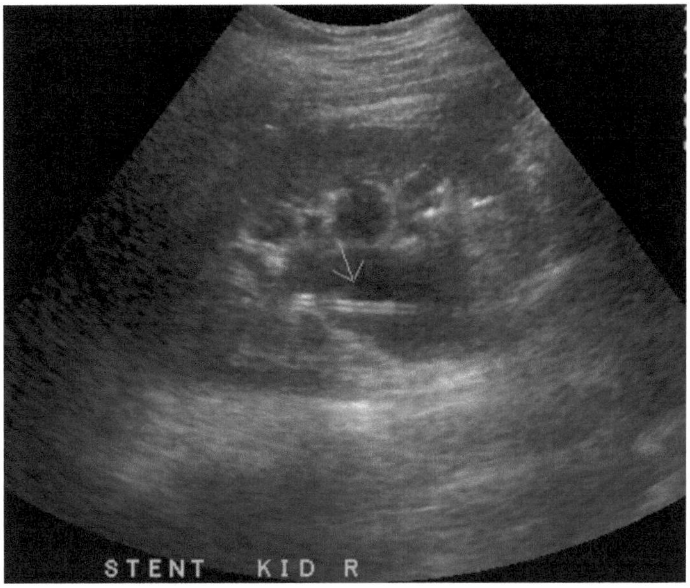

Fig. 32.2 Intraoperative ultrasound appearance of stent within renal collecting system

to have the narrowest margin of tissue safety, with unproven but queried effects on fetal hearing and uterine contractions [28].

Pneumatic lithotripsy has been successfully employed for intracorporeal lithotripsy during pregnancy. However, it must be used with a semirigid ureteroscope, leaving no option for lithotripsy if flexible scopes are required for navigation to stone or stone fragments. Furthermore, retropulsion of stone fragments is a well-recognized effect of this device and in one series, 27% of pregnant patients had stones pushed back to the renal pelvis and required postpartum SWL [32, 33].

The holmium:YAG laser best meets the demands of the ideal lithotripter in this situation and has emerged as a first line lithotripsy device, with excellent safety profile [28]. The holmium:YAG laser's small diameter fibers allow passage through flexible scopes with preservation of irrigant flow. It has also been demonstrated to have significantly less retropulsion than pneumatic lithotrites [34].

Stent Placement

After ureteroscopic inspection confirms all ipsilateral stone fragments have been removed, a stent is typically placed. A retrospective review detailing a single institution's experience in ureteroscopy in seven pregnant women noted that both of the two who did not have stents placed returned postoperatively with severe colic requiring hospitalization of 48 and 72 h. A third whose stent was removed the day of placement also returned with severe colic and premature uterine contractions requiring stent replacement. These authors thus recommended that all pregnant women have stents placed for at least 72 h postoperatively [35].

Over the previously placed safety wire, a stent of appropriate length is passed. Real-time ultrasound confirms the tram-track appearance of the hollow stent in the renal pelvis (Fig. 32.2), and as the wire is withdrawn, the deployed curl is visualized. Direct visualization of the distal curl confirms adequate coil in the bladder.

Note well, care must be taken to ensure timely removal of the stents. Encrusted stents may be encountered. Cystolitholopaxy, ureteroscopic lithotripsy and stent extraction, postpartum PCNL, and ureterolithotomy all may be potentially required to address these encrusted stents [1, 26, 33]. Tethers left attached to the distal curl may be utilized to aid timely removal of the stents in appropriately selected patients.

Complications

With unique anatomic and physiologic characteristics, the pregnant woman is different than the nongravid patient undergoing ureteroscopy. In light of this, a systematic review of the literature and meta-analysis was performed to assess the endoscopic safety of ureteroscopy in pregnancy. The overall complication rate was 8.3%—2 Claiven 1, 6 Claiven 2, and 1 Claiven 3 complications were noted. These were then compared with the complication rates derived from the AUA/EAU ureteral stone guidelines and specifically revealed no statistical difference in the rate of ureteral injury or UTI [36].

In order to better define the risk of obstetric complications, a multicenter retrospective review was performed of 46 ureteroscopies performed during pregnancy [37]. There were two obstetric complications of preterm labor in this series for an incidence of 4.3%. One was managed with tocolytics and the other required cesarean section. There were no pregnancies lost. The reported 4.3% incidence of obstetric complication is no more than that observed in women simply admitted with renal colic during pregnancy. Nonetheless, their occurrence emphasizes the need for a multidisciplinary team prepared to manage preterm labor expediently if it occurs.

Summary

When expectant management fails and temporizing measures are not tolerated or unacceptable, ureteroscopy has been shown to be an effective method for treating stones during pregnancy. Obstetric consultation should be obtained. Fetal heart monitoring, obstetric services, and a neonatal team may be required and thus should be available. If all of the recommended services are available, the experience and expertise of the urologist and anesthesiologist serve as final determinants as to whether it is prudent to proceed or whether transfer to another center should be considered.

Ureteroscopy may be performed as typically described, although intraoperative radiation exposure should be minimized. Techniques to reduce or eliminate this exposure have been outlined and should be utilized. Lithotripsy may be safely performed if required, ideally with holmium:YAG laser. Brief postoperative stenting has been recommended. Endoscopic complications are no more common in the gravid patient, although preterm labor is a complication unique to and observed in this cohort, underscoring the need for the coordination of a team with the necessary expertise to ensure safety of both the mother and child in the intra- and postoperative period.

References

1. Rodriguez PN, Klein AS. Management of urolithiasis during pregnancy. Surg Gyn Obstet. 1988;166:103–6.
2. Lewis DF, Robichaux AG, Jaekle RK, et al. Urolithiasis in pregnancy-diagnosis, management, and pregnancy outcome. J Reprod Med. 2003;48:28–32.
3. Swartz MA, Lydon-Rochelle MT, Simon D, et al. Admission for nephrolithiasis in pregnancy and risk of adverse birth outcomes. Obstet Gynecol. 2007;109:1099–104.
4. Stothers L, Lee LM. Renal colic in pregnancy. J Urol. 1992;148:1383–7.
5. Coe FL, Parks JH, Lindheimer MD. Nephrolithiasis during pregnancy. N Engl J Med. 1978;298:324–6.
6. Mhuireachtaigh RN, O'Gorman DA. Anesthesia in pregnant patients for nonobstetric surgery. J Clin Anesth. 2006;18:60–6.
7. Loughlin KR. Management of urologic problems during pregnancy. Urology. 1994;44:159–69.
8. Smith CL, Kristensen MD, Abraham PA. An evaluation of the physiochemical risk for renal stone disease during pregnancy. Clin Nephrol. 2001;55:205–11.
9. Maikranz P, Holley JL, Parks JH, et al. Gestational hypercalciuria causes pathological urine calcium oxalate supersaturations. Kidney Int. 1989;36:108–13.
10. Maikranz P, Lindheimer M, Coe F. Nephrolithiasis in pregnancy. Baillieres Clin Obstet Gynaecol. 1994;8(2):375–86.
11. Yatzidis H. Gestational urinary hyperthiosulfaturia protects hypercalciuric normal pregnant women from nephrolithiasis. Int Urol Nephrol. 2004;36:445–9.
12. Parulkar BG, Hopkins TB, Wollin MR, et al. Renal colic during pregnancy: a case for conservative treatment. J Urol. 1998;159:365–8.

13. Travassos M, Amselem I, Filho NS, Miguel M, Sakai A, Consolmagno H, Nogueira M, Fugita O. Ureteroscopy in pregnant women for ureteral stone. J Endourol. 2009;23(3):405–7.
14. Burgess KL, Gettman MT, Rangel LJ, et al. Diagnosis of urolithiasis and rate of spontaneous passage during pregnancy. J Urol. 2011;186:2280–4.
15. Preminger GM, Tiselius HG, Assimos DG, et al. Guideline for the management of ureteral calculi. J Urol. 2007;178:2418–34.
16. Semins MJ, Matlaga BR. Management of stone disease in pregnancy. Curr Opin Urol. 2010;20(2):174–7.
17. Khoo L, Anson K, Patel U. Success and short-term complication rates of percutaneous nephrostomy during pregnancy. J Vasc Interv Radiol. 2004;15:1469.
18. ACOG Committee on Obstetric Practice. ACOG Committee opinion no. 474. Non-obstetric surgery during pregnancy. Obstet Gynecol. 2011;117:420–1.
19. Rosen MA. Management of anesthesia for the pregnant surgical patient. Anesthesiology. 1999;91:1159–63.
20. Wolf JS, Bennett CJ, Dmochowski RR, et al. Best practice policy statement on urologic surgery antibiotic prophylaxis. J Urol. 2008;179:1379–90.
21. Bar-Oz B, Moretti ME, Boskovic R, et al. The safety of quinolones-a meta-analysis of pregnancy outcomes. Eur J Obstet Gynecol Reprod Biol. 2009;143:75–8.
22. Davis SM, Branch DW. Thromboprophylaxis in pregnancy: who and how. Obstet Gynecol Clin North Am. 2010;37:333–43.
23. Forrest JB, Clemens JQ, Finamore P, et al. AUA best practice statement for the prevention of deep venous thrombosis in patients undergoing urologic surgery. J Urol. 2009;181:1170–7.
24. ACOG Committee on Obstetric Practice. ACOG Committee opinion no. 299. Guidelines for diagnostic imaging during pregnancy. Obstet Gynecol. 2004;104:647–51.
25. Loughlin KR. Urologic radiology during pregnancy. Urol Clin North Am. 2007;34:23–6.
26. Lifshitz DA, Lingeman JE. Ureteroscopy as a first line intervention for ureteral calculi in pregnancy. J Endourol. 2002;16:19.
27. Cocuzza M, Colombo JR, Lopes RI, et al. Use of Inverted fluoroscope's c-arm during endoscopic treatment of urinary tract obstruction in pregnancy: a practicable solution to cut radiation. Urology. 2010;75: 1505–8.
28. Watterson JD, Girvan AR, Beiko DT, et al. Ureteroscopy and holmium: yag laser lithotripsy: an emerging definitive management strategy for symptomatic ureteral calculi in pregnancy. Urology. 2002;60:383–7.
29. Tawfiek ER. Ureteroscopy during pregnancy with follow-the-wire technique. Afr J Urol. 2009;15: 245–9.
30. Clayman M, Uribe CA, Eichel L, et al. Comparison of guidewires in urology. Which, when, and why? J Urol. 2004;171:2146–50.
31. Bakke A, Ulvik NM. Ureterorenoscopy in pregnancy. Scand J Urol Nephrol Suppl. 1988;110: 243–4.
32. Polat F, Suleyman Y, Kirac M, et al. Treatment outcomes of semi rigid ureterorenoscopy and intracorporeal lithotripsy in pregnant women with obstructive ureteral calculi. Urol Res. 2011;39:487–90.
33. Rana AM, Aquil S, Khawaja AM. Semirigid ureteroscopy and pneumatic lithotripsy as definitive management of obstructive ureteral calculi during pregnancy. Urology. 2009;73:964–7.
34. Marguet CG, Sung JC, Springhart WP, et al. In vitro comparison of stone retropulsion and fragmentation of the frequency doubled, double pulse nd:yag laser and holmium: yag laser. J Urol. 2005;173: 1797–800.
35. Akpinar H, Tufek I, Alici B, Kural AR. Ureteroscopy and holmium laser lithotripsy in pregnancy: stents must be used postoperatively. J Endourol. 2006;20: 107–10.
36. Semins MJ, Trock BJ, Matlaga BR. The safety of ureteroscopy during pregnancy: a systematic review and meta-analysis. J Urol. 2009;181(1):139–43.
37. Johnson EB, Krambeck AE, White WM, et al. Obstetric complications of ureteroscopy during pregnancy. J Urol. 2012;188(1):151–4.

Complex Anatomy: Horseshoe, Pelvic, and Malrotated Kidneys

33

Naeem Bhojani and James E. Lingeman

Anatomy and Embryology

During the development of the kidney, ascension occurs between the 6th and 9th weeks of life. By the end of this period the kidney is positioned in the upper lumbar area just below the adrenal gland. As the kidney ascends it is vascularized by a succession of transient aortic blood vessels that develop at sequentially higher levels [1]. If this ascension does not occur, the kidney remains in the pelvis and is then referred to as a pelvic kidney. In certain circumstances, abnormal fusion of the metanephric blastema at the midline results in the formation of a horseshoe kidney [1]. The fusion occurs between the lower poles of the kidneys on the ventral aspect of the aorta. Due to this fusion, ascension is interrupted as the fused lower poles of the kidney become trapped under the inferior mesenteric artery. Therefore the kidney lies more caudad in position compared to normal kidneys [2, 3].

Ascension of the normal kidney begins with the renal pelvis facing anteriorly while the calyces point posteriorly [1]. As the kidney ascends, the kidney rotates in order for the calyces to reach their final position facing laterally, while the pelvis faces medially [2]. Normally, the kidney starts to rotate at about 6 weeks of gestation soon after it leaves the true pelvis. It completes this process after having rotated 90° and this occurs by the time ascension is complete. If rotation of the kidney is anomalous, different renal positions are realized, including incomplete, hyper, or reverse rotation. In horseshoe kidneys, due to incomplete rotation, the renal pelvis is anterior to all the calyces and the calyces point posteriorly [3].

Impact of Anatomy on Stone Disease

Renal anatomic changes are associated with an increased risk of stone disease [2]. At the end of gestation the horseshoe kidney presents with its renal pelvises and ureters facing anteriorly and with the ureters crossing ventral to the isthmus (fibrous tissue connecting the lower poles of the horseshoe kidney) [2]. As the inferior poles of horseshoe kidneys are fused, the calyces, although normal in number, point posteriorly as opposed to laterally. This is secondary to the incomplete rotation of the kidneys. Furthermore, the ureters usually insert more superiorly and laterally on the renal pelvis [2]. Finally, the blood supply to [AU1]
the horseshoe kidney, including the lower poles and the isthmus, is especially variable. These factors can often lead to a situation similar to a ureteropelvic junction (UPJ) obstruction [4]. Up to 1/3 of horseshoe kidney patients will have a UPJ obstruction [5–7]. This is caused not only by the variable blood supply but also because of the high insertion of the ureter into the renal pelvis

N. Bhojani, M.D. • J.E. Lingeman, M.D. (✉)
Urology, Indiana University Health, 1801 North Senate Blvd, Suite 220, Indianapolis, IN 46202, USA
e-mail: jlingeman@iuhealth.org

M. Monga (ed.), *Ureteroscopy: Indications, Instrumentation & Technique*, Current Clinical Urology,
DOI 10.1007/978-1-62703-206-3_33, © Springer Science+Business Media New York 2013

and its abnormal course anterior to the isthmus. Due to these anomalies, urinary drainage is impaired and stasis ensues which is hypothesized to contribute to stone formation [8]. The incidence of stones in horseshoe kidneys is as high as 20% [1]. The most common locations of stones within a horseshoe kidney are in the posterior medial lower pole calyx followed by the renal pelvis [1].

Pelvic kidneys have possibly been associated with malrotation as well as a higher than normal insertion of their ureters into their renal pelvises [1]. These anatomic changes, which are similar to horseshoe kidneys, are believed to be associated with calculus formation.

Ureteroscopic Outcomes

The ureteroscopic treatment of stones associated with horseshoe, pelvic, and malrotated kidneys is a relatively young and evolving field. There are very few studies that have looked at this innovative procedure in patients with renal anomalies. The first report was by Andreoni et al. in 2000, who treated one horseshoe kidney containing three renal calculi (12 × 10 mm, 8 × 5 mm, and 3 mm) with a ureteral access sheath, a holmium laser, and a flexible ureteroscope. Three residual fragments of 1–2 mm were seen at 1 week post-op [9].

A study by Weizer et al. focused on eight patients, four with horseshoe kidneys and four with pelvic kidneys, all treated with flexible ureteroscopy. In this study all renal calculi required repositioning with nitinol graspers or baskets as well as the use of a holmium laser. The mean stone size was 1.4 cm (range 0.3–2 cm) and the mean operative time was 126 min (range 90–185 min). A ureteral access sheath was used in 50% of the patients and a ureteral stent was placed in all patients at the completion of each procedure. Overall, six patients (three horseshoe and three pelvic kidneys) had complete stone clearance after a single ureteroscopic session [10].

Another study by Symons et al. looked at the treatment of renal calculi in horseshoe kidneys. They reported a total of 55 patients but only 2 were treated with flexible ureteroscopy. One patient had a single stone with a digitized surface area (width × length) of 63 mm^2 and the other patient had four stones with a digitized surface area of 281 mm^2. In both patients stone fragmentation/clearance was complete [11].

The largest study was done by Molimard et al. in which they had a total of 17 patients with horseshoe kidneys that were treated with flexible ureteroscopy. In this study the average stone burden was 16 mm (range 7–35 mm). The mean number of procedures was 1.5 per patient. 41.2% of patients required more than 1 procedure and the mean operative time was 92 min (range 45–140 min). 88.2% of patients were successfully treated (residual fragments <3 mm) at follow-up using only flexible ureteroscopy and a holmium laser. Interestingly, all patients with initial stone burden ≤1 cm were successfully treated with a single session; however, those with stone burden ≥1.3 cm had an 88% chance of requiring at least one additional procedure [12].

These ureteroscopic outcomes demonstrate the feasibility and effectiveness of flexible ureteroscopy for the treatment of renal calculi in horseshoe, pelvic, and malrotated kidneys.

Important Equipment/Techniques

Using flexible ureteroscopy to treat patients with horseshoe, pelvic, and malrotated kidneys can be challenging. However, the use of various adjunct modalities and techniques can reduce this challenge. Adjunct modalities include the use of a holmium laser, nitinol baskets, ureteral access sheaths, and newer flexible ureteroscopes with improved secondary deflection.

The advent of smaller laser fibers (200 μm) has allowed for their use with flexible ureteroscopes. This has been instrumental in the application of flexible ureteroscopy in the treatment of nearly every type of renal calculi. Along with their ability to fragment any type of stone, holmium lasers allow for the production of small residual fragments that can be removed through a ureteral access sheath using nitinol baskets. Ureteral access sheaths permit continuous

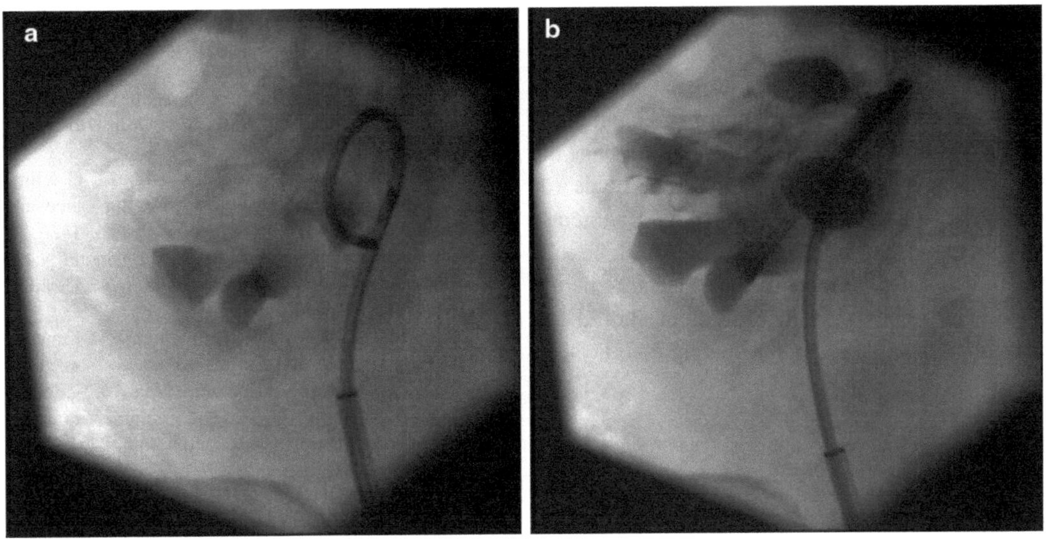

Fig. 33.1 Display of flexibility of flexible fiber-optic ureteroscope (**a**) 180°, (**b**) 360°

drainage of the renal pelvis, which facilitates irrigation and allows for the drainage of smaller stone fragments. As well, ureteral access sheaths allow repeat, rapid, atraumatic passage of the flexible ureteroscope to and from the renal pelvis. Finally, in cases in which the ureter is tortuous, as is the case with pelvic kidneys, ureteral access sheaths straighten the ureter, which permits rapid and easy access to the renal pelvis. This straightening of the ureter also improves the deflectability of the flexible ureteroscope.

Another important piece of equipment is the nitinol basket, which can be used to remove smaller stone fragments. In addition the nitinol basket can be used to reposition larger stones from the lower pole calyces to the upper pole calyces for fragmentation with a laser. Finally, the use of flexible ureteroscopes with secondary deflection is advantageous as they have a greater propensity to reach calculi in the lower pole even in horseshoe kidneys that have high ureteral insertions and bizarre or very dilated renal collecting systems. As well, fiber-optic ureteroscopes have slightly better deflectability compared to digital ureteroscopes and therefore, these scopes can add some benefit in the treatment of calculi in patients with renal anomalies (Fig. 33.1).

Our Approach

Preoperative

Although ureteroscopic treatment is planned, the possibility of percutaneous nephrolithotomy and/or laparoscopy should always be considered. Therefore, before embarking on the ureteroscopic treatment of horseshoe, pelvic, or malrotated kidneys, a CT scan of the abdomen is prudent. This allows for the examination of not only the kidney and the orientation of its calyces but also of the adjacent structures, including the colon. The patient should be made aware that if at the time of surgery it is determined that a ureteroscopic approach is not feasible, then an alternative approach (percutaneous) will be used at the same setting.

Operative

Once a guide wire is placed into the kidney a ureteral access sheath should be introduced. This will not only help with irrigation and drainage of the renal pelvis, but it will also straighten the ureter and facilitate the repeat passage of the flexible ureteroscope. Once the stone is identified and if it is small, it should be removed with a nitinol basket. However, if the stone is larger it should be moved into an upper pole calyx for fragmentation with a holmium laser. Due to the poor drainage of these kidneys, every effort should be made to remove all stone fragments, as residual fragments will increase the risk of recurrence of stones in the future. Finally, once all the stone fragments have been removed, a ureteral stent should be placed for a period of approximately 3–7 days.

Postoperative

A full metabolic analysis should be completed in these patients. Most will be found to have at least one metabolic anomaly [13]. As well, prevention is paramount in this population to minimize recurrences and prevent growth of residual fragments.

References

1. Gupta M, Lee MW. Treatment of stones associated with complex or anomalous renal anatomy. Urol Clin North Am. 2007;34(3):431–41.
2. Stein RJ, Desai MM. Management of urolithiasis in the congenitally abnormal kidney (horseshoe and ectopic). Curr Opin Urol. 2007;17(2):125–31.
3. Wein AJ, Kavoussi LR, Partin AW, Peters CA, Novick AC. Campbell-Walsh urology, vol. 1. 10th ed. New York: Elsevier Inc; 2011.
4. Ganpule AP, Desai MR. Urolithiasis in kidneys with abnormal lie, rotation or form. Curr Opin Urol. 2011; 21(2):145–53.
5. Jabbour ME, Goldfischer ER, Stravodimos KG, Klima WJ, Smith AD. Endopyelotomy for horseshoe and ectopic kidneys. J Urol. 1998;160(3 Pt 1):694–7.
6. Bellman GC, Yamaguchi R. Special considerations in endopyelotomy in a horseshoe kidney. Urology. 1996;47(4):582–5. discussion 585–586.
7. Keeley Jr FX, Bagley DH, Kulp-Hugues D, Gomella LG. Laparoscopic division of crossing vessels at the ureteropelvic junction. J Endourol. 1996;10(2):163–8.
8. Yohannes P, Smith AD. The endourological management of complications associated with horseshoe kidney. J Urol. 2002;168(1):5–8.
9. Andreoni C, Portis AJ, Clayman RV. Retrograde renal pelvic access sheath to facilitate flexible ureteroscopic lithotripsy for the treatment of urolithiasis in a horseshoe kidney. J Urol. 2000;164(4):1290–1.
10. Weizer AZ, Springhart WP, Ekeruo WO, et al. Ureteroscopic management of renal calculi in anomalous kidneys. Urology. 2005;65(2):265–9.
11. Symons SJ, Ramachandran A, Kurien A, Baiysha R, Desai MR. Urolithiasis in the horseshoe kidney: a single-centre experience. BJU Int. 2008;102(11): 1676–80.
12. Molimard B, Al-Qahtani S, Lakmichi A, et al. Flexible ureterorenoscopy with holmium laser in horseshoe kidneys. Urology. 2010;76(6):1334–7.
13. Raj GV, Auge BK, Assimos D, Preminger GM. Metabolic abnormalities associated with renal calculi in patients with horseshoe kidneys. J Endourol. 2004;18(2):157–61.

34 Complex Ureteral Access: Transplants, Diversions, and Duplications

John D. Denstedt and Andrew Fuller

Ureteral Access Following Renal Transplantation

As the surgical techniques of renal transplantation have evolved over the past 60 years, the method of urinary tract reconstruction has changed from cutaneous ureterostomy or ureteroureterostomy to ureteroneocystostomy. The intravesical (Leadbetter-Politano) technique of ureteroneocystostomy (Fig. 34.1) was first utilized in the context of renal transplant by Murray and colleagues in 1954 [1]. This technique requires exposure via an anterior cystotomy to allow submucosal tunneling of the ureter and placement of the neo-orifice in a near anatomic location.

An extravesical approach was described by Lich and Gregoir (Fig. 34.2) in 1961 [2, 3]. With this simplified technique, a single small cystotomy is created at the bladder dome and the distal ureter is anastomosed to the bladder mucosa. An antireflux mechanism is created by closure of the detrusor muscular fibers over the distal ureter. The extravesical approach has emerged as the preferred method in many centers worldwide as it avoids the need for a second cystotomy, requires less ureteral length, is generally associated with less postoperative complications, is faster, and technically less challenging to perform [4, 5].

The location of the ureteric neo-orifice at the bladder dome after the extravesical technique may make subsequent transurethral ureteric access difficult or impossible in the event of a postoperative complication. Advocates of the intravesical technique have proposed that the higher rate of postoperative complications with this technique is offset by easier endoscopic access to the ureter due to its location in proximity to the native ureteric orifice on the posterolateral bladder wall. Tillou and associates [4] evaluated the success of endoscopic management for each of the two common ureteroneocystostomy techniques in a retrospective series of 43 patients requiring endoscopic management of complications following transplantation. Successful endoscopic management was achieved in 75% of those who underwent an intravesical technique as compared with 53% for those who had a Lich–Gregoir extravesical reimplantation. Although ureteric access is simplified by the intravesical technique, one must be mindful that this technique is generally associated with a higher rate of complications, particularly ureterovesical stenosis. A study comparing complications related to the two techniques demonstrated that the rate of urological complications was 9.4% and 3.4% for the intravesical and extravesical approach, respectively [5].

Ureteral obstruction, whether intrinsic or extrinsic occurs in up to 10% of renal transplant recipients [6, 7]. In a meta-analysis considering the role of routine stenting following transplantation,

J.D. Denstedt, M.D., F.R.C.S.C., F.A.C.S. (✉)
A. Fuller, M.B.B.S.
Division of Urology, Department of Surgery,
The University of Western Ontario, London, ON, Canada
e-mail: john.denstedt@sjhc.london.on.ca

M. Monga (ed.), *Ureteroscopy: Indications, Instrumentation & Technique*, Current Clinical Urology,
DOI 10.1007/978-1-62703-206-3_34,

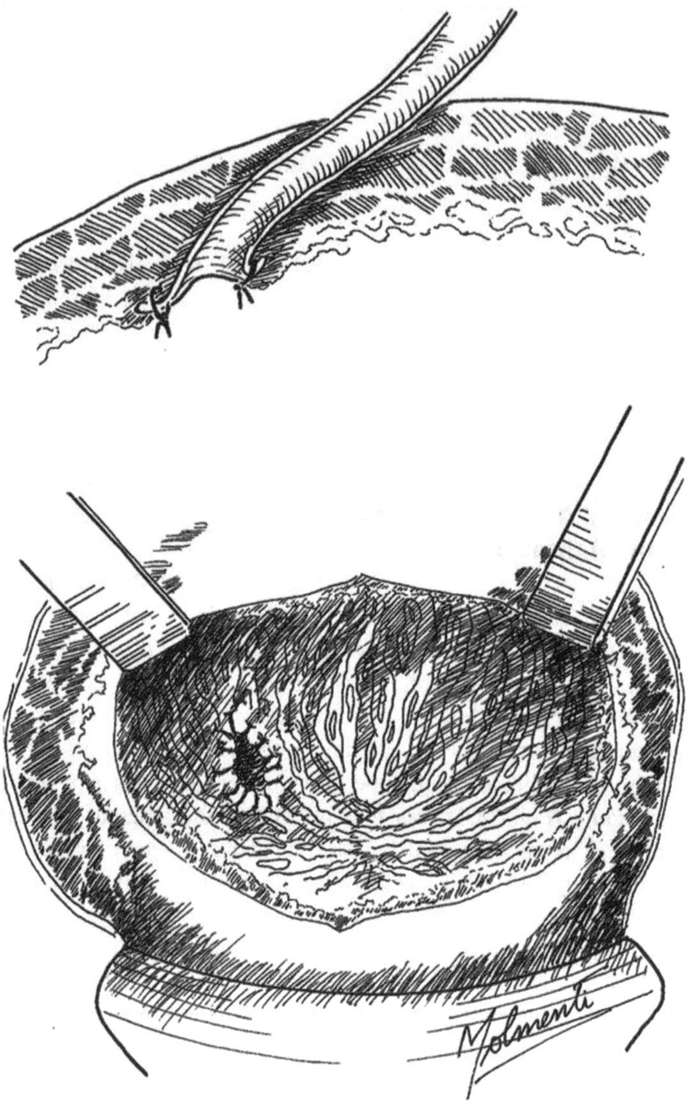

Fig. 34.1 Leadbetter-Politano intravesical ureteral reimplantation. From Kayler L, Kang, Molmenti E et al. Kidney transplant uretero-neocystostomy techniques and complications: review of the literature. Transplant Proc 2010;42:1413–1420. Reprinted with permission from Elsevier Inc

Wilson and colleagues [8] found stent placement to be associated with reduced rates of both urinary obstruction and leakage. The beneficial effect of routine stenting needs to be balanced against a higher rate of urinary tract infection in this group. Additionally, although stents are generally well tolerated, longer stents (≥20 cm) for longer periods (>6 weeks) may be associated with higher rates of encrustation and migration [8]. Particularly in the immediate postoperative period, complications may compromise graft function and result in significant clinical deterioration for patients who are immunosuppressed and have preexisting renal and cardiovascular comorbidities. When recognized and managed in timely manner, such complications are associated with a negligible effect on graft or patient survival [9].

While there remains an important role for open surgical exploration in select cases, improvements in endoscopic equipment and ancillary devices have lead to excellent outcomes with minimally invasive endoscopic techniques. All such techniques require ureteric access, either retrograde or antegrade. Percutaneous antegrade techniques are now generally regarded as the preferred first line approach to ureteric

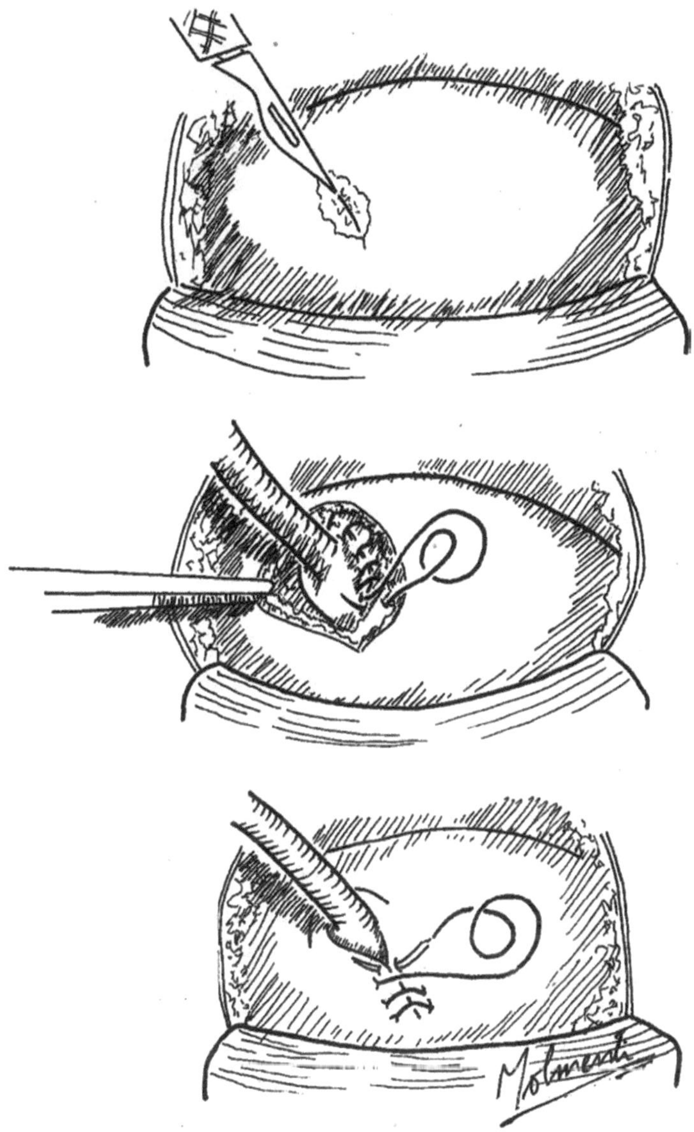

Fig. 34.2 Lich–Gregoir extravesical ureteral reimplantation. From Kayler L, Kang, Molmenti E et al. Kidney transplant ureteroneocystostomy techniques and complications: review of the literature. Transplant Proc 2010;42:1413–1420, reprinted with permission from Elsevier Inc

pathology following transplant [10]. With appropriate imaging facilities and interventional radiology expertise, percutaneous allograft nephrostomy can be achieved with minimal morbidity [11]. Advocates for an antegrade approach argue that compared with retrograde transurethral ureteric access, the antegrade technique affords the opportunity to perform a nephrostogram to evaluate the entire renal collecting system and ureter. The location, length, and nature of ureteric obstruction can be evaluated, and intervention in the form of dilatation, endoureterotomy, and/or stent placement can occur. Following such intervention, a percutaneous tube may be left in place to maximize drainage and to allow confirmation that the obstruction has resolved prior to tube removal.

Although the published experience with the retrograde approach is less, Gerrard and colleagues suggested that in many cases, a percutaneous approach may be avoided by an attempt at transurethral access [12]. The likelihood of success with the retrograde technique depends on the location of the ureteroneocystostomy.

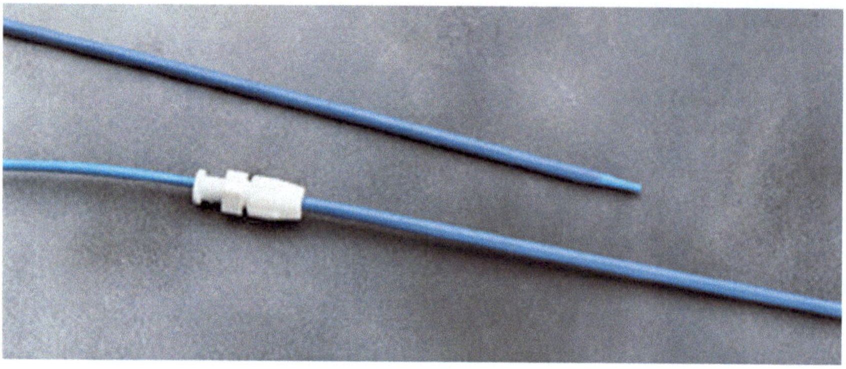

Fig. 34.3 8/10 Fr coaxial dilator

When an extravesical (Lich–Gregoir) ureteroneocystostomy is performed, the neo-orifice is located at the bladder dome. In recognition of the difficulties accessing the orifice in this location, several investigators have described techniques for ureteric access [12]. There should be a low threshold to utilize flexible instrumentation. A guidewire should be passed if possible to the level of the renal pelvis. Because of the acute angle between the bladder neck and neo-orifice on the bladder dome this wire should be exchanged for an Amplatz extra-stiff wire prior to contemplated intervention to minimize the likelihood of losing the wire and access to the ureter. There remains a lack of data with regard to the role for a ureteral access sheath in this context. Although it is not our practice to utilize a sheath in this scenario, a short sheath placed carefully under fluoroscopic guidance may in some cases facilitate repeated passage of flexible instruments, reduce intra-pelvic pressure, and maximize irrigant flow. In a series of 52 patients with posttransplant ureteric obstruction over a period of 12 years, Gerrard et al. [12] were able to successfully access the ureter and place a ureteric stent in a retrograde fashion in 54% of cases utilizing the above technique. The authors proposed that the retrograde approach may be an appropriate first line management option and a means of avoiding the morbidity associated with percutaneous antegrade renal access.

The usual technique of passing a ureteral stent under direct vision over a wire through the working channel of a rigid cystoscope can be accomplished only when the neo-orifice is visible with rigid instrumentation. When flexible cystoscopy is required, alternative techniques utilizing fluoroscopy have been described [13]. In particular, we advocate the use of an 8/10-Fr coaxial dilator (Fig. 34.3). This device may be passed under fluoroscopy over a guidewire until the 10-Fr outer component is located within the distal ureter. The 8 Fr component is then removed, and a stent may be advanced through the 10-Fr sheath which acts as a buttress to augment subsequent stent passage. A stent pusher with a radiopaque marker is used to position the distal end of the stent. The 10-Fr sheath is then removed along with the wire and the distal coil of the stent should be located within the bladder. The ureteric stent should be removed with a flexible cystoscope at 1 week postoperatively unless a longer duration of stent placement is indicated in scenarios such as ongoing obstruction or intraoperative ureteric perforation. Where ureteric access has been achieved to evaluate and treat obstruction, it is prudent to reevaluate the patient with renal ultrasonography after stent removal to confirm that there is no evidence of persistent hydroureteronephrosis.

Although the superficial location of the transplant kidney makes it amenable to imaging with ultrasound, antegrade access to the transplant kidney is complicated by anomalies in orientation, vascular supply, and location of the graft. Additionally, due to challenges in retrograde access to the ureter and intolerance of intravenous contrast due to the potential effect on graft function, it may not be possible in some cases to opacify the collecting system with contrast. The abnormal orientation of the allograft collecting system complicates puncture in several ways [14]. As compared with the usual approach in a native kidney where access is achieved via a posteriorly oriented calyx, access in the transplant kidney is usually via an anterior calyx. It may be challenging to enter the collecting system at the tip of the calyx and puncture of the infundibulum or renal pelvis may occur. Both of these factors increase the risk of hemorrhagic complications such as pseudoaneurysm and AV fistula. Peri-graft fibrosis may also increase the difficulty of tract dilatation once guidewire access is achieved [15].

With appropriate image guidance in the form of ultrasound or computerized tomography (CT), the interventional radiologist may avert many of the abovementioned factors after making a thorough assessment of the paranephric anatomy prior to tract placement. Additionally, particularly for unstable patients, image-guided percutaneous renal access has the advantage of being able to be performed under local or neurolept anesthesia in most cases.

In exposing the patient to the risks of percutaneous access, one must ensure that the nephrostomy provides appropriate access to the collecting system and ureter. Acute angulation, particularly between the tract and the ureter may make subsequent passage of wires, stents, angiographic catheters, and dilating balloons challenging [16].

Figure 34.4 demonstrates successful antegrade stent placement for treatment of a proximal ureteric stricture in a transplant kidney. After ultrasound-guided access was achieved, a nephrostogram was performed to define the location and length of the ureteric obstruction. A 0.035 in. guidewire was passed through the level of obstruction and a stent placed in satisfactory position with distal and proximal coils in the urinary bladder and transplant renal pelvis, respectively.

In summary, access to the ureter in the transplant patient offers unique challenges. When performed correctly, both the retrograde and antegrade approaches are viable, safe options in this patient cohort.

Urinary Tract Duplication

Duplication of the urinary tract is a common congenital abnormality with a reported incidence of 0.8% in autopsy series [17]. Ureteral duplication may be partial or complete. In a bifid system, the collecting systems of the upper and lower moieties join at the uretero-pelvic junction (UPJ). When the confluence of the ureters occurs below the UPJ and above the bladder, a partial or incomplete duplication results. In the case of complete duplication, two ureters enter the bladder at separate locations. As compared with partial duplication, where the ureteric orifice is usually orthotopic, the rates of pathology associated with complete duplication are much higher due to associated vesico-ureteric reflux, ectopia, and ureterocele formation [18]. The right and left kidneys are affected equally. There does appear to be a genetic component, with a 12.5% incidence of duplication in parents or siblings of an affected child [19].

A detailed understanding of the embryologic development of this condition forms the basis of successful identification and management of subsequent ureteric pathology. During normal development, the ureteric bud arises from the mesonephric (Wollfian) duct at 4 weeks and extends cranially to fuse with the metanephric blastema. Complete duplication occurs when two separate ureteral buds arise from the mesonephric duct. The upper and lower pole ureteric buds fuse caudally with the urogenital sinus (UGS) at different time points, leading to the classic configuration of the ureteric orifices as described by Carl Weigert and Robert Meyer [20, 21]. The lower ureteric bud associated with the lower moiety is the first to incorporate into the UGS and hence migrates more laterally on the trigone. The Weigert–Meyer rule states that the upper pole ureter is medial and caudal in relation to the lateral and cranially positioned lower pole ureter. By convention, the bud which drains the lower pole generally represents the normal bud. One must be cognizant of the potential for the upper pole ureter to insert ectopically. In females, an ectopic ureter may enter anywhere from the bladder neck to the perineum and may also insert into

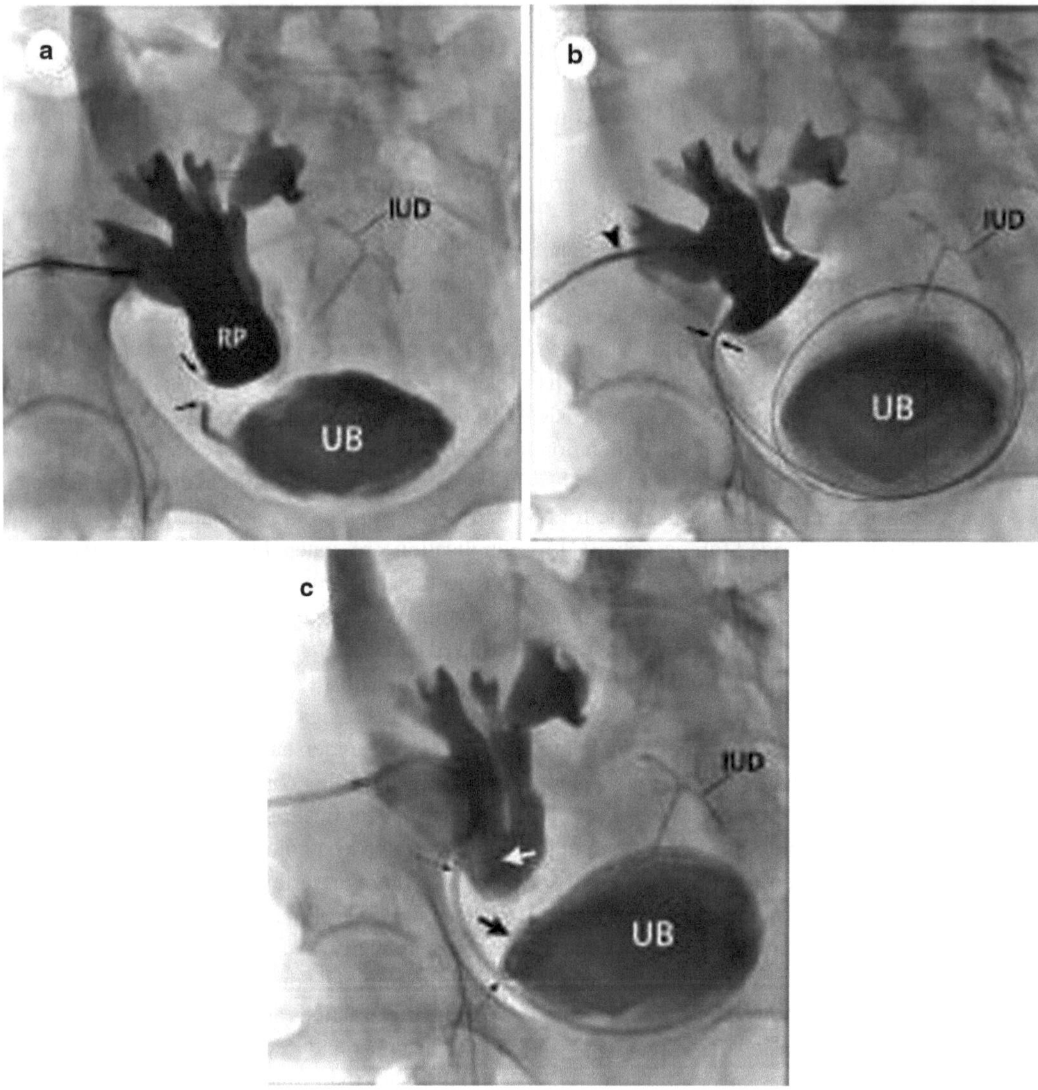

Fig. 34.4 Placement of a nephroureteral stent in a transplant kidney. Ultrasound guidance was used to obtain access (**a**). A guidewire has been placed across the proximal ureteric stricture (**b**) (*arrow*) with subsequent placement of a ureteric stent in satisfactory position (**c**). From [16], reprinted with permission from W.B./Saunders Co

the vagina, uterus, or rectum. In males, the ectopic insertion occurs above the external sphincter and involves the Wolffian derived structures such as the seminal vesicles, ejaculatory ducts, and vas deferens.

The likelihood of successful endourologic management in the context of ureteric duplication hinges on preoperative delineation of the anomalous anatomy with appropriate imaging. Prior to the widespread availability and use of noncontrast CT scanning, the urinary system was routinely evaluated with excretory urography (IVP). This technique effectively identified cases of asymptomatic duplication. CT offers many benefits over IVP including speed, accuracy of stone identification and allows detailed assessment of surrounding structures [22]. It also obviates the need for administration of intravenous contrast. While this may be beneficial in the vast majority of cases, Eisner and associates [23]

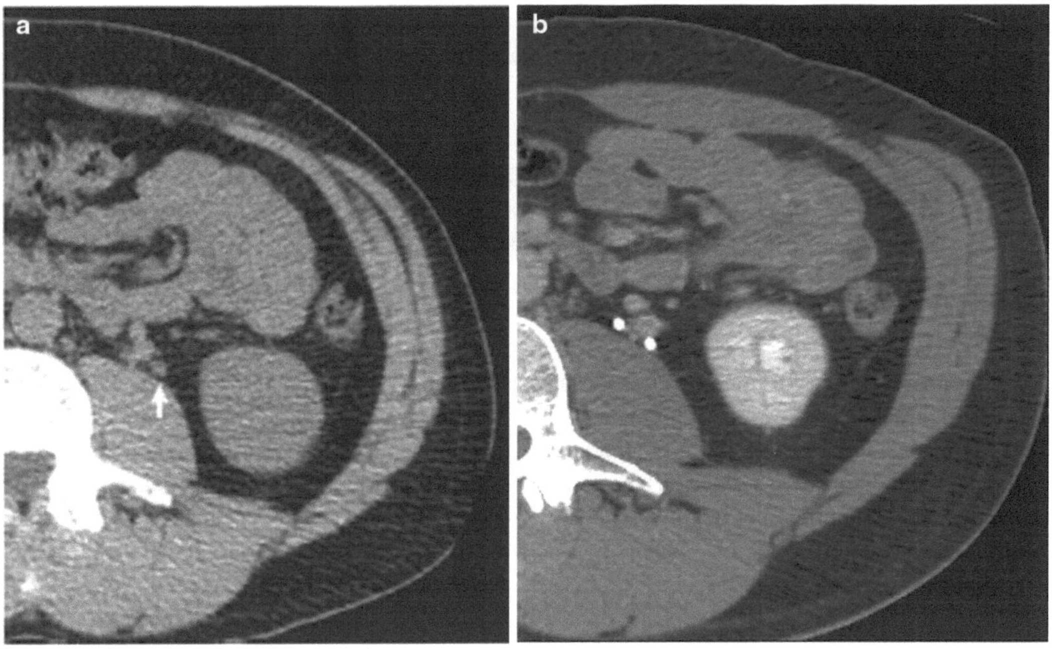

Fig. 34.5 Contrast (**b**) and noncontrast (**a**) enhanced images indicating the potential for missed duplication based on noncontrast imaging. From [23], reprinted with permission from Elsevier

demonstrated that axial noncontrast CT was only 59% sensitive for detecting ureteral duplication when interpreted by specialized genitourinary radiologists. When contrast was administered and a delayed excretory phase was performed, the sensitivity increased to 96% (Fig. 34.5). This study reinforces the importance of carefully evaluating a noncontrast scan. Where doubt exists, further assessment of the collecting system with contrast-enhanced imaging is recommended to identify the location of the ureteric orifice in a completely duplicated system and to demonstrate the branch point of a partially duplicated ureter [23]. Failure to appreciate a partial or complete duplication preoperatively and instrumentation of the wrong ureter may lead to the erroneous conclusion that a stone has passed or is inaccessible with potential clinical consequences.

Access to the duplex ureter can usually be achieved in a retrograde manner. Either flexible or rigid cystoscopy can be utilized to identify and cannulate the ureteric orifice with a guidewire. Particularly when preoperative imaging is limited to a noncontrast scan, we would advocate for the routine performance of retrograde pyelography using a 5 Fr ureteric catheter. This can be advanced over the guidewire to the level of the renal pelvis and slowly withdrawn while injecting contrast. This assists in localizing the branch point of the partially duplicated system. An angled tip angiographic catheter (Fig. 34.6) can be inserted over the guidewire to the level of the branch point to assist with wire cannulation at this level. Rotation at the tip of this device allows manipulation through a tortuous section of ureter. This catheter also allows injection of contrast as necessary to further clarify anomalous anatomy. Additionally, the use of angled tip guidewires in this scenario alone, or in combination with an angled tip angiographic catheter may assist in achieving ureteric access.

Although the ureteric caliber may be smaller in the context of duplication, it is normally possible to pass flexible instruments under fluoroscopy to the level of the renal pelvis. Likewise, an access sheath may be passed gently under image guidance once the anatomy of the duplication has been clearly defined. Intraoperative imaging also facilitates placement of a ureteric stent where required into the correct moiety.

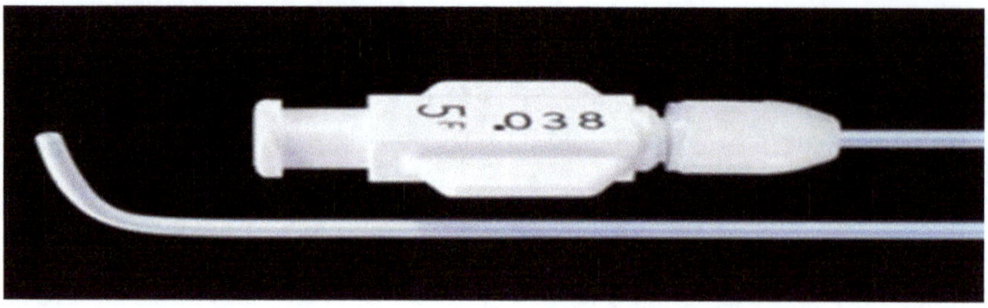

Fig. 34.6 Angled tip angiographic catheter

In summary, successful ureteric access in the context of ureteral duplications requires a high index of suspicion and attention to preoperative planning with delineation of the urinary tract anatomy. When identified preoperatively, a successful intervention can be planned and implemented.

Urinary Diversion

The use of intestinal segments in reconstruction of the urinary tract results in a number of structural and metabolic alterations. In combination, these factors may result in upper urinary tract pathology necessitating intervention [24]. In particular, metabolic alterations increase the risk of stone disease and include hyperchloremic metabolic acidosis, hypercalciuria, enteric hyperoxaluria, and hypocitraturia [25]. The increased incidence of struvite calculi in this patient population is due to the high rate of bacterial colonization with urease producing organisms. Urinary stasis within a chronically dilated urinary tract, reflux, excess mucous production, and foreign bodies including nonabsorbable surgical materials such as staples may also contribute to stone formation. Although stone disease is the most common indication for intervention, ureteric strictures, particularly at the site of the ureterointestinal anastomosis are often managed with ureteric stenting, endoureterotomy, or balloon dilatation.

Endourological management of upper tract pathology after urinary diversion is associated with satisfactory outcomes in experienced hands [26, 27]. It offers an attractive alternative to open surgery which is often complicated by scar formation and altered anatomical relations. While the ureter may be approached in either an antegrade or retrograde fashion, retrograde ureteric access presents several advantages. In particular, the potential morbidity of percutaneous renal access including hemorrhage and damage to adjacent organs is avoided. In the context of recurrent malignancy, retrograde access may also reduce the likelihood of tumor spread to non-urothelial surfaces [28]. Many cases necessitate a combined antegrade and retrograde approach and particularly for uretero-enteric stricture management, an antegrade approach may be advantageous [29, 30].

Irrespective of the technique adopted, preoperative planning is essential to maximize the likelihood of a successful procedure. A thorough review of the surgical records and consultation with colleagues involved in the original surgery is helpful to define the nature of the urinary diversion. Altered anatomical relations after reconstruction of the urinary tract can make localization of the ureteric orifices very challenging. Preoperative cross-sectional imaging is a useful adjunct particularly in assessing the site of ureteric pathology, relation of the ureter to surrounding structures, and site of uretero-enteric anastomosis [25]. The intraoperative availability of fluoroscopy, flexible instrumentation, and a full range of ancillary devices including guidewires and ureteric catheters should be confirmed prior to surgery.

Urinary diversions can be broadly classified as either continent or incontinent. Ileal conduit remains the most common form of incontinent diversion. Developments in surgical technique

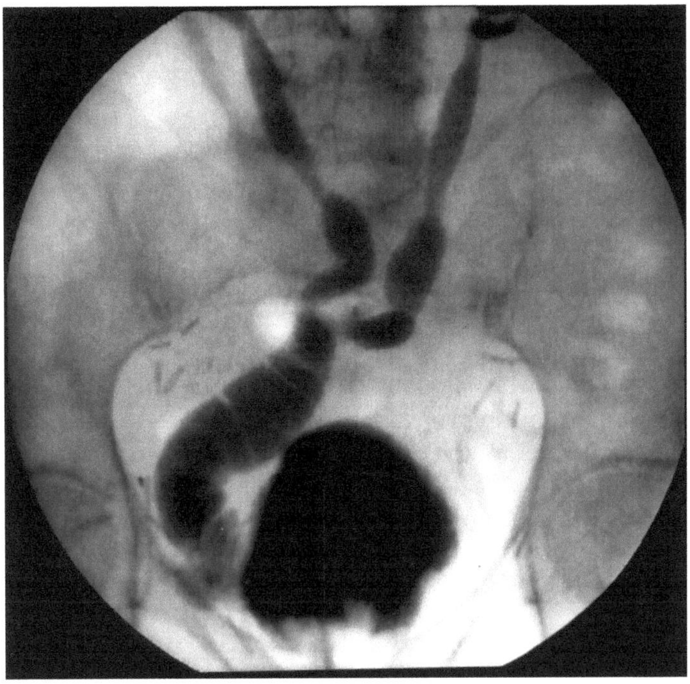

Fig. 34.7 Intraoperative cystogram demonstrating reflux of contrast into the afferent limb and ureters in an orthotopic urinary diversion. From [26], reprinted with permission from Elsevier

have led to the increased adoption of continent diversions, initially with continent cutaneous diversions and more recently in the form of orthotopic urinary diversion. Each form of diversion presents unique challenges in obtaining ureteric access, particularly in a retrograde fashion. Despite these challenges, retrograde endourologic techniques have been shown to be feasible and safe, with success rates of up to 75% [27].

Nelson and associates [26] described their experience with retrograde access in the context of continent orthotopic urinary diversion. In demonstrating the feasibility of this approach, several technical points were reinforced. In particular, clear delineation of the afferent limb to which the ureters are anastomosed is essential. Utilizing the working channel of the flexible cystoscope, one may inject contrast to outline the neobladder and afferent limb. Where a refluxing form of uretero-enteric anastomosis has been performed, it may also be possible to outline the ureters and renal pelvis using this technique (Fig. 34.7). A combination of fluoroscopy and direct visualization may then be used to access the afferent limb and localize the ureteric orifices. Where localization of the ureteric orifice proves difficult, intravenous administration of indigo carmine may facilitate access [27].

Under direct vision, the ureteric orifice may be cannulated with a guidewire. Angulation between the working channel of the cystoscope and the orifice may be overcome with the use of an angled tip guidewire and/or ureteric catheter. Once access is achieved, it may be prudent to exchange the initial access wire for an extra-stiff wire, particularly where a hydrophilic wire has been used to minimize the likelihood of losing access due to inadvertent distal migration of the wire. As the relationship of the right and left ureteric orifice is not consistent at the level of the afferent limb, fluoroscopy is essential to clarify that the correct side has been accessed before proceeding with further instrumentation [26].

Although access is transstomal rather than transurethral in the case of ileal conduit diversion, retrograde ureteric access techniques are similar for the two diversions. Conduitoscopy should be performed with a flexible cystoscope. Particularly in redundant conduits, fluoroscopy with injection of contrast through the flexible cystoscope may help to define the location of the uretero-enteric anastomosis allowing cannulation with a guidewire under direct vision. At the completion of conduitoscopy and ureteroscopy, a double J ureteric stent is routinely placed across the uretero-ileal anastomosis. This can be easily accessed and removed with flexible cystoscopy at a later date.

Retrograde ureteric access following continent cutaneous diversion presents unique challenges. Hyams and associates [27] demonstrated a 33% success rate in accessing the ureter in a retrograde manner after this form of urinary diversion and cited difficulties in negotiating the relationship between the catherizable stoma and ureteric orifices. A transstomal approach in this patient population is also complicated by the potential for stomal stenosis and damage to the delicate continence mechanism, particularly after repeated instrumentation [25]. While antegrade percutaneous access is the preferred method of ureteric access in this patient population, retrograde injection of contrast through the stoma is often helpful in outlining the pouch, ureters, and renal collecting system to direct percutaneous access.

Although associated with a high rate of success, percutaneous antegrade renal access after urinary diversion may present several challenges. Retrograde injection of contrast media to direct fluoroscopic-guided puncture may not be possible. In this scenario, image-guided puncture with ultrasound or CT in consultation with interventional radiology is required. Such access can be used to perform a nephrostogram. Particularly where access has been placed by image guidance, one should confirm placement of the tube at the tip of a posteriorly oriented calyx prior to tract dilatation to minimize the likelihood of segmental arterial injury. When location of percutaneous renal access is deemed inadequate, one should have a low threshold to repuncture in a more suitable location. Access via an upper pole calyx often provides optimal access to the ureter in this context.

It has been suggested that an antegrade approach is most suitable in a number of clinical scenarios. As outlined previously, an antegrade approach obviates the need for repeated instrumentation across the catherizable continence mechanism after continent cutaneous diversion, which may predispose to incontinence or stomal stenosis [25]. Several investigators have also suggested that endoureterotomy for ureteroenteric strictures is more effectively performed in an antegrade fashion [29, 30].

The standard technique of percutaneous renal access has been described previously and involves puncture of the collecting system under fluoroscopic guidance with placement of a 30 Fr working sheath after balloon or sequential dilatation [31]. Winter and colleagues described access sheath-aided percutaneous antegrade ureteroscopy as a useful alternate technique in the context of urinary diversion [32]. An upper or midpole puncture is used to manipulate a guidewire down the ureter. To avoid the need for balloon dilation, a 12–14 Fr access sheath is passed directly over the guidewire to the level of the pathology. Direct visualization with a flexible ureteroscope can then direct subsequent laser lithotripsy, balloon dilatation, or endoureterotomy as dictated by the nature of the obstruction.

Conclusion

Ureteric access in the context of congenital and acquired anatomical abnormalities of the urinary tract can be challenging even for the experienced endourologist. Despite this, the ability to intervene in a minimally invasive manner may offer excellent outcomes with considerably reduced morbidity compared with traditional open reconstructive techniques. With appropriate preoperative planning, equipment, and expertise, ureteric access can be achieved safely and effectively in the majority of individuals to facilitate appropriate endourologic management of ureteric and renal pathology.

References

1. Murray JE, Merrill JP, Harrison JH. Renal homotransplantations in identical twins. J Am Soc Nephrol. 2001;12:201–4.
2. Lich R, Howerton LW, Davis LA. Recurrent urosepsis in children. J Urol. 1961;86:554.

3. Gregoir W. Le reflux vesico-ureteral congenital. Acta Urol Belg. 1962;30:286.
4. Tillou X, Raynal G, Demailly M, et al. Endoscopic management of urologic complications following renal transplantation: impact of ureteral anastomosis. Transplant Proc. 2009;41:3317–9.
5. Thrasher JB, Temple DR, Spees EK. Extravesical versus Leadbetter-Politano ureteroneocystostomy: a comparison of urological complications in 320 renal transplants. J Urol. 1990;144:1105–9.
6. Sigman DB, Del Pizzo JJ, Sklar GN. Endoscopic retrograde stenting for allograft hydronephrosis. J Endourol. 1999;13:21–5.
7. Kim JA, Banner MP, Ramchandani P, et al. Balloon dilation of ureteral strictures after renal transplantation. Radiology. 1993;186:717–22.
8. Wilson CH, Bhatti AB, Rix DA, et al. Routine intraoperative ureteric stenting for kidney transplant recipients. Cochrane Database Syst Rev. 2005;(4):CD004925. doi: 10.1002/14651858.CD004925.pub2.
9. Streeter EH, Little DM, Cranston DW, et al. The urological complications of renal transplantation: a series of 1535 patients. BJU Int. 2002;90:627–34.
10. Hobart MG, Streem SB, Gill IS. Renal transplant complications: minimally invasive management. Urol Clin North Am. 2000;27:787–98.
11. Bhagat VJ, Gordon RL, Osorio RW, et al. Ureteral obstructions and leaks after renal transplantation—outcome of percutaneous antegrade ureteral stent placement in 44 patients. Radiology. 1998;209:159–67.
12. Gerrard Jr ER, Burns JR, Young CJ, et al. Retrograde stenting for obstruction of the renal transplant ureter. Urology. 2005;66:256–60.
13. Mendez-Probst CE, Razvi H, Denstedt JD. Fundamentals of instrumentation and urinary tract drainage. In: Wein AJ, Kavoussi LR, Novick AC, Partin AW, Peters CA, editors. Campbell-Walsh urology. 10th ed. Philadelphia: Elsevier Saunders; 2012. p. 177–91.
14. Oliveira M, Branco F, Martins L, et al. Percutaneous nephrolithotomy in renal transplants: a safe approach with a high stone-free rate. Int Urol Nephrol. 2011;43:329–35.
15. Benoit G, Blanchet P, Eschwege P, et al. Occurrence and treatment of kidney graft lithiasis in a series of 1500 patients. Clin Transpl. 1996;10:176–80.
16. Saad WEA, Moorthy M, Ginat D. Percutaneous nephrostomy: native and transplanted kidneys. Tech Vasc Inter Radiol. 2009;12:172–92.
17. Bauer SB, Perlmutter AD, Retik AB. Anomalies of the upper urinary tract. In: Walsh PC, Retik AB, Stamey TA, et al., editors. Campbell's urology. Philadelphia: WB Saunders; 1992. p. 1357–442.
18. Decter RM. Renal duplication and fusion anomalies. Paediatr Clin North Am. 1997;44:1323–41.
19. Whitaker J, Danks DM. A study of the inheritance of duplication of the kidney and ureters. J Urol. 1966;95:176–8.
20. Weigert C. Ueber einige Bilddunsfehler der Ureteren. Virchows Arch. 1877;70:490.
21. Meyer R. Normal and abnormal development of the ureter in the human embryo—a mechanistic consideration. Anat Rec. 1946;96:355.
22. Ripolles T, Agramunt M, Errando J, et al. Suspected ureteral colic: plain film and sonography vs unenhanced helical CT. A prospective study in 66 patients. Eur Radiol. 2004;14:129–36.
23. Eisner BH, Shaikh M, Uppot RN, et al. Genitourinary imaging with noncontrast computerized tomography—are we missing duplex ureters? J Urol. 2008;179:1445–8.
24. El-Nahas AR, Eraky I, El-Assmy AM, et al. Percutaneous treatment of large upper tract stones after urinary diversion. Urology. 2006;68:500–4.
25. Okhunov Z, Duty B, Smith AD, et al. Management of urolithiasis in patients after urinary diversions. BJU Int. 2011;108:330–6.
26. Nelson CP, Wolf Jr JS, Montie JE, et al. Retrograde ureteroscopy in patients with orthotopic ileal neobladder urinary diversion. J Urol. 2003;170:107–10.
27. Hyams ES, Winer AG, Shah O. Retrograde ureteral and renal access in patients with urinary diversion. Urology. 2009;74:47–50.
28. Kulp DA, Bagley DH. Does flexible ureteropyeloscopy promote local recurrence of transitional cell carcinoma? J Endourol. 1994;8:111–3.
29. Gerber GS, Kuznetzov D, Leef JA, et al. Holmium:YAG laser endoureterotomy in the treatment of ureteroenteric strictures following orthotopic urinary diversion. Tech Urol. 1999;5:45–8.
30. Delvecchio FC, Kuo RL, Iselin CE, et al. Combined antegrade and retrograde endoscopic approach for the management of urinary diversion-associated pathology. J Endourol. 2000;14:251–6.
31. Ko R, Soucy F, Denstedt JD, et al. Percutaneous nephrolithotomy made easier: a practical guide, tips and tricks. BJU Int. 2007;101:535–9.
32. Winter M, Lynch C, Appu S, et al. Surgery illustrated—focus on details. Access sheath-aided percutaneous antegrade ureteroscopy; a novel approach to the ureter. BJU Int. 2011;108:620–2.

Medical Comorbidities: Anticoagulation and Obesity

35

Elias S. Hyams and Brian R. Matlaga

Introduction

Retrograde ureteroscopy (URS) is used routinely for treatment of urolithiasis as well as evaluation and treatment of other upper urinary tract pathology, such as ureteral stricture disease and upper tract urothelial carcinoma. The utility of endoscopic approaches for these disease processes has been established [1–3]. Certain patient populations, however, require special technical considerations to maximize the safety and efficacy of URS. In this chapter, we review the technical considerations for use of URS in two specific patient populations: those with significant clinical obesity and those with bleeding diathesis.

Ureteroscopy in Obese Patients

Background

Obesity has been rapidly increasing in the United States and abroad, with an associated rise in related comorbidities. Indeed, obesity is associated with such problems as diabetes mellitus, cardiovascular disease, hyperlipidemia, and general disability [4]. There has been growing recognition of the association between obesity and stone disease as well. Indeed, epidemiological studies have shown an up to twofold increased risk for kidney stones among obese patients. Lithogenic risk factors associated with obesity have included hyperinsulinemia, hyperoxaluria, hypocitraturia, low urinary volume, hypercalciuria, and high sodium consumption [5].

Obese patients, then, represent a growing proportion of kidney stone patients seen in clinical practice. These patients may present treatment dilemmas based on technical challenges due to large habitus. Importantly, there are varying degrees of obesity based on body mass index, including "obesity" (>30 kg/m^2), "morbid obesity" (>35 kg/m^2), and "severe morbid obesity" (>40 kg/m^2). As such, not all patients with colloquial "obesity" are equivalent, either in clinical practice or in the academic setting, and it is critical to evaluate these subgroups independently. Additionally, height and distribution of body mass can impact the risk/benefit evaluation of stone treatment for a given patient, thus not all patients with a given degree of obesity will have similar surgical risks.

Traditionally kidney stones are treated by URS, shock wave lithotripsy (SWL), or percutaneous nephrolithotomy (PNL). There have been multiple studies evaluating the safety and efficacy of these approaches in obese patients. Unfortunately, these studies have been primarily retrospective in nature with small patient numbers, and have included patients with variable stone sizes and variable degrees of obesity.

E.S. Hyams, M.D. (✉) • B.R. Matlaga, M.D., M.P.H.
Brady Urological Institute, Johns Hopkins
Medical Institutions, 600 N. Wolfe Street, Park 221,
Baltimore, MD 21287, USA
e-mail: elias.s.hyams@hitchcock.org

M. Monga (ed.), *Ureteroscopy: Indications, Instrumentation & Technique*, Current Clinical Urology,
DOI 10.1007/978-1-62703-206-3_35, © Springer Science+Business Media New York 2013

Overall, though, there has been concern about the limited efficacy of SWL in obese patients [6, 7], as well as concern regarding safety of PNL in this population [8, 9]. As such, URS has been investigated as an option for patients whose habitus may be prohibitive or limiting for alternative procedures, particularly for larger stone burdens for which PNL is the traditional standard of care.

What are the limitations of PNL in the obese population? For patients with very large body habitus, an increased distance may need to be traversed on the flank to reach the kidney, which may be prohibitive even with longer instruments. Indeed, these patients frequently have increased subcutaneous fat and increased mobility of the kidney because of greater retroperitoneal fat. Anatomical landmarks may be obscured, and there may be an increased risk of nephrostomy tube dislodgement. Furthermore, there may be concerns regarding prone positioning and cardiopulmonary issues related to anesthesia. Supine and flank positioning, as well as use of conscious sedation, have been studied to obviate these difficulties [10–12] but these are infrequently utilized and present their own technical and anesthesia-related challenges.

Interestingly, there are several studies that demonstrate similar efficacy and safety of PNL in obese vs. nonobese patients [13–17]. However, these studies have primarily represented small retrospective series. Also, these series have been reported primarily by tertiary centers with high volume and efficiency of PNL, thus the results are not necessarily generalizable to other centers. Other studies have demonstrated a higher rate of complications in obese patients, including a higher risk of blood transfusion in those with morbid obesity [8], and increased complication rate and length of hospital stay [9]. In our experience, PNL is feasible in patients with varying degrees of obesity, however tolerability of the prone position has been the major limiting factor in patients with large body habitus. As such, URS may be the preferred option in selected patients with larger stone burdens.

For smaller ureteral and renal stones (<2 cm), SWL is the most commonly performed procedure in clinical practice [18]. However, multiple studies have demonstrated that SWL has limited efficacy in patients with obesity [6, 7]. Limitations of SWL in these patients are thought to pertain to increased skin-to-stone distance, causing attenuation of the shock wave and limiting one's ability to center the stone within the focal point of the lithotripter [19]. Also, fluoroscopy may be less effective at targeting the stone in obese patients, and obesity may necessitate increased radiation doses. Finally, patients with more severe obesity may not be able to be placed on the SWL table based on weight limits and table capacity. Because of these concerns, SWL may be inferior to URS in patients with larger body habitus, though patients should be counseled regarding their treatment options and their relative merits.

URS, then, may be the preferred treatment approach for stones in certain obese patients. For certain large (>2 cm) stones, URS may be a reasonable alternative to PNL, thereby avoiding anesthetic risk associated with PNL in the very obese. Advantages of URS vs. PNL include positioning in dorsal lithotomy rather than a flank or prone position, the possibility of sedation rather than general anesthesia, absence of a skin incision or puncture of the kidney, lack of a need for nephrostomy drainage, and surgery on an outpatient basis [20]. There are several studies of URS for larger stones that include subsets of obese patients, for whom body habitus was the deterrent to pursuing PNL. Safety and efficacy of URS in these patients have been demonstrated, though frequently with a staged approach [21–24]. Smaller caliber flexible ureteroscopes with improved optics, as well as improvements in intracorporeal lithotripsy, have improved the efficacy of URS for treatment of larger stone sizes in both obese and nonobese patients, making this a viable alternative to PNL. In many cases, though, these larger volume stones may require staged treatment approaches.

URS for treatment of stone disease in the obese population has been the subject of multiple studies in the literature. Despite methodological limitations, i.e., small retrospective series with variable distributions of obesity and diverse stones sizes, these studies have, in general, demonstrated safety and efficacy of URS in obese patients. In one retrospective comparative study, Natalin and colleagues evaluated treatment outcomes for 34 normal, 39 overweight, and 34 obese patients undergoing URS for treatment of renal or ureteral stones [25]. Mean stone size was not given but stones were stratified into <1 cm or 1 cm or greater; rigid URS was used for distal stones, while flexible URS was used for proximal ureteral and renal stones. The authors used a ureteral access sheath for proximal stones as well as Holmium:YAG laser lithotripsy. They found no difference in operating times or stone-free rate between groups; neither stone size nor location affected outcomes. However, the limited number of morbidly obese patients limited conclusions in this subgroup.

Several studies provide findings instructive on the need for multistaged approaches in patients with larger stones, which appears to be the tradeoff for a lower complication rate compared with percutaneous surgery. Bultitude and colleagues reported treatment of 18 kidneys in 17 morbidly obese patients [26]. Mean BMI was 46.8 kg/m^2, and mean stone size was 16 mm (5–50). The authors noted that stones >15 mm were more likely to require multiple treatment sessions. Nguyen and colleagues also found in a series of 48 morbidly obese patients that stone-free rate was significantly better following staged procedures [27]. Best and Nakada, interestingly, found that for more moderate stone burdens (mean size 9.1mm), the non-obese actually required a greater number of procedures to achieve a stone-free outcome compared with the obese, suggesting likely equivalence in outcomes between these populations [28].

Operative times, also an important indicator of surgical complexity, have been reported to be comparable among the obese and nonobese. Dash and colleagues performed a retrospective comparison of 16 morbidly obese and 38 nonobese patients matched by stone size and location [29], finding no significant differences in stone-free rate, operative times, and complications.

Technical Considerations

There are several important considerations regarding URS in patients with large body habitus. Preoperative evaluation is required to identify comorbid conditions that may impact the safety of anesthesia care. Obesity is associated with cardiopulmonary disease and obstructive sleep apnea that can affect anesthetic management and necessitate additional monitoring postoperatively. While conscious sedation may be considered in some patients, those requiring endotracheal intubation may require a team approach to anesthesia care based on a difficult airway. Indeed, fiberoptic intubation may be required, and LMA or spinal may be contraindicated depending on airway anatomy.

Perioperatively, there are several important considerations in patients with large habitus. For those with severe morbid obesity, standard operating room tables may be insufficient and special tables or two brought together may be necessary. Positioning in dorsal lithotomy requires careful padding to minimize risk of nerve compression injury. Deep venous thrombosis prophylaxis with sequential compression devices +/− subcutaneous heparin, depending on the duration of the procedure, is warranted. As prolonged positioning with obesity may increase risk of rhabdomyolysis, prolonged procedures should generally be avoided and staging may be necessary. Access to the genital region may be challenging in patients with severe morbid obesity, and the pannus may need to be elevated and suspended with surgical tape. An access sheath can be used for repeat access if there is difficulty accessing the groin based on habitus. There have been reports of simultaneous bilateral URS to reduce the need for multiple anesthesias, or prolonged single anesthesia; one report included an obese (BMI 38.4 kg/m^2) and a superobese (BMI 58.2 kg/m^2) patient without complications, though this is an experimental approach [30]. Care to minimize fluoroscopy time, including using "spot" images rather than continuous fluoroscopy, is important in treating obese patients, as visualization of radiopaque stones may be limited by habitus, and increased body mass leads to radiation scatter that can dramatically increase radiation exposure to providers.

Postoperatively obese patients may require more intense monitoring based on comorbid details. Those with severe obstructive sleep apnea may require overnight observation [30]. Patients may be at increased risk of cardiovascular events, atelectasis, and venous thromboembolism, necessitating inpatient monitoring as well [31].

Anticoagulation

Background and Review of the Literature

Patients with bleeding diathesis, either medical or pharmacological, are at increased risk for bleeding complications related to stone treatment. It is generally accepted that active ongoing anticoagulation or bleeding disorders are contraindications to SWL or PNL [32, 33]. In these patients, URS is the preferred therapy as it can be performed under direct vision and with minimal trauma. Urologists may be confronted with patients who require continued antiplatelet therapy or anticoagulation (e.g., those with drug-eluting stents, metallic heart valves), or for whom there is strong preference to continue these agents perioperatively (e.g., severe coronary artery disease, recent thrombosis). For patients with absolute indications for warfarin, bridging with low molecular weight or unfractionated heparin may enable treatment during a window in which bleeding risk is decreased. Additionally, those with relative indications may have their agents safely held for 5–7 days preoperatively. These patients have varying degrees of risk for bleeding, and a detailed discussion of the risks/benefits/alternatives of different treatment approaches is warranted. However, in those with high bleeding risk, or for whom a bleeding event would be catastrophic (e.g., solitary kidney), URS should be strongly considered. Importantly, significant bleeding complications have been reported during stone treatment even in patients with held or bridged anticoagulation [34], thus these patients should be treated with extreme care.

URS may be the preferred treatment option in this patient population. The development of smaller and more flexible ureteroscopes, dual deflection, and digital imagery has enabled access to all calyces with decreased manipulation. Improvements in working tools such as flexible wires and tipless nitinol baskets have also been useful for this purpose, as have ureteral access sheaths that enable repeated atraumatic access to the collecting system. Advances in intracorporeal lithotrites have minimized the "collateral damage" of lasering; in particular, Holmium:YAG laser has become widely utilized based on low depth of penetration but sufficient power for stone fragmentation, tumor ablation, or stricture incision. As Holmium laser energy is rapidly absorbed in water, there is minimal mucosal damage provided there is no direct contact with tissue.

There have been four published studies of URS in patients who are anticoagulated or with bleeding diathesis. Overall these studies have demonstrated safety and efficacy of these interventions. Kuo and colleagues retrospectively reviewed nine cases of URS in patients with bleeding diathesis, including eight patients with stone disease and one with UT-TCC [35]. Six patients were on warfarin with a mean INR of 2.1, two had thrombocytopenia, and one had von Willebrand's disease. Either semirigid or flexible URS was performed with Holmium laser lithotripsy or tumor ablation. There were no perioperative complications, including no perioperative bleeding. Postoperatively, one patient had transient oliguria secondary to a small ureteral clot that passed with lasix administration, and one patient developed epistaxis after ketorolac dosing for pain. Short-term outcomes were excellent for stone clearance (six of seven patients were stone free on intravenous urogram at 1 month) and tumor recurrence (negative at 4 months), though these were secondary outcomes.

Turna and colleagues retrospectively reviewed their experience with 37 patients on anticoagulation or antiplatelet agents (warfarin, clopidogrel, or aspirin) in whom this therapy was not discontinued prior to flexible URS/Holmium laser lithotripsy for renal stones [36]. These authors matched these patients with 37 control patients who were not anticoagulated and who underwent similar procedures. There were no early terminations of procedures for poor visibility, though there was a minor increased drop in hemoglobin among anticoagulated patients (0.6 g/dl vs. 0.2 g/dl,

$p<0.0001$). There were comparable stone-free rates and low incidence of intraoperative and postoperative complications in the two groups. Furthermore no bleeding or thromboemobolic events occurred. Ureteral balloon dilation and access sheath use was performed at the discretion of the surgeon. Notably, stones were repositioned if they were in challenging locations to decrease risk of intrarenal trauma.

Watterson and colleagues performed another retrospective review of 25 patients at two centers with bleeding diathesis treated with URS/Holmium laser lithotripsy for upper tract calculi [37]. Specific etiologies of diathesis included chronic warfarin therapy (17), liver dysfunction (3), thrombocytopenia (4), and von Willebrand's disease (1). There was one bleeding complication in one of the two patients simultaneously treated with electrohydraulic lithotripsy; this patient developed a retroperitoneal bleed requiring blood transfusion. Thirty-seven percent of patients had ureteral dilation either with a coaxial sheath, balloon dilator, or access sheath. The authors concluded that electrohydraulic lithotripsy has a narrower safety margin; as such this technique is not recommended in patients who are at increased risk for bleeding.

In a study of patients with bleeding diathesis who were bridged, reversed, or had their anticoagulation held prior to surgery, Klingler and colleagues retrospectively examined 35 such patients undergoing treatment for stone disease (SWL, URS, or PCNL) [34]. Known bleeding disorders were corrected either with low molecular weight heparin bridging, or vitamin K administration. Aspirin therapy was stopped at a mean 3.6 days prior to surgery. URS was performed in eight patients, specifically semirigid ureteroscopy and pneumatic (6) or Holmium (2) laser lithotripsy. Two of eight patents developed hematuria postoperatively and had clot obstructing their stents, and thus required earlier stent removal than planned. Intravenous urography performed 2 weeks after stent removal showed normal function and excretion bilaterally. Interestingly, among 59 SWL treatments in this study, there was an overall complication rate of 33.3 % despite normal clotting parameters at the time of treatment. There were four cases of severe thrombocytopenia, and >1 cm renal hematoma in three patients. Two of these three patients had no sequelae after monitoring, though one required delayed URS for persistent stone disease and hydronephrosis. One of three patients treated with PNL had severe gross hematuria 5 days postoperatively after resumption of heparin therapy. These data indicate that patients with held or reversed anticoagulation may still be at increased risk of bleeding complications, and resumption of therapy can be associated with bleeding depending on patient risk factors.

Technical Considerations

Meticulous effort to minimize upper and lower urinary tract trauma is essential during URS in patients with bleeding diathesis. Male patients with benign prostatic enlargement may be at risk for prostatic bleeding during cystoscopy, exacerbated by anticoagulation. Care to place the cystoscope under direct vision during initial access, and to avoid torquing on the prostate when possible, reduces the risk of significant bleeding. Flexible cystoscopy may be necessary for ureteral access when a large friable median lobe is present. A foley catheter may be required at the end of the case if there is persistent oozing from the prostate for tamponade effect.

Minimizing ureteral and intrarenal trauma requires careful advancement of flexible wires during retrograde access; avoiding redundancy of wires in the kidney may be helpful, and a retrograde pyelogram can be performed to ensure that the collecting system anatomy is well understood. If a ureteral orifice is anatomically tight, it can be actively dilated. An 8/10 French coaxial catheter can be passed over a wire with fluoroscopic guidance to enable passage of a ureteroscope through the orifice. Balloon dilators can also be utilized, as reported in the literature (Kuo [35]), although there is still a concern that this technique may increase the risk for hemorrhage. Placing a ureteral stent and allowing for passive dilation with scheduling of a second stage procedure may be a less traumatic alternative. During laser lithotripsy, constant visualization of the tip of the fiber is necessary with strict avoidance of the mucosa. The lowest power setting that enables stone fragmentation should be utilized. Ureteral access sheaths can be utilized for repeated access, and stone clearance provided the sheath passes easily. A safety wire can be helpful in this population should visualization become obscured, and there should be a low threshold to terminate the procedure if there is poor visibility, placing a stent and scheduling a second stage. URS and tumor ablation can also be performed in patients with bleeding disorders, though there are no published series of these patients. Indeed, these patients may have lower risk from endoscopic treatment than with extirpative surgery given their bleeding/thrombosis risks, though it is important that patients be carefully selected with low volume, low grade urothelial disease.

References

1. Wang AJ, Preminger GM. Modern applications of ureteroscopy for intrarenal stone disease. Curr Opin Urol. 2011;21(2):141–4.
2. Bader MJ, Sroka R, Gratzke C, et al. Laser therapy for upper urinary tract transitional cell carcinoma: indications and management. Eur Urol. 2009;56(1):65–71.
3. Patel RC, Newman RC. Ureteroscopic management of ureteral and ureteroenteral strictures. Urol Clin North Am. 2004;31(3):107–13.
4. Ogden CL, Yanovski SZ, Carroll MD, et al. The epidemiology of obesity. Gastroenterology. 2007;132: 2087–102.
5. Duffey BG, Pedro RN, Kriedberg C, et al. Lithogenic risk factors in the morbidly obese population. J Urol. 2008;179:1401–6.
6. Delakas D, Karyotis I, Daskalopoulos G, et al. Independent predictors of failure of shockwave lithotripsy for ureteral stones employing a second-generation lithotripter. J Endourol. 2003;17(4):201–5.
7. El-Nahas AR, El-Assmy AM, Mansour O, et al. A prospective multivariate analysis of factors predicting stone disintegration by extracorporeal shock wave lithotripsy: the value of high-resolution noncontrast computed tomography. Eur Urol. 2007;51(6): 1888–93.
8. Pearle MS, Nakada SY, Womack S, et al. Outcomes of contemporary percutaneous nephrostolithotomy in morbidly obese patients. J Urol. 1998;160:669–73.
9. Faerber GJ, Goh M. Percutaneous nephrolithotripsy in the morbidly obese patient. Tech Urol. 1997;3: 89–95.
10. Manohar T, Jain P, Desai M. Supine percutaneous nephrolithotomy: effective approach to high-risk and morbidly obese patients. J Endourol. 2007;21(1): 44–9.
11. Kerbl K, Clayman RV, Chandhoke PS, et al. Percutaneous stone removal with the patient in a flank position. J Urol. 1994;151(3):686–8.
12. Kanaroglou A, Razvi H. Percutaneous nephrolithotomy under conscious sedation in morbidly obese patients. Can J Urol. 2006;13(3):3153–5.
13. El-Assmy AM, Shokeir AA, El-Nahas AR, et al. Outcome of percutaneous nephrolithotomy: effect of body mass index. Eur Urol. 2007;52:199–204.
14. Tomaszewski JJ, Smaldone MC, Schuster T, et al. Outcomes of percutaneous nephrolithotomy stratified by body mass index. J Endourol. 2010;24(4):547–50.
15. Koo BC, Burtt G, Burgess NA. Percutaneous stone surgery in the obese: outcome stratified according to body mass index. BJU Intl. 2004;93:1296–9.
16. Bagrodia A, Gupta A, Raman JD, et al. Impact of body mass index on cost and clinical outcomes after percutaneous nephrostolithotomy. Urology. 2008;72: 756–60.
17. Sergeyev I, Koi PT, Jacobs SL, et al. Outcome of percutaneous surgery stratified according to body mass index and kidney stone size. Surg Laparosc Endosc Percutan Tech. 2007;17(3):179–83.
18. Turney BW, Reynard JM, Noble JG, et al. Trends in urological stone disease. BJU Int. 2012;109(7): 1082–7.
19. Patel T, Kozakowski K, Hruby G, et al. Skin to stone distance is an independent predictor of stone-free status following shockwave lithotripsy. J Endourol. 2009;23(9):1383–5.
20. Andreoni C, Afane J, Olweny E, et al. Flexible ureteroscopic lithotripsy: first-line therapy for proximal ureteral and renal calculi in the morbidly obese and superobese patient. J Endourol. 2001;15(5):493–8.
21. Fabrizio MD, Behari A, Bagley DH. Ureteroscopic management of intrarenal calculi. J Urol. 1998; 159:1139–43.
22. Ricchiuti DJ, Smaldone MC, Jacobs BL, et al. Staged retrograde endoscopic lithotripsy as alternative to PCNL in select patients with large renal calculi. J Endourol. 2007;21(12):1421–4.
23. Hyams ES, Munver R, Bird VG, et al. Flexible ureterorenoscopy and Holmium laser lithotripsy for the management of renal stone burdens that measure 2 to 3 cm: a multi-institutional experience. J Endourol. 2010;24(10):1583–8.
24. Grasso M, Conlin M, Bagley D. Retrograde ureteropyeloscopic treatment of 2 cm or greater upper urinary tract and minor staghorn calculi. J Urol. 1998;160:346–51.
25. Natalin R, Xavier K, Okeke Z, et al. Impact of obesity on ureteroscopic laser lithotripsy of urinary tract calculi. Int Braz J Urol. 2009;35(1):36–42.
26. Bultitude MF, Tiptaft RC, Dasgupta P, et al. Treatment of urolithiasis in the morbidly obese. Obes Surg. 2004;14(3):300–3004.

27. Nguyen TA, Belis JA. Endoscopic management of urolithiasis in the morbidly obese patient. J Endourol. 1998;12(1):30–5.
28. Best SL, Nakada SY. Flexible ureteroscopy is effective for proximal ureteral stones in both obese and nonobese patients: a two-year, single surgeon experience. Urology. 2011;77:36–9.
29. Dash A, Schuster TG, Hollenbeck BK, et al. Ureteroscopic treatment of renal calculi in morbidly obese patients: a stone-matched comparison. Urology. 2002;60:393–7.
30. Chung SY, Chon CH, Ng CS, et al. Simultaneous bilateral retrograde intrarenal surgery for stone disease in patients with significant comorbidities. J Endourol. 2006;20(10):761–5.
31. Flancbaum L, Choban PSA. Surgical implications of obesity. Annu Rev Med. 1998;49:215–34.
32. Pliskin MJ, Wikert GA, Dresner ML. Hemorrhagic complications of extracorporeal shock wave lithotripsy in an anticoagulated patient. J Endourol. 1989;3:405–9.
33. Ruiz H, Saltzman B. Aspirin-induced bilateral renal hemorrhage, after extracorporeal shock wave lithotripsy therapy: implicatiosn and conclusions. J Urol. 1990;143:791–2.
34. Klingler HC, Kramer G, Lodde M, et al. Stone treatment and coagulopathy. Eur Urol. 2003;43:5–9.
35. Kuo RL, Aslan P, Fitzgerald KB, et al. Use of ureteroscopy and Holmium:YAG laser in patients with bleeding diatheses. Urology. 1998;52:609–13.
36. Turna B, Stein RJ, Smaldone MC, et al. Safety and efficacy of flexible ureterorenoscopy and Holmium:YAG lithotripsy for intrarenal stones in anticoagulated cases. J Urol. 2008;179:1415–9.
37. Watterson JD, Girvan AR, Cook AJ, et al. Safety and efficacy of Holmium:YAG laser lithotripsy in patients with bleeding diatheses. J Urol. 2002;168:442–5.

36 Intrarenal Stenosis and Stones: Calyceal Diverticulum and Infundibular Stenosis

Steven G. Koopman and Gerhard J. Fuchs

Introduction

Calyceal diverticula of the kidney, first described in 1841 by Rayer, are nonsecretory, urothelial-lined cavities containing urine that passively originates from the adjacent collecting system [1]. The prevalence is similar in the adult and pediatric population and is observed in approximately 4.5/1,000 intravenous pyelograms [2]. Calyceal diverticula do not appear to show laterality and they occur equally in males and females.

As described more recently by Dretler, the opening and neck of the diverticulum may range from wide and short to long and narrow [3]. As the opening becomes narrower, the risk of infection and stone formation increases. The prevalence of stones associated with a calyceal diverticula ranges from 10 to 50% [4]. Most commonly, these lesions are found in the upper and midcalyceal group of the renal collecting system.

Open surgery has been historically employed for treatment of calyceal diverticula, but minimally invasive approaches including percutaneous, ureteroscopic, and laparoscopic techniques are now almost exclusively used. Although shock wave lithotripsy offers a noninvasive treatment option, stone-free rates are low (4–58%) [5–7] and the underlying condition, the poorly draining diverticulum is not addressed. While percutaneous nephrolithotomy (PCNL) has proven to have the highest success rate (>80%) for treatment of calyceal diverticula, access can be difficult in anteriorly located and in small lesions [8–10]. Also, percutaneous surgery provides the additional advantage of allowing for expeditious ablation of the diverticulum cavity and reduces the risk of recurrence [11–13]. As fiberoptic and laser technology have evolved, retrograde ureteroscopic surgery in the kidney (Retrograde Intrarenal Surgery = RIRS) for calyceal diverticula and other intrarenal stenoses associated with and precluding passage of stone or disintegrated stone gravel has become an effective, minimally invasive management strategy [14–16]. RIRS for these pathologic conditions has been proven safe and efficacious when performed on the properly selected patient, using appropriate instrumentation and technique.

Infundibular stenosis, technically a similar entity, is defined as a dilated calyx that drains through a narrow infundibulum into the renal pelvis. The difference between infundibular stenosis and calyceal diverticulum is the presence of collecting tubules within the dilated calyx. This rare condition may be congenital or acquired after previous stone treatments of infection. Usually, these lesions appear as a dilated calyx on radiographic imaging or a hydrocalyx [17].

The indications for treatment are the same as for the calyceal diverticulum. These lesions are both managed identically at our institution [18].

S.G. Koopman, M.D. • G.J. Fuchs, M.D, F.A.C.S. (✉)
Urology Division, Surgery Department,
Cedars-Sinai Medical Center, 8635 W. 3rd Street,
Suite 1070W, Los Angeles, CA 90048, USA
e-mail: gerhard.fuchs@cshs.org

M. Monga (ed.), *Ureteroscopy: Indications, Instrumentation & Technique*, Current Clinical Urology,
DOI 10.1007/978-1-62703-206-3_36, © Springer Science+Business Media New York 2013

A third entity of intrarenal pathology promoting stone disease and/or preventing stone passage is found in patients presenting with medullary sponge kidneys (MSK) and in cases where, after extracorporeal shockwave lithotripsy (E-SWL), stone gravel is retained in a blood clot and eventually becomes encased in fibrous scar tissue.

In patients with MSK stone formation is a frequent complication [19, 20]. Stone formation is promoted as the collecting ducts in the renal pyramids are dilated and cavities, clefts, and cysts form in the medulla. Rommel and Pirson described MSK as tubular ectasia and cystic dilation. Although the exact factors that lead to stone formation are not clearly understood, recurrent infection and urinary stasis within the ectatic tubules are felt to contribute to stone formation [20]. Symptomatic renal calculi are frequent complications of MSK and often these stones are also harboring bacteria resulting in relapsing UTI [20].

While these anatomic anomalies contribute to stone formation, up to greater than 80% of these patients have been found to have metabolic anomalies as well. Therefore, these patients must have metabolic evaluation and treatment to optimize stone clearance and reduce the risk of recurrence. E-SWL has long been considered as a noninvasive treatment option, but reported success rates have been as low as 18–24% [21]. At our institution we utilize RIRS with Holmium laser incision of the intrarenal "stenoses" to liberate all accessible stone in the surgical management of these problematic anatomic variants.

Similarly, stone particles retained after E-SWL can be not infrequently found trapped in fibrinous scar tissue precluding their passage. This condition can be found when the mild bleeding caused by E-SWL energy encases the stone gravel with a blood clot before the stone gravel can be discharged from the—often dependent—calyx. The blood then gets organized in a fibrinous scar encasing the stone gravel and thus preventing passage.

In this chapter, we review the indications for treatment of renal stones complicated by different conditions of intrarenal stenosis, specifically discuss the technical aspects of retrograde ureteroscopic intrarenal surgery for the minimally invasive management of these complex conditions, and present results for calyceal diverticulum and infundibular stenosis.

Indications and Patient Selection

Treatment indications for calyceal diverticula and other forms of intrarenal stenoses relate to the associated complications. Many calyceal diverticula are asymptomatic and may not require intervention. Pain is the most common complaint and occurs in approximately 50% of patients [17, 22, 23]. Calculi occur within diverticula in 11–50% of patients [17, 22, 23]. Other symptoms requiring intervention include recurrent infection and hematuria related to the diverticulum.

While E-SWL is the first treatment of choice for greater than 80% of renal calculi, patients with stones trapped behind narrow intrarenal segments such as stones in a calyceal diverticulum or stones behind a stricture are not ideal candidates for E-SWL, since passage of the fragmented debris will not clear in most and symptoms may persist or recur. Therefore, endoscopic surgeries such as RIRS, percutaneous renal surgery (PRS) with PCNL, and laparoscopic surgery are preferred to remove such stones and provide the opportunity to also repair the underlying anatomical abnormality [10–13, 24].

Clinical decision-making for the treatment of stones contained in a calyceal diverticulum or trapped behind a stenotic segment of the renal collecting system is based on (1) symptoms requiring intervention, (2) location and orientation of the diverticulum, (3) size of the diverticulum, (4) stone burden within the diverticulum, and (5) outcome of initially chosen treatment.

Upper and midrenal location are ideal for the RIRS approach, whereas for lower pole diverticula PRS (with PCNL) is used if RIRS is not readily feasible; usually under the same anesthesia. Anterior or posterior locations are likewise suited for the RIRS approach, whereas for PRS the posterior location is ideal as it allows for a direct approach and for anterior locations the indirect approach is preferable to avoid a longer trajectory through parenchyma and increased risk of bleeding complications.

Diverticulum size of less than 2 cm (and stone burden less than 1.5 cm) are well suited for the RIRS approach. For larger intact stones (up to 1.5 cm) intracorporeal (Holmium laser) and extracorporeal (SWL) energy sources can be employed simultaneously to accelerate the fragmentation process. Diverticulum size of greater than 2 cm (and larger stone burden) favor the PRS (PCNL) approach and with diverticulum size greater than 3 cm PRS fulguration is best performed after stone removal (especially for a diverticulum in a dependent location) [12, 13]. Failure of RIRS to achieve anatomical repair and/or stone clearance may require PRS as a secondary procedure if stones or symptoms persist or recur (principle of increasing invasiveness). In such cases of a lower pole location with posterior location PRS with subsequent fulguration of the mucosa is the first choice, and for anterior lower pole location PRS with indirect (upper pole) access or laparoscopic surgery. For larger diverticulum sizes between 2 and 4 cm, laparoscopic surgery can be employed for anterior orientation and lower pole locations, whereas PRS is an option for posterior orientation in upper and midpolar location. Diverticulum size of greater than 4 cm usually is managed primarily with laparoscopic surgery.

MSK stones and stone gravel trapped in fibrinous encasement can be accessed and treated successfully by RIRS usually in the entire renal collecting system and PRS is only employed when there is a very large stone burden in the collecting system as well.

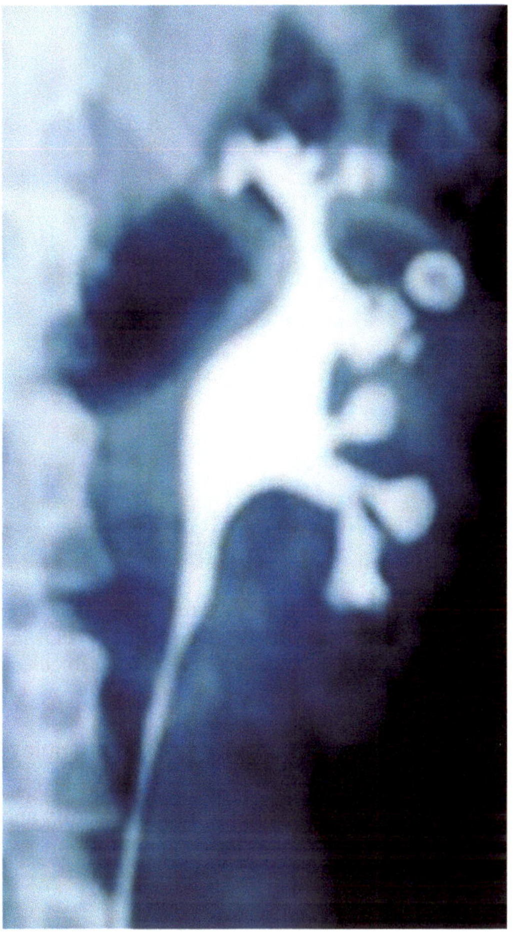

Fig. 36.1 Retrograde pyelogram showing midrenal calyceal diverticulum; stone seen as filling defect

Preoperative Preparation

Contrast imaging with an intravenous pyelogram or a CT urogram should be obtained to provide information on potential anatomic difficulties and serve as an anatomic guide (Figs. 36.1 and 36.2a, b).

Before performing RIRS, an existing urinary infection must be treated with culture-directed antibiotics. A sterile urine culture should be confirmed within 5 days of the planned surgery. Broad-spectrum or culture-specific antibiotics should be utilized preoperatively for prophylaxis. In patients with relapsing UTI antibiotic coverage should be started prior to the procedure even when the preoperative urine is found to show no growth.

RIRS is best performed in the intubated patient under general anesthesia in the lithotomy position. Occasionally, a procedure can be performed with regional anesthesia or even local anesthesia but kidney movement with extensive breathing excursion may increase the technical difficulty of performing the delicate instrumentation. At our institution, the procedure is performed as a day-surgery case, with plans for the patient to return home under supervision the same evening. The procedure is performed on a multipurpose endoscopy and lithotripsy table (Modulith, Karl Storz Medical; Kreuzlingen, Switzerland), which allows for endoscopic surgery with real-time

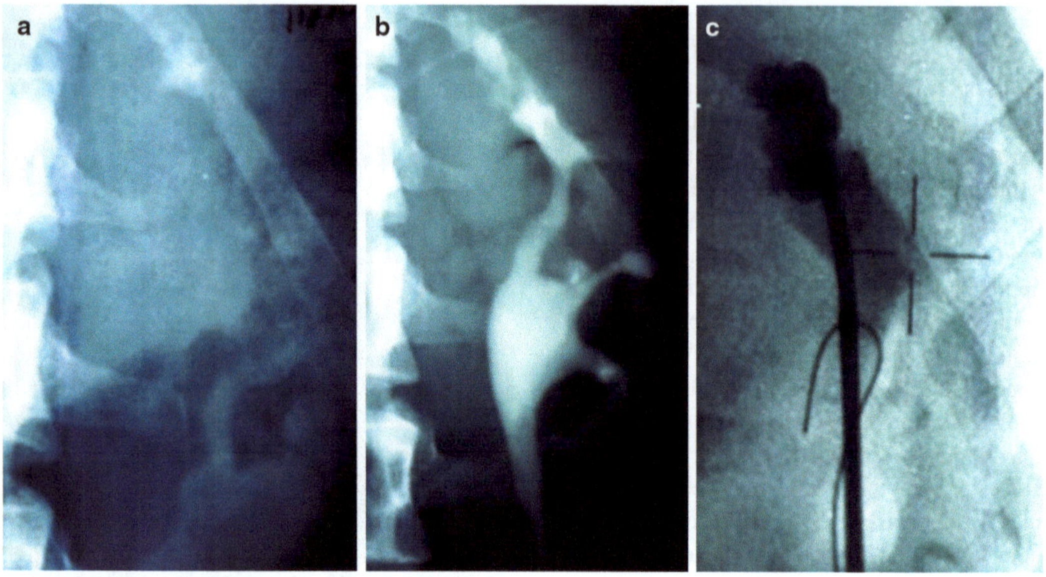

Fig. 36.2 (**a**) KUB depicting well fragmented stone after E-SWL in upper pole of left kidney. (**b**) IVP showing the stone gravel in an upper pole calyceal diverticulum. (**c**) Flexible ureteroscope at the mouth of a stone-bearing diverticulum. Contrast injection delineates the spacious diverticulum cavity

fluoroscopy as well as the simultaneous employment of E-SWL during RIRS for larger stone burden or stone portions which cannot be readily and safely accessed with the flexible endoscope.

Equipment

Table 36.1 lists the equipment commonly used at our institution for RIRS and the treatment of calyceal diverticulum and infundibular stenosis (Table 36.1).

Access to the Kidney

After cystoscopy, a retrograde pyelography is performed under fluoroscopic control; the film is stored for further reference during the procedure. After a safety 0.038-in. guide wire is placed into the renal pelvis, diuresis is induced with furosemide (weight adjusted; 0.25 mg/kg) to reduce the risk of pyelorenal reflux and infectious complications.

If there is no previous stenting, we routinely use a graduated 9.5-Fr semirigid ureteroscope to optically dilate the ureter in preparation for flexible upper tract endoscopic surgery. The semirigid instrument is advanced over a second 0.038-in. working wire under direct vision as far as the scope can reach and then is withdrawn. In cases where the semirigid ureteroscope cannot be advanced into the ureter, an indwelling stent is placed to allow the narrow ureter to passively dilate for 10–14 days. Access to the kidney is then usually possible without difficulty.

If a stent was placed previously, it is removed after a safety wire has been placed into the kidney. A flexible ureterorenoscopy (7.5-Fr) is then advanced into the kidney alongside the safety wire. If difficulty engaging the orifice is encountered, the scope can be railroaded over a second working wire and up into the renal pelvis. Access sheaths are rarely used in a straightforward case, but they can be helpful in cases of patients with coagulopathy (reduced risk of bleeding), in cases of larger stone burden in the kidney (improved visibility and more expeditious removal of stone particles), and occasionally for increasing fulcrum to negotiate a tight access of the scope into a stenotic area in the kidney.

Table 36.1 Equipment for retrograde intrarenal surgery for calyceal diverticula and intrarenal stenoses

Basic equipment (manufacturer)	Alternatives
21-F rigid cystoscope (Karl Storz)[a]	Wolf[b], Olympus[c], ACMI[d] scopes
9.5-F semirigid ureteroscope (Karl Storz)[a]	Ureteral balloon dilator set
	Ureteral serial dilator set (Cook, Microvasive)
7.5-F flexible ureteroscope (FleXX2, Karl Storz) (Olympus-ACMI[d])[a]	
Holmium laser system w/200 μm fiber (ACMI-Dornier)	3-Fr EHL (Calcutript, Storz)
	1.6-Fr EHL (Storz)[a]
	3-Fr Bugbee electrode
Nitinol tipless basket (Cook)	4 wire baskets
	2/3 pronged grasper (Cook, Microvasive)
5-F angiographic catheter (Cook)	
0.038-in. Bentson wire (Cook)	0.038-in. or 0.035-in. straight wire
Double-J stent (Cook, Microvasive)	
Xenon light source, irrigation tubing, suction apparatus	
Optional equipment (manufacturer)	
0.035-in. Glide wire (Microvasive)	
8-Fr or 10-Fr coaxial catheters (Cook, Microvasive)	
Multi-purpose endoscopy table with fluoroscopy and simultaneous E-SWL (Storz Modulith , Dornier MFL5000, Siemens Lithostar)	

[a]Karl Storz Endoscopy-America, Inc, Culver City, CA
[b]Wolf Medical Instruments Corp, Thousand Oaks, CA
[c]Olympus America, Inc, Melville, NY
[d]Circon ACMI Corp, Stamford, CT

RIRS for Intrarenal Stenoses

Flexible upper tract endoscopy with analog—and more recently digital—ureterorenoscopes allows selective and complete evaluation of the entire renal collecting system in all but rare cases of severely abnormal intrarenal anatomy. Using a camera system with up to 15 times magnification, the intrarenal pathology such as the entry point to the narrow diverticulum or stenosed calyceal neck, the area of MSK stones protruding from under the papilla, or the area of stone gravel encased in fibrinous matrix can be identified. The access point to a diverticulum usually presents itself as a small dimple, anywhere from the fornix of the calyx to the infundibulum. Dilute contrast is injected through the scope directly into the area of the perceived opening to identify and confirm the diverticulum fluoroscopically (Fig. 36.2c). If a diverticulum or stenotic segment fills with contrast but the entry point is not clearly identifiable, the so-called "Blue Spritz" technique can be used. Saline colored by methylene blue is instilled through the work channel of the flexible scope into the collecting system. The whole system then is decompressed by suction. Residual blue dye trapped in the diverticulum then slowly trickles out from the stenotic area thus allowing the identification of the entry point.

Once the access into the diverticulum is identified, a 0.038-in. guide wire is advanced through the 7.5-Fr flexible ureteroscope past the neck into the diverticulum, and an attempt is made to coil as much of the wire as possible inside. The instrument is cautiously withdrawn, leaving the guide wire coiled in the diverticulum. The instrument then is reintroduced alongside the guide wire and advanced back up into the kidney. At this point, access of the ureteroscope into the diverticulum is negotiated. Depending on the length and width of the "infundibulum" access is gained either by advancing the scope over a second guide wire in case of a wider, accommodating "infundibulum" or by performing a Holmium laser incision of the intrarenal stricture with a 200 μm laser fiber in case of a short "infundibulum." In case of a longer, narrow access a 3-Fr zero-tip dilating balloon (Microvasive) which dilates up to 12 Fr can be inserted through the work channel of the 7.5-Fr flexible ureteroscope and is inflated under fluoroscopic or endoscopic control [18]. So incision of the neck with the Holmium laser is used for short connections into a wide diverticulum or when the diverticulum presents as an area of bulging mucosa. Balloon dilation is preferred for longer connections as the use of the laser incision in such circumstances would have a higher risk of bleeding and extravasation. The flexible ureteroscope is then advanced into the diverticulum, while the surgeon inspects the neck for adequacy of dilatation and the stone/s can then be treated.

RIRS for Stones in a Diverticulum

If the neck accommodates a Nitinol tipless basket (Cook), stones less than 5 mm may be removed intact with the basket. The tipless basket reduces risk of mucosal trauma with forward basketing. Stones that are too large for direct removal are fragmented and vaporized with the Holmium laser using a 200 μm laser fiber. Larger stones can be treated expeditiously by simultaneously employing intracorporeal laser lithotripsy and E-SWL. Fragments are then removed actively with the Nitinol basket if they are larger than 3 mm; the rest are flushed out of the diverticulum and are left for spontaneous passage from the renal collecting system.

In a first time treatment of a diverticulum containing stone usually no attempt is made to fulgurate the mucosa of the diverticulum since there is no data to suggest that this maneuver reduces stone recurrence or infection.

Once stone treatment is completed we place a double-J pigtail stent across the widened infundibulum and coil it in the diverticulum cavity if space permits this. Otherwise, the upper curl may be placed in the renal pelvis. The distal placement of the stent then is checked endoscopically. A Foley catheter is placed in the bladder and withdrawn in recovery before patient discharge.

RIRS for Stones Associated with MSK or Retained in Fibrinous Matrix after E-SWL

In patients with MSK and stones, the first step of RIRS is to assess the renal collecting system and to "take inventory" of all stones freely mobile in the collecting system (target 1) and of the stones trapped partially under mucosa (target 2). The target 2 areas are marked on a stored retrograde pyelogram film with a marker so as to assure eventual complete removal of all accessible stone. Depending on the overall stone burden in the kidney simultaneous E-SWL can be utilized to accelerate stone fragmentation. If simultaneous E-SWL is performed the Holmium laser incision of tissue trapping the partially exposed stones is performed first to ascertain optimal visibility as the use of E-SWL will cause some minor oozing from the parenchyma which may compromise visibility for precise and safe Laser incision. The laser incision itself basically does not result in any bleeding as the tissue covering the stones is thin and rarely vascularized. "Liberation" of trapped MSK stones is usually started in the lower pole region as access and treatment of the lower pole is technically more challenging and therefore is best undertaken first. Using the roadmap retrograde pyelogram we approach all calyces from the bottom up until all are accessible, i.e., visible stone has been addressed.

In patients with stone gravel retained in fibrinous matrix after E-SWL usually only one calyx is involved and this is mostly in the lower pole or an otherwise dependent calyx. Careful inspection of the renal collecting system using the plain KUB film and the retrograde pyelogram for guidance will allow identification of the stone-bearing calyx. In most cases a small piece of stone may be seen poking through the matrix or the irregular appearance of the occluded calyx will identify the location (Fig. 36.3a). Holmium laser incision is then cautiously performed to liberate the stones which usually are found well fragmented and can be removed completely with Nitinol baskets (Figs. 36.3b–d and 36.4).

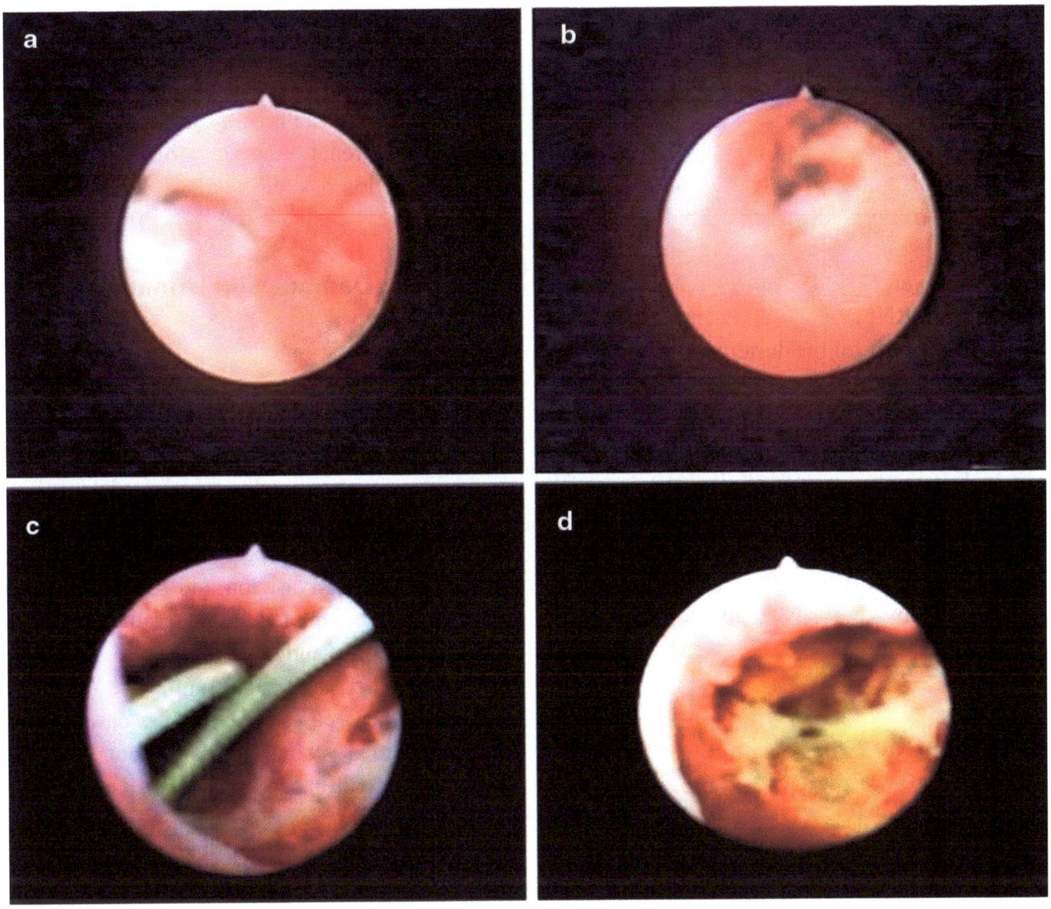

Fig. 36.3 (**a**) Retained stones after E-SWL with calyx occluded by fibrinous matrix. (**b**) Retained stone seen through fibrinous tissue after initial Holmium laser incision. (**c**) The fibrinous tissue entrapping the stone gravel has been incised and a wire keeps the calyx open to allow for wash out of the stone gravel. (**d**) The last residual stone piece before basketing from the now widely patent calyx

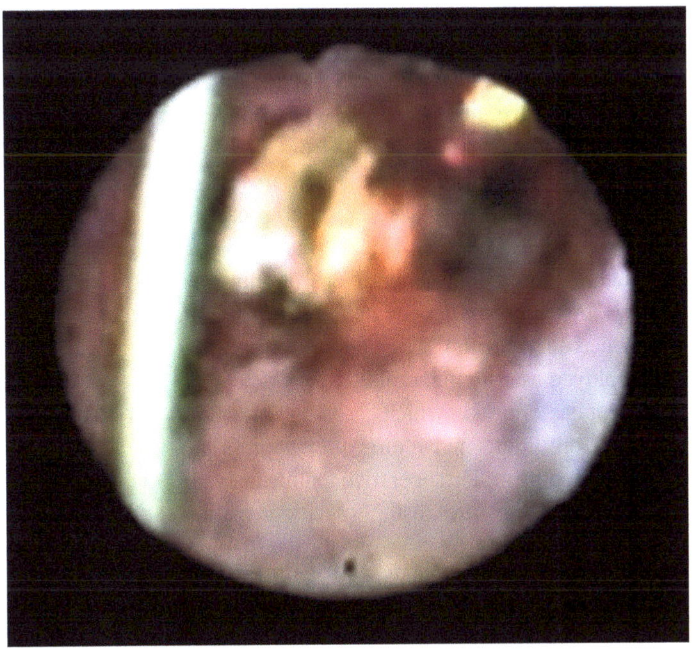

Fig. 36.4 Depicts Holmium laser incision of stone partially exposed in MSK kidney

Postoperative Care

Most patients can be discharged on the day of surgery barring medical comorbid conditions requiring observation after anesthesia. Discharge medications are usually Pyridium TID × 3 days and Norco PRN; as long as a stent remains, we prescribe Flomax for the duration to reduce stent-related discomfort. Oral antibiotic coverage is routinely continued for 3 days, in patients with previous infection for 7 days or until after stent removal. Patients return to clinic 7–10 days after the procedure for reevaluation and possible stent removal. Once a renal ultrasound confirms no residual stone or hydronephrosis, the indwelling stent is removed cystoscopically under local anesthesia.

Complications

Infection

As urinary tract infection is often found in patients with stones and intrarenal stenosis, special attention has to be placed on ruling out infection preoperatively and if present treat appropriately prior to proceeding with RIRS. Untreated bacteriuria is an absolute contraindication to RIRS. Ideally, the urine should be sterile at the time of surgery; if previous cultures were positive, appropriate antibiotic therapy for at least 5 days before the procedure should have been instituted. If persistent infection is suspected, especially from the contents of the diverticulum or stone/s harboring bacteria, a stent should be placed and the procedure deferred for at least 1 week with further antibiotic coverage. At times, intraoperative urine-dipstick analysis to check for leucocytes and nitrites or urine microscopy with Gram staining for bacteria are employed as a simple, rapid ways of detecting persistent bacteriuria in which case it is prudent to abort the procedure and return after appropriate antibiotic treatment. Intraoperative maintenance of low intrarenal pressures using gravity irrigation only (no pressurized irrigation) and the use of intravenous diuretics are important measures to decrease the risk of pyelovenous reflux and infectious complications. In cases of prolonged intrarenal surgery the use of an access sheath is also helpful to keep intrarenal pressures low and thereby reduce infection risk.

Iatrogenic Damage and Urinary Extravasation

Laser incision of the stenotic calyceal or diverticulum neck or a perforation through a diverticulum may result in extravasation into the renal parenchyma or perirenally, which is detected on retrograde pyelography. In such cases maintenance of low intrarenal pressures reduces the risk of significant extravasation and some cases can be cautiously completed but generally it is better to abort the case and place a stent to minimize extravasation. Postoperative antibiotic coverage is used in these cases. Usually, the case can be completed in a second session about 2 weeks later. Ultrasound is used postoperatively to rule out significant extravasation.

Bleeding

Infundibular vessels may be disturbed with incision of a stenotic intrarenal segment or neck of a diverticulum. Therefore, laser incision is only performed for short strictures to avoid visually uncontrolled incision and higher risk of bleeding. Any amount of bleeding may impede vision and jeopardize the procedure. In this scenario, the procedure should be terminated and a stent placed. Expectant management is usually successful and transfusion is rare. If bleeding persists, arteriography and embolization should be considered. When the hematuria has ceased, a second elective procedure may be planned.

Treatment Results

The technique of flexible ureterorenoscopy for treatment of stones retained in calyceal diverticula after E-SWL was described in 1989 as one of the early complex RIRS procedures (Table 36.2) [14]. Access to the diverticulum was identified, a

Table 36.2 Results of retrograde intrarenal surgery for calyceal diverticula

Author	No.	Diverticula management	Lithotripsy	Symptom free (%)	Stone-free rate (%)	Complications (%)
Fuchs et al. [14]	15	Balloon	EHL, SWL	87	73	
Batter and Dretler [16]	26	Balloon	EHL, dye laser	100	95	15
Grasso et al. [15]	2	Balloon or incision			50	0
Chong et al. [18]	96	Balloon or Incision	EHL, Holmium, SWL	95	90	
Auge et al. [25]	17	Balloon or incision	Holmium	35	18	10
Sejiny et al. [26]	15		Holmium	90	55	

guide wire placed and dilation of the diverticular neck was performed initially with a 7-Fr balloon under fluoroscopic control. Stones were fragmented with the electrohydraulic lithotriptor or E-SWL under the same anesthesia. Fragments were removed under direct endoscopic vision with a basket or grasper, or (if <1 mm) were left to pass spontaneously. A double-J stent was left for 3 weeks. Of 15 patients treated in this way, 13 had upper- or midpolar diverticula. Eleven patients (73%) became **stone-free at a mean follow-up of 7.4 months. There were no stone recurrences during this time [14].

Grasso et al. in 1995 described an approach combining retrograde, percutaneous access in two patients with large stone burdens. Four patients were treated. Two patients were managed only with flexible URS. The remaining patients required a combined percutaneous and retrograde approach. In the retrograde only group, a flexible ureteroscope was passed into the kidney over a guide wire. The diverticulum was then intubated with a hollow-core injectable guide wire. Contrast was injected to opacifiy the diverticulum. The diverticular neck was then dilated with a 3-Fr, 2 cm balloon passed through the ureteroscope. In those requiring both percutaneous and retrograde approach, a wire was placed percutaneously into the diverticulum then retrieved by an ensnaring device placed retrograde. The wire was pulled into the urethra. The remainder of the procedure was primarily a percutaneous with dilatation of the tract, ultrasonic lithotripsy, and then fulguration of the mucosa. All three cases were treated successfully this way (Table 36.2) [15].

Batter and Dretler performed URS on 26 patients with symptomatic diverticula. The neck was dilated with a 3-F Bagley balloon. Pulsed-dye laser or EHL was used for stone fragmentation. Three patients required secondary percutaneous treatment and one had a partial nephrectomy. Overall, 18 (69%) cases were treated successfully. The remainder required adjunctive E-SWL. At a mean follow-up of 45 months, 1 of the 18 cases treated successfully with URS had residual stones, but all remained asymptomatic. Lower pole diverticula only had a 29% success rate. Four patients were hospitalized for complications related to pain control, bleeding, and sepsis (Table 36.2) [16].

Chong et al. reviewed 96 patients with stone containing calyceal diverticula. 10% had lower pole diverticula. The neck was either balloon dilated or incised with a Bugbee electrode or Holmium laser. Stones were fragmented with Holmium laser or electrohydraulic energy and E-SWL. Stones were removed with basket. The diverticular neck was identified and incised in 95% of cases and 90% were considered stone-free. The failures occurred in the lower pole diverticula. These patients had percutaneous access performed in the same session. Only 8% had stone or symptom recurrence over an 8 year period (Table 36.2) [18].

Auge et al. reviewed 17 patients with symptomatic stone-bearing calyceal diverticula treated with RIRS. Four patients required PCNL because diverticula were not able to be identified by URS. Three had PCNL because of persistent pain and retained stones. Of the ten treated only with URS, three were stone-free and seven were symptom-free (Table 36.2) [25].

Finally, Sejiny et al. recently reviewed 38 patients with symptomatic stone-bearing calyceal diverticula. URS was used in 30 patients as an alternative after failed E-SWL. Two patients required repeat URS. In one patient, the diverticulum was not initially identified, and the other had incomplete stone fragmentation. Thirty-one patients were considered successful (21 were stone free and 10 had clinically insignificant fragments), and 34 were symptom-free (Table 36.2) [26].

Conclusions

Calyceal diverticula and infundibular stenosis have traditionally required invasive techniques for management. With the evolution of flexible ureteroscopy technique and advances in the instrumentation, RIRS offers a safe, minimally invasive technique in the appropriately selected patients. While there is still a role for percutaneous, laparoscopic and open surgery, RIRS appears to have equal success in the appropriately selected patient with low complication rate. Other intrarenal conditions preventing stone passage such as stones associated with MSK and stones retained in fibrinous matrix after E-SWL can be readily treated also with the RIRS technique.

References

1. Rayer. P. Traits des maladies des reins. Bailliere: Paris 1841; 3: 407.
2. Timmons Jr JW, Malek RS, Hattery RR, Deweed JH. Calyceal diverticulum. J Urol. 1975;114:6–9.
3. Dretler SP. A new useful classification of calyceal diverticula. J Endourol 1992; 6 (suppl): 81.
4. Middleton Jr AW, Pfister RC. Stone-containing pyelocalyceal diverticulum: embryogenic, anatomic, radiologic, and clinical characteristics. J Urol. 1974;111:2.
5. Jones JA, Lingeman JE, Steidle CP. The role of extracorporeal shock wave lithotripsy and percutaneous nephrostolithotomy in the management of pyelocaliceal diverticula. J Urol. 1991;146:724.
6. Psihramis KE, Dretler SP. Extracorporeal shock wave lithotripsy of caliceal diverticula calculi. J Urol. 1987;138:707.
7. Hendrikx AJ, Bierkens AF, Bos R, et al. Treatment of stones in caliceal diverticula: extracorporeal shockwave lithotripsy versus percutaneous nephrolitholapaxy. Br J Urol. 1992;70:478.
8. Bellman GC, Silverstein JL, et al. Technique and follow-up of percutaneous management of caliceal diverticula. Urology. 1993;42:21.
9. Gluckman GR, Stoller M, Irby P. Laparoscopic pyelocaliceal diverticula ablation. J Endourol. 1993;7:315.
10. Shalhav AL, Soble JJ, Nakada SY, et al. Long-term outcome of caliceal diverticula following percutaneous endosurgical management. J Urol. 1998;160(5): 1635–9.
11. Al-Basam S, Bennett JD, Layton ZA, Denstedt JD, Razvi H. Treatment of caliceal diverticular stones: transdiverticular percutaneous nephrolithotomy with creation of neoinfundibulum. J Vascular Intervent Radiol. 2000;11(7):885–9.
12. Monga M, Smith R, Ferral H, Thomas R. Percutaneous ablation of caliceal diverticulum: long-term follow-up. J Urol. 2000;163(1):28.
13. Schwartz BF, Stoller ML. Percutaneous management of caliceal diverticula. Urol Clinics of N Am. 2000;27(4):635–45.
14. Fuchs GJ, David RD. Flexible ureterorenoscopy, dilation of narrow caliceal neck and ESWL: a new minimally invasive approach to stones in calicealdiverticulua. J Endourol. 1989;3:255–63.
15. Grasso M, Lang G, Loisides P, et al. Endoscopic management of the symptomatic caliceal diverticular calculus. J Urol. 1878;1995:153.
16. Batter SJ, Dretler SP. Ureteroscopic approach to the symptomatic caliceal diverticulum. J Urol. 1997;158: 709–13.
17. Abeshouse BS. Serous cysts of the kidney and their differentiation from other cystic diseases of the kidneys. Urol Cutaneous Rev. 1950;54:582–602.
18. Chong T, Bui M, Fuchs G. Calyceal diverticula ureteroscopic management. Urol Clin North Am. 2000;27(4):647–54.
19. Rommel D, Pirson Y. Medullary sponge kidney—part of a congenital syndrome. Nephrol Dial Transplant. 2001;16(3):634–6.
20. Ginalski JM, et al. Does medullary sponge kidney cause nephrolithiasis? AJR Am J Roentgenol. 1990;155:299–302.
21. Gallucci M, et al. Extracorporeal shock wave lithotripsy in ureteral and kidney malformations. Urol Int. 2001;66(2):61–5.
22. Hsu TH, Streem SB. Metabolic abnormalities in patients with caliceal diverticular calculi. J Urol. 1998;160:1640.
23. Liatsikos EN, Bernardo NO, Dinlenc CZ, et al. Caliceal diverticular calculi: is there a role for metabolic evaluation ? J Urol. 2000;164(1):18–20.
24. Hoznek A, Herard A, Ogiez N, et al. Symptomatic caliceal diverticula treated with extraperitoneal laparoscopic marsupialization, fulguration and gelatin resorcinol formaldehyde glue obliteration. J Urol. 1998;160:352.
25. Auge BK, Munver R, Kourambas J, Newman GE, Preminger GM. Endoscopic management of symptomatic caliceal diverticula: a retrospective comparison of percutaneous nephrolithotripsy and ureteroscopy. J Endourol 2002;16:557–63.
26. Senjiny M, Al-Qahtani A, Elhaous A, Molimard B, Traxer O. Efficacy of flexible ureterorenoscopy with holmium laser in the management of stone-bearing caliceal diverticula. J Endourol 2010;24 (6): 961–67.

Part VI

Complications of Ureteroscopy

Complications of Ureteroscopy

37

David A. Leavitt, J. Kyle Anderson, and Sean P. Elliott

Introduction

The first documented ureteroscopy occurred in 1912 when Hugh Hampton Young advanced a pediatric cystoscope into the dilated ureter of a child with posterior urethral valves [1]. Ureteroscopy for upper tract urolithiasis disease took hold in the 1980s. Since then, significant advances in technology have allowed for the application of ureteroscopy in the diagnosis and management of myriad upper urinary tract pathology including surveillance and treatment of upper tract urothelial carcinoma. Small caliber ureteroscopes, improved optics, and refinement in surgical technique have made ureteroscopy incredibly safe in the modern era (Table 37.1).

Nonetheless, ureteroscopy is not without its complications and overall major complications of ureteroscopy, either for diagnostic or therapeutic purposes range between 0 and 2% [2–5]. Currently, there exists no standardization for reporting complications of ureteroscopy and this must be kept in mind when evaluating the literature. At least one recent study used the modified Clavien morbidity score to classify complications of ureteroscopy and suggested this as a means to standardize reporting [6].

D.A. Leavitt, M.D. • J.K. Anderson, M.D. (✉)
S.P. Elliott, M.D.
Department of Urology, University of Minnesota, MMC 394 Mayo, 420 Delaware St SE, Minneapolis, MN 55455, USA
e-mail: ande1821@umn.edu; jka42@hotmail.com

Most reports on the complications of ureteroscopy tend to follow a similar classification schema and organize complications by chronology and by severity. A similar approach will be followed here and complications will be classified as intraoperative, early postoperative, or late postoperative. The significance of the complication will be classified as major if significant further surgical or medical therapy is required or if the complication is life-threatening and minor if nonoperative management or minimal intervention will be corrective.

Intraoperative Complications

Minor Complications

Failure to Access the Upper Tract

Inability to safely access the upper urinary tract for diagnostic or therapeutic purposes is not well reported. Problems with access range from 1.6 to 8.4% [4, 7, 8]. Common locations that may present access challenges include the ureteral orifice, a narrow intramural ureter, and unfavorable calyceal anatomy with acute angles and long narrow infundibula [9]. Ureteral strictures or impacted ureteral wall stones, which may present at any location, can preclude ureteroscopic advancement. Anatomic anomalies and variations such as severe spinal column angulation, external ureteral compression, renal and ureteral ectopia, prior ureteral reimplantation, cystoceles in women, and benign prostatic enlargement in

M. Monga (ed.), *Ureteroscopy: Indications, Instrumentation & Technique*, Current Clinical Urology,
DOI 10.1007/978-1-62703-206-3_37, © Springer Science+Business Media New York 2013

Table 37.1 Reported complications[a] from ureteroscopy series comprising ≥200 ureteroscopies

Author	No. of ureteroscopies	Avulsion	Major perforation[b]	Minor perforation	Mucosal abrasion	Stricture
Netto [44]	483	0.8%	–	5.8%	0.2%	0.6%
Grasso [12]	1,000	0%	0%	0.4%	–	0.4%
Abdel-Razzak [10]	290	–	0%	1.7%	–	0.7%
Harmon [29]	209	0%	0%	1%	–	0.5%
Puppo [45]	378	0.26%	0%	1.3%	–	0%
Butler [30]	2,273	0.04%	0.08%	0.79%	0.3%	–
Blute [11]	346	0.6%	–	4.6%	0.3%	1.4%
Jeromin [31]	1,575	–	0.3%	0.3%	1.3%	0.4%
Totals	6,554	0.28%	0.06%	1.99%	0.52%	0.58%

[a]Complication rates refer to total number of ureteroscopies
[b]Major perforation is defined by requiring open surgical repair
From [19] with permission from Elsevier

men may also pose access difficulties. Ureteral injury such as mucosal flaps or ureteral perforation can also limit safe retrograde access.

When access problems are encountered, the safest option is to place a ureteral stent and allow for passive ureteral dilation over 1–2 weeks with an attempt at repeat ureteroscopy thereafter. This can reduce the risk of avoidable ureteral injury. In one single-institution retrospective review of 322 ureteroscopies which sought to determine factors predictive of ureteroscopic complications, one third of the ureteral perforations were associated with balloon dilation of the ureteral orifice or trying to manipulate a wire past an obstructing stone [7]. When access to the upper urinary tract is still not possible despite passive ureteral dilation with a stent, a percutaneous antegrade approach may be considered as well.

Bleeding

Bleeding during ureteroscopy is rarely of significant concern and it is only in the exceptional case that intervention is necessary beyond procedure termination and possibly ureteral stenting. Procedure termination is a result of compromised visualization from intraluminal bleeding. Most often bleeding is encountered with ureteral orifice dilation, mucosal, or calyceal injury from wire or ureteroscope trauma, or during stone lasing and manipulation. The incidence of bleeding severe enough to cause premature termination of ureteroscopy has been reported between 0.1 and 2.1% [4, 10–12]. Abdel-Razzak and Bagley reviewed 290 flexible ureteroscopies performed in the late 1980s and early 1990s for urolithiasis and upper tract urothelial carcinoma. They experienced two aborted procedures secondary to bleeding severe enough to limit vision. Geavlete et al., the largest of these series, retrospectively reviewed 2,735 semirigid ureteroscopies at a single center between 1994 and 2005 with three cases prematurely aborted because of bleeding limiting visualization. In all cases a ureteral stent was placed and the bleeding resolved. None of these cases required a blood transfusion.

A single case report described a significant delayed bleed after uncomplicated ureteroscopy and holmium laser lithotripsy for a 0.8 × 0.9 cm right proximal ureteral stone. The patient required a transfusion of 4 units of packed red blood cells and eventual angioembolization of a lower pole arteriovenous fistula [13]. Interestingly, the patient had undergone failed shockwave lithotripsy (SWL) 2 months prior. Endoureterotomy or endopyelotomy is another instance where significant bleeding may be encountered if a crossing vessel is injured. Prevention of this serious complication is through analysis of preoperative cross-sectional imaging such as computed tomography angiogram, careful selection of incision location away from likely artery location, and thorough ureteroscopic inspection for arterial pulsation at the incision site prior to incision. If bleeding does occur, placement of a large ureteral balloon dilator (24–30 Fr) can help temporize the bleeding to all for further intervention such as angioembolization.

In general, careful technique and fastidious use of lasers and other instruments can help minimize potential bleeding and allow for successful ureteroscopy even in anticoagulated patients and those with bleeding diatheses [14].

Thermal Tissue Damage

Modern ureteroscopes are well insulated and if maintained properly should not cause ureteral thermal injury. Some of the instruments commonly used during uretersocopy, such as lasers and electrohydraulic lithotripters can cause thermal damage to the ureter. This complication is rarely reported. The Holmium:YAG laser was reported to cause a ureteral perforation in 1 patient out of 598 patients (0.2%) undergoing laser lithotripsy in a large prospective study between 1993 and 1999 [15]. Ureteral mucosal spark damage from the electrohydraulic lithotripter was reported to cause ureteral perforations in 2 patients out of 198 patients (1%) with ureteral or renal stones in a separate study between 1985 and 1991 [16]. Three cases (0.1%) of mucosal thermal injury were reported in a more contemporary series of 2,275 semirigid ureteroscopies [4]. Comparisons between the two instruments have shown no difference in complication rates [17].

Proper technique during lithotripsy including avoiding direct contact with the ureteral wall and aiming the energy source parallel rather than perpendicular to the ureteral wall, should minimize thermal tissue damage. If there is concern for thermal injury, ureteral stent placement is prudent. Four to six weeks after ureteral stent removal, renal ultrasound can be used as a screen for ureteral stricture formation, as this has been reported after thermal injuries [18].

Instrument Malfunction

Successful ureteroscopy depends on the proper function of multiple instruments and technologies including the endoscope, light source, lithotripsy device, stone basket, biopsy forceps, and digital camera. Any of these may be damaged during surgical use or during processing and sterilization. Baskets may break when extracting larger stone fragments that become lodged within the ureter or within the calyces when acute angles are present. Laser fibers may crack within the sheath of the ureterscope and cause unintentional damage to the scope or patient. On very rare occasions the ureteroscope may fracture within the ureter [9].

Broken or entrapped baskets can be challenging problems. This is most often encountered during stone basket extraction of larger stones or fragments. Tipped baskets that break often have wire fragments extending out toward the ureteral wall [19]. Tipless baskets have less of a tendency to do this and are safer from this perspective. Many strategies have been suggested. Clearing the engaged stone first can allow safer manipulation of the basket. Cutting or lasering the remaining intact basket wires can help disengage most of the basket. Then grasping the remaining portion of the basket may be easier. The remaining portion of the basket can also be carefully manipulated so that the tip of the basket is angled down the ureter and then removed tip first. In this orientation ureteral injury is less likely. Alternatively, trying to backload a small catheter over the basket may sheath the broken wire fragments and protect the ureter with basket removal through the catheter [19].

Ureteroscopy accessories such as basket retrieval devices and laser fibers are usually easily replaced. Malfunctioning or damaged ureteroscopes often require manufacturer repair, which are expensive and can represent a majority of the cost of a flexible ureteroscopy program over time [20]. Instrument malfunction is likely underreported, and has ranged in incidence from 0.7 to 1.9% [4, 7, 10]. Unfortunately all ureteroscopes require repair at some point, and a prospective comparison of four contemporary ureteroscopes showed three of the four to have relatively similar durability with approximately 17–18 uses before repair was necessary [21]. However, the fourth ureteroscope required repair after only approximately five uses, though the authors did not comment further as to the differences.

Proper technique during ureteroscope use is important to reducing preventable damage to instruments. The ureteroscope should be straight when advancing and removing instruments through the working channel. Ureteral access sheaths and small laser fibers and baskets can minimize deflexion strain on ureteroscopes and improve longevity [22].

Ureteroscope processing, sterilization, and storage is another source of preventable damage and has been of increased interest recently. Specific causes of ureteroscope damage include overcurling of the scope during storage, improper cleansing techniques, and closing the storage case onto the ureteroscope shaft [23]. Developing a dedicated and well educated team responsible for ureteroscope cleansing and storage has been shown to reduce ureteroscope damage and increase ureteroscope lifespan [24].

When broken or damaged instruments are detected they should be removed from the surgical field and no longer used. In some cases this may require early termination of the current procedure and a repeat procedure at a later time. This approach is preferred to the possible major complications that may occur when continuing with poorly functioning or broken equipment.

Mucosal Abrasion

Some degree of ureteral mucosal abrasion occurs routinely with most ureteroscopy cases. It is rarely of clinical significance and because of this likely underreported. Moreover, no standard definition of mucosal abrasion exists further complicating the understanding and impact of this problem.

A recent retrospective series of 2,275 semirigid ureteroscopies reported ureteral abrasions in 1.5% of cases while using a variety of ureteroscopes between 6 and 10 F [4]. An older series compared the complications of 248 rigid ureteroscopies using ureteroscope diameters between 9.5 and 11.5 F to 49 semirigid ureteroscopies with ureteroscope diameters between 6 and 7 F. Ureteral mucosal abrasions were reported in 24% of the rigid ureteroscopies and in only 6% of the cases using the smaller caliber semirigid ureteroscopes [25]. Principles to help minimize abrasions includes careful technique, avoiding rapid jerky movements while in the ureter, keeping the ureteral lumen in view when advancing and withdrawing the ureteroscope, and not advancing the ureteroscope with accessories protruding from the working channel. The use of ureteral access sheaths when expecting multiple passes with the ureteroscope should also help minimize mucosal injuries.

Submucosal Tunneling (False Passage)

This occurs when an instrument passes across the ureteral mucosal and tunnels submucosally for some distance, but does not completely perforate through the outer layers of the ureter. The incidence is reported between 0.4 and 1% [4, 11, 12]. Ureteral strictures, considerable ureteral tortuosity, and impacted ureteral stones all may increase the risk of submucosal tunneling. Small, short submucosal tunnels infrequently lead to termination of ureteroscopy and can be managed with short-term ureteral stenting. Unrecognized submucosal tunneling over a long distance with subsequent dilation or passage of large instruments can lead to devastating ureteral injury and loss [26].

Resistance to easy guidewire or instrument advancement is a clue to possible submucosal tunneling. Some have described guidewire passage through a submucosal tunnel as "tachy." [18]. Retrograde ureteropyelograms can help expose submucosal tunnels or confirm intraluminal wire placement if any concerns arise. If a wire is detected submucosally, retrogression of the wire followed by intraluminal placement is recommended. This can also be done under direct vision with a ureteroscopy placed just distal to the false passage. Utilizing floppy tipped guidewires, especially when trying to negotiate past ureteral stones, strictures or severe tortuosity can help minimize this complication.

Extravasation

Extravasation refers to the migration of intraluminal contents outside of the upper collecting system. This most commonly occurs through an iatrogenic perforation in the collecting system, but may also occur through a forniceal rupture. Fluids such as urine, irrigant, blood, and contrast as well as solids such as tissue and stone fragments may extravasate. Fluid extravasation has a reported incidence of 1% or less [10, 11]. As with ureteral perforation, the true incidence of fluid extravasation is likely underreported because routine evaluation (such as with retrograde ureteropyelograms) is not usually done. Stone or stone fragment extravasation has been reported to occur between approximately 0.2 and 2% [4, 27, 28].

Extravasation of small fluid volumes is often insignificant. However, large volume extravasation can have clinically important consequences. Urine extravastion can lead to urinoma formation and subsequent mass effect if large, abscess formation if infected, and possibly periureteral fibrosis [18]. Hypervolemia and hyponatermia can result from the extravasation and absorption of large amounts of hypotonic irrigant. Thus as a rule, water should be avoided during ureteroscopy.

Extravasation of noninfected stones or stone fragments into the retroperitoneum usually has no adverse long-term effects and this complication can be managed similar to a ureteral perforation. Attempts should not be made to retrieve the stone because this often enlarges the ureteral perforations, increases the associated inflammation, and may increase the long-term stricture risk. Documenting stone location with perioperative imaging and informing the patient should help reduce misdiagnosis and unnecessary future procedure [28]. Limiting high pressure irrigation and the use of ureteral access sheaths can also help reduce the risk of extravasation.

Ureteral Perforation

Ureteral perforation occurs when a hole is created across all layers of the ureteral wall. The reported incidence of this complication varies but overall has become less frequent in recent years. Contemporary series report the incidence of ureteral perforation to be approximately 2% or less, with the incidence of major perforations requiring further surgical repair to be approximately 0.1–0.6% [4, 12, 18, 29, 30]. Older series found perforation rates between 6.1 and 15% of cases, however many of these were done with large caliber ureteroscopes (>9.5 Fr) [3]. Larger stones or impacted stones, retroperitoneal fibrosis, and prolonged operative time all increase the risk of perforation.

The increasing use of small caliber ureteroscopes and safer intraluminal lithotripters are both likely responsible for the decreasing rate of ureteral perforations despite increasing utilization of ureteroscopy. The true incidence of ureteral perforation is likely underreported. This may in part be due to the fact that small, clinically insignificant perforations may not be detected at the time of ureteroscopy. Along similar reasoning, the true incidence of large perforations may be more accurate because these are more readily detected intraoperatively.

Small ureteral perforations, such as small puncture holes from guidewires or laser fibers, are most often of little consequence. Larger perforations often require premature termination of the procedure and in rare circumstances necessitate further surgical repair. In all instances when a ureteral perforation is detected ureteral stent placement and antibiotics are advised. Duration of stenting can be as short as 1 week for small perforations to closer to 6 weeks for larger perforations, as is commonly done after endopyelotomy [18, 31]. Careful technique, ureteral access sheaths, and never advancing the ureteroscope with accessories protruding from the end can minimize ureteral perforation.

Major Complications

Ureteral Intussusception

An infrequent but devastating complication of ureteroscopy, ureteral intussusception, occurs when the ureteral mucosa circumferentially tears away from the underlying submucosa and then invaginates as a sleeve along the intact ureteral lumen. Described another way, it can be thought of as avulsion of the ureteral mucosa while the underlying ureteral layers remain intact. It has only rarely been described, and has been associated with stone manipulation, retrograde pyelography, and during diagnostic endoscopic management of urothelial cell carcinoma [32–34].

In the case of intussusception after retrograde diagnostic ureteroscopy, ureteral dilation with a 12 Fr peel-away sheath was believed to be the inciting factor.

Prompt recognition requires a high index of suspicion, and should be considered in cases of ureteral obstruction after recent instrumentation or stone extraction. Inability to place a ureteral stent after stone extraction or ureteral dilation should serve as an alert to possible intussusception. Retrograde pyelogram may show a "bell-shaped" ureter [35]. If not found intraoperatively, it can present as ureteral obstruction at a later time. Cross-sectional imaging with contrast can show an inner contrast-filled lumen surrounded concentrically by the intussuscepted ureteral mucosa and an outer ring of contrast. On coronal sections a narrow line of contrast, recently dubbed the "line sign," can be appreciated [36].

If possible, a ureteral stent should be placed once the injury is identified. If retrograde stenting is unsuccessful, then percutaneous nephrostomy tube placement is advised. These are only temporizing measures to drain the kidney, as the intussuscepted segment can be expected to fibrose and stricture off rather than heal with any meaningful lumen. Ultimately, resection of the intussuscepted nonviable segment is required with ureteroneocystotomy, ureteroureterostomy, ureteropyelostomy, or ureteral substitution depending on the location and length of intussuscepted ureter.

Ureteral Avulsion

Arguably the most severe intraoperative complication of ureteroscopy is ureteral avulsion. This occurs when the ureter circumferentially tears apart resulting in total discontinuity of the ureter. Immediate operative intervention to rectify the avulsion is usually the rule if recognized intraoperatively. Post-ureteroscopic reconstruction of the avulsed ureter can be quite challenging and may ultimately lead to loss of the affected kidney.

The most common cause of avulsion is attempted basket extraction of stones or stone fragments too large to safely pass down the ureter. Other risk factors include stone basketing in the proximal ureter, retrieval of impacted stones, ureteral anatomic anomalies, and diseased ureters [19]. Many of the early reports of ureteral avulsion from the 1980s and 1990s occurred in the setting of blind stone basket extraction, and in particular with the Dormia stone basket. The ureteropelvic junction was the most frequent site of avulsion and can be explained by the local anatomy. The ureteral muscular wall and urothelium is the thinnest at the ureteropelvic junction and proximal ureter. Additionally, the renal pelvis is relatively fixed compared to the rest of the ureter which has considerable mobility within the retroperitoneum. The avulsion is often recognized intraoperatively as the ureter intussuscepts into the bladder or out of the urethra was the stone and basket are withdrawn [18]. The injury may also be detected by retrograde pyelography.

Thankfully, this is a very rare occurrence with a documented incidence less well than 1% in most reports and appears to be occurring less often as experience with ureteroscopy increases (Table 37.2). Five large reviews each evaluating between 1,000 and 5,000 patients reported a ureteral avulsion rate of 0.3, 0.1, 0.18, 0 and 0% respectively [2–5, 37]. More recent reports of ureteral avulsion are scarce despite increasing use of ureteroscopy. This is likely a result of improved technology leading to endoscope miniaturization, smaller more mobile stone baskets,

Table 37.2 Incidence of ureteral avulsion through time

Author	Date	Period	Review	Patients	Incidence
Weinberg [27]	1987	1982–1986	28 institutions	941	5 (0.5%)
Soller [3]	1996	1984–1992	33 series	5,117	17 (0.3%)
Grasso [2]	2001	1992–1998	3 series	1,059	0 (0%)

From [19], with permission from Elsevier

wide-spread adoption of fine holmium laser fibers that are deployable alongside stone baskets and better ureteroscopic visualization.

A contemporary small series evaluated three cases of a unique type of avulsion where the ureter was avulsed both at the level of the ureterovesical junction (UPJ) and the ureteropelvic junction (UVJ) [38]. Two of these cases occurred during stone manipulate using semirigid ureteroscopes that were 8 F at the distal shaft and 9 or 9.5 F at the proximal shaft. Passage of the ureteroscope in each case was difficult with a "give" of pressure with scope removal. The entire avulsed ureter was withdrawn encasing the ureteroscope shaft with the UVJ and distal ureter tightly wedged around the proximal ureteroscope sheath. The third case occurred during diagnostic ureteroscopy for a filling defect seen on retrograde pyelogram in a woman with a large pelvic mass. The filling defect turned out to be a ureteral stricture and the scope became stuck within the ureter during scope extraction and resulted in ureteral avulsion proximally and distally.

Excessive force during ureteroscope advancement appears to be an underlying causative factor in each of these cases. In addition, no ureterovesical junction dilation was carried out prior to ureteroscope placement, though routine balloon dilation has been shown to be safe from prior evaluation [39]. Interestingly use of ureteral access sheaths, commonly 12 F or 14 F in size, have not been reported to cause ureteral avulsion and this may be due to their hydrophilicity and frequent use of copious lubrication.

Ureteroscopic experience, good technique, and sound judgment are crucial to minimizing the risk for ureteral avulsion. Retrograde passage of a ureteroscope should not require excessive force, and if not passing easily then attempts to pass the ureteroscopy should be abandoned. Ureteral dilation and switching to a narrower caliber ureteroscope may help reduce avulsion risk. Application of copious lubrication along the entire working length of the ureteroscope, not just at the tip, can also be helpful. Alternatively, repeating ureteroscopy after ureteral stent placement for 1–2 weeks of passive ureteral dilation is always a safe approach.

In terms of stone extraction, avoiding extraction of large stones or stone fragments and limiting excessive force during stone extraction are core principles in minimizing ureteral avulsion. Additionally, the use of ureteral access sheaths may help minimize distal and mid-ureteral avulsions. Use of safety wires should be considered a must. Another option is the use of three-pronged graspers which are designed such that excessive force will cause the stone to dislodge from the basket and should avoid avulsion [19]. If a stone fragment becomes stuck within the ureter during basket retrieval, concomitant laser lithotripy can be used to fragment the stone or laser the basket wires to help disengage the basket. Depending on the ureteroscope used, small diameter laser fibers frequently can be passed through the same working port alongside the basket sheath. Though no successful technique to dislodge a wedged ureteroscopy has been reported, one potential strategy employing the use of a second ureteroscopy passed into the bladder alongside the first and allowing for possible ureteral meatotomy has been described [38].

Ureteral avulsions are usually recognized intraoperatively and can be repaired immediately if the patient is stable. This can be done open or laparoscopically with re-anastomosis of the ureter. The specific type of repair depends on the location and nature of the avulsion and considerations are discussed later in this chapter. Alternatively, a percutaneous nephrostomy tube can be placed to temporarily drain the kidney and definitive repair undertaken at a later time.

Early Postoperative Complications

Minor Complications

Post-ureteroscopy Ureteral Obstruction and Pain

Some degree of pain can be expected after any ureteroscopy. Mucosal trauma during scope and instrument manipulation may lead to transient ureteral obstruction from ureteral spasm, blood clot, or tissue edema. The placement of ureteral stents may also cause significant renal colic symptoms in some patients. The incidence of significant postoperative pain has been reported between 2 and 9% [4, 18].

This is usually self-limited and can initially be managed with pain medications, hydration, and observation if necessary. Imaging can evaluate for hydronephrosis, but this may be misleading if significant hydronephrosis was present prior to ureteroscopy or if a ureteral stent was placed during the procedure. In instances when no ureteral stent was left, the need for subsequent ureteral stent placement to relieve presumed ureteral obstruction and pain has been reported between 2.6 and 8.3% [29, 40]. Harmon et al. [29] preformed ureteroscopies in 209 patients of which 7 (3.5%) developed renal colic following ureteral stent removal. Of these, five patients (2.6%) had the ureteral stent replaced. Tanriverdi et al. [40] performed 276 uncomplicated ureteroscopies for ureteral calculi, and 23 patients (8.3%) required ureteral stenting within 24 h postprocedure for severe renal colic. Longer operative times, repeated upper tract access, larger stones, impacted calculi, and recent urinary tract infections were all associated with a high likelihood of needing postoperative stent placement.

The need for routine ureteral stenting after "umcomplicated" ureteroscopy remains controversial, with two recent meta-analyses evaluating this issue [41, 42]. Pengfei et al. [41] preformed a systematic meta-analysis comparing outcomes of stented and non-stented patients after ureteroscopy. They reviewed 16 randomized controlled trials involving a total of 1,573 patients. Those in the stented group had significantly more pain and lower urinary tract symptoms compared to those with no stent. No difference was found between the groups in terms of postoperative complications, need for analgesia, infections, or unplanned readmission. Nabi et al. [42] also performed a systematic review and meta-analysis of nine randomized controlled trials including 831 patients. Similarly, there was no significant difference in postoperative analgesia requirement, infections, stone-free rate, or ureteral strictures. A trend toward fewer unplanned admissions was seen in the stented group.

Vesicoureteral Reflux

Vesicoureteral reflux after ureteroscopy has been described in up to 10% of patients and has only been documented as low grade [3, 43]. The pre-ureteroscopy prevalence of vesicoureteral reflux in the study populations was not known or evaluated. Given the similar prevalence in the adult population and lack of clinical consequence from low-grade sterile reflux, postoperative screening for reflux should not be performed [3, 18].

Major Complications

Steinstrasse

Steinstrasse, which is German for "street of stones," is a well-described complication after stone lithotripsy where a column of obstructing stone fragments accumulates within the ureter. This was originally described after SWL, but can also occur after ureteroscopy. Steinstrasse is infrequently seen after ureteroscopy and intracorporeal lithotripsy because a number of the fragments are either basket extracted, irrigated out, or broken into small enough stone gravel thought not to cause steinstrasse. Frequent stent placement after ureteroscopy may postpone the clinical presentation of steinstrasse until after ureteral stent removal [18].

Initial descriptions after SWL classified steinstrassen into various types including a column of large stone fragments, a single obstructing large leading stone fragment with finer fragments stacked behind, and a column of only fine stone fragments [46]. Fragment accumulation can lead to ureteral wall edema with subsequent luminal narrowing and further impede spontaneous passage.

Steinstrasse may develop anywhere along the ureter, with the areas of anatomic narrowing most commonly involved including the ureterovesical junction, where the ureter crosses the iliac vessels, and where the ureter crosses anteriorly over the psoas muscle. The distal ureter is the most commonly affected site with the leading stone fragment located here up to 75% of the time [47, 48]. The mid-ureter is involved between 3 and 10% of the time, making it the least affected site.

Though not specifically evaluated for ureteroscopy some of the risk factors for steinstrasse during SWL may apply to ureteroscopy such as increasing stone size (especially >2 cm) and stone location (renal>ureteral) [48–50]. Radiographically, hydronephrosis often accompanies steinstrasse if there is associated obstruction of urine flow. A spontaneous resolution rate of around 60–80% can be expected and often occurs within a few days, thought occasionally requires several weeks [47, 48, 50, 51]. The remainder of patients often requires intervention.

Indications for intervention of steinstrassen include poorly controlled pain, fever, severe nausea, and vomiting or other signs of urinary infection, bilateral obstruction, obstruction of a solitary kidney, and failure of spontaneous passage of obstructing fragments. Asymptomatic steinstrasse can be reasonably followed for a number of weeks with serial imaging, given the majority of these patients will eventually spontaneously pass the fragments. Up to a third of patients may develop silent obstruction [47, 48].

For clinically symptomatic or persistent steinstrasse, a number of management options exist such as percutaneous nephrostomy tube placement, ureteroscopy, and in very rare circumstance laparoscopic or open stone removal. Percutaneous nephrostomy tube placement alone can be effective in allowing the obstructing stone fragments to pass almost 75% of the time [46]. SWL, with particular focus on the leading or most distal fragment, has proven efficacious in up to 80% of cases and ureteroscopy with laser lithotripsy has and efficacy approaching 100% [50]. If steinstrasse occurs with considerable stone burden remaining in the kidney, percutaneous nephrolithotomy with antegrade ureteroscopy is a good option. Open or minimally invasive ureterolithotomy is usually reserved as a salvage procedure if shock wave and endoscopic approaches fail.

Infection and Fever

Urinary tract infection after ureteroscopy can range from routine and uncomplicated to life-threatening sepsis. The presence of calculi in the urinary tract, which are often the reason for ureteroscopy in the first place, can serve as a nidus for infection. Moreover, despite appropriate preoperative antibiotics and a negative urine culture, urinary calculi can still harbor bacteria that may cause serious infection during lithotripsy. The placement of ureteroscopes and instruments across the urethral meatus or skin can introduce bacteria into an otherwise sterile urinary tract. Pressurized irrigation can facilitate pyelovenous and pyelosinus translocation of uropathogens and promote sepsis.

The incidence of post-ureteroscopic fever has been reported between 1.2 and 22%, and fever may occur in the absence of infection [18]. Interestingly, the vast majority of patients did not receive peri-procedural antibiotics in the single study that reported a postprocedure fever rate of 22%. In the same study, the infection rate was only 3.7% [31]. The incidence of urinary tract infection after contemporary ureteroscopy varies between 1 and 4% [4, 7, 31]. The incidence of sepsis has been reported between 0.3 and 2% [7, 39]. Fungal sepsis has been seen after ureteroscopy in patients with advanced liver cirrhosis, but this is rare [52].

Many strategies exist to reduce urinary tract infections after ureteroscopy. Sterilizing the urine with culture-directed antibiotics prior to ureteroscopy should be considered a must. Peri-ureteroscopic antibiotics for up to 24 h are recommended by the American Urological Association [53]. Using low pressure irrigation and only as much irrigation as necessary for adequate visualization can help minimize pyelovenous and pyelosinus backflow. Ureteral access sheaths and continuous or intermittent bladder drainage can help reduce renal collecting system pressures subsequent microbial translocation.

Late Postoperative Complications

Major Complications

Silent Hydronephrosis

Asymptomatic, or "silent," hydronephrosis after ureteroscopy has been described by a number of different groups [54–56]. The incidence has been reported to be approximately 2–5%. The concern in these patients is ongoing silent obstruction that may eventually lead to loss of the affected renal

Table 37.3 Incidence of stricture formation in patients undergoing ureteroscopic treatment of upper tract urothelial carcinoma

Author	Renoureteral units	No. of strictures	Mean follow-up (months)
Martinez-Pineiro [61]	39	5 (13%)	30.5
Elliot [62]	37	6 (16.2%)	37
Kelley [64]	41	2 (4.9%)	35.1
Chen [63]	23	2 (8.7%)	35
Elliot [60]	21	0 (0%)	72
Total	161	15 (9.3%)	44.5

From [18], with permission from Elsevier

unit. Routine postoperative imaging may capture these patients at a time when intervention would be useful. Imaging in these studies was via many different modalities including computed tomography, intravenous pyelogram, renography, or renal ultrasound.

Routine imaging after uncomplicated ureteroscopy may not be mandatory and many feel this is unnecessary in asymptomatic patients [19, 55, 57]. However, routine imaging may be more useful after complicated ureteroscopy, such as cases with impacted stones, postoperative pain, intraoperative ureteral injury, or when ureteral balloon-dilation was necessary. Renal ultrasound 4–6 weeks after complicated ureteroscopy is a good screening test and poses no known risks to patients. If hydronephrosis is detected, further function imaging studies and diagnostic studies can be considered.

Ureteral Stricture

The incidence of ureteral strictures after routine ureteroscopy is between 0 and 4% [18]. The incidence in more contemporary series is less than 1%, and usually less than 0.4% [2, 4, 7, 29, 30]. Risk factors believed to predispose to ureteral strictures include larger caliber instruments, stone impaction, and ureteral injury during ureteroscopy. The exact etiology for stricture formation is unclear but may be a combination of direct instrument trauma, thermal injury, and possibly relative ischemia from larger diameter instruments. A ureteral stricture rate of 24% (5 of 21 patients) at 7 months mean follow-up was observed in a series of patients with impacted ureteral stones [58]. In four of the five patients with a ureteral stricture, ureteral perforation at the site of the stone impaction also occurred and was believed to be the primary risk factor for stricture formation. Another group found a 5.9% ureteral stricture rate on subgroup analysis of patients with documented ureteral perforations [3].

In addition to impacted ureteral stones, fragments embedded within the ureteral wall may predispose to stone granuloma formation and subsequent ureteral stricture [2, 59]. Some evidence suggests the closer the embedded stone fragment is to the ureteral lumen, the more likely the chance of developing a ureteral stricture with stones more than 4 mm from the ureteral lumen unlikely to be clinically significant [59].

Patients with upper tract urothelial carcinoma managed primary by ureteroscopic measures appear to be at high risk for ureteral strictures than those undergoing ureteroscopy for urinary stone disease (Table 37.3). The incidence of ureteral stricture in this setting is closer to 9% over a mean follow-up of 44.5 months. The reason is likely multifactorial including repeated screening and therapeutic ureteroscopies, direct laser ablation of ureteral tissue, and upper tract BCG exposure.

Advances and miniaturization in instrument design and improvements in ureteroscopic technique are likely the reason for reduced stricture rates in more recent series. However, some concern has been generated by the increasing use of ureteral access sheaths, which commonly have outer diameters of 12–14 Fr. Though no robust reviews exist, at least two series have evaluated this question. The earlier series reported a single ureteral stricture (1.4%) in 71 ureteroscopies done with a ureteral access sheath [65]. Mean follow-up was 322 days. The more recent series evaluated 194 cases in which a uretereal access sheath was deployed and no ureteral strictures were found at a mean follow-up of 41 months [66].

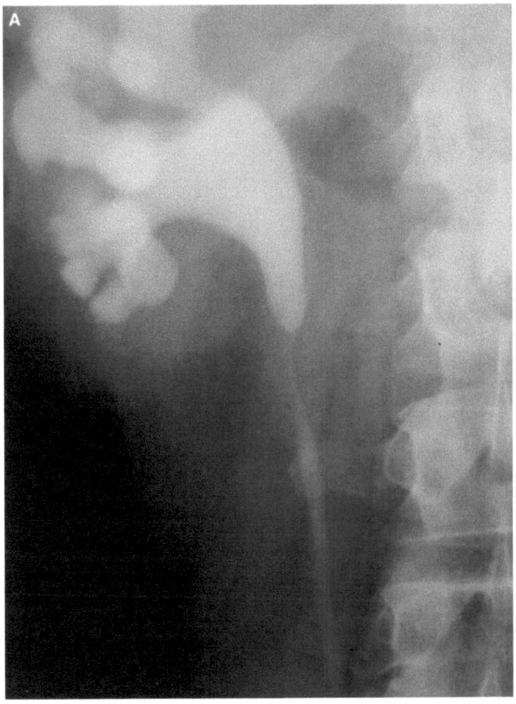

Fig. 37.1 Intravenous urogram demonstrating proximal ureteral stricture. From [18], with permission from Elsevier

Careful technique, gentle ureteral manipulation during stone basket extraction or tumor ablation, and avoidance of excessive force when advancing instruments should help minimize ureteral trauma and subsequent ureteral stricture formation. Using Nitinol baskets, especially ones with the ability to articulate, may help minimize the risk [19]. If difficulty advancing the ureteroscope or access sheath is encountered, temporary ureteral stenting for 1–2 weeks almost always allows for successful access at repeat ureteroscopy and is considered the safest option and the least likely to lead to late ureteral stricture formation. Balloon dilation of the intramural ureter to 12–15 Fr is another reasonable strategy to navigate past a narrow ureteral orifice, however balloon dilation in other segments of the ureter should be discouraged [18]. Ureteral strictures after ureteroscopy are often narrow and rarely ischemic making them favorable to initial endoscopic management (Figs. 37.1 and 37.2). Recurrent strictures, long strictures, and segments with multiple strictures are usually repaired in an open fashion by one of the techniques described later in this chapter.

Management of Major Ureteroscopic Ureteral Injuries

Major intraoperative complications of ureteroscopy such as significant ureteral perforations, ureteral avulsion, and ureteral intussusception requiring timely surgical repair may occur in up to 1.1% cases [3]. Large, more contemporary series report a lower rate of ureteroscopic complications requiring further open or laparoscopic surgery to be closer to 0.2% [4, 30, 31]. It is recommended that these injuries be immediately repaired transabdominally [67]. The most likely places for ureteral injury during ureteroscopy include the ureterovesical and ureteropelvic junction because the muscular component of the ureteral wall is the least developed in these areas. The angulation of the ureter as it traverses over the pelvic brim puts this area at higher risk for injury as well.

Strategies for open repair depend on the length and location of the ureteral injury, patient age and stability, surgeon experience, and kidney function. Principles of ureteral injury repair include adequate mobilization of the injured segment with careful preservation of the ureteral adventitia, complete debridement of any devitalized ureter, spatulation of the ureteral end prior to repair, and anastomosis over a ureteral stent to minimize urine leak and facilitate healing over a wet anastomosis. In the modern era, most ureteral avulsions are associated with mechanical shear forces rather than thermal injury. Therefore, most of these injuries have little devitalized tissue, require minimal debridement, and ureterureterostomy is often all that is required to bridge the short gap (Fig. 37.3). Intussusception injury may involve significantly longer segments of ureter and can require vesico-psoas hitch, Boari flap, ileal interposition, autotransplant, or nephrectomy.

Short distal ureteral injuries are best managed with ureteroneocystotomy (Fig. 37.4). The new ureteral hiatus should be located superiomedial to

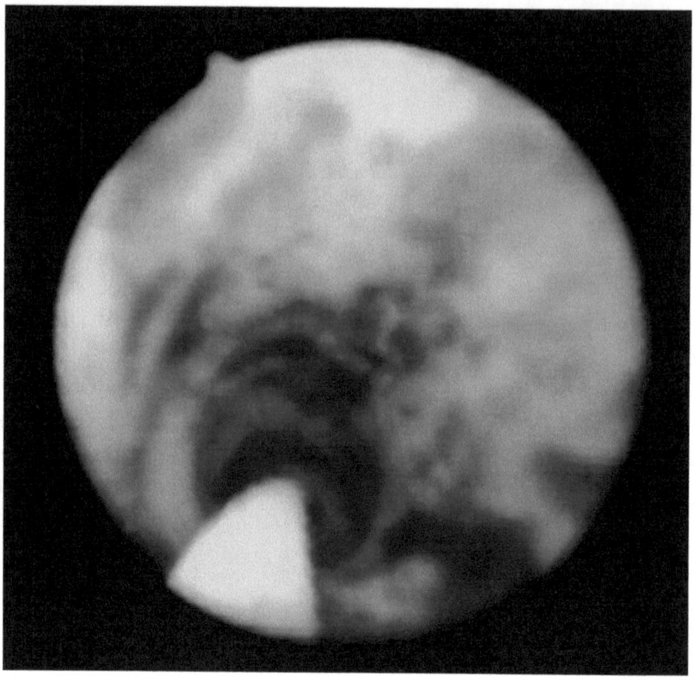

Fig. 37.2 Intraoperative view of the ureteral stricture crossed by a guidewire. From [18], with permission from Elsevier

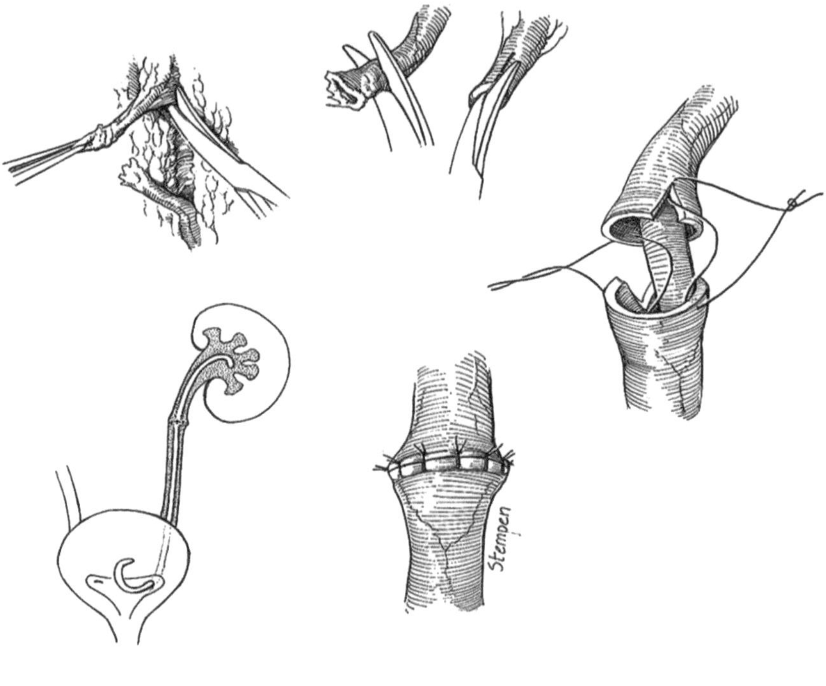

Fig. 37.3 Ureteroureterostomy demonstrating the principles of debridement, spatulation and end-to-end repair using interrupted, absorbable, fine sutures over an indwelling stent. From Presti JC, Jr and Carroll PR. Interoperative management of the injured ureter. In: Schrock TR, editor. Perspectives in colon and rectal surgery. St. Louis (MO): Quality Medical Publishing; 1988, with permission from Thieme Publishers, New York

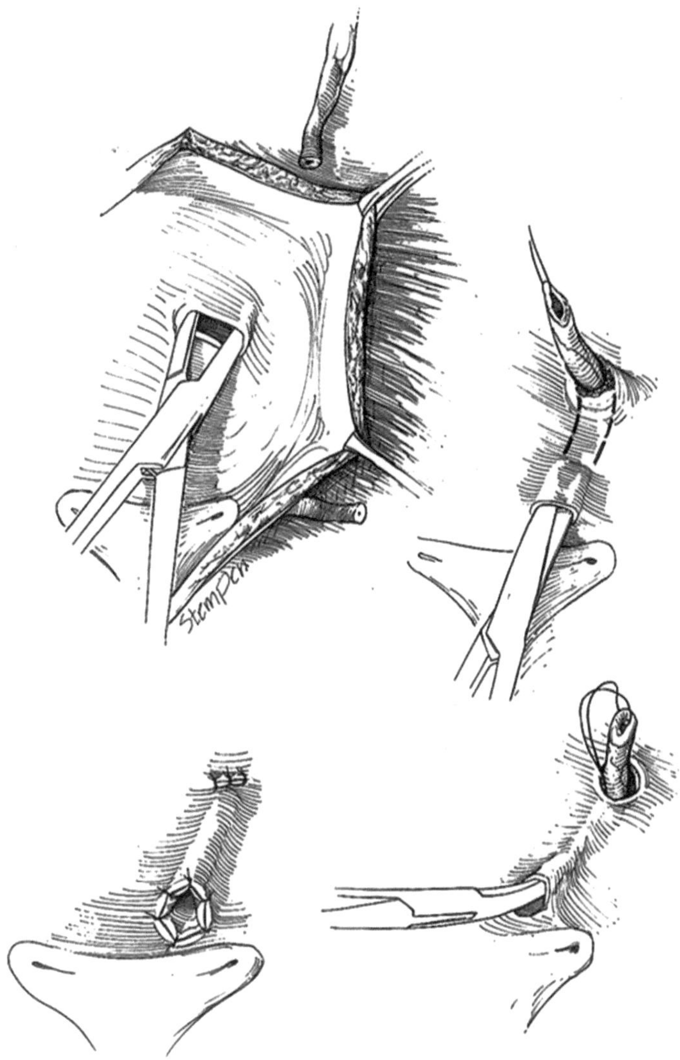

Fig. 37.4 Ureteroneocystostomy in a fashion modified from Politano and Leadbetter. From Presti JC, Jr and Carroll PR. Intraoperative management of the injured ureter. In: Schrock TR, editor. Perspectives in colon and rectal surgery. St. Louis (MO): Quality Medical Publishing; 1988, with permission from Thieme Publishers, New York

the native ureteral orifice. If placed too laterally on the bladder wall, the reimplanted ureter is subject to kinking and intermittent obstruction. A 3:1 detrusor tunnel to ureteral lumen ratio is recommended for nonrefluxing anastomoses [67]. Alternatively, a refluxing anastomosis can be created. The distal ureteral segment does not need to be tied off or resected unless there is known significant vesicoureteral reflux.

Longer distal and some mid-ureteral segments may be best repaired by combining a number of procedures depending on the length of the defect. Bladder mobilization within the space of Retzius may be all that is necessary, and sacrificing the contralateral superior vesicle pedicle can provide extra length. A psoas hitch will provide extra length. This is performed by making a vertical cystotomy and then securing the bladder to the psoas muscle ipsilateral to the side of the injury. Care must be taken to avoid injuring the genitofemoral nerve when securing the bladder.

The majority of mid and proximal ureteral avulsion injuries create a short defect that is usually best repaired with primary ureteroureterostomy (Fig. 37.4). Careful ureteral mobilization and tension-free primary anastomosis is preferred to bridging the defect with nonurothelial lined tissue such as buccal mucosa, ileum, or appendix. Primary anastomosis is the most frequently used approach to repair mid and proximal ureteral injuries [68]. Ureteropelvic junction or high proximal ureteral avulsion may be accompanied by loss of proximal ureteral blood supply which can limit successful pyeloplasty or proximal ureteroureterostomy. Transureteroureterostomy is an alternative approach, but is relatively contraindicated in this patient population as most have urolithiasis disease or upper tract urothelial carcinoma.

Larger ureteral defects such as those created by ureteral intussusception or long and severe submucosal tunnels may be bridged through bladder mobilization and Boari flap creation, ileal interposition, or autotransplant. In these instances where the reconstructive options are complex and not without significant potential morbidity, the ureteral segment in continuity with the affected kidney may be tied off and a percutaneous nephrostomy tube placed. This will temporize the situation and allow adequate time to discuss reconstructive options with the patient and adequate time for the patient to choose a treatment course. In the case of marginal function of the affected kidney and strong contralateral renal function, consideration may be given to nephrectomy, but again only after full discussion and weighing of the risks and benefits with the patient. Between 11 and 53% or ureteral repairs will have complications of their own that can be managed with either open repair or endoscopically [18, 69].

Conclusion

Complications during ureteroscopy are occurring less frequently as a result of improved instrumentation and technique. Most complications can be safely handled with ureteral stenting and time. Major complications are rare but can pose significant risk to the patient and can be challenging to manage. A complete understanding of the possible complications, approaches to minimize their occurrence, and strategies to manage them deftly as they arise are central to ensuring safe and successful ureteroscopy.

References

1. Young HH, McKay RW. Congenital valvular obstruction of the prostatic urethra. Surg Gynecol Obstet. 1929;48:509–35.
2. Grasso M. Complications of ureteropyeloscopy. In: Taneja SS, Smith RB, Ehrlich RM, editors. Complications of urologic surgery. 3rd ed. Philadelphia: WB Saunders; 2001. p. 268–76.
3. Stoller ML, Wolf JS. Ensoscopic ureteral injuries. In: McAninch JW, editor. Traumatic and reconstructive urology. Philadelphia: WB Saunders; 1996. p. 199–211.
4. Geavlete P, Georgescu D, Niţa G, Mirciulescu V, Cauni V. Complications of 2735 retrograde semirigid ureteroscopy procedures: a single-center experience. J Endourol. 2006;20(3):179–85.
5. Krambeck AE, Murat FJ, Gettman MT, Chow GK, Patterson DE, Segura JW. The evolution of ureteroscopy: a modern single-institution series. Mayo Clin Proc. 2006;81(4):468–73.
6. Rioja J, Mamoulakis C, Sodha H, Suwijn S, Laguna P, de la Rosette J. A Plea for centralized care for ureteroscopy: results from a comparative study under different conditions within the same center. J Endourol. 2011;25(3):425–9.
7. Schuster TG, Hollenbeck BK, Faerber GJ, Wolf JS. Complications of ureteroscopy: analysis of predictive factors. J Urol. 2001;166(2):538–40.
8. Cetti RJ, Biers S, Keoghane SR. The difficult ureter: what is the incidence of pre-stenting? Ann R Coll Surg Engl. 2011;93(1):31–3.
9. Flam TA, Malone JM, Roth RA. Complications of ureteroscopy. Urol Clin North Am. 1988;15(2): 167–81.
10. Abdel-Razzak OM, Bagley DH. Clinical experience with flexible ureteropyeloscopy. J Urol. 1992;148(6): 1788–92.
11. Blute ML, Segura JW, Patterson DE. Ureteroscopy. J Urol. 1988;139(3):510–2.
12. Grasso M. Ureteropyeloscopic treatment of ureteral and intrarenal calculi. Urol Clin North Am. 2000;27(4): 623–31.
13. Tiplitsky SI, Milhoua PM, Patel MB, Minsky L, Hoenig DM. Case report: intrarenal arteriovenous fistula after ureteroscopic stone extraction with holmium laser lithotripsy. J Endourol. 2007;21(5): 530–2.

14. Watterson JD, Girvan AR, Cook AJ, Beiko DT, Nott L, Auge BK, Preminger GM, Denstedt JD. Safety and efficacy of holmium: YAG laser lithotripsy in patients with bleeding diatheses. J Urol. 2002;168(2):442–5.
15. Sofer M, Watterson JD, Wollin TA, Nott L, Razvi H, Denstedt JD. Holmium:YAG laser lithotripsy for upper urinary tract calculi in 598 patients. J Urol. 2002;167(1):31–4.
16. Başar H, Ohta N, Kageyama S, Suzuki K, Kawabe K. Treatment of ureteral and renal stones by electrohydraulic lithotripsy. Int Urol Nephrol. 1997;29(3):275–80.
17. Teichman JM, Rao RD, Rogenes VJ, Harris JM. Ureteroscopic management of ureteral calculi: electrohydraulic versus holmium:YAG lithotripsy. J Urol. 1997;158(4):1357–61.
18. Johnson DB, Pearle MS. Complications of ureteroscopy. Urol Clin North Am. 2004;31(1):157–71.
19. de la Rosette JJ, Skrekas T, Segura JW. Handling and prevention of complications in stone basketing. Eur Urol. 2006;50(5):991–8.
20. Landman J, Lee DI, Lee C, Monga M. Evaluation of overall costs of currently available small flexible ureteroscopes. Urology. 2003;62(2):218–22.
21. Knudsen B, Miyaoka R, Shah K, Holden T, Turk TM, Pedro RN, Kriedberg C, Hinck B, Ortiz-Alvarado O, Monga M. Durability of the next-generation flexible fiberoptic ureteroscopes: a randomized prospective multi-institutional clinical trial. Urology. 2010;75(3):534–8.
22. Pietrow PK, Auge BK, Delvecchio FC, Silverstein AD, Weizer AZ, Albala DM, Preminger GM. Techniques to maximize flexible ureterscope longevity. Urology. 2002;60(5):784–8.
23. Sung JC, Springhart WP, Marguet CG, L'Esperance JO, Tan YH, Albala DM, Preminger GM. Location and etiology of flexible and semirigid ureteroscope damage. Urology. 2005;66(5):958–63.
24. Semins MJ, George S, Allaf ME, Matlaga BR. Ureteroscope cleaning and sterilization by the urology operating room team: the effect on repair costs. J Endourol. 2009;23(6):903–5.
25. Francesca F, Scattoni V, Nava L, Pompa P, Grasso M, Rigatti P. Failures and complications of transurethral ureteroscopy in 297 cases: conventional rigid instruments vs. small caliber semirigid ureteroscopes. Eur Urol. 1995;28(2):112–5.
26. Lytton B, Weiss RM, Green DF. Complications of ureteral endoscopy. J Urol. 1987;137(4):649–53.
27. Weinberg JJ, Ansong K, Smith AD. Complications of ureteroscopy in relation to experience: report of survey and author experience. J Urol. 1987;137(3):384–5.
28. Evans CP, Stoller ML. The fate of the iatrogenic retroperitoneal stone. J Urol. 1993;150(3):827–9.
29. Harmon WJ, Sershon PD, Blute ML, Patterson DE, Segura JW. Ureteroscopy: current practice and long-term complications. J Urol. 1997;157(1):28–32.
30. Butler MR, Power RE, Thornhill JA, Ahmad I, McLornan I, McDermott T, Grainger R. An audit of 2273 ureteroscopies–a focus on intra-operative complications to justify proactive management of ureteric calculi. Surgeon. 2004;2(1):42–6.
31. Jeromin L, Sosnowski M. Ureteroscopy in the treatment of ureteral stones: over 10 years' experience. Eur Urol. 1998;34(4):344–9.
32. Bernhard PH, Reddy PK. Retrograde ureteral intussusception: a rare complication. J Endourol. 1996;10(4):349–51.
33. Park J, Siegel C, Moll M, Konnak J. Retrograde ureteral intussusception. J Urol. 1994;151(4):997–8.
34. Compton JS, Drummond M. Intussusception of the ureter by a polypoid transitional cell carcinoma. Br J Urol. 1986;58(6):725–6.
35. Mazer MJ, Lacy SS, Kao L. "Bell-shaped ureter", a radiographic sign of antegrade intussusception. Urol Radiol. 1979;1(1):63–5.
36. Xu W, Yu CS, Yang L, Li KC. Ureteral intussusception due to a polyp. Abdom Imaging. 2007;32(5):675–7.
37. Alapont JM, Broseta E, Oliver F, Pontones JL, Boronat F, Jiménez-Cruz JF. Ureteral avulsion as a complication of ureteroscopy. Int Braz J Urol. 2003;29(1):18–22.
38. Ordon M, Schuler TD, Honey RJ. Ureteral avulsion during contemporary ureteroscopic stone management: "the scabbard avulsion". J Endourol. 2011;25(8):1259–62.
39. Stoller ML, Wolf Jr JS, Hofmann R, Marc B. Ureteroscopy without routine balloon dilation: an outcome assessment. Urol. 1992;147(5):1238–42.
40. Tanriverdi O, Yencilek F, Koyuncu H, Yencilek E, Sarica K. Emergent stenting after uncomplicated ureteroscopy: evaluation of 23 patients. Urology. 2011;77(2):305–8.
41. Pengfei S, Yutao L, Jie Y, Wuran W, Yi D, Hao Z, Jia W. The results of ureteral stenting after ureteroscopic lithotripsy for ureteral calculi: a systematic review and meta-analysis. J Urol. 2011;186(5):1904–9.
42. Nabi G, Cook J, N'Dow J, McClinton S. Outcomes of stenting after uncomplicated ureteroscopy: systematic review and meta-analysis. BMJ. 2007;334(7593):572.
43. Richter S, Shalev M, Lobik L, Buchumensky V, Nissenkorn I. Early postureteroscopy vesicoureteral reflux–a temporary and infrequent complication: prospective study. J Endourol. 1999;13(5):365–6.
44. Netto Jr NR, de Almeida Claro J, Esteves SC, Amdrade EFM. Ureteroscopic stone removal in the distal ureter. Why Change? J Urol. 1997;157(6):2081–3.
45. Puppo P, Ricciotti G, Bozzo W, Introini C. Primary endoscopic treatment of ureteral calculi. A review of 378 cases. Eur Urol. 1999;36(1):48–52.
46. Coptcoat MJ, Webb DR, Kellet MJ, Whitfield HN, Wickham JE. The steinstrasse: a legacy of extracorporeal lithotripsy? Eur Urol. 1988;14(2):93–5.
47. Fedullo LM, Pollack HM, Banner MP, Amendola MA, Van Arsdalen KN. The development of steinstrassen after ESWL: frequency, natural history, and

radiologic management. AJR Am J Roentgenol. 1988;151(6):1145–7.
48. Madbouly K, Sheir KZ, Elsobky E, Eraky I, Kenawy M. Risk factors for the formation of a steinstrasse after extracorporeal shock wave lithotripsy: a statistical model. J Urol. 2002;167(3):1239–42.
49. Al-Awadi KA, Abdul Halim H, Kehinde EO, Al-Tawheed A. Steinstrasse: a comparison of incidence with and without J stenting and the effect of J stenting on subsequent management. BJU Int. 1999;84(6):618–21.
50. Sulaiman MN, Buchholz NP, Clark PB. The role of ureteral stent placement in the prevention of steinstrasse. J Endourol. 1999;13(3):151–5.
51. Kim SC, Oh CH, Moon YT, Kim KD. Treatment of steinstrasse with repeat extracorporeal shock wave lithotripsy: experience with piezoelectric lithotriptor. J Urol. 1991;145(3):489–91.
52. Beck SM, Finley DS, Deane LA. fungal urosepsis after ureteroscopy in cirrhotic patients: a word of caution. Urology. 2008;72(2):291–3.
53. Wolf Jr JS, Bennett CJ, Dmochowski RR, Hollenbeck BK, Pearle MS, Schaeffer AJ. Urologic Surgery Antimicrobial Prophylaxis Best Practice Policy Panel. Best practice policy statement on urologic surgery antimicrobial prophylaxis. J Urol. 2008;179(4):1379–90.
54. Manger JP, Mendoza PJ, Babayan RK, Wang DS. Use of renal ultrasound to detect hydronephrosis after ureteroscopy. J Endourol. 2009;23(9):1399–402.
55. Adiyat KT, Meuleners R, Monga M. Selective postoperative imaging after ureteroscopy. Urology. 2009;73(3):490–3.
56. Weizer AZ, Auge BK, Silverstein AD, Delvecchio FC, Brizuela RM, Dahm P, Pietrow PK, Lewis BR, Albala DM, Preminger GM. Routine postoperative imaging is important after ureteroscopic stone manipulation. J Urol. 2002;168(1):46–50.
57. Bugg Jr CE, El-Galley R, Kenney PJ, Burns JR. Follow-up functional radiographic studies are not mandatory for all patients after ureteroscopy. Urology. 2002;59(5):662–7.
58. Roberts WW, Cadeddu JA, Micali S, Kavoussi LR, Moore RG. Ureteral stricture formation after removal of impacted calculi. J Urol. 1998;159(3):723–6.
59. Dretler SP, Young RH. Stone granuloma: a cause of ureteral stricture. J Urol. 1993;150(6):1800–2.
60. Elliott DS, Segura JW, Lightner D, Patterson DE, Blute ML. Is nephroureterectomy necessary in all cases of upper tract transitional cell carcinoma? Long-term results of conservative endourologic management of upper tract transitional cell carcinoma in individuals with a normal contralateral kidney. Urology. 2001;58(2):174–8.
61. Martinez-Pineiro JA, Garcia Matres MJ, Martinez-Pineiro L. Endourological treatment of upper tract urothelial carcinomas: analysis of a series of 59 tumors. J Urol. 1996;156(2 Pt 1):377–85.
62. Elliott DS, Blute ML, Patterson DE, Bergstralh EJ, Segura JW. Long-term follow-up of endoscopically treated upper urinary tract transitional cell carcinoma. Urology. 1996;47(6):819–25.
63. Chen GL, Bagley DH. Ureteroscopic management of upper tract transitional cell carcinoma in patients with normal contralateral kidneys. J Urol. 2000;164(4):1173–6.
64. Keeley Jr FX, Bibbo M, Bagley DH. Ureteroscopic treatment and surveillance of upper urinary tract transitional cell carcinoma. J Urol. 1997;157(5):1560–5.
65. Delvecchio FC, Auge BK, Brizuela RM, Weizer AZ, Silverstein AD, Lallas CD, Pietrow PK, Albala DM, Preminger GM. Assessment of stricture formation with the ureteral access sheath. Urology. 2003;61(3):518–22.
66. Ayyathurai R, Kanagarajah P, Shields J, Young E, Alvarez A, Bird VG. Single-center clinical comparison of two reinforced ureteral access sheaths for retrograde ureteroscopic treatment of urinary lithiasis. Int Urol Nephrol. 2012;44(2):409–14.
67. Elliott SP, McAninch JW. Ureteral injuries: external and iatrogenic. Urol Clin North Am. 2006;33(1):55–66.
68. Perez-Brayfield MR, Keane TE, Krishnan A, Lafontaine P, Feliciano DV, Clarke HS. Gunshot wounds to the ureter: a 40-year experience at Grady Memorial Hospital. J Urol. 2001;166(1):119–21.
69. Ghali AM, El Malik EM, Ibrahim AI, Ismail G, Rashid M. Ureteric injuries: diagnosis, management, and outcome. J Trauma. 1999;46(1):150–8.

Part VII

The Future

38 Robotics

Dennis J. Lee and Mihir M. Desai

Introduction

The first ureteroscopic evaluation was performed using a pediatric cystoscope in the dilated ureter of an infant with posterior urethral valves [1]. Since that time, significant technologic advancements have been made in flexible ureteroscopy, including improved scope design, optics, and deflection capability. Ureteroscopic accessory development, such as laser lithotripsy, wires, baskets, and access sheaths, have paralleled advancements in flexible ureteroscopic technology [2]. These advances allow experienced surgeons to perform a wide variety of diagnostic and therapeutic procedures [3]. In the treatment of urinary stone disease, ureteroscopic treatment has advanced sufficiently to replace shock wave lithotripsy as the primary therapy for ureteral and renal stones at many institutions [4, 5].

Despite significant progress, currently available endoscopic equipment continues to have limitations inherent to manual flexible ureteroscopy. The movement of the distal tip of the flexible ureteroscope is achieved by passive conformity to the ureteral contour and inserting, rolling, and deflecting maneuvers using a proximal hand piece. From an engineering perspective, these maneuvers provide suboptimal control and stability at the distal tip of the flexible ureteroscope, which is further complicated by patient respiration. In addition, advanced manipulations require the aid of a skilled assistant [3]. Thus, there is a potential opportunity in developing a computer-controlled robotic platform to manipulate flexible endoscopes.

A robotic flexible catheter system has several potential advantages. It allows for the translation of the advantages of a rigid robotic system into the endoscopic environment, enhancing the capabilities of conventional flexible ureterorenoscopy by providing a stable, easily maneuverable, and ergonomically superior platform [2, 3]. The application of robotic technology has the potential to allow a level of precision that even the expert cannot achieve with manual control [5].

Flexible Robotic System

The flexible Sensai® (registered trademark) robotic catheter system developed by Hansen Medical System (Mountain View, California, USA) is the only flexible robotic system to have been applied to ureteroscopic purposes, to the author's knowledge. The system was initially developed for cardiovascular applications, such as endocardial ablation for arrythmia. The system's hardware and software has been adapted and modified for ureterorenoscopy.

D.J. Lee, M.D. • M.M. Desai, M.D. (✉)
USC Institute of Urology, University of Southern California, 1441 Eastlake Avenue, Suite 7416, Los Angeles, CA 90089, USA
e-mail: adityadesai2003@gmail.com

M. Monga (ed.), *Ureteroscopy: Indications, Instrumentation & Technique*, Current Clinical Urology,
DOI 10.1007/978-1-62703-206-3_38, © Springer Science+Business Media New York 2013

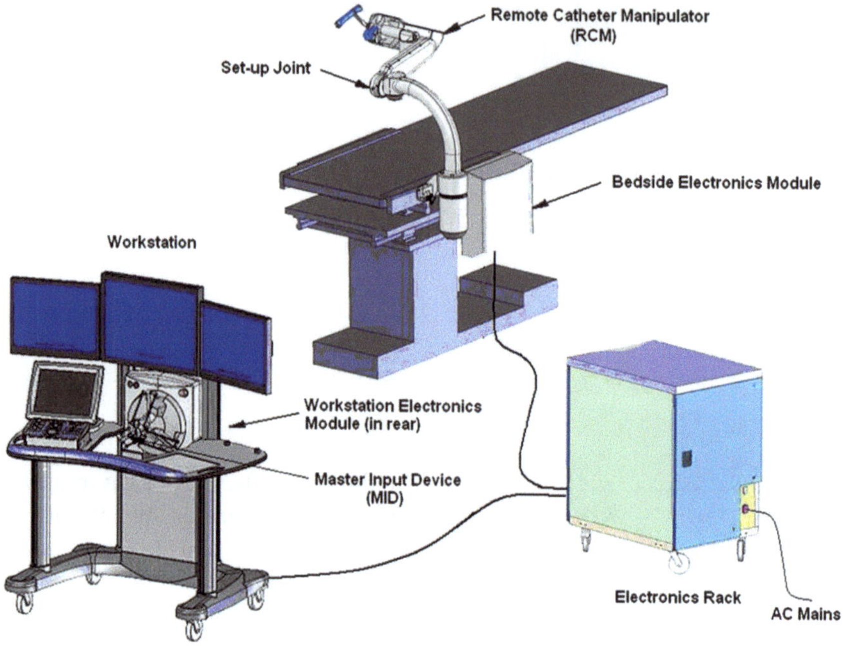

Fig. 38.1 Schematic representation of flexible robotic catheter control system (courtesy of Hansen Medical, Mountain View, CA. Used with permission)

The Sensei robotic catheter is based on a remote master–slave control system and consists of four components (Fig. 38.1): (1) the surgeon console (Fig. 38.2), which consists of the master input device (MID) and display monitors; (2) the flexible catheter system; (3) the remote catheter manipulator (RCM); and (4) the electronics rack, which contains all the video and computer hardware. The MID is a three-dimensional joystick that the surgeon uses to remotely manipulate the catheter tip. Movement of the catheter tip mimics the surgeon's hand manipulation of a motion controller joystick. The display monitor is a multi-panel display station showing endoscopic visualization and real-time fluoroscopic views. The display monitor is equipped to incorporate and synchronously display other imaging modalities, such as computed tomography. In addition, a catheter animation on the LCD display allows the surgeon to determine the location and orientation of the ureteroscope tip in the collecting system [2, 3, 6, 7].

The functional remote element consists of the RCM, an arm that attaches to the operating table on which the steerable catheter sheath and guide catheter are attached. The steerable catheter system (Fig. 38.3) contains an outer catheter sheath (14 F/12 F), which is used to stabilize the catheter at the level of the ureteropelvic junction and an inner catheter guide (12 F/10 F), which is controlled remotely by the MID. A custom-designed flexible ureteroscope is fixed to and guided by the inner catheter. The space between the inner guide catheter and the flexible ureteroscope allows for inflow and efflux of irrigation fluid. The working channel of the ureteroscope provides additional drainage. Maximum deflection of the flexible catheter system is 270° and is not decreased by placement of accessory instruments through the working channel [2, 7].

Preliminary Experience

The preliminary animal studies using the flexible robotic system were performed by Desai et al. in the swine model [2]. Flexible robotic ureteroscopy was performed in five swine kidneys bilaterally. In two animals (four kidneys) 4 mm human stones were placed in the collecting system and fragmented using a Ho:YAG laser. In one animal

Fig. 38.2 Setup of surgeon console

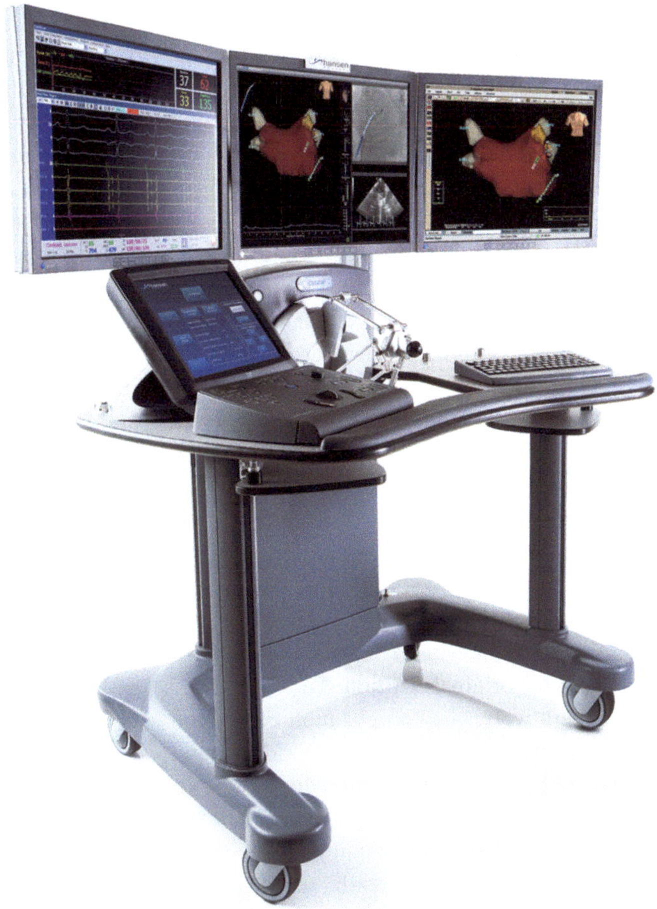

Fig. 38.3 RCM with steerable guide catheter and sheath (courtesy of Hansen Medical, Mountain View, CA. Used with permission)

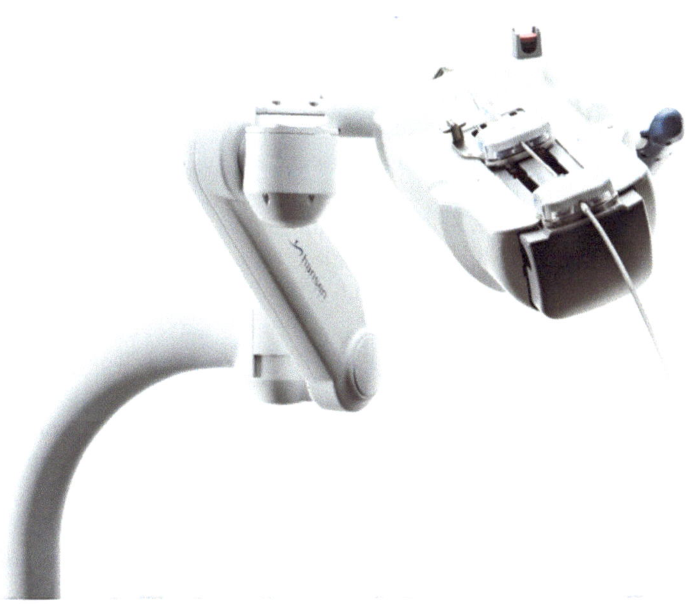

(two kidneys) one papilla from each caliceal group was laser fulgurated. Diagnostic ureteropyeloscopy was performed in the other two pigs (four kidneys).

Balloon dilation of the ureter was required in two of the ten kidneys (20%) to accommodate the robotic catheter system. 83 of 85 (98%) calices could be adequately inspected in the ten kidneys. Two lower pole minor calices could not be accessed due to small ostial size. The mean time to inspect the entire collecting system was 4.6 min (range 49 s to 15 min), but decreased considerably with experience.

A Visual analog scale (VAS; 1=worst, 10=best) was completed by the surgeon at the end of each procedure to evaluate the performance of the system. The flexible catheter was rated 10 out of 10 for ureteroscope tip stability, 10 out of 10 for reproducibility of access in each calyx, and 8 out of 10 for reproducibility of the auto-retract mechanism to retract the ureteroscope tip to the original position.

Intraoperatively, one complication of ureteral perforation was observed in one kidney unit (10%) at the ureteropelvic junction due to the surgeon retracting the robotic catheter in the flexed position. On histologic examination of the injured ureter, changes consistent with acute dilation were found, but no necrosis was observed.

On necropsy, significant irrigation extravasation was observed in the retroperitoneum and peritoneal cavity of all five animal subjects. Subsequently, the diameter of the prototype ureteroscope was reduced in size from 8.5 to 7.5 F to increase the space between the ureteroscope and the catheter guide and improve drainage of irrigant fluid. The changes improved drainage sufficiently to eliminate irrigant fluid extravasation on a mechanical and an ex vivo animal study.

Early Clinical Data

After successful application of the flexible robotic system to treat nephrolithiasis in the swine model, improvements were made based on findings from the preliminary animal studies. Applying lessons learned from the animal studies, the authors performed the first clinical study in urology using a flexible robotic system for ureteroscopy [7]. The prospective trial treated 18 patients with renal calculi using a modified Sensei robotic catheter system. All patients had a preexisting ureteral stent in place for approximately 2 weeks prior to the procedure. The robotic catheter system was manually inserted and advanced under fluoroscopic guidance to position the tip of the outer sheath, marked by a radiopaque marker, at the ureteropelvic junction. Stones were fragmented using a Ho:YAG laser with a 365 μm (micron) laser fiber. A ureteral stent was left in place for 2 weeks postoperatively.

The inclusion criteria included patients with 5–15 mm renal stones. The exclusion criteria excluded patients with concomitant ipsilateral ureteral calculi, ipsilateral ureteral stricture or obstruction, documented active urinary tract infection (UTI), baseline renal insufficiency, a solitary kidney, or any anatomical renal anomalies.

Flexible robotic catheter ureteroscopy and laser lithotripsy were performed successfully in 18 patients. The mean operative time was 91 min (range 60–130), stone size was 11.8 mm (range 9–25), stone localization time was 8.7 min (range 1–36), robot docking time was 7.3 min (range 4–18), and total robot time including docking time was 41.4 min (range 21–70). No intra-operative complications were observed and retrograde contrast injection confirmed the absence of perforation at the end of each case. Fluid absorption was clinically insignificant and volume negligible, based on ethanol and fluid absorption testing.

Complete stone clearance was achieved in 10 patients (56%) at 2 months based on CT imaging and 15 patients (89%) at 3 months based on intravenous pyelogram. One patient required a secondary surgical procedure for clearance of symptomatic residual stone burden. All patients were found to have stable renal function and no evidence of ureteral stricture on follow-up at 3 months.

Complications from the procedure included transient upper extremity paresis in one patient with severe scoliosis and a febrile UTI in two patients that responded to antibiotics. The mean length of hospital stay was 2.3 days (range 2–7).

In the clinical experience with robotic ureteroscopy and laser lithotripsy, the surgeon evaluation using the mean VAS Rating (1 = worst, 10 = best) was 8.5 out of 10 for ease of maneuvering, 9.0 out of 10 for ureteroscopic tip stability, and 9.2 out of 10 for ease of stone fragmentation.

The results from the initial clinical trial are promising, but there exists much room for improvement. Hardware improvements such as a narrower catheter system may reduce the need for prestenting and the incorporation of accessories (baskets/lasers) with control from the surgeon console can improve efficiency and eliminate the need for a bedside assistant. The incorporation of haptic feedback may prevent inadvertent injury to tissue. Refinements in software can also improve surgical efficiency by providing benefits such as automated movements and surgical navigation. Further development and studies are necessary to determine the role of flexible robotics in urologic surgery.

Discussion

Advances in flexible ureteroscopic technology allow endourologists to perform a wide range of diagnostic and therapeutic procedures, but there is still scope for improvement. Flexible robotics builds upon the manual ureteroscope platform and enhances technical precision, stability, and range of motion. Developments in flexible robotic technology have the potential to be applied across surgical disciplines and warrant further investigation [7].

One of the key benefits to precision in flexible robotic ureteroscopy stems from motion scaling. In the treatment of stone disease fine scaling can be used for the management of small fragments. Scaling in conjunction with improved stability of the catheter tip has the potential to be useful for precise targeting and management of stones and upper tract lesions.

A remote surgical system provides surgeon-specific benefits in addition to technical benefits. Over the course of their careers, urologists can be exposed to chronic low doses of ionizing radiation from procedures requiring fluoroscopy. Radiation exposure is cumulative and has been shown to lead the development of cataracts, neoplastic disease, and a shortened life span (California Department of Public Health). The use of a remote master–slave control system console provides an ergonomic advantage over manual ureteroscopy and protects the surgeon from exposure to radiation [3].

Although preliminary results from studies are encouraging, the costs associated with the institution of the robotic ureteroscopic platform require evaluation. Given the high level of expertise using current flexible ureteroscope technology, a clinical benefit is necessary in order to justify the initial financial investment costs and necessary surgeon learning curve in equipping centers with flexible robotic systems [8]. Ultimately, further trials comparing manual ureteroscopy to the flexible robotic catheter system are necessary to evaluate potential economic feasibility and clinical benefits.

Summary

The robotic flexible catheter system has shown promising results in preliminary animal and clinical studies. The technology has the potential to provide improved precision, better ergonomics, and reduced occupational radiation exposure. However, further studies are necessary to determine if there is a clinical advantage and if the benefits outweigh the potentially increased cost of the system.

References

1. Young H, McKay R. Congenital valvular obstruction of the prostatic urethra. Surg Gynecol Obstet. 1929; 48:509.
2. Desai MM, Aron M, Gill IS, Pascal-Haber G, Ukimura O, Kaouk JH, et al. Flexible robotic retrograde renoscopy: description of novel robotic device and preliminary laboratory experience. Urology. 2008;72(1):42–6.
3. Aron M, Desai MM. Flexible robotics. Urol Clin North Am. 2009;36(2):157–62.
4. Eisner BH, Kurtz MP, Dretler SP. Ureteroscopy for the management of stone disease. Nat Rev Urol. 2010; 7(1):40–5.

5. Canes D, Desai M. New technology in the treatment of nephrolithiasis. Curr Opin Urol. 2008;18(2):235–40.
6. Crouzet S, Gill IS. Robotic surgery: considerations for the future. In: Palmer JS, editor. Pediatric robotic urology. Humana Press: New York; 2009. p. 69–87.
7. Desai MM, Grover R, Aron M, Ganpule A, Joshi SS, Desai MR, et al. Robotic flexible ureteroscopy for renal calculi: initial clinical experience. J Urol. 2011;186(2):563–8.
8. Matlaga B. Robotic flexible ureteroscopy. J Urol. 2011;186(2):569.

Surgical Simulation

39

Amy E. Krambeck, Matthew T. Gettman, and Mitra R. de Cógáin

The Utility of Surgical Simulation

Endoscopic training has traditionally followed a Halstedian approach, with initial observation, increased operative responsibility, and finally surgical autonomy, with residents and fellows participating in supervised surgical cases [1–5]. The surgical opportunities afforded to the trainee are random and rely solely upon presentation of patients to the office or hospital setting [2, 3]. Until recently, techniques were taught either in the office setting or operating room, on actual patients. Instruction in ureteroscopic cases presents a unique challenge, as visual cues and tactile feedback are altered as compared to open surgical procedures. Furthermore, the visual field is quite limited both for the resident surgeon and the supervisor [1]. A novel skill set is required to perform these cases safely, and a significant learning curve is associated with some procedures, contributing to longer operative times and increased patient morbidity.

Early training in ureteroscopic procedures required educators and trainees to alternate looking through the eye-piece. The advent of the duplicate viewing lens allowed residents to directly observe surgical technique and later, the use of videoendoscopy provided simultaneous viewing to the consultant and trainee, allowing for direct instruction and supervision [6]. However, a training gap still exists, as procedures must be undertaken in an independent fashion, with a unique armamentarium of skills only acquired through repetition. Also, the breadth of minimally invasive procedures has expanded significantly over the recent past, increasing training demands on residents and consulting staff [6–8].

In addition to the difficulties faced in endoscopic education resulting from the unique procedural requirements, there are fewer opportunities for mentoring residents in the operating room due to multiple factors. Recent mandates have limited resident duty hours and have resulted in decreased time for training in the operating room [6]. Medicolegal issues have also impacted surgical training, as consulting staff, fearful of litigation, tend to restrict the procedural autonomy allowed to residents and fellows. Finally, budget-conscious programs may emphasize efficiency in the operating room, possibly to the detriment of trainee education [4, 5]. These factors have resulted in decreased resident-patient contact in the office setting and in the operative suite.

All of the aforementioned issues have resulted in the need for endourological teaching opportunities outside of the cystoscopy suite. Simulation, i.e., the use of any device that recreates situations encountered in practice, has long been used in training in other technically demanding fields, including the airline industry and the military

A.E. Krambeck, M.D. (✉) • M.T. Gettman, M.D.
M.R. de Cógáin, M.D.
Department of Urology, Mayo Clinic, 200 1st SW, Rochester, MN 55905, USA
e-mail: Krambeck.amy@mayo.edu

M. Monga (ed.), *Ureteroscopy: Indications, Instrumentation & Technique*, Current Clinical Urology, DOI 10.1007/978-1-62703-206-3_39, © Springer Science+Business Media New York 2013

[1, 6, 9]. However, only over the past two decades has simulation come to the forefront of surgical training. Both the American Council for Graduate and Medical Education (ACGME) and the American College of Surgeons (ACS) have recently imposed new mandates regarding the use of surgical simulation for accreditation of various residency programs and medical institutions [10, 11]. In fact, the ACS Accredited Education Institutes' motto reads "Enhancing patient safety through simulation" [12].

Simulation provides a low-stress environment for trainees to grasp a basic skill set, and to explore complex surgical situations without the repercussions of a technical error in a live patient [10]. Repetition afforded by simulation provides the resident increased comfort and technical ability with a particular procedure, and allows surgical errors with exploration of all possible outcomes, without incurring harm, shame, or liability [10]. Sweet and McDougall, in their recent analysis of training programs incorporating simulation activities, note that in the clinical setting, consultants must prioritize their goals, with care of the patient being at the forefront, and education of the resident a secondary concern [13]. Simulation allows educators to focus all of their attention on instructing the resident and improving their performance. In addition, simulators allow for objective evaluation of a particular skill set, minimizing procedural variability and the impact of exogenous factors, which may be encountered in the operating room [13]. It is, however, important to mention the limitations of simulators. Not only can appropriate technique be taught by these novel training tools; poor procedural skills can also be reinforced without proper instruction and guidance from experts in the field.

The use of animal and cadaveric models has fallen out of favor due to ethical concerns, maintenance costs, and the inaccurate representation of human systems [6–8]. Over the past 5–10 years, new endoscopic simulators have been introduced to aid in Urology resident education. However, no consensus exists as to the optimal simulation training program, as each individual residency program has various technologies available to them and employs available resources differently. A 2006 survey of Urology residency program directors found unanimous agreement regarding the utility of simulation in training programs; however, only 16% of programs had such resources available to residents [2, 7]. In addition, program directors felt that simulation may have a role in providing an objective, ongoing assessment of the progression of endoscopic skills during residency or fellowship. Although most program directors felt strongly about the use of simulation for various reasons, a majority also expressed hesitation that simulators provide an adequate substitute for hands-on training. While simulation provides a significant compliment to surgical training, it may not be a direct substitute for operating room experiences.

A variety of factors have contributed to the need for adjunct surgical instruction, above and beyond what can be offered through a traditional Halstedian format. Rising concern over resident duty hours, medicolegal issues and rapidly evolving technologies have limited resident experiences in the operating room. The novel skill set required to perform ureteroscopy safely presents a significant challenge with regards to intraoperative teaching, however, it ideally lends itself to instruction through simulation.

Validation of Surgical Simulators

In urology, simulators have been primarily developed for endoscopic procedures including cystoscopy and ureteroscopy [8]. Prior to initiating the use of simulators in resident training to either teach or assess a particular skill set, the construct must go through a rigorous subjective and objective evaluation process to assess validity and reliability [6, 15]. Validity refers to how well a simulator measures and teaches the procedure it is designed to simulate [6, 14–17]. Reliability refers to the uniform reproducibility of a desired simulated situation [17]. Validation of a simulator is a multifaceted task, which requires the input of trainees and experts alike, in addition to analytical evaluation of the simulation activity [6, 15–17].

Table 39.1 Global rating score (adapted from Wilhelm et al. [21])

Task	1	3	5
Identify anatomy	No knowledge	Moderate identification	100% identification
Endoscopic maneuvers	Significant trauma, trouble with luminal view	Rare trauma, reasonable luminal view	No trauma, excellent luminal view
Employment of adjunct instrumentation	Required multiple attempts with guidewire, basket, or laser	Relatively good use guidewire, basket, or laser	Smooth use of guidewire, basket, or laser
Procedural autonomy	Needed significant assistance, frequent pauses	Minimal assistance required	No assistance
Overall proficiency	Poor	Average	Excellent

When introducing a proposed simulator for educational purposes, rigorous studies to establish multiple forms of validity must be carried out [17, 18]. Subjective validity refers to the assessment of simulators for appropriateness of content and is comprised of two subsets, face and content validity. Face validity refers to how well a simulator represents the reality of the procedure it is designed to teach, as assessed by nonexperts, ensuring that subject matter is appropriate [6, 15, 18]. Content validity requires the evaluation of the content and construct of the simulator by experts in the field, ensuring that simulation covers important surgical concepts [6, 15, 18]. Objective validity is also comprised of multiple components, including construct validity and criterion validity, which can be further broken down into concurrent validity and predictive validity. Construct validity refers to the ability of a simulator to differentiate a novice from an expert or to identify progression of skill in a particular individual [18]. Concurrent validity compares a new simulation activity to an established "gold standard" [18]. Lastly, predictive validity refers to the ability of a simulation activity to portend the future performance of a specific surgical task in a real-life setting [18].

One commonly used measure of operative performance is an Objective Structured Assessment of Technical Skills (OSATS) protocol for a particular procedure, which employs a scoring system for achieving certain tasks and also for the quality of maneuvers performed [19]. This provides a structured assessment of simulation, which can be followed over time, and also has been shown to differentiate between novice and expert surgeons [19]. In addition, objective measures such as OSATS can provide criteria for concurrent and predictive validity, correlating a new simulation activity with existing models or looking at intraoperative resident achievement as compared to OSATS scores [18]. Also, a subjective assessment can be performed using a global rating score for ureteroscopic procedures, validated by Matsumoto and colleagues and adapted by a number of researchers, with points awarded for a trainee's performance in a number of categories (Table 39.1) [4, 20].

Simulators

Simulators are commonly categorized as low or high fidelity. Low-fidelity simulators are defined as those inanimate models that have decreased similarity to real-life situations, such as suture tying boards and laparoscopic box trainers [6]. These trainers allow the improvement of certain surgical skills, but not the ability to practice or evaluate the completion of an entire procedure [6]. Low-fidelity simulators also require a mentor to instruct in and observe for appropriate technique. One benefit of low-fidelity simulators is that they tend to be low cost and easily accessible. High-fidelity simulators are those that more closely mimic reality, traditionally with the use of cadaveric or animal models, but more recently with the use of accurate inanimate constructs, computer-aided technology, and the creation of simulators which may also include virtual instruction. The highest fidelity simulation is achieved by maximizing representation of visual, physical, psychological, and tactile reality [21]. Changes in the model and environment are designed to elicit trainee responses that would mimic those in real-life operative situations [13].

Early reports of endoscopic simulation were made by Trindade and colleagues in 1981, when they described the use of a cadaveric dog model for cystoscopic and ureteroscopic procedures [18]. Subsequently, the development of low fidelity of bench-top models and virtual reality simulators has provided an accessible training alternative, avoiding ethical issues and high costs of using cadaveric models. Preminger and colleagues first described the use of a VR simulator for ureteroscopy in 1996, and over the past 10–15 years, other high-fidelity simulators have become available for ureteroscopic instruction [22]. However, low fidelity models have also been studied and found to be efficacious in resident training, with similar improvement in surgical technique as what is observed with high-fidelity simulators [6]. Schout and colleagues performed a systematic review of the literature on endourologic simulators in 2008 [23]. Of the 26 validation studies reviewed for this publication, they found that high fidelity models (as described below) generally had construct validity. However, they note that relatively few studies have been performed to look that the transfer of skills, from simulator to real patient.

Low-Fidelity Simulators

Matsumoto and colleagues advocate the use of a cost-effective, low fidelity bench model for ureteroscopy, with a 2002 study demonstrating that a model constructed from readily available materials provided equitable improvement in performance, provided that the model is constructed thoughtfully, with specific maneuvers required to successfully complete the task at hand [4]. Their model was comprised of a Styrofoam cup to mimic the bladder, two straws to replicate ureters, and a Penrose drain to act as the urethra, and cost $20 to build. Importantly, in designing the low-fidelity model, expert consensus of the key steps of ureteroscopy was obtained, with the construction of the simulator intended to replicate these steps [4]. The authors were able to confirm construct validity, with low-fidelity and high-fidelity trainees with statistically significant superior performance as compared to didactic-only trainees [4]. However, predictive validity of this model was not established, as the medical student subjects could not be ethically allowed to operate autonomously on a real patient [4, 18].

Although some low cost simulators have been described for other endoscopic procedures, often times incorporating the use of standard surgical equipment and substitute tissue (i.e., chicken breast for a prostate tissue), few low-fidelity ureteroscopic simulators have been described [6]. This is likely due to the significant variability in procedural steps encountered in upper tract interrogation, due to both patient and operative factors [6]. The primary advantages of low-fidelity simulators include low cost and easy portability [6]. However, low-fidelity simulators cannot generally replicate entire procedures and will have a decreased relationship to real-life situations encountered in the operating room [6].

High-Fidelity, Non-virtual Reality Simulators

High-fidelity, non-VR simulators used in surgical training are currently constructed using materials such as latex and silicone to replicate human tissues and often employ the use of standard endoscopic equipment [8, 24]. Significant advances in available materials have allowed more accurate representation, allowing for a more realistic simulation experience. These models can be manipulated to introduce procedural variability that may be encountered in the operating room, in real-life situations. Some authors argue that use of the high-fidelity bench models is preferable to virtual reality models, as they use real surgical equipment and can be placed in the operating theater to most closely approximate a true surgical case [8]. Several simulators have been described and validated, incorporating the use of objective testing, including OSATS criteria, and subjective measures with global rating scores.

Uro-Scopic Trainer

The Uro-Scopic Trainer™ (Limbs and Things, Bristol, UK) is one high-fidelity bench model that incorporates a mannequin replica of the adult male genitourinary tract, with model urethra, bladder, ureters, and intrarenal collecting systems. It is designed to be used with standard endoscopic flexible and rigid equipment. Multiple simulation activities can be carried out with this model, including urethroscopy and cystoscopy, in addition to therapeutic and diagnostic ureteroscopy. Irrigation can be used with this system. The simulator incorporates built-in ports that can be used to place calculi into the urinary tract, and realism can be reinforced with simulated blood [18]. The simulated ureters are transparent to allow for direct observation of instrument placement during the training activity.

Matsumoto and colleagues evaluated this simulator, with validation studies including 11 junior and 6 senior urology residents [4]. All subjects underwent a pretest, a didactic training session, a post-didactic test, a simulation hands-on training session, and a final posttest. Hands-on skills were assessed using a global rating score and checklist. Senior residents outperformed juniors on the global rating score, establishing construct validity and simulation training appeared to have a direct association with overall performance [18].

Scope Trainers

The Scope Trainer™ and Advanced Scope Trainer™ (Mediskills Ltd, Edinburgh, UK), are high-fidelity bench models, with a distensible bladder and anatomic representation of the location of the ureteral orifices, the course of ureters, and orientation of the collecting systems of an adult male [18]. The Advanced Scope Trainer also has a see-through dome to allow for direct visualization of endoscopic instruments. Irrigation can be used with these models, and is emptied through the bladder. These models can also be used with a percutaneous access trainer, to teach percutaneous nephrolithotomy. In addition, the simulators contain both an upper tract calculus and an upper tract tumor, to teach both lithotripsy and endoscopic tumor management, and can be used with fluoroscopy [18].

In Brehmer's initial validation studies of the Scope Trainer, performed in 2002, the model was prepared in the operating room, and draped as a live patient, to maximally replicate a real-life operative case [25]. Fourteen urologists were tested on rigid ureteroscopy, including nine consultants and five residents. All participants were studied on the model once and on live patients twice, to account for intraoperative variability. The mean score on a task-specific checklist was identical between the model and live patients, loosely suggesting predictive validity, and did not vary between trainees and attendings; however, subspecialists in endourology scored higher, demonstrating construct validity. Content validity was demonstrated as well, as individuals felt that the activity accurately replicated real surgery [18].

Brehmer's group expanded the initial study of the Scope Trainer to include residents with little endourologic experience [16]. The performance of all resident groups with rigid ureteroscopy for a distal ureteral calculus, as assessed by a task-specific and global checklist, including those who had never performed ureteroscopy before, improved following instruction and 2 days of simulation training [16]. Residents who had never before performed ureteroscopy improved somewhat more than those with some endoscopic experience. All residents assessed had improved confidence with the technique following the educational program [16].

Adult Ureteroscopy Trainer

The Adult Ureteroscopy Trainer™ (Ideal Anatomic Modeling, Holt, Michigan) is a novel, high-fidelity model that was developed by a Urology resident as an affordable alternative to commercially produced simulators [24]. A computerized tomography study from a patient who had difficulty with spontaneous stone passage was used to recreate the urinary collecting system in silicone using rapid prototyping technology. This model can be used with standard ureteroscopic and fluoroscopic technologies.

White and colleagues performed validation studies of the Adult Ureteroscopy Trainer, the first with 19 consultant urologists, 11 Urology residents, 10 medical students, and 6 biotechnology industry representatives performing both ureteroscopy and nephroscopy, with questionnaires completed before and after the procedures [24]. The groups' second study assessed construct validity with two, ten-person groups, one of which had never performed ureteroscopy and the second who performed more than 30 cases per year [24]. The first study established face and content validity, with all participants rating the simulator as a realistic training tool that was easy to use, while the second demonstrated construct validity, with consultant urologists outperforming trainees, as evaluated by a task-based scoring system [24].

High Fidelity Virtual Reality Simulators

The UroMentor™ (Simbionix, Lod, Israel) is a high fidelity, commercially available virtual reality cystoscopic and ureteroscopic simulator. It employs the use of standard semirigid and flexible endoscopic instruments and a mannequin shell, with computer-generated graphics and haptic technology to simulate anatomical structures and intraoperative situations [8, 18, 26, 27]. A database of real-life cases is available, allowing the trainee exposure to a variety of patient and surgical factors, including situations with decreased visualization and difficult anatomic configurations. This high fidelity, virtual reality model is linked to teaching modules and the simulator itself has the ability to evaluate the practitioner and record the performance history for a particular individual [18, 27].

The UroMentor has undergone numerous validation studies, looking at content, realism, and the predictive ability of simulation activities [1, 8, 20, 27–30]. Watterson and colleagues assert that content and face validity are established in this model, as it incorporates high-fidelity graphics, the use of real endoscopic instruments, and has multiple real surgical cases available for training [8]. Two studies, one by Wilhelm and colleagues and the other by Watterson and colleagues, evaluated medical students with randomization to control groups or instruction with UroMentor simulation [20, 28]. Both studies demonstrated significant improvement in a subjective global rating score following UroMentor training. Further studies by Jacomides and associates evaluated the performance of simulation-trained medical students as compared to nonsimulation-trained residents [1]. The performance of the simulation-trained medical students paralleled that of first-year Urology residents, who had performed 14 ureteroscopic procedures on average, while more senior residents performed better overall than the aforementioned groups, establishing construct validity. The medical students demonstrated significant reduction in operative time following UroMentor training as compared to their preoperative assessments. Ogan and colleagues also performed initial studies establishing predictive validity of this model, with medical students who performed well in simulation activities demonstrating higher proficiency in cadaveric models [29]. Interestingly, resident scores between the simulation activities and cadaveric procedures were not well correlated, perhaps indicating that simulation activities are most useful in instructing and evaluating the clinically inexperienced surgeon [29].

High Fidelity, Biological Models

A number of various live and cadaveric animal models have been used historically to study the upper urinary tract, namely dog, rabbit, and more recently, swine [11, 31–33]. The use of a live porcine model is favored, due to the similarity of the anatomical structure to that of humans, including multi-papillary kidney architecture [31]. Sampaio and associates conducted morphologic studies of the porcine kidney and found that, despite some minor differences, they are similar to human kidneys with regard to length, caliceal orientation, and variability and urinary drainage, making them ideal representative models. This model was also advocated as an accurate model for the study of urological procedures by Paterson and colleagues, although they noted the lack of perinephric fat in swine (causing increased kidney mobility), tortuosity of the ureters, and location of the ureteral orifices at the bladder neck, all of which may make ureteroscopic procedures more

Table 39.2 Comparison of various simulators (adapted from Wignall et al. [4])

Category	Examples	Advantages	Disadvantages
Low fidelity	Suture tying board, laparoscopic box trainers	Inexpensive, reusable	Require mentor presence, cannot evaluate entire procedure
High fidelity			
Non-virtual reality	Uro-Scopic Trainer, Scope Trainers, Adult Ureteroscopy Trainer	Procedural representation, reusable, can be placed in OR to recreate real-life situations	Unrealistic representation of human tissues
Virtual reality	URO Mentor	Feedback not requiring mentor presence, variable cases, reusable	Expensive, maintenance costs
Biological	Cadavers, animal models	Real anatomy with tissue responsiveness, complete procedure possible	Poor tissue quality, deterioration or poor representation of human tissues, ethical concerns, expensive, not reusable

difficult and decrease the content validity [32]. The main concerns regarding the use of live animals include ethical considerations, the high cost required to maintain the research subjects as well as issues related to animal–human disease transmission, including bovine encephalopathy [15].

An alternative option is the employment of cadavers or cadaveric tissues for endourological instruction, which has long been utilized and reported [26, 34–37]. The primary advantage of cadaveric instruction is the obvious accurate anatomical representation and the ability to perform a complete procedure. However, the high cost, ethical concerns, and deterioration of tissues may impede the common use of this model [29]. A summary of the simulators discussed is included in this chapter for easy comparison (Table 39.2).

Curriculum Development and Implementation

As reviewed above, ureteroscopic simulation employing a variety of models appears to provide realistic and potentially transferrable training that can be used as an adjunct to traditional Halstedian teaching practices. When devising an educational curriculum, simulation or otherwise, it is imperative to understand the fundamentals of human learning [17]. Kolb constructivist theory describes "experiential learning" or acquisition of knowledge through activities, and encompasses a learning cycle of concrete experience, reflective observation, abstract conceptualization, and active experimentation. Carter and colleagues describe the integration of surgical simulation into this construct, with residents performing repetition of a particular task (concrete experience), self-reflection with external feedback from a supervising consultant (reflective observation), self-determination of methods to improve performance (abstract conceptualization), and finally tests of these ideas to see if improved outcomes are achieved (active experimentation) [17]. The available simulation technologies must be complimented by expert feedback, which can be accomplished through computerized training modules or through direct observance by consulting staff [8].

Thus, in order to implement a simulation curriculum, it is imperative to understand adult learners and transfer this educational construct into a series of simulation modules designed to teach specific procedures. In a survey of Urology residency program directors, they unanimously agreed that surgical simulation should play a role in trainee education [2]. However, no consensus as to the content or the method of implementation of such a training program exists.

A recent study by Ahmed and associates discusses the practical aspects of designing a sustainable teaching program and implementation of this type of instruction in current Urology residency programs [38]. The authors describe the "6 P's," which provide the fundamental framework to design a functional simulation curriculum: "Place," i.e., geographic accessibility, "People" or faculty in leadership positions, "Pounds" or funding, "Programs/Products," i.e., a curriculum composed by experts with evidence-based endpoints and "Positioning," or appropriate location of simulation within the rest of the surgical training program [38]. The authors do note significant impediments in the initiation of simulation programs, including poor funding, decreased acceptability, lack of evidence, and the limited research in the area.

Grantcharov and colleagues have described a simulation curriculum, first with an initial introduction to relevant instrumentation along with discussion of surgical theory, followed by the use of a simulation curriculum until proficiency is achieved, with ongoing assessment of surgical skill progression, either by an observer or computerized feedback using a validated assessment [39]. Hammond and colleagues review a comprehensive simulation curriculum, which has a provided syllabus with concrete learning objectives and a presimulation instructional session led by an expert followed by a simulation activity using cadaveric porcine urinary tracts (which were locally donated and thus inexpensive) [11]. In the realm of simulation in general surgery, Aggarwal and colleagues studied the learning curve of laparoscopic cholecystectomy, evaluating both novice and expert surgeons, and based on the skill progression and learning curves, proposed a stepwise simulation training module for laparoscopic cholecystectomy [40, 41]. Perhaps similar studies in ureteroscopic simulation could be used to devise a standardized ureteroscopic simulation curriculum. In summary, an ideal curriculum for ureteroscopy simulation should incorporate a syllabus describing the tasks at hand, an appropriately graded set of simulation activities to perform under expert supervision, with a posttest to ensure competence.

Conclusions

In light of increasingly stringent resident duty hours, decreased operating room opportunities, medicolegal concerns, and difficulty in endoscopic instruction in the operative suite, simulation has come to the forefront as a potential way to enhance endourological training. Although multiple studies have been performed to assess the validity of various simulators, those establishing predictive validity, or the transferability of skills acquired in the simulation lab to the operating room, are small in number. However, it appears that surgical simulation is a useful adjunct to traditional surgical instruction, and this transition of experience should be investigated further. In order to fully maximize the possibilities of the use of simulation in ureteroscopic training, a structured, stepwise curriculum must be designed by experts, and should incorporate adult learning styles, ACGME requirements, and a valid assessment of proficiency. Only in this way will simulation activities fulfill their potential in resident instruction.

References

1. Jacomides L, Ogan K, Cadeddu JA, Pearle MS. Use of a virtual reality simulator for ureteroscopy training. J Urol. 2004;171(1):320–3.
2. Le CQ, Lightner DJ, VanderLei L, Segura JW, Gettman MT. The current role of medical simulation in American urological residency training programs: an assessment by program directors. J Urol. 2007;177(1):288–91.
3. Wallack MK, Chao L. Resident work hours: the evolution of a revolution. Arch Surg. 2001;136(12):1426–31.
4. Matsumoto ED, Hamstra SJ, Radomski SB, Cusimano MD. The effect of bench model fidelity on endourological skills: a randomized controlled study. J Urol. 2002;167(3):1243–7.
5. Bridges M, Diamond DL. The financial impact of teaching surgical residents in the operating room. Am J Surg. 1999;177(1):28–32.
6. Wignall GR, Denstedt JD, Preminger GM, Cadeddu JA, Pearle MS, Sweet RM, McDougall EM. Surgical simulation: a urological perspective. J Urol. 2008;179(5):1690–9.
7. Gettman MT, Le CQ, Rangel LJ, Slezak JM, Bergstralh EJ, Krambeck AE. Analysis of a computer based simulator as an educational tool for cystoscopy: subjective and objective results. J Urol. 2008;179(1):267–71.
8. Watterson JD, Denstedt JD. Ureteroscopy and cystoscopy simulation in urology. J Endourol. 2007;21(3):263–9.
9. Fairhurst K, Strickland A, Maddern GJ. Simulation speak. J Surg Educ. 2011;68(5):382–6.
10. Sutton E and Park A. Minimally invasive surgery training: theories, methods, outcomes [Internet].

Washington: Department of Health & Human Services (US), National Institutes of Health, National Library of Medicine; 2010. Chapter 7, Simulation's Role in Surgical Training. Available from: http://mastri.umm.edu/NIH-Book/index.html
11. Hammond L, Ketchum J, Schwartz BF. Accreditation council on graduate medical education technical skills competency compliance: urologic surgical skills. J Am Coll Surg. 2005;201(3):454–7.
12. Listing of ACS Accredited Education Institutes [Internet]. 2011 [cited 2011 Dec 2]; Available at: www.facs.org/education/accreditationprogram/list.html
13. Sweet RM, McDougall EM. Simulation and computer-animated devices: the new minimally invasive skills training paradigm. Urol Clin North Am. 2008;35(3):519–31.
14. Schout BM, Hendrikx AJ, Scheele F, Bemelmans BL, Scherpbier AJ. Validation and implementation of surgical simulators: a critical review of present, past, and future. Surg Endosc. 2010;24(3):536–46.
15. McDougall EM. Validation of surgical simulators. J Endourol. 2007;21(3):244–7.
16. Brehmer M, Swartz R. Training on bench models improves dexterity in ureteroscopy. Eur Urol. 2005; 48(3):458–63.
17. Carter FJ, Schijven MP, Aggarwal R, Grantcharov T, Francis NK, Hanna GB, Jakimowicz JJ. Consensus guidelines for validation of virtual reality surgical simulators. Surg Endosc. 2005;19(12):1523–32.
18. Olweny EO, Pearle MS. Update on resident training models for ureteroscopy. Curr Urol Rep. 2011;12(2): 115–20.
19. Chou DS, Abdelshehid C, Clayman RV, McDougall EM. Comparison of results of virtual-reality simulator and training model for basic ureteroscopy training. J Endourol. 2006;20(4):266–71.
20. Wilhelm DM, Ogan K, Roehrborn CG, Cadeddu JA, Pearle MS. Assessment of basic endoscopic performance using a virtual reality simulator. J Am Coll Surg. 2002;195(5):675–81.
21. Shah J, Mackay S, Vale J, Darzi A. Simulation in urology–a role for virtual reality? BJU Int. 2001; 88(7):661–5.
22. Preminger GM, Babayan RK, Merril GL, Raju R, Millman A, Merril JR. Virtual reality surgical simulation in endoscopic urologic surgery. Stud Health Technol Inform. 1996;29:157–63.
23. Schout BM, Hendrikx AJ, Scherpbier AJ, Bemelmans BL. Update on training models in endourology: a qualitative systematic review of the literature between January 1980 and April 2008. Eur Urol. 2008;54(6): 1247–61.
24. White MA, Dehaan AP, Stephens DD, Maes AA, Maatman TJ. Validation of a high fidelity adult ureteroscopy and renoscopy simulator. J Urol. 2010; 183(2):673–7.
25. Brehmer M, Tolley D. Validation of a bench model for endoscopic surgery in the upper urinary tract. Eur Urol. 2002;42(2):175–9.
26. Michel MS, Knoll T, Köhrmann KU, Alken P. The URO Mentor: development and evaluation of a new computer-based interactive training system for virtual life-like simulation of diagnostic and therapeutic endourological procedures. BJU Int. 2002;89(3): 174–7.
27. Matsumoto ED, Pace KT, D'A Honey RJ. Virtual reality ureteroscopy simulator as a valid tool for assessing endourological skills. Int J Urol. 2006; 13(7):896–901.
28. Watterson JD, Beiko DT, Kuan JK, Denstedt JD. Randomized prospective blinded study validating acquistion of ureteroscopy skills using computer based virtual reality endourological simulator. J Urol. 2002;168(5):1928–32.
29. Ogan K, Jacomides L, Shulman MJ, Roehrborn CG, Cadeddu JA, Pearle MS. Virtual ureteroscopy predicts ureteroscopic proficiency of medical students on a cadaver. J Urol. 2004;172(2):667–71.
30. Shah J, Montgomery B, Langley S, Darzi A. Validation of a flexible cystoscopy course. BJU Int. 2002;90(9): 833–5.
31. Sampaio FJ, Pereira-Sampaio MA, Favorito LA. The pig kidney as an endourologic model: anatomic contribution. J Endourol. 1998;12(1):45–50.
32. Paterson RF, Lingeman JE, Evan AP, Connors BA, Williams Jr JC, McAteer JA. Percutaneous stone implantation in the pig kidney: a new animal model for lithotripsy research. J Endourol. 2002;16(8): 543–7.
33. Evan AP, Connors BA, Lingeman JE, Blomgren P, Willis LR. Branching patterns of the renal artery of the pig. Anat Rec. 1996;246(2):217–23.
34. Cervantes L, Keitzer WA. Endoscopic training in urology. J Urol. 1960;84:585–6.
35. Trindade JC, Lautenschlager MF, de Araujo CG. Endoscopic surgery: a new teaching method. J Urol. 1981;126(2):192.
36. Habib HN, Berger J, Winter CC. Teaching transurethral surgery using a cow's udder. J Urol. 1965;93: 77–9.
37. Narwani KP, Reid EC. Teaching transurethral prostatic resection using cadaver bladder. J Urol. 1969; 101(1):101.
38. Ahmed K, Amer T, Challacombe B, Jaye P, Dasgupta P, Khan MS. How to develop a simulation programme in urology. BJU Int. 2011;108(11):1698–702.
39. Grantcharov TP, Reznick RK. Teaching procedural skills. BMJ. 2008;336(7653):1129–31.
40. Aggarwal R, Grantcharov TP, Eriksen JR, Blirup D, Kristiansen VB, Funch-Jensen P, Darzi A. An evidence-based virtual reality training program for novice laparoscopic surgeons. Ann Surg. 2006;244(2): 310–4.
41. Aggarwal R, Grantcharov T, Moorthy K, Hance J, Darzi A. A competency-based virtual reality training curriculum for the acquisition of laparoscopic psychomotor skill. Am J Surg. 2006;191(1): 128–33.

Ferromagnetics in Ureteroscopy

40

Yung Khan Tan and Jeffrey A. Cadeddu

This chapter contains video segments that can be found on the accompanying DVD

Introduction

Urolithiasis is an increasing medical problem in the United States. Pearle et al. found that between 1994 and 2000 there was approximately a 40 % increase in medical visits for stone-related disorders and 2.1 billion US dollars was spent in 2000 alone for the management of these conditions. This represented a 50 % increase in expenditure compared with 1994 [1]. Further studies have noted that the previous preponderance for males has slowly shifted towards a more equal distribution among the sexes [2].

Management of urolithiasis has largely evolved through advancements in surgical technology as medical management of this disease has been difficult to accomplish due to its limited effectiveness and poor patient compliance with medication regimes. New technologies, like shockwave lithotripsy (SWL), percutaneous nephrolithotomy (PCNL), and more recently flexible ureteroscopy and lasers, have supplanted the need for invasive procedures like an open nephrolithotomy. Unfortunately, these newer technologies, though orders of magnitude less invasive, have not necessarily meant better stone clearance rates.

Y.K. Tan, M.B.B.S(Melbourne), M.R.C.S(Edin.) (✉)
J.A. Cadeddu, M.D.
Department of Urology, University of Texas Southwestern Medical Center at Dallas, Dallas, TX, USA
e-mail: yungkhan@gmail.com

Current Stone-Free Success Rates

Recent SWL results quote a stone-free rate of 60–80 % at 3 months [3]. The data on flexible ureteroscopy is not much better. Macejko et al. [4] reported stone-free rates after flexible ureteroscopy using computed tomography of only 50.4 % increasing to 84.1 % success if they accepted residual fragments less than 4 mm as being successful. Even in more invasive procedures like PCNL, Altunrende et al. [5] noted a stone-free rate of 74.5 % with a 22 % clinically insignificant residual fragment (CIRF) rate.

There are a number of reasons for the failure of these procedures to completely eradicate the calculi. In SWL this can include improper patient selection. It is widely recognized that SWL for lower pole stones yields low success rates of around 67 % in stones less than 1 cm in diameter [6]. This success falls further as the stone size increases. In PCNL and flexible ureteroscopy, failure of success stems from difficult anatomy, poor visualization, limited maneuverability of instruments, and operator fatigue from long surgical times.

M. Monga (ed.), *Ureteroscopy: Indications, Instrumentation & Technique*, Current Clinical Urology,
DOI 10.1007/978-1-62703-206-3_40, © Springer Science+Business Media New York 2013

Clinically Insignificant Residual Fragments

In the arena of SWL for renal calculi an entity known as CIRF emerged to try and improve the success rates of SWL. Stones less than 4 mm in diameter were classified as CIRF as it was believed that though these fragments remained in the kidney they had an excellent chance of passage without causing significant clinical symptoms. CIRF was also used in the flexible ureteroscopy and PCNL data to determine success rates of treatment. The issue with such a classification of course was the possibility that a number of these stone fragments will not pass but instead would act as a nidus for stone formation. Osman et al. found that in patients post SWL with CIRF, up to 20 % would have stone recurrence necessitating retreatment [7]. Rebuck et al. [8] found that in patients with CIRF after ureteroscopy up to 20 % would develop stone-related events over the following 1.6 years. Similarly, Altunrende et al. [5] noted that in patients post PCNL with CIRF, up to 26 % would develop symptomatic stone episodes requiring treatment. Raman et al. found that post PCNL stones greater than 2 mm or located in the renal pelvis or ureter independently predicted for future stone-related events [9].

Recognizing the problems of residual fragments, there have been a number of attempts at reducing these fragments. With proximal ureteric stones, the use of stone cones [10] and dissolvable gels [11] has been shown to reduce the retropulsion of fragments into the kidney. In retrograde intrarenal surgery, practices such as upper pole displacement of lower pole stones have been used to try and overcome difficulties of lower calyceal anatomy and improve fragmentation and clearance rates. In SWL, practices such as mechanical inversion and percussion have been shown to improve stone clearance [12]. Ultimately, the ideal situation would be a single procedure that would be able to achieve stone-free status.

Ferromagnetic Extraction of Stone Fragments

A novel concept to improve stone-free rates in a single procedure was thus developed to remove stone fragments with a magnet during flexible ureteroscopy or PCNL. In 2010, Tracy et al. [13] first described the proof of concept of stone fragment extraction with a magnetic tool. The surface characteristics of calcium-based stones, which are the predominant form of urinary stones, were investigated (data not published). It was found that carboxyl-functionalized polymers inhibited the growth of calcium oxalate crystals in vitro by binding to the crystals. One micron microparticles with an iron oxide core (Invitrogen, Carlsberg, USA) were then coated with the polymer to facilitate their binding to calcium-based stones. When human calcium oxalate stone fragments (between 1 and 3 mm diameter) were exposed to a solution of these microparticles, the microparticles bound to the surface of stone fragments rendering them supraparamagnetic. Tracy et al. placed the coated stone fragments in a bladder model and an 8 F magnet rod was passed through the working channel of a rigid cystoscope to attract the stone fragments. A comparison was made between magnetic extraction of stone fragments versus a 2.4 F tipless nitinol basket. They found that there was a 53 % reduction in extraction time favoring the magnetic tool (Table 40.1). They also reported that less passes were required for the extraction (average of 3.7 passes for the magnet vs. 9.4 for the basket) with a mean of 2.7 stones extracted per pass with the magnetic tool. The basket on the other hand did not manage to extract more than one stone per pass. Tests were also done on the performance envelope of the magnetic system. Incubation studies were performed and it was found that at a concentration of 1 mg/ml of microparticles with an incubation of 10 min, 100 % of stones less than 3 mm could be retrieved in vitro with the magnetic tool.

One of the reasons for failure of complete stone extraction during PCNL and flexible

Table 40.1 Time (s) required to extract ten fragments in a bladder model

Trial	Magnetic removal (s)	Basket removal (s)	Difference (s)	Stones in ureteral orifice (magnetic, basket)
1	257	555[a]	298	1, 1
2	413	410	−3	2, 1
3	235	730	495	2, 2
4	174	298	124	0, 0
5	228	265	37	0, 0
6	46	250	204	0, 0
7	150	320	170	0, 0
Mean*	215	404	189	0, 0

[13], reprinted with permission from Elsevier Limited
*$P < 0.009$, Mann–Whitney *U* test
[a]One stone fragment could not be removed from ureter with basket but was easily removed with the prototype magnetic device

ureteroscopy is of course the issue of poor visualization. This is often due to bleeding in the collecting system. Mir et al. [14] thus studied the effect of urine and blood on the binding of these novel microparticles to calcium oxalate stone fragments and the ability to attract the functionalized stones to the magnetic tool in these environments. In vitro urine concentrations of 5, 20, and 50 % were combined with microparticles (1 mg/ml) and stone fragments for a 10-min incubation period. Similarly blood concentrations of 0.5, 1, and 2 % (on visual inspection one cannot see through a test tube of 2 % concentration blood) were used. In both experiments, the investigators were able to achieve 100 % stone extraction, of fragment sizes of up to 3 mm, at all concentrations indicating a negligible interference of urine and blood in the clinical environment.

Mir et al. [14] also performed initial investigations of the in vitro toxicity of these microparticles on murine fibroblast, human urothelium, and human transitional cell carcinoma cell lines. Each cell line was plated at three different concentrations of cells and exposed uniformly to 1 mg/ml concentration of microparticles. No toxicity was seen in any of the three cell lines after 48 h of exposure except in urothelial cells at the lowest concentration of cells. Further biotoxicity tests have since been conducted in mice (data not published). The animals were exposed to these novel microparticles intravesically or intravenously. The systemic exposure was for a worst-case scenario where microparticles breached the urothelial membrane and entered the systemic circulation. Each group was further subdivided and given concentrations of the microparticles at 0.5, 1, and 5 mg/ml. We found that when particles were intravesically instilled, they did not translocate across the urothelial layer, regardless of the concentration used, with no associated systemic toxicity. In the mice that had intravenous injections of microparticles, there was a dose-dependent distribution of the particles to the liver, lung, and spleen. There was minimal inflammation seen on histology, and all the mice survived and gained weight appropriately indicating minimal toxicity.

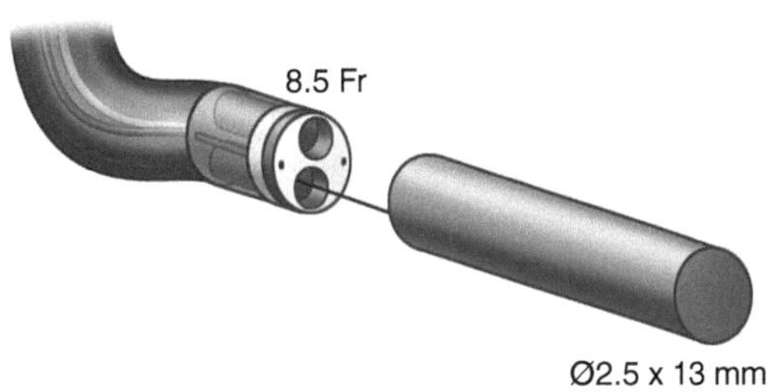

Fig. 40.1 Schematic of magnet mounted on guidewire and backloaded on flexible ureteroscope. Fernandez R, Tan YK, Kaberle W, et al. Determining a Performance Envelope for Capture of Kidney Stones. Journal of Endourology, in press

Since the tests of the technology utilized an 8 F magnetic rod, new tool design is required for the intended use during flexible ureteroscope. As such, we have recently developed a ureteroscopic tool consisting of a magnet attached to a 0.038 in. guidewire (Fig. 40.1). This tool has undergone

Table 40.2 Number of fragments extracted in 5 min in ureteroscopic model

Stone size	No. of stone fragments retrieved in 5 min						
	Trial	1	2	3	4	Median	*P*-value
1–1.5 mm	Magnet	5	9	10	10	9.5	0.03
	Basket	3	5	3	4	3.5	
1.5–2 mm	Magnet	3	9	10	10	9.5	0.19
	Basket	3	7	5	4	4.5	
2–2.5 mm	Magnet	2	8	6	6	6	1
	Basket	7	7	5	5	6	

Tan YK, McLeroy SL, Faddegon Stephen et al. In vitro comparison of prototype magnetic tool with conventional nitinol basket for ureteroscopic retrieval of stone fragments rendered paramagnetic with iron oxide microparticles Journal of Urology, in press

preliminary, non-published evaluation in an in vitro model of the pelvicollecting system. Access was gained via a ureteric access sheath and the magnetic tool was backloaded onto the flexible ureteroscope. Trials were performed comparing the magnetic tool against a standard 2.4 F nitinol basket in the extraction of stone fragments ranging from 1 to 2.5 mm in greatest diameter. Timed trials found that the magnetic tool outperformed the basket in the extraction of stones less than 2 mm in size but was of equal efficacy for fragments larger than 2 mm (Table 40.2). Nevertheless, there were a number of issues encountered with the current itineration of the tool. The size of the magnet affected the visibility of the system and it was easy to dislodge stones from the magnet as they were being trawled out of the pelvicollecting system (data unpublished).

Future Developments

The functionalizing of stone fragments for magnetic extraction is still in its infancy. As a proof of concept, it has shown promise but as with any new technology further development is required before it can be considered for use in patients.

The main issues are the relatively weak attractive forces that were generated. In the current itineration, with a 10-min incubation time limit, no fragments larger than 3 mm can be attracted by a magnetic tool [13]. The strength of a magnetic field deteriorates exponentially with distance such that we can capture stones at a maximum distance of 2 mm. There are a number of factors that can affect this attractive force. First the density of iron oxide microparticles binding to the stone fragments will affect the supraparamagnetic forces that can be generated in a magnetic field. This iron oxide density is a function of both the number of particles per surface area of stone and the concentration of iron oxide in each microparticle. Further research should go into finding microparticle surface proteins that will have a greater affinity to calcium stones across a wide spectrum of pH and temperatures. This would increase the density of particles binding to stone fragments and also shorten the incubation times for adherence to occur. In addition the current microparticles are only 30 % iron oxide. Increasing the concentration of iron in the microparticles should increase the paramagnetic forces generated. It is also planned that in its final itineration, the microparticles can be run as part of the irrigant during ureteroscopy. How the fluid dynamics might affect the binding of the microparticles to the stones has as yet to be determined.

The current microparticles in use are not biodegradable though their components are suitable for human use. If they were to enter the systemic circulation, their deposition in different tissues could have unknown long-term sequelae. An option may be to use biodegradable iron oxide microparticles. Of note, ultrasmall iron oxide microparticles have been developed and are used in MRI for lymph node metastasis [15] and brain inflammation [16]. Of course, this could mean a potential iron load to the body, though it would in all probability be of such a small volume that the body could easily cope with it. Further studies will also be needed to study the safety profiles of the microparticles when used in a human.

Lastly, further development will have to continue to develop a more suitable magnetic tool. The shape of the tool will have to be altered to improve maneuverability and visibility. The issues of relatively weak attractive forces could also potentially be addressed by a tool with a combination magnet and basket.

Conclusion

Intrarenal stone fragments after laser lithotripsy continue to pose a health problem to the patient with a relatively high incidence of recurrent symptoms requiring treatment. The magnetic extraction of intrarenal stone fragments is a novel approach to the clearance of small stone fragments during treatment. Currently the technology is in the proof-of-concept stage with further work needed to improve its reliability and ensure its safety in humans.

References

1. Pearle MS, Calhoun FA, Curhan GC. Urologic diseases in America project: urolithiasis. J Urol. 2005;173(3):848–57.
2. Strope SA, Wolf Jr JS, Hollenbeck BK. Changes in gender distribution of urinary stone disease. Urology. 2010;75(3):543–54. 546 e541.
3. Zehnder P, Roth B, Birkhauser F, et al. A prospective randomised trial comparing the modified HM3 with the MODULITH(R) SLX-F2 lithotripter. Eur Urol. 2011;59(4):637–44.
4. Macejko A, Okotie OT, Zhao LC, Liu J, Perry K, Nadler RB. Computed tomography-determined stone-free rates for ureteroscopy of upper-tract stones. J Endourol. 2009;23(3):379–82.
5. Altunrende F, Tefekli A, Stein RJ, et al. Clinically insignificant residual fragments after percutaneous nephrolithotomy: medium-term follow-up. J Endourol. 2011;25(6):941–5.
6. Preminger GM. Management of lower pole renal calculi: shock wave lithotripsy versus percutaneous nephrolithotomy versus flexible ureteroscopy. Urol Res. 2006;34(2):108–11.
7. Osman MM, Alfano Y, Kamp S, et al. 5-year-follow-up of patients with clinically insignificant residual fragments after extracorporeal shockwave lithotripsy. Eur Urol. 2005;47(6):860–4.
8. Rebuck DA, Macejko A, Bhalani V, Ramos P, Nadler RB. The natural history of renal stone fragments following ureteroscopy. Urology. 2011;77(3):564–8.
9. Raman JD, Bagrodia A, Gupta A, et al. Natural history of residual fragments following percutaneous nephrostolithotomy. J Urol. 2009;181(3):1163–8.
10. Eisner BH, Dretler SP. Use of the Stone Cone for prevention of calculus retropulsion during holmium:YAG laser lithotripsy: case series and review of the literature. Urol Int. 2009;82(3):356–60.
11. Mirabile G, Phillips CK, Edelstein A, et al. Evaluation of a novel temperature-sensitive polymer for temporary ureteral occlusion. J Endourol. 2008;22(10): 2357–9.
12. Chiong E, Hwee ST, Kay LM, Liang S, Kamaraj R, Esuvaranathan K. Randomized controlled study of mechanical percussion, diuresis, and inversion therapy to assist passage of lower pole renal calculi after shock wave lithotripsy. Urology. 2005;65(6):1070–4.
13. Tracy CR, McLeroy SL, Best SL, Gnade BE, Pearle MS, Cadeddu JA. Rendering stone fragments paramagnetic with iron-oxide microparticles improves the efficiency and effectiveness of endoscopic stone fragment retrieval. Urology. 2010;76(5). 1266 e1210-1264.
14. Mir SA, Best SL, McLeroy S, et al. Novel stone-magnetizing microparticles: in vitro toxicity and biologic functionality analysis. J Endourol. 2011;25(7):1 203–7.
15. Will O, Purkayastha S, Chan C, et al. Diagnostic precision of nanoparticle-enhanced MRI for lymph-node metastases: a meta-analysis. Lancet Oncol. 2006;7(1):52–60.
16. Stoll G, Bendszus M. New approaches to neuroimaging of central nervous system inflammation. Curr Opin Neurol. 2010;23(3):282–6.

Index

M. Monga (ed.), *Ureteroscopy: Indications, Instrumentation & Technique*, Current Clinical Urology,
DOI 10.1007/978-1-62703-206-3, © Springer Science+Business Media New York 2013

V

X

MIX
Papier aus verantwortungsvollen Quellen
Paper from responsible sources
FSC® C105338

If you have any concerns about our products,
you can contact us on
ProductSafety@springernature.com

In case Publisher is established outside the EU,
the EU authorized representative is:
Springer Nature Customer Service Center GmbH
Europaplatz 3, 69115 Heidelberg, Germany

Printed by Libri Plureos GmbH
in Hamburg, Germany